CANCER ETIOLOGY, DIAGNOSIS AND TREATMENTS

FIELD CANCERIZATION: BASIC SCIENCE AND CLINICAL APPLICATIONS

Cancer Etiology, Diagnosis and Treatments

Additional books in this series can be found on Nova's website under the Series tab.

Additional E-books in this series can be found on Nova's website under the E-books tab.

CANCER ETIOLOGY, DIAGNOSIS AND TREATMENTS

FIELD CANCERIZATION: BASIC SCIENCE AND CLINICAL APPLICATIONS

GABRIEL D. DAKUBO
EDITOR

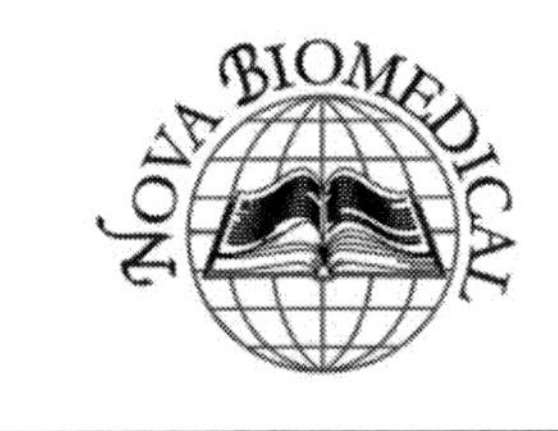

Nova Science Publishers, Inc.
New York

For permission to use material from this book please contact us:
Telephone 631-231-7269; Fax 631-231-8175
Web Site: http://www.novapublishers.com

Library of Congress Cataloging-in-Publication Data

Field cancerization : basic science and clinical applications / editor,
Gabriel D. Dakubo.
p. ; cm.
Includes bibliographical references and index.
ISBN 978-1-61761-006-6 (hardcover)
1. Carcinogenesis. 2. Cancer invasiveness. I. Dakubo, Gabriel D.
[DNLM: 1. Neoplasms, Multiple Primary--genetics. 2. Antibodies,
Monoclonal. 3. Neoplasm Metastasis--genetics. 4. Neoplasm
Metastasis--pathology. 5. Neoplasms, Multiple Primary--pathology. QZ 202]
RC268.5.F54 2010
616.99'4071--dc22
2010027276

Published by Nova Science Publishers, Inc. † New York

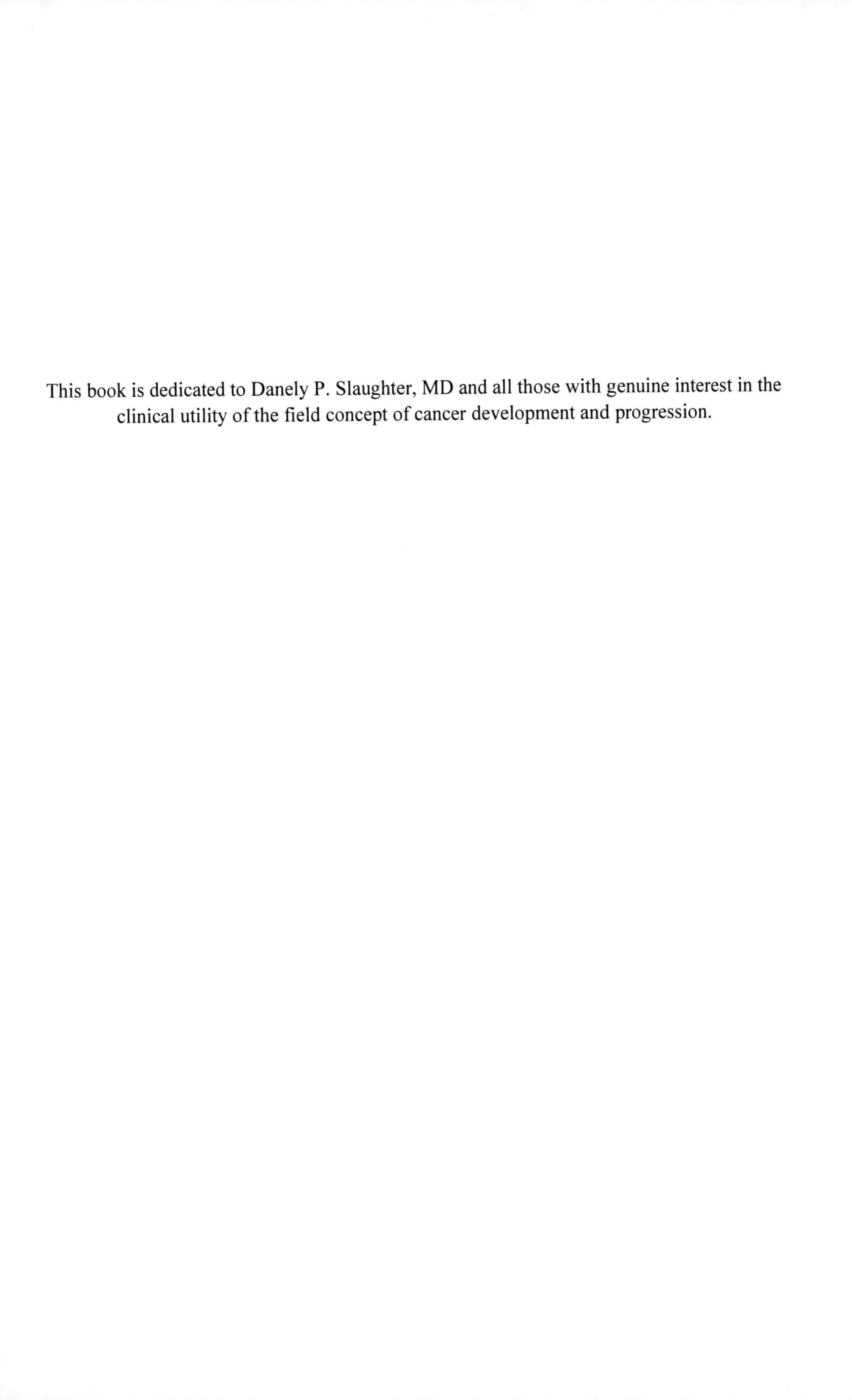

This book is dedicated to Danely P. Slaughter, MD and all those with genuine interest in the clinical utility of the field concept of cancer development and progression.

Contents

Preface

Field cancerization was conceived by D. P. Slaughter at the era of the Second World War following detailed examination of the histopathologic features of multiple cancers. With recent advancement in new molecular biologic technologies, ample evidence is provided that confirms the presence of molecular genetic changes in precancerous lesions, and in tissues exposed to carcinogens but without overt histologic features of cancer. Whereas the mechanism(s) of "cancer-field" formation may differ between different cancers, a fundamental concept shared by all is the occurrence of these genetic changes before the development of cancer and/or in the vicinity of cancer. There is an important need to clinically harness such molecular signatures for early cancer detection, diagnosis, chemoprevention, and monitoring their progressive pattern and therapy response. Several documentations of the field concept of carcinogenesis are available, but these are scattered in the literature. *Field Cancerization: Basic Science and Clinical Applications* is the first book to make accessible in a composite form, evidences for, and utility of biologic signatures in "cancer-fields", and it will serve as an easy reference for oncologists, cancer researchers, or industry experts interested in the field mechanism of carcinogenesis. Hopefully, this treatise by distinguished authorities in their various disciplines will stimulate discussion, attract researchers and accelerate translational research.

Authored by over fifty international experts, the book is organized into four parts. Part I addresses the current conceptual mechanistic framework of field cancerization, including expanding super-competitors, multistep carcinogenesis, and our emerging view of stem cell models of cancer fields. Part II details epidemiologic evidences of field changes. Part III comprises of chapters primarily focused on field changes in several cancers, inclusive of hematologic and pediatric cancers. A common theme emphasized throughout each of these chapters is the basic science component and the clinical importance of field biomarkers in cancer management. Finally, part IV is a critical synthesis of the processes required to harness, confirm, standardize and hence clinically translate cancer signatures. This section concludes with a discussion on therapeutic targeting of epigenetic changes in cancer fields as a viable chemoprevention strategy.

I am grateful to the authors for their shared enthusiasm, time and efforts in preparing the various excellent chapters that make this a unique book indeed. It is my hope that readers will find your knowledge valuable in the various aspects of their work. I thank my wife Crescentia, and children, Collins, Ethan, Bernard, and Zaneta for their patience and understanding during the editorial process.

Gabriel D. Dakubo, March 2010

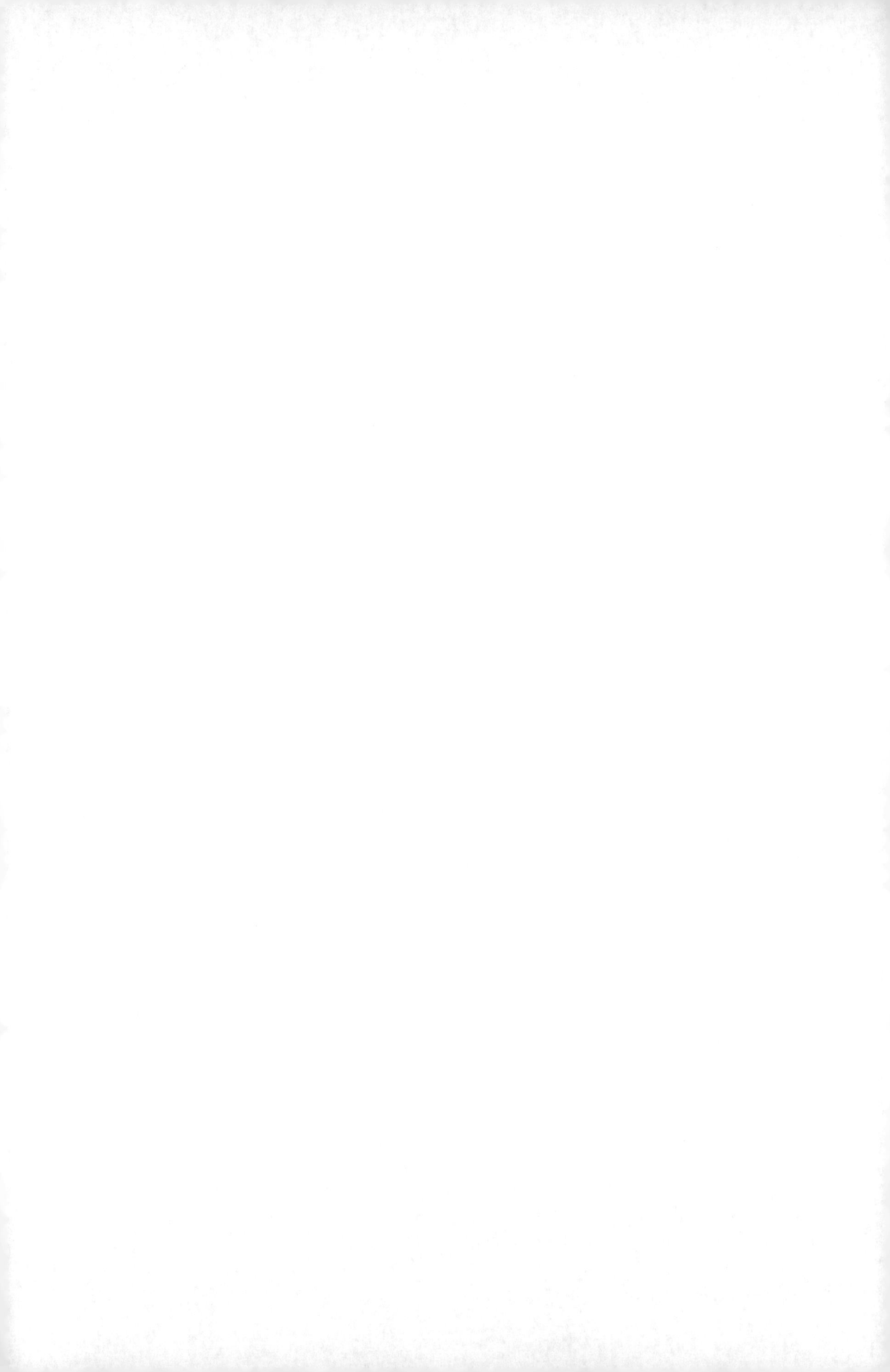

Part I - Mechanisms of Field Cancerization

In: Field Cancerization: Basic Science and Clinical Applications ISBN 978-1-61761-006-6
Editor: Gabriel D. Dakubo

Chapter 1

Expanding Supercompetitors as a Mechanism of Field Cancerization

Eduardo Moreno, Christa Rhiner and Davide Soldini

Abstract

Field cancerization describes the proliferative advantage and expansion of a clone of genetically altered cells at the expense of normal tissue. Initially, neither invasive growth nor aberrant histology are present, but as the field becomes larger, additional genetic hits give rise to various subclones that eventually evolve into primary tumours and later into "second field tumours" that share a common clonal origin. Herein we present recent data suggesting a relationship between field cancerization and the phenomenon called cell competition, providing a novel interpretation of early stages of tumourigenesis.

1.1. Introduction: Cancer Is a Multi-Step Process Caused by Several Mutations in a Cell

The concept of "early steps of carcinogenesis" in solid tumours is not well defined and studies focusing on this topic have addressed a wide range of issues, such as the characterization of mutations in oncogenes and tumour suppressor genes in benign precursor lesions of the gastrointestinal tract and the genetic analysis of different grades of dysplasia in squamous epithelia. At the stage when early lesions become clinically detectable, they may already comprise a mass of up to 10^9 transformed cells and, following a very simplistic model of exponential tumour cell growth, only 10 further doubling cycles would be required to produce a tumour mass of 10^{12} cells, usually considered a tumour size incompatible with life [1]. This observation implies that these late-stage doubling cycles, which occur in the phase where the tumour is clinically detectable, represent merely the tip of the iceberg. Many of the molecular alterations underlying the initial neoplastic events are not well-known and currently few molecular markers are available able to detect a cancerous process at such early stages. In this respect, the concept of multistep carcinogenesis postulates that a tumour does not arise from a single mutation, but from the accumulation of several genetic lesions. Thus, at the point when the tumour becomes clinically detectable, its cells will have already acquired several genetic and epigenetic changes or hits [2,3,4]. Initial supporting evidence came from epidemiologic studies, in particular from the observation that the incidence of most human cancers increases exponentially with age, which could be explained by the need to accumulate a certain number of hits for cancer to arise [5]. Therefore, improving the understanding of the early phases could potentially lead to the development both of new diagnostic tools and targeted therapeutic agents enabling an improvement of prognosis.

1.2. Stem Cells Are Prone to Accumulate Mutations

Recent estimations propose that the number of mutations necessary to give rise to a malignant tumour ranges from 3 to 12, depending on the cancer type, and that organs with rapid turnover of cells might require even more mutations [6]. Some of the most frequent types of cancer occur in tissues with a very high cell turnover (e.g. the skin and the epithelia of the gastrointestinal tract) and in these cases, stem cells, which are defined by their ability to self-renew, are the only ones with sufficient life span to acquire the required number of genetic abnormalities for malignant transformation. In this regard, cancer can also be considered as a disease originating from deregulated stem cells [7,8]. In the two-stage experimental model of mouse skin carcinogenesis, a classic example supporting the role of stem cells in cancer, initial mutations in squamous epithelial cells are induced by the administration of 7,12-dimethylbenz(a)anthracene (the initiator), followed by exposure to phorbol ester (the promoter), which drives them to tumourigenesis. Since increasing the time interval between the administration of initiator and promoter to a time point where the initiated cells are expected to have been already eliminated due to turnover has no impact on subsequent tumour incidence, the origin of the cancerous event is thought to occur in the long-lived epidermal stem cells [9]. This supports the notion of cancer stem cell model, in which a small subset of so-called cancer stem cells constitutes a reservoir of self-sustaining cells with the ability to self-renew and maintain the tumour. According to this model, cancer stem cells have the capacity not only to divide and expand the cancer stem cell pool, but also to differentiate into heterogeneous non-tumour propagating cancer cell types that in most cases appear to constitute the bulk of cancer cells within the tumour [10]. This tumour heterogeneity is thought to derive from aberrant differentiation and epigenetic changes [11,12] rather than from general genetic instability [13,14,15] and proteins that control chromatin organization have been recently shown to regulate stem cell pluripotency by maintaining repression of alternative lineage genes that are necessary for the differentiation of stem or progenitor cells into various tissue types [17].

Although cancer stem cells may share properties with their normal counterparts, it is not yet clear whether they originate from mutant stem cells or from cancerous cells that have acquired certain stem cell characteristics by reactivating a developmental program [18]. Recent studies carried out with genetically engineered mice for direct genetic labelling of adult stem cells of the intestinal epithelium suggest, however, that cancer stem cells are indeed mutated stem cells [19,20]. Additional studies will be necessary to define whether this is specific for the intestine or a phenomenon of general validity.

1.3. Clonal Expansion Can Compensate or Low Mutation Rates

An intriguing question in tumourigenesis is connected to the rate of somatic mutations. Some data suggest that the spontaneous rate of somatic mutations is not high enough to account for the accumulation of several tumourigenic mutations in a cell and, moreover, most of them are neutralized by effective DNA-repair mechanisms.

A hypothesis has been put forward in order to explain the elevated number of mutations in cancer cells based on the existence of a "mutator phenotype" [21,22], caused by mutations in genes encoding DNA polymerases and DNA repair enzymes, which decreases the ability of cells to remove potentially mutagenic DNA lesions [23], as well as in genes involved in chromosomal, microsatellite, and checkpoint stability [24]. Such mutations would increase genomic instability and increase the overall frequency of mutations including those associated with cancer. The fact that malignancies are characterized by a high number of mutations, which are not consistent with the low mutation rates exhibited by normal human cells, supports the mutator phenotype model [22]. However, several arguments against the mutator phenotype hypothesis have been raised. On the one hand, increasing mutagenesis would reduce cellular fitness as most non-neutral mutations are thought to be deleterious [25], so that overall a mutator phenotype would be detrimental [22]. On the other hand, in bacterial experiments, mutator phenotypes have been observed with an evolutive significance [26]. Finally, despite leading to an increased cancer risk through genomic instability when two mutant alleles are present in the germline, genes involved in excision repair mechanisms are rarely mutated in sporadic cancers [27].

An alternative hypothesis suggests that the acquisition of several mutations could be explained by the occurrence of an increased number of cells with a first mutation and susceptible to accumulate further mutations. Such "pre-neoplastic fields", i.e. lesions with genetically altered cells [3], would be sufficiently large to increase the likelihood of subsequent genetic hits occurring in this population [27,28,29]. So far, few models have been proposed to explain how these pre-neoplastic fields could arise.

In a first model, the creation of some field changes could occur during organogenesis, when some altered cells proliferate to generate a vast area of pre-conditioned epithelial surface [27]. In fact, many human cancers occur in renewing epithelial tissues, in which cellular lineages typically go through two distinct phases: early in life, when cell populations expand exponentially to form the tissue, and in later stages, when the tissue is renewed by stem cells dividing to create an almost linear cellular history [30]. The idea that mutations which arise during the exponential phase probably seed tissues with stem cells carrying mutations that may predispose to cancer was supported by a simple mathematical model [31]. According to this model, the risk imparted by a mutation during embryo-foetal development could vary widely, depending on when the mutation occurs, and individuals with several predisposing mutations are likely to develop multiple independent tumours relatively early in life, whereas those with few predisposing mutations should develop few tumours relatively late in life. Such developmental mutations could be therefore one source of the considerable heterogeneity of risks of cancer observed in human populations.

In another model proposed to explain the origin of pre-neoplastic fields, prolonged exposure of a certain tissue to a particular carcinogen (e.g. smoke) could simultaneously induce several genetic alterations in different cells of the tissue resulting in polyclonal preneoplastic lesions from which multiple tumours develop.

We favour a third model which argues that, in rapidly dividing tissues, successive rounds of clonal selection can account for the multiple mutations found in human cancers in the absence of an increase in mutation rate [27]. Tumourigenesis would thus be an evolutionary process driven by selection and an increased mutation rate would not be necessary. In colorectal cancer, for example, *APC* mutations lead to growth advantage, so that when both *APC* alleles are mutated, expansion of the colorectal tumour clone is observed [32] and a second mutation (e.g. *K−ras*) could occur more likely on this expanded population without necessarily requiring an increased mutation rate [33]. Subsequent rounds of clonal expansion, mutation and selection would lead to the stepwise progression of colorectal tumours. Interestingly, mathematical models which have shown that the number of mutations found in cancers is too high to be explained without increased mutation rates [23] do not take into account clonal expansion, i.e. the fact that increased number of cells can compensate for low mutation rates [21] and that the rate of cell turnover exceeds the net rate of tumour growth, so that a raised mutation rate does not seem to be necessary to explain carcinogenesis in general [33,34]. Carcinogenic progression as an evolutionary process driven by selection would also account for long lag periods without having to assume slow exponential growth rates or improbable conditions like dormancy. In this regard, experiments in a mouse model of skin cancer were performed with the use of UVB [35], known to generate C → T mutations at dipyrimidine sites [36], notably affecting *p53* and *PTCH* tumour suppressor genes [37,38]. They started from the observation that mutation frequencies after UVB irradiation are 10^{-5} - 10^{-3} per gene per cell division. Supposing that six mutations in key genes are needed for a tumour to develop, the chances of consecutively achieving these in a single cell are at best 10^{-18}. Genomic instability will not suffice, but expansion of the single mutant cell to a clone of thousands of cells, however, would increase the likelihood that one of the mutant cells would acquire a further mutation and so on. Clonal expansion may therefore be a rate-limiting step in tumour development.

Interestingly, in the human epidermis of sun-exposed skin it is possible to observe clones with p53 mutation ranging in size from 3 to 3000 cells, which are completely normal by conventional hematoxylin-eosin staining [39]. In the skin of UV-exposed mice, detailed counts of clone sizes revealed that they occurred in quantized sizes, which were multiples of the size of one stem cell compartment consisting of about 12–14 nucleated cells [40]. These data indicate that a limiting step in clonal expansion is the ability to expand beyond the first stem cell compartment, and that stem cells are restricted in their ability to proliferate outside their own compartment, which might represent a safety mechanism [30]. Zhang et al. performed some experiments in order to explain the clonal expansion [41]. They observed that p53 mutant clones regress in the absence of UVB [42] and that the longer the mice are irradiated, the larger the average clone size [41]. This suggests that UVB is indeed driving clonal expansion. Moreover, in a mouse with impaired apoptosis (transgenic mice that overexpresses survivin in the epidermis) UVB creates more, but smaller *p53*-mutant clones, which can be explained by a role of UVB in the induction of apoptosis in the cells surrounding the clone, possibly involving reactive oxygen species [43].. These findings reveal that the process of clonal expansion is not simply one of hyperproliferation and that tissue proliferation is limited at least in part by neighbouring cells of the same cell type.

1.4. Cell Competition Provides a Mechanism for Clonal Expansion

The model proposed so far shows many similarities with the phenomenon called "cell competition". The phenomenon of cell competition was first discovered in Drosophila where several genetic tools are available to generate patches of mutant cells in an otherwise wild-type tissue [44,45]. The first evidence of competition between cells was obtained in an experiment where cells mutant for ribosomal genes (*Minutes*) were apposed with wild-type cells and the proliferation of both cell types was monitored over time [46]. *Minute* homozygous cells did not survive because they lacked functional ribosomes. Surprisingly however, *Minute* heterozygous cells, which were viable on their own and gave rise to normal-sized flies in a homotypic background, proliferated less and were replaced by surrounding wild-type cells when both cell types were mixed [47,48]. These experiments showed that the active purging of the slower growing "losers" was dependent on the presence of the wild-type cells and therefore reflected a true case of cell competition (reviewed in [49]). It has been shown later that a similar process takes place during the development of chimeric mice, partly generated with *Minute* cells. When wild-type cells were injected into blastocysts heterozygous for a ribosomal mutation, the wild-type cells showed a growth advantage and ultimately contributed to a greater extent to diverse tissues of the adult mouse [50].

More recently, the transcription factor and proto-oncogene myc was identified as a key mediator of cell competition. Analogous to the Minute cells, clones mutant for Drosophila myc (dmyc) were outcompeted by wild-type cells when both cell types were confronted in the epithelial tissue of the developing wing imaginal discs [51,52]. Even more intriguing was the finding that cells overexpressing dMyc were able to eliminate "optimal" wild-type cells (therefore named "supercompetitors") and take over the entire wing epithelia [52,53]. Detailed analysis revealed that dMyc-overexpressing supercompetitor cells proliferated at higher levels, but remarkably this excess growth was compensated by the concomitant death of wild-type cells, and the overall cell numbers were not altered. Hence, no morphological malformations appeared, neither in the developing larval discs nor later in the adult wing structure. Mutations inactivating the conserved Salvador-Hippo-Warts pathway, implicated in growth control, were also proposed to trigger supercompetition [54,55,56,57] and the fact that deregulation of both Myc and the Hippo pathway is associated with tumourigenesis points to a possible link between cell supercompetition and cancer.

One important observation characteristic of cell competition is the disappearance of the "loser" cell population, which is characterized by continuous apoptosis of "loser" cells along the borders, where "winners" and "losers" physically interact [52,53,58,59]. If the apoptotic machinery is blocked, however, the supercompetitor behaviour of the "winner" cells is restricted and both groups co-exist, suggesting that cell competition relies on the killing of surrounding cells to allow the expansion of potential competitors. Interestingly, this has many similarities with the observations made in the mouse model of skin cancer [35], and suggests the possibility that cell competition might be involved in the expansion of mutated clones in mammals (see figure 1-1).

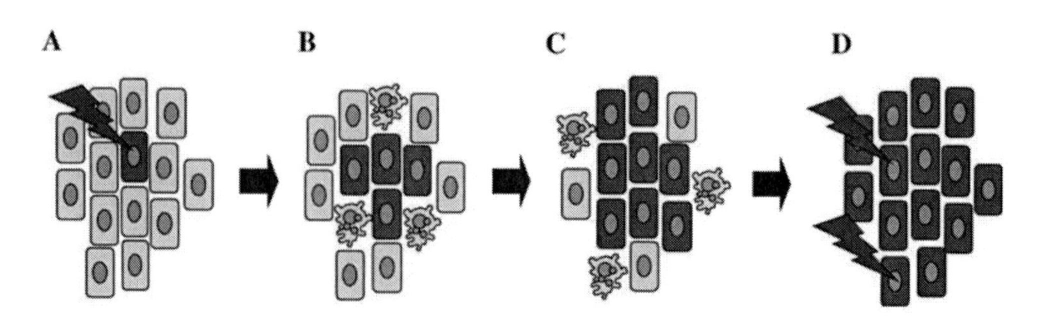

Figure 1-1. Supercompetition could contribute to early cancer progression. A mutation of a myc proto-oncogene could transform a normal epithelial cell into a ''supercompetitor'' (A), able to undergo clonal expansion at the expense of the normal surrounding tissue without any morphological alterations (B and C). Secondary mutations in a supercompetitor background could initiate tumour formation (D).

Finally, it was shown that the expansion of supercompetitors depends on the ability of dMyc to maximally activate the protein synthesis machinery [60]. dMyc-overexpressing supercompetitors that are heterozygously mutant for a ribosomal protein gene are no longer able to outcompete surrounding cells [52]. This demonstrates that the highly competitive behaviour of dMyc supercompetitors depends on increased metabolic activity, which probably allows highly efficient endocytosis of survival factors such as Dpp/BMP.

Taken together, the work in the Drosophila imaginal discs over the last few years has shown that cell competition is a multistep process, characterized by at least six distinguishable events. At first, an insult (i.e. mutation in *Minute* or *dmyc* genes) alters the fitness of a particular cell or subpopulation within the imaginal disc epithelium. Second, this gain or loss of fitness translates into imbalances in morphogen and survival factor signalling (i.e. differences in uptake or signal transduction of the BMP2/4 homolog Dpp). Third, through an unknown mechanism, cells are able to monitor the signalling levels of their neighbouring cells and recognize distortions in the morphogen gradient (i.e. the Dpp gradient). Fourth, several lines of evidence suggest that once such discrepancies in signalling levels are detected, a signal is sent by the "winner" cells in order to kill the "loser" cells. Such a signalling molecule might be expressed at the cell surface or secreted to allow communication between cells. Recently, the conditioned medium of co-cultured "winner" and "loser" cells was found to contain factors able to trigger apoptosis when transferred to naïve cells [61], whereas the factors were not produced in homogenous cell populations. This indicates that a secreted molecule might be involved in conveying information, at least in vitro. Fifth, this cell-to-cell communication ultimately leads to JNK signalling and weak caspase activation in the "loser" cell. Last, weak caspase activation in the "loser" cell activates an engulfment response in the "winner" cell, which helps kill and finally removes the corpse of the outcompeted "loser" cell and/or accompanies its extrusion from the epithelial layer [59] (see figure 1-2). Ultimately, this process results in a novel type of proliferation, where the "winner" cells proliferate by replacing (killing) the "loser" cells. Consequently, this type of proliferation requires the killing of the surrounding cells and has been termed "apoptosis-dependent proliferation".

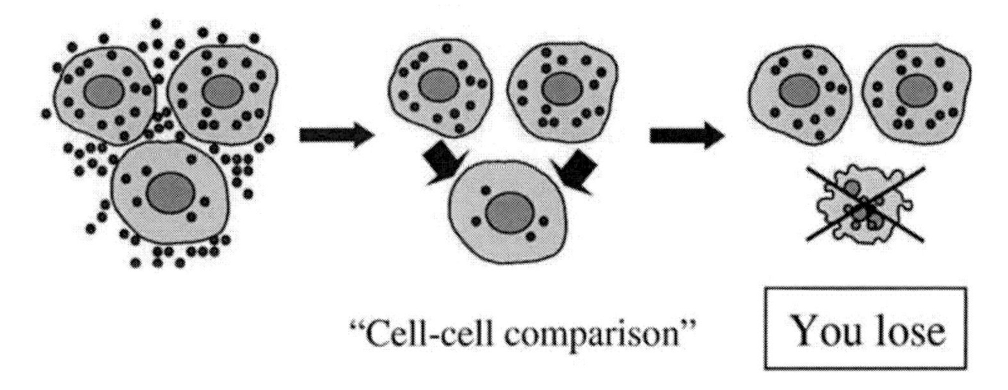

Figure 1-2. Different levels of endocytosis of morphogen lead to an imbalance of survival factor signalling. As a consequence, cells monitor the signalling levels of their neighbouring cells and a signal is sent by the "winner" cells in order to kill the "loser" cells which undergo apoptosis.

1.5. Field Cancerization and Expanding Supercompetitors

Cell competition might be the basic mechanism of clonal expansion in the very first step of tumourigenesis and be related to a clinical phenomenon known as field cancerization, in which a field of genetically altered cells of monoclonal origin is associated with a proliferative advantage and expands at the expense of normal tissue. Initially, neither invasive growth nor aberrant histology are present, but as the field becomes larger, additional genetic hits give rise to various subclones that eventually evolve into primary tumours and later into "second-field tumours" that share a common clonal origin [52,62,63].

The concept of field cancerization was developed by Slaughter and colleagues based on histological examinations. In their classic paper, the term field cancerization was used for the first time in a study of 783 patients with oral cancer [64]. They observed that oral cancer develops in multifocal areas of pre-cancerous change and that histologically abnormal tissue surrounds the tumours. Finally, they suggested that the persistence of abnormal tissue after surgery may explain second primary tumours and local recurrences. Since then, the term has been used to describe multiple patches of pre-malignant disease, a higher-than-expected prevalence of multiple local primary tumours, as well as the presence of synchronous distant tumours [65]. Molecular data accrued from studies of head and neck, oesophagus, and bladder cancers support a clonal expansion model [67], in which in an initial phase a cell acquires a mutation that allows it to multiply and form a patch of altered daughter cells. Molecular signatures of field cancerization have also been documented for several epithelial tumours including those of the stomach, lungs, skin, cervix, vulva, colon, breast, ovary, pancreas, prostate and it has even been proposed in brain and haematological malignancies [67].

Based on the observations described herein we propose that cell competition would provide a possible explanation for this mechanism. In particular, when mutations conferring a growth advantage occur in stem cells, a "patch", i.e. a clonal unit consisting of the stem cell and its daughter cells which share the alteration, is formed. This initial phase of tumour formation is characterized by the presence of two cell populations which are confronted in a "habitat" of limited dimensions and resources. Variations among them and possible intercellular communication lead to competition, which is reminiscent of an evolutionary process during carcinogenesis [68]. Cell populations with favourable mutations tend to expand and out-compete surrounding cells, and clonal expansion implies that some mutations are able to confer means to breach the barriers between proliferative units. For this step to occur, apoptosis of the out-competed population needs to occur, as demonstrated in a mouse model [35].

Conclusion

In a short-lived fly, the consequences of replacing most tissue with dMyc-overexpressing clones might be small. In humans, however, the successful expansion of such supercompetitor cells could create patches and eventually large fields of pre-cancerous cells, where the probability of secondary and tertiary genetic hits will be more likely [66]. In most cases, it is unknown how clones expand through a neoplasm and if there are population sub-structures that inhibit those expansions. The most challenging aspect of this process is that the conquest of the supercompetitors is accompanied by the loss of neighbouring cells that give way to the invaders in a form that no disturbance of the tissue becomes visible. This feature is clinically relevant, since it leads to a macroscopically and microscopically undetectable lesions, which, when not removed, would be the cause of multi-focal and locally recurrent cancers [3].

It is evident that many key mediators of cell competition are still unknown. Current efforts in the field are centred on the identification of upstream players, such as the receptors that might allow cells to compare their signalling levels or the killing signal produced by the "winners". Recent approaches include genetic screens and microarray techniques, which allow detection of genes specifically up-regulated (or down-regulated) during cell competition [69,70]. The discovery of such cell competition-dedicated components might yield useful markers to trace early expansion of pre-cancerous clones, enabling early diagnosis, as well as offer novel targets for cancer therapy blocking the expanding pre-neoplastic clones at very early stages or avoiding recurrence in the adjuvant setting.

References

[1] Moreno E (2008) Is cell competition relevant to cancer? *Nat. Rev. Cancer* 8: 141-147.

[2] Fearon ER, Vogelstein B (1990) A genetic model for colorectal tumourigenesis. *Cell* 61: 759-767.

[3] Braakhuis BJ, Brakenhoff RH, Leemans CR (2005) Second field tumours: a new opportunity for cancer prevention? *Oncologist* 10: 493-500.

[4] Vogelstein B, Kinzler KW (1993) The multistep nature of cancer. *Trends Genet.* 9: 138-141.

[5] Miller DG (1980) On the nature of susceptibility to cancer. The presidential address. *Cancer* 46: 1307-1318.

[6] Merlo LM, Pepper JW, Reid BJ, Maley CC (2006) Cancer as an evolutionary and ecological process. *Nat. Rev. Cancer* 6: 924-935.

[7] McDonald SA, Graham TA, Schier S, Wright NA, Alison MR (2009) Stem cells and solid cancers. *Virchows Arch.* 455: 1-13.

[8] Radtke F, Clevers H (2005) Self-renewal and cancer of the gut: two sides of a coin. *Science* 307: 1904-1909.

[9] Berenblum I (1949) The carcinogenic action of 9,10-dimethyl-1,2-benzanthracene on the skin and subcutaneous tissues of the mouse, rabbit, rat and guinea pig. *J. Natl. Cancer Inst.* 10: 167-174.

[10] Clarke MF, Dick JE, Dirks PB, Eaves CJ, Jamieson CH, et al. (2006) Cancer stem cells--perspectives on current status and future directions: AACR Workshop on cancer stem cells. *Cancer Res.* 66: 9339-9344.

[11] Warner JK, Wang JC, Hope KJ, Jin L, Dick JE (2004) Concepts of human leukemic development. *Oncogene* 23: 7164-7177.

[12] Hess AR, Margaryan NV, Seftor EA, Hendrix MJ (2007) Deciphering the signaling events that promote melanoma tumor cell vasculogenic mimicry and their link to embryonic vasculogenesis: role of the Eph receptors. *Dev. Dyn.* 236: 3283-3296.

[13] Jones S, Zhang X, Parsons DW, Lin JC, Leary RJ, et al. (2008) Core signaling pathways in human pancreatic cancers revealed by global genomic analyses. *Science* 321: 1801-1806.

[14] Cancer Genome Atlas Research Network (2008) Comprehensive genomic characterization defines human glioblastoma genes and core pathways. *Nature* 455: 1061-1068.

[15] Parsons DW, Jones S, Zhang X, Lin JC, Leary RJ, et al. (2008) An integrated genomic analysis of human glioblastoma multiforme. *Science* 321: 1807-1812.

[16] Jones PA, Baylin SB (2002) The fundamental role of epigenetic events in cancer. *Nat. Rev. Genet.* 3: 415-428.

[17] Lee TI, Jenner RG, Boyer LA, Guenther MG, Levine SS, et al. (2006) Control of developmental regulators by Polycomb in human embryonic stem cells. *Cell* 125: 301-313.

[18] Sparmann A, van Lohuizen M (2006) Polycomb silencers control cell fate, development and cancer. *Nat. Rev. Cancer* 6: 846-856.

[19] Barker N, Ridgway RA, van Es JH, van de Wetering M, Begthel H, et al. (2009) Crypt stem cells as the cells-of-origin of intestinal cancer. *Nature* 457: 608-611.

[20] Zhu L, Gibson P, Currle DS, Tong Y, Richardson RJ, et al. (2009) Prominin 1 marks intestinal stem cells that are susceptible to neoplastic transformation. *Nature* 457: 603-607.

[21] Loeb LA (1991) Mutator phenotype may be required for multistage carcinogenesis. *Cancer Res.* 51: 3075-3079.

[22] Loeb LA, Bielas JH, Beckman RA (2008) Cancers exhibit a mutator phenotype: clinical implications. *Cancer Res.* 68: 3551-3557; discussion 3557.

[23] Loeb LA, Springgate CF, Battula N (1974) Errors in DNA replication as a basis of malignant changes. *Cancer Res.* 34: 2311-2321.

[24] Paulovich AG, Toczyski DP, Hartwell LH (1997) When checkpoints fail. *Cell* 88: 315-321.

[25] Sniegowski PD, Gerrish PJ, Johnson T, Shaver A (2000) The evolution of mutation rates: separating causes from consequences. *Bioessays* 22: 1057-1066.

[26] Sniegowski PD, Gerrish PJ, Lenski RE (1997) Evolution of high mutation rates in experimental populations of E. coli. *Nature* 387: 703-705.

[27] Tomlinson I, Bodmer W (1999) Selection, the mutation rate and cancer: ensuring that the tail does not wag the dog. *Nat. Med.* 5: 11-12.
[28] Abrams JM (2002) Competition and compensation: coupled to death in development and cancer. *Cell* 110: 403-406.
[29] Moolgavkar SH, Luebeck EG (2003) Multistage carcinogenesis and the incidence of human cancer. *Genes Chromosomes Cancer* 38: 302-306.
[30] Cairns J (1975) Mutation selection and the natural history of cancer. *Nature* 255: 197-200.
[31] Frank SA, Nowak MA (2003) Cell biology: Developmental predisposition to cancer. *Nature* 422: 494.
[32] Nowell PC (1976) The clonal evolution of tumor cell populations. *Science* 194: 23-28.
[33] Tomlinson IP, Novelli MR, Bodmer WF (1996) The mutation rate and cancer. *Proc. Natl. Acad. Sci. USA* 93: 14800-14803.
[34] Loeb LA (1997) Transient expression of a mutator phenotype in cancer cells. *Science* 277: 1449-1450.
[35] Brash DE, Zhang W, Grossman D, Takeuchi S (2005) Colonization of adjacent stem cell compartments by mutant keratinocytes. *Semin Cancer Biol.* 15: 97-102.
[36] Glickman BW, Schaaper RM, Haseltine WA, Dunn RL, Brash DE (1986) The C-C (6-4) UV photoproduct is mutagenic in Escherichia coli. *Proc. Natl. Acad. Sci. USA* 83: 6945-6949.
[37] Ziegler A, Jonason AS, Leffell DJ, Simon JA, Sharma HW, et al. (1994) Sunburn and p53 in the onset of skin cancer. *Nature* 372: 773-776.
[38] Gailani MR, Stahle-Backdahl M, Leffell DJ, Glynn M, Zaphiropoulos PG, et al. (1996) The role of the human homologue of Drosophila patched in sporadic basal cell carcinomas. *Nat. Genet.* 14: 78-81.
[39] Jonason AS, Kunala S, Price GJ, Restifo RJ, Spinelli HM, et al. (1996) Frequent clones of p53-mutated keratinocytes in normal human skin. *Proc. Natl. Acad. Sci. USA* 93: 14025-14029.
[40] Potten CS, Morris RJ (1988) Epithelial stem cells in vivo. *J. Cell Sci. Suppl.* 10: 45-62.
[41] Zhang W, Remenyik E, Zelterman D, Brash DE, Wikonkal NM (2001) Escaping the stem cell compartment: sustained UVB exposure allows p53-mutant keratinocytes to colonize adjacent epidermal proliferating units without incurring additional mutations. *Proc. Natl. Acad. Sci. USA* 98: 13948-13953.
[42] Berg RJ, van Kranen HJ, Rebel HG, de Vries A, van Vloten WA, et al. (1996) Early p53 alterations in mouse skin carcinogenesis by UVB radiation: immunohistochemical detection of mutant p53 protein in clusters of preneoplastic epidermal cells. *Proc Natl Acad Sci U S A 93*: 274-278.
[43] Chedekel MR, Smith SK, Post PW, Pokora A, Vessell DL (1978) Photodestruction of pheomelanin: role of oxygen. *Proc. Natl. Acad. Sci. USA* 75: 5395-5399.
[44] Golic KG (1991) Site-specific recombination between homologous chromosomes in Drosophila. *Science* 252: 958-961.
[45] Struhl G, Basler K (1993) Organizing activity of wingless protein in Drosophila. *Cell* 72: 527-540.
[46] Morata G, Ripoll P (1975) Minutes: mutants of drosophila autonomously affecting cell division rate. *Dev. Biol.* 42: 211-221.

[47] Simpson P, Morata G (1981) Differential mitotic rates and patterns of growth in compartments in the Drosophila wing. *Dev. Biol.* 85: 299-308.

[48] Lambertsson A (1998) The minute genes in Drosophila and their molecular functions. *Adv. Genet.* 38: 69-134.

[49] Diaz B, Moreno E (2005) The competitive nature of cells. *Exp. Cell Res.* 306: 317-322.

[50] Oliver ER, Saunders TL, Tarle SA, Glaser T (2004) Ribosomal protein L24 defect in belly spot and tail (Bst), a mouse Minute. *Development* 131: 3907-3920.

[51] Johnston LA, Prober DA, Edgar BA, Eisenman RN, Gallant P (1999) Drosophila myc regulates cellular growth during development. *Cell* 98: 779-790.

[52] Moreno E, Basler K (2004) dMyc transforms cells into super-competitors. *Cell* 117: 117-129.

[53] de la Cova C, Abril M, Bellosta P, Gallant P, Johnston LA (2004) Drosophila myc regulates organ size by inducing cell competition. *Cell* 117: 107-116.

[54] Hariharan IK, Bilder D (2006) Regulation of imaginal disc growth by tumor-suppressor genes in Drosophila. *Annu. Rev. Genet.* 40: 335-361.

[55] Harvey K, Tapon N (2007) The Salvador-Warts-Hippo pathway - an emerging tumour-suppressor network. *Nat Rev Cancer* 7: 182-191.

[56] Saucedo LJ, Edgar BA (2007) Filling out the Hippo pathway. *Nat. Rev. Mol. Cell Biol.* 8: 613-621.

[57] Tyler DM, Li W, Zhuo N, Pellock B, Baker NE (2007) Genes affecting cell competition in Drosophila. *Genetics* 175: 643-657.

[58] Moreno E, Basler K, Morata G (2002) Cells compete for decapentaplegic survival factor to prevent apoptosis in Drosophila wing development. *Nature* 416: 755-759.

[59] Li W, Baker NE (2007) Engulfment is required for cell competition. *Cell* 129: 1215-1225.

[60] Grewal SS, Li L, Orian A, Eisenman RN, Edgar BA (2005) Myc-dependent regulation of ribosomal RNA synthesis during Drosophila development. *Nat. Cell Biol.* 7: 295-302.

[61] Senoo-Matsuda N, Johnston LA (2007) Soluble factors mediate competitive and cooperative interactions between cells expressing different levels of Drosophila Myc. *Proc. Natl. Acad. Sci. USA* 104: 18543-18548.

[62] Donaldson TD, Duronio RJ (2004) Cancer cell biology: Myc wins the competition. *Curr. Biol.* 14: R425-427.

[63] Secombe J, Pierce SB, Eisenman RN (2004) Myc: a weapon of mass destruction. *Cell* 117: 153-156.

[64] Slaughter DP, Southwick HW, Smejkal W (1953) Field cancerization in oral stratified squamous epithelium; clinical implications of multicentric origin. *Cancer* 6: 963-968.

[65] Ha PK, Califano JA (2003) The molecular biology of mucosal field cancerization of the head and neck. *Crit. Rev. Oral. Biol. Med.* 14: 363-369.

[66] Braakhuis BJ, Tabor MP, Kummer JA, Leemans CR, Brakenhoff RH (2003) A genetic explanation of Slaughter's concept of field cancerization: evidence and clinical implications. *Cancer Res.* 63: 1727-1730.

[67] Dakubo GD, Jakupciak JP, Birch-Machin MA, Parr RL (2007) Clinical implications and utility of field cancerization. *Cancer Cell Int.* 15;7:2.

[68] Tarafa G, Tuck D, Ladner D, Topazian M, Brand R, Deters C, Moreno V, Capella G, Lynch H, Lizardi P, Costa J (2008) Mutational load distribution analysis yields metrics reflecting genetic instability during pancreatic carcinogenesis. *Proc Natl Acad Sci U S A.* 18;105(11):4306-11

[69] Portela M, Casas-Tinto S, Rhiner C, López-Gay JM, Domínguez O, Soldini D, Moreno E (2010) Drosophila SPARC is a self-protective signal expressed by loser cells during cell competition. *Dev Cell.* 19(4):562-73.

[70] Rhiner C, López-Gay JM, Soldini D, Casas-Tinto S, Martín FA, Lombardía L, Moreno E (2010) Flower forms an extracellular code that reveals the fitness of a cell to its neighbors in Drosophila. *Dev Cell.* 18(6):985-98.

In: Field Cancerization: Basic Science and Clinical Applications ISBN 978-1-61761-006-6
Editor: Gabriel D. Dakubo

Chapter 2

The Multistep Field Cancerization Theory of Carcinogenesis

Sabrina L. Spencer and Miguel H. Bronchud

Abstract

The transformation of a normal cell to a cancerous cell is thought to require four to six random mutations to occur in the lineage of a single cell. As each mutation is a rare event, this process is more likely to occur in a tissue with a high background of genetic alterations, perhaps due to exposure to environmental mutagens, than in a tissue with a low background of such alterations. Both modelling and experiment have shown that the order in which mutations are acquired can dramatically change the dynamics of tumor formation. Computational models of cancer progression can bring current empirical observations into a defined framework and can make testable predictions. Technological advances, such as the combination of histology with molecular cancer markers, time-lapse imaging of tumors in mice, and longitudinal genetic and epigenetic measurements of cancer progression in patients will allow key model parameters to be measured and will aid in turning cancer detection and treatment into a rational, predictive science.

2.1. Introduction

Cancer progression can be viewed as a form of somatic evolution where the acquisition of certain mutations provides a proliferation advantage for a cell [1]. Tumor formation is thought to require four to six stochastic mutational events along the lineage of a single cell [2-4]. In a landmark paper 10 years ago, Hanahan and Weinberg [5] proposed six hallmark features that a normal cell must acquire to become a cancer cell: (i) *self-sufficiency in growth signals,* (ii) *insensitivity to antigrowth signals,* (iii) *evasion of apoptosis,* (iv) *limitless replicative potential,* (v) *sustained angiogenesis,* and (vi) *tissue invasion and metastasis*. Genetic instability is defined as an "enabling characteristic" that facilitates the acquisition of other mutations due to defects in DNA repair [5]. These hallmarks provide a framework for understanding the steps a normal cell takes as it becomes a cancer cell and can be modeled quantitatively. It remains open to question whether a better knowledge of molecular changes in tissues along the process of human carcinogenesis can truly translate into more effective preventive measures in human populations and target groups. Nevertheless, it seems a very reasonable pathway to explore, considering that earlier detection of cancers and more effective chemopreventive therapies can potentially lead to improved clinical outcomes.

2.2. Modeling Carcinogenesis

Agent-based modeling approaches are becoming increasingly common for simulating the behavior of a population of cells. In this type of simulation, each cell is modeled as an "agent" that behaves according to certain encoded rules. One implementation of such a model [6] began with a single normal cell that divided in three-dimensional space to build a normal tissue and accompanying vasculature. This normal tissue was bounded in size by angiogenic and growth factor constraints. At each cell division, the cell had a chance of acquiring a mutation in one of six hallmark categories, each of which conferred some benefit to the cell and brought it one step closer to becoming a cancer cell. Several stochastic elements were incorporated into this model, including a probabilistic mutational event as a cell's "genome" is copied from mother cell to daughter cells, a probabilistic waiting period between cell divisions, a probability of random death, and a probability of death due to the cell's detection of acquired mutations.

The simulation of single cells through time and the tracking of key events in the cells' history allowed for the monitoring of mutated cell populations that are successful or unsuccessful in tumor formation. With six hallmark mutations, there are 1956 distinct sequences of mutation history, and both simulation [6] and experimental results [7] have shown that the order in which mutations are acquired significantly alters the dynamics and the likelihood of tumor formation. Thus, it is important to consider the ordered pathway of mutation accumulation rather than the lumped set of mutations disregarding order.

Additionally, the modeling of single cells allows for the examination of tumor heterogeneity and genetic diversity, which are considered important predictors of cancer progression [8]. One unexpected finding from the single cell simulations of cancer progression [6] is the dynamic balance between the selective advantage of diversity and the selective pressure to homogenize as the fittest and most aggressive clone becomes dominant. Thus in tumors driven by a clonal population with an extreme selective advantage, homogeneity of the tumor might correlate better with progression than heterogeneity.

The main limitations for developing predictive models of multi-step cancer progression involve the lack of quantitative measurements. Technological advances allow for measurements of key parameters to be made. Below, we outline three types of data that would provide the greatest benefit, as wells as two specific numbers whose measurement would improve the accuracy of cancer modeling efforts.

The importance of accumulating multiple advantageous mutations in an individual cell underscores the need to consider cancer progression at the single cell level. With single-cell PCR techniques available and DNA sequencing becoming ever more inexpensive, it should be possible to examine the number and types of mutations in populations of single cells rather than in pooled populations that obscure the single cell heterogeneity.

Second, simulation predicts that the early pre-cancerous mutations (before a tumor is clinically detectable) can be important in setting the dynamics of tumor progression [6]. For example, the acquisition of a mutation in DNA damage detection/response can drastically change the rate at which other mutations appear. Animal models of cancer and early biopsies in human cancer pre-disposition conditions such as Barrett's esophagus can be used to detect the appearance of mutations before a cancer has developed and to determine the impact on the timing of cancer development.

Third, and most importantly for understanding the evolutionary pressures that drive tumorigenesis, is the need to acquire longitudinal data of a developing cancer in the same patient through time. This can be accomplished through serial biopsies in diseases such as Barrett's esophagus or hematopoietic malignancies. Moreover, animal models of cancer could be periodically biopsied throughout the development of a tumor rather than at a single time point when the animal is sacrificed. Statisical analysis of such longitudinal studies will also aid in our understanding of conditional mutant phenotypes (i.e. when mutation 'x' only affects proliferation or survival in the presence or absence of mutation 'y'), which may be more common than expected and will demand more complex models.

Several specific model parameters are in need of experimental measurement. One is the net tumor volume doubling time for various types of cancers, which can now be measured using tumor luminescence assays in living mice [9]. On a cellular level, the cell division and death rates that produce the net tumor-doubling rate would benefit from direct measurement. This measurement would allow dissection of which tumors have a normal proliferation rate and depend on evasion of apoptosis to increase in size versus those that depend on increased proliferation. Additionally, the net effect of cytostatic and cytotoxic drugs could be assessed. The technology to image single cell divisions inside a tumor *in vivo* is advancing rapidly; such imaging typically involves multiphoton microscopy of fluorescent reporters inside living cells through a tumor window chamber in an anesthetized mouse [10].

2.3. Field Cancerization

Patients with a head and neck squamous cell carcinoma (HNSCC) often develop multiple premalignant lesions, ranging from leucoplakia to other cancers. This led Slaughter *et. al* [11] to postulate the concept of "field cancerization" (the development of multiple primary tumors due to a high background of genetic mutations in a tissue) in 1953. The incidence rate of second primary tumors following a first diagnosis of HNSCC is 10-35%, depending on both the location of the first primary tumor and the age of the patient. The carcinogens associated with HNSCC (alcohol and tobacco smoking) are thought to induce mucosal changes in the entire upper aerodigestive tract (UADT), causing multiple genetic abnormalities in the whole tissue region. Similar arguments apply also to other tobacco-related cancers, like transitional cell carcinomas of the urogenital tract or bronchogenic carcinomas [12, 13].

An alternative theory for these observations is based on the premise that any transforming event is rare and that the multiple lesions arise due to the widespread migration of transformed cells through the whole UADT [14, 15]. This alternative theory that multiple tumors arise due to the migration of cancerous cells, if true, probably applies to cancer(s) more than to 'pre-malignant' cells. Most pre-malignant field changes in smokers, for example, appear to be induced by smoking itself, supporting the theory of carcinogen-induced field cancerization rather than field cancerization due to migrated transformed cells.

Additional causes of "field carcinogenic events" can involve hormonal factors (e.g. changes in the ovaries, breasts or prostate), inflammation and hyperemia (increased proliferative and angiogenic activity in chronic cystitis, gastritis, esophagitis or colitis), chronic viral infections (e.g. Hepatitis B virus for hepatocarcinomas, Epstein-Barr virus for nasopharyngeal carcinomas or some lymphomas), aberrant methylation linked to ageing, free-radical induced DNA damage (e.g. for cancers of the gastrointestinal tract), skin exposed to ultraviolet irradiation (e.g. actinic keratosis and squamous cell carcinomas), ionizing radiation-induced damage, or aberrant morphogenetic pathways. It is also possible that different carcinogenic pathways operate in different tissue fields belonging to the same organ. For example, adenocarcinomas of the right side of the colon are often associated with different clinical and molecular characteristics than adenocarcinomas of the colorectal region. Even in breast cancer, the reported incidence of multicentric or multifocal lesions in areas away from the primary tumor in mastectomy specimens ranges from 9% to 75%, depending on the definition of multicentricity, the extent of tissue sampling and different histological techniques of examination [16, 17]. Thus, multifocality or multicentricity of breast cancers may in fact be a lot more common than currently acknowledged.

If, as proposed by Hanahan and Weinberg [5], it does require some six sequential carcinogenic "genetic hits" in a single cellular clone for a malignant tumor to develop, it is more likely to occur in a tissue with a high background of genetic alterations in neighbouring cellular clones, than in a tissue with a low background of such alterations, or with no detectable carcinogenic mutations at all (figure 2-1). The probability of a single clone accumulating six independent but sequential genetic alterations leading to a malignant phenotype, without any similar events occurring in neighbouring cells would seem to be lower than the probability of similar changes in a tissue field exposed to the same carcinogens and/or promoters and with detectable epigenetic or genetic changes. Our ability to measure "background carcinogenesis" in different parts of the body might lead to several unexpected implications. Technology is just beginning to be sufficiently sensitive to start detecting such background carcinogenesis. However, one potential technical problem is that in pre-malignant tissue, the "signal" (e.g. relevant oncogenetic lesions) might be diluted by the "noise" (normal genome of most of the cells in the tissue), until the pre-malignant clones have expanded enough to become more numerous locally than normal cells.

A molecular understanding of cancer now allows us to bring together the "Field Cancerization" theory by Slaughter [11] and the more recent "Multi-step Carcinogenesis" model by Fearon and Vogelstein [18] into a single framework: Sequential Field Cancerization [19].

This framework can be easily incorporated into the agent-based model of multi-step carcinogenesis described earlier. For example, the "normal" cell population could actually be modeled as having one or two latent mutations which do not provide any advantage until the environment changes or other mutations are acquired as the tissue ages. The implementation of this effect would simply be a matter of updating the model's initial conditions.

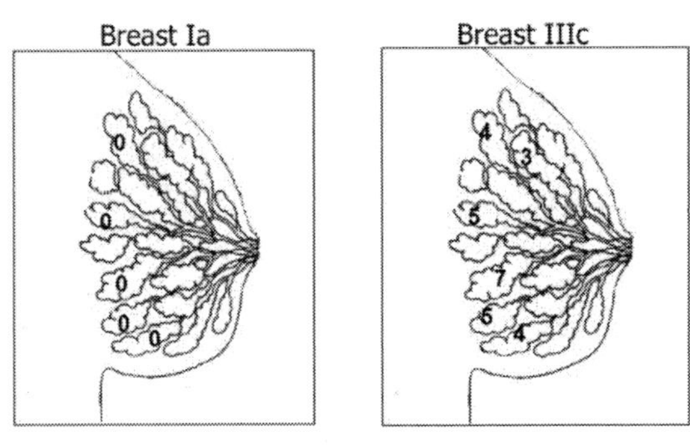

	NORMAL MUCOSA	PROFILERATIVE	DYSPLASTIC
No Mutations	I a	I b	I c
< 3 Mutations	II a	II b	II c
> 3 Mutations	III a	III b	III c

Figure 2.1. Combined histological and molecular staging system of pre-malignant changes. Breast Ia is considerably less likely to develop a malignant tumor than breast IIIc. This combined approach might be helpful to determine relative risks of malignancy for benign but suspicious mammograms, for example in the BIRAD 3 or 4 categories. (Figure taken from Bronchud, 2008; ref. 20).

2.4. Toward a Combined Histological and Molecular Staging of Cancer

Gradually, in the process of human cancer formation, a given target tissue experiences a transition from normal histology, to proliferative and/or dysplastic changes, to so-called "intraepithelial neoplasia" (IEN), which can be early or severe, to superficial cancers ("in situ"), and finally to invasive disease. In some instances, the process may be aggressive and relatively rapid (e.g. in the presence of a DNA repair-deficient genotype or an aggressive human papilloma virus), but in general these changes occur over a long period of time. In the breast, for example, it is estimated that progression from atypical hyperplasia through ductal carcinoma "in situ" (DCIS) to adenocarcinoma may require 30 years or more [21, 22]. Similar observations have been made in other tissues, such as lung, head and neck, prostate, bladder and colorectal tissue [23-26].

However, it would be a mistake to believe that all common epithelial human cancers follow these clear-cut histological sequential patterns from adenoma to carcinoma. In fact, only a minority of the most common type of breast cancers (infiltrating ductal carcinomas, or IDC) arise from ductal carcinoma in situ. Thus, the molecular changes leading to IDC that account for almost 70% of all breast cancers, can happen before the histological features associated with DCIS become evident. DCIS is characterized by a proliferation of malignant epithelial cells confined to the mammary ducts without light microscopic evidence of invasion through the basement membrane into the surrounding stroma; but IDC, by definition, shows signs of invasion of stromal tissue, often with vascular and/or lymphatic vessel involvement. In other words, conventional histological and radiological techniques (e.g. bilateral mammograms) are not sensitive enough to detect with precision on-going carcinogenic risk in many cases of women at risk.

A possible future objective is the development of a combined histological and molecular staging system (figure 2-1). For example, after a follow up of 5-10 years, one would expect more new cancers to develop in group IIIc of figure 2-1 (dysplastic changes and three or more than three "significant mutations" identified), than in group Ia (normal histology and no mutations identified). "Mutations" in this model could also mean non-mutational epigenetic changes, such as changes in DNA methylation, altered chromatin structure, or misregulation of protein chaperones or transcription factors, including the expression of microRNAs.

This, if confirmed, could lead to a more specific and meaningful method to classify individual risk of breast cancer than simply the conventional Breast Imaging Reporting and Data System (BIRAD) scoring of mammograms. This indicates the radiologist's subjective (but experienced) opinion of the absence or likelihood of breast cancer. A low score (<3) does not require special follow up because the risk of cancer is considered too low; a score of 3, 4 or 5 will require follow up; a score of 6 is given only after a biopsy has been examined and found to be cancerous. In those cases where the score is 3 to 5, an additional histological and molecular score based on a fine-needle aspirate might prove more indicative of breast cancer risk, and might indicate the need for specific chemopreventive measures or more intensive follow ups.

Similarly, dysplastic changes in the oropharyngeal mucosa of smokers (including leukoplakia) can lead to laser surgery and aggressive resection, but none of these approaches is of clear clinical benefit. Tailor-made chemopreventive methods based on a combined histological and molecular score might help improve the outlook of these conditions. Other clinical situations where a combined histological and molecular scoring system should be attempted as cancer predictor include almost any clinical non-malignant condition with dysplastic (e.g. chronic gastritis), metaplastic (e.g. Barrett's esophagus), proliferative or proliferative-dysplastic features.

Longitudinal studies in target high-risk populations, like heavy smokers and drinkers, are needed to further verify the dynamics of cancer progression in head and neck cancers. Ethanol is a synergistic carcinogen in smokers, markedly increasing the incidence of squamous cell carcinomas of the head and neck, perhaps because it enhances the uptake of potent tobacco carcinogens by epithelial cells, and acts as a tumor promoter through tissue damage and resultant chronic regenerative proliferation, overwhelming the repair capacity of the cell for the ongoing genetic damage introduced by tobacco mutagens.

The clinical application of this concept and technology should then help to classify patients into various relative risk groups early on in the development of a malignant disease, allowing a tailor-made program for follow-up and screening, as well as more appropriate therapeutic and chemopreventive interventions [27, 28]. In another example, a suitable combination of relevant biomarkers might help clinicians to identify smokers at high risk of developing lung cancers (approximately 10%-15% of frequent smokers) [29, 30]. Confrontation with personal cancer risk rather than general statistical risk is a potent motivation to quit smoking and to undergo more frequent health checks (like the still controversial high-resolution CT-scans to detect isolated pulmonary nodules). Some smokers might be protected because of genetic polymorphisms of enzymes involved in the molecular activation of pre-carcinogens present in tobacco, whereas others may be more vulnerable to the carcinogenic effects because of genetic defects in DNA repair enzymes.

The problem has dramatic public health implications, and could lead to far reaching clinical implications. It has been estimated that in the USA alone some 30% of people above the age of 60 can be found to have adenomas of the colon by colonoscopy, 70% or more of men above the age of 80 will have IEN of the prostate, 30% of people aged 60 or more have actinic keratosis on their skin, 20% of sexually active women above the age of 40 may have some degree of cervical IEN, at least 40% of heavy smokers can show metaplastic or dysplastic changes in their bronchial mucosa, and some 20% of women over age 50 with dense mammograms may show atypical cells on ductal washings from the nipple or ultrasound-guided fine-needle aspirates. The use of a battery of genetic or protein biomarkers relevant to each of the main cancer types may soon help us to better define individual cancer risks, and to measure background carcinogenesis in individual tissue samples. Perhaps, not too long from now, oncology units will be devoted to the treatment of carcinogenesis just as much as to the treatment of cancer.

It has been said that current research efforts against cancer have made some fundamental mistakes, like stressing 'curative treatments' instead of specific measures to lower cancer incidence in target populations [31]. One example is the control of classical cardiovascular risk factors (hypertension, high cholesterol levels, diabetes, obesity and sedentarism) in the case of heart disease - the age-specific death rates for cardiovascular disease have gone down by some 40% to 60% in the past 50 years, whereas those for cancer have gone down by only some 5%, in spite of a huge increase in expenditure on new cancer treatments [32]. By analogy, efforts to reduce cancer risk (for example, the choice to quit smoking) might therefore be a cheaper and more successful method to lower the incidence of many cancers. The American Society of Clinical Oncology (ASCO) has recently proposed a number of guidelines and initiatives to increase the role of clinical oncologists in cancer prevention and risk assessment [33].

2.5. The Importance of Non-Genetic Factors

One caveat to modeling cancer progression as a series of acquired genetic mutations is the emerging awareness that not all cancer cell phenotypes require a genetic alteration. In biology, the term "epigenetics" refers to changes in phenotype (appearance) or gene expression caused by mechanisms other than changes in the underlying DNA sequence. Probably the best example of epigenetic changes is the process of cellular differentiation and morphogenesis, whereby totipotent stem cells become pluripotent cell lines and committed progenitor cells with increasingly specialized features until they become fully differentiated cells. Cancer, in many ways, represents a failure of this normal differentiation process, and it is not surprising that epigenetic molecular changes - like abnormal DNA methylation, histone protein modifications, microRNA up or down regulation, and chromatin remodeling – have been described as an integral part of the carcinogenesis process [34].

Andrew Feinberg's group [35, 36] at Johns Hopkins University School of Medicine has recently focused on cancer predisposing epigenetic alterations. They have, for example, linked loss of imprinting (LOI) of the autocrine growth factor gene IGF2 to cancer risk, suggesting an epigenetic progenitor model of cancer, in which epigenetically altered stem cells (or progenitor cells) precede other cancerous mutations. This model differs from the classical clonal mutational model, and is quite compatible with the multistep field cancerization theory of carcinogenesis. Epigenetic changes, like mutations, are often associated with specific places on DNA and are only relevant insofar as they are also similarly heritable. Just as mutation of a transcription factor can affect many genes, so can alteration of a gene product involved in the epigenetic control of gene expression. Perhaps the most significant difference is the more likely reversal of an epigenetic state as a cancer develops.

Aging is the single major risk factor for most common human cancers. The exact mechanisms responsible for the effect of aging on tumor incidence are poorly understood, in part because very few model systems are available to study age-dependent genomic or epigenomic instability. The intuitive role of DNA mutations in 'normal aging' and 'life-span extension' is unclear and it is very important to develop powerful experimental systems to identify genetic and epigenetic modifications that regulate genomic stability or instability in aging. How does aging affect DNA stability? Is there a genetic or epigenetic molecular clock that somehow protects the genome until the fourth or fifth decade of human life but that goes progressively wrong thereafter? In women, aging-associated menopause can have a protective effect against female breast cancer. This phenomenon is demonstrated by the characteristic shape of age-specific incidence rates plotted on a log-log scale: around age 50 in women (but not in men) there is a distinct slowing in the rate of increase for breast cancer incidence. This is probably because estradiol (and perhaps progesterone) can be regarded as a tumor promoter in breast carcinogenesis. This age-specific risk of breast cancer differs by hormone-receptor status (ER/PR) to the extent that the large international variation of breast cancer incidence rates may to some extent be explained by the risk difference for the ER+/PR+ subtype [37].

Beyond classical epigenetic modification is the growing realization that non-genetic/non-epigenetic cell-to-cell variation in the levels of proteins and other biomolecules can have dramatic phenotypic consequences that may be relevant to cancer. Recent research tracking the fates of single cells using time-lapse microscopy has revealed non-genetic heterogeneity in the ability of cells to avoid chemotherapy-induced apoptosis [38, 39, 40]. Even members of a genetically identical population of cancer cells grown in an identical environment exhibit variability in their sensitivity to apoptosis to the extent that some cells die while others live on indefinitely after a death-inducing stimulus. Neighbor effects, position in the culture dish, and cell cycle effects were ruled out as possible causes of heterogeneity, while both experimental and computational methods implicated cell-to-cell variability in protein levels as the source of variability in cell fate [38]. Stochasticity in gene expression has been shown to give rise to cell-to-cell variation in protein concentrations, resulting in "outlier" cells that have much higher than average or much lower than average levels of key proteins involved in apoptosis. This natural heterogeneity allows some cells to survive the apoptotic insult (and thus re-grow the tumor) and is believed to relate to the "fractional killing" of tumor cells following exposure to chemotherapy [38]. Similarly, cell-to-cell variation in protein levels could allow for the existence of a population of outlier cells that possess other capabilities. For example, variability in the tumorigenicity of cancer cells is a commonly observed phenomenon. In many studies, individual cells or subpopulations of cells obtained from tumors are assayed for tumorigenicity, revealing large variability in the malignancy of individual cancer cells [41]. These observations have traditionally been explained by genetic differences among cells within a tumor. More recently, such observations have been considered evidence for the existence of cancer stem cells. Cancer stem cells have been defined as "rare cells with indefinite potential for self-renewal that drive tumorigenesis" [42]. However, it is also possible that stochasticity in gene expression could transiently create subpopulations of cells that express a specific set of initial conditions and cell surface markers that favor tumor formation. In summary, while mutation to genes that are critical to the checks and balances of cellular proliferation have been shown time and again to drive carcinogenesis, transiently heritable non-genetic heterogeneity in the levels of proteins and other biomolecules could provide the extra push that allows a cell to form a tumor.

Conclusions

There are still vast gaps in our knowledge of the natural history of most common human cancers in spite of the great achievements of molecular oncology and epidemiology in the past three decades. Our understanding of human cancer 'pre-history' (the often long and clinically silent premalignant evolution of a cancer) is even more limited. Yet, in our view, both increasing molecular evidence and recent conceptual advances point toward a model of "sequential field cancerization': a premalignant carcinogenic evolution of some cells in any given tissue, or tissue field. The process of carcinogenesis is by nature progressive but not necessarily irreversible. In most epithelial tissues, progression means the sequential accumulation of genetic somatic mutations. In some cases of familial predisposition to cancer some of these mutations are inherited. Epigenetic changes in the progenitor or stem cell compartment of proliferating tissues might precede genetic mutations, and some of these epigenetic changes can also be inherited. Unlike genetic changes, such as chromosomal translocations or gene mutations, epigenetic changes are 'reversible' but can initiate irreversible genetic changes. By uncovering variants that might be deleterious to the whole organism and suppressed epigenetically in familial transmission, cancer cells might also gain a selective growth advantage. Although not inherently mutagenic, chronic cell injury and inflammation is a major cause of cancer. A relevant clinical example could be Barrett's esophagus, a condition of intestinal metaplasia of the esophagus associated with chronic gastric fluid reflux and an increased risk of adenocarcinoma. Close clinical and endoscopic follow up of these patients is mandatory and recent evidence from a randomized study in 127 patients, stratified according to the grade of dysplasia and the length of Barrett's esophagus, has shown that radiofrequency ablation of the dysplastic mucosa can lead to a high rate of complete eradication of both dysplasia and intestinal metaplasia, and a reduced risk of disease progression towards cancer [43]. More longitudinal studies of this kind, preferably also associated with molecular (genetic and epigenetic) screening methods, promise a new era in oncology.

References

[1] Cahill DP, Kinzler KW, et al. (1999). Genetic instability and darwinian selection in tumours. *Trends Cell Biol.*, 9(12):M57-60.

[2] Armitage P, and Doll R. (1954). The age distribution of cancer and a multi-stage theory of carcinogenesis. *Br. J. Cancer*, 8(1):1-12.

[3] Nowell PC. (1976). The clonal evolution of tumor cell populations. *Science*, 194(4260): 23-28.
[4] Renan MJ. (1993). How many mutations are required for tumorigenesis? Implications from human cancer data. *Mol. Carcinog.*, 7(3):139-146.
[5] Hanahan D, and Weinberg RA. (2000). The hallmarks of cancer. *Cell,* 100(1):57-70.
[6] Spencer SL, Gerety RA, et al. (2006). Modeling somatic evolution in tumorigenesis. *PLoS Comput. Biol.*, 2(8):e108.
[7] Kinzler KW, and Vogelstein B. (1996). Lessons from hereditary colorectal cancer. *Cell,* 87(2):159-170.
[8] Maley CC, Galipeau PC, et al. (2006). Genetic clonal diversity predicts progression to esophageal adenocarcinoma. *Nat. Genet.*, 38(4):468-473.
[9] Blow N. (2009). In vivo molecular imaging: the inside job. *Nat. Methods* 6(6):465-469.
[10] Weissleder R, and Pittet MJ. (2008). Imaging in the era of molecular oncology. *Nature,* 452(7187):580-589.
[11] Slaughter DP, Southwick HW, and Smejkal W. (1953) "Field cancerization" in oral stratified squamous epithelium. *Cancer* (Phila.), 6:963-968.
[12] Knowles MA. (1999). The genetics of transitional cell carcinoma: progress and potential clinical applications. *Br. J. Urol. International*, 84:412-427.
[13] Ahrendt SA, Chow JT, Xu LH, et al. (1999). Molecular detection of tumor cells in bronchioalveolar lavage fluid from patients with early stage lung cancer. J Natl Cancer Inst, 91:332-339.
[14] Bedi GC, Westra WH, Gabrielson E, et al. (1996). Multiple head and neck tumors: evidence for a common clonal origin. *Cancer Res.,* 56:2484-2487.
[15] Partridge M, Emilion G, et al. (1997). Field cancerisation of the oral cavity: comparison of the spectrum of molecular alterations in cases presenting with both dysplastic and malignant lesions. *Oral. Oncol.*, 33(5):332-337.
[16] Lagios MD, Westdahl PR, Rose MR. (1981). The concept and implications of multicentricity in breast carcinoma. *Pathol. Annu.*, 16:83-102.
[17] Lagios MD, Richards VE, Rose MR, Yee E. (1983). Segmental mastectomy without radiotherapy: short term follow-up. *Cancer,* 52:2173-2179.
[18] Fearon ER, and Vogelstein B. (1990). A genetic model for colorectal tumorigenesis. *Cell,* 61:759-767.
[19] Bronchud MH. (2002). Is cancer really a "local" cellular clonal disease? *Medical Hypotheses*, 59:560-565.
[20] Bronchud MH. Selecting the right targets for cancer therapy. In: Principles of Molecular Oncology. Bronchud M.H., Foote M.A., Giaccone G., Olopade O., and Workman P. (2008); *Humana Press* NJ: 1-26.
[21] Frykberg ER, and Bland KI. (1993). "In situ" breast carcinoma. *Adv. Surg.*, 26:29-72.
[22] Page DL, Dupont WD, Rogers LW, and Rados MS. (1985). Atypical hyperplastic lesions of the female breast. A long-term follow-up study. *Cancer* (Phla.), 55:2698-2708.
[23] Day DW, and Morson BC. The adenoma-carcinoma sequence. In: "The Pathogenesis of Colorectal Cancer", 1978, Bennington J.L. (ed.) vol 10, chapter 6:58-71; Saunder and Co., Philadelphia.
[24] Bostwick DG. (1992). Prostatic intraepithelial neoplasia (PIN): current concepts. *J. Cell. Biochem.*, 16H:10-19.

[25] Califano J, van der Riet P, Westra W, et al. (1996). Genetic progression model for head and neck cancer: implications for field cancerization. *Cancer Res.*, 56:2488-2492.
[26] Sidransky D, Messing E. (1992). Molecular genetics and biochemical mechanisms in bladder cancer. Oncogenes, tumor suppressor genes and growth factors. *Urol. Clin. North Amer*, 19:629-639.
[27] Kelloff GJ, Sigman CC, Johnson KM, et al. (2000). Perspectives on surrogate end points in the development of drugs that reduce the risk of cancer. *Cancer Epid. Biomark. and Prevention*, 9:127-137.
[28] Miller AB, Bartsch H, Boffetta P, Dragsted L, and Vainio H. (2001). Biomarkers in Cancer Chemoprevention. IARC Scientific Publications, 154.
[29] Moolgavkar S, Krewski D, Zeise L, Cardis E, and Moller H. (1999). Quantitative estimation and prediction of human cancer risks. IARC Scientific Publications, 131.
[30] Kersting M, Friedl C, Kraus A, et al. (2000). Differential frequencies of p16 (INK4a) promoter hypermethylation, p53 mutation, and K-ras mutation in exfoliative material mark the development of lung cancer in symptomatic chronic smokers. *J. Clin. Oncol.*, 18:3221-3229.
[31] Gina Kolata. Advances elusive in the drive to cure cancer. Published in
[32] The New York Times, April 23, 2009.
[33] Gina Kolata. As other death rates fall, cancer's scarcely moves.
[34] Published in The New York Times, April 24, 2009.
[35] Zon RT, Goss E, Vogel VG, et al. (2009). American Society of Clinical Oncology Policy Statement: the role of the oncologist in cancer prevention and risk assessment. *J. Clin. Oncol.* 27(6):986-993.
[36] Issa JP. (2000). The epigenetics of colorectal cancer. *Ann. N. Y. Acad. Sci.*, 910:140-153.
[37] Feinberg A.P. (2004). The epigenetcis of cancer etiology. *Seminars in Cancer Biology,* 14:427-432.
[38] Feinberg AP. (2006). Ohlsson R, and Henikoff S. The epigenetic progenitor origin of human cancer. *Nature Reviews Genetics*, 7:21-33.
[39] Yutaka Y, and Potter JD. (1999). The shape of age-incidence curves of female breast cancer by hormone-receptor status. *Cancer Casues and Control*, 10:431-437.
[40] Spencer, S. L., S. Gaudet, et al. (2009). Non-genetic origins of cell-to-cell variability in TRAIL-induced apoptosis. *Nature,* 459(7245):428-32.
[41] Gascoigne KE, Taylor SS. (2008). Cancer cells display profound intra- and interline variation following prolonged exposure to antimitotic drugs. *Cancer Cell*, 14:111-22.
[42] Cohen AA, Geva-Zatorsky N, Eden E, et al. (2008). Dynamic proteomics of individual cancer cells in response to a drug. *Science*, 322:1511-1516.
[43] Brock A, Chang H, and Huang S. (2009). Non-genetic heterogeneity - a mutation-independent driving force for the somatic evolution of tumours. *Nat. Rev. Genet.* 10(5):336-42.
[44] Reya T, Morrison SJ, et al. (2001). Stem cells, cancer, and cancer stem cells. *Nature* 414(6859):105-11.
[45] Shaheen NJ, Sharma P, Overholt BF, et al. (2009). Radiofrequency ablation in Barret's esophagus with Dysplasia. *NEJM*, 360(22):2277-2288.

In: Field Cancerization: Basic Science and Clinical Applications ISBN 978-1-61761-006-6
Editor: Gabriel D. Dakubo

Chapter 3

Development of Tumor Stem Cells: Implication in Field Cancerization

Jian-Xin Gao

Abstract

Field cancerization is a generalized phenomenon of cancers but usually exhibits as occult precancerous lesions surrounding cancers. It appears to be associated with recurrence and metastasis of cancers after treatment. However, the mechanisms underlying the field cancerization are not yet clear. With the identification of various stages of developing tumor stem cells (TSCs), an innovative TSC theory is emerging to emphasize that a developing cancer is evolutionarily mediated by developing TSCs. The TSCs may be hierarchically developed from tumor-initiating stem cells (TISCs) to precancerous stem cells (pCSCs) and cancer stem cells (CSCs), regulated by environmental cues. The composition of TSC subpopulations determines tumor malignancy or the stage of cancerization, which manifests clinically and histopathologically as benign proliferation, precancer or cancer. The field cancerization might be associated with sporadic seeding of TSCs. In this chapter, we will review and discuss current understanding on TSCs and propose a potential model of TSC-mediated field cancerization, which might lead to novel strategies for effective detection and intervention of cancers.

3.1. Introduction

Cancerization or carcinogenesis is a long process, including the stages of benign but abnormal proliferation, precancer and cancer. Relatively to cancerization, the concept of "field cancerization" reflects the late, multicentric recurrence surrounding primary cancers [1-5]. The concept of "field cancerization" was initially described by Slaughter *et al.* in 1953, based on the contiguous pathology of oral carcinoma, in which microscopic multicentric precancerous lesions were found in the grossly normal epithelial mucosa surrounding the cancers [1]. These precancerous lesions are occult and not easily removed by surgery. Thus, these lesions rather than preexisting malignant lesions were considered as the origin of recurrent cancers [1]. Since then, organ systems in which field cancerization has been described include head and neck (oral cavity, oropharynx, and larynx), lung, vulva, esophagus, cervix, breast, skin, colon, and bladder [1-4,6]. However, the lack of understanding of the mechanisms underlying the field cancerization hinders prevention and treatment of cancer in practice.

Recently, the concept of "field cancerization" has been extended from histologically abnormal tissue to histologically normal appearing tissue surrounding or distant from primary carcinomas, in which cancer-like epigenetic and genetic changes were observed and referred as to "field effect" [3,4,7-9]. The discovery of tumor stem cells (TSCs) provides a cellular basis of field cancerization. The TSC model of field cancerization emphasizes that TSCs play a central role for the field cancerization; the interaction between TSCs and the carcinogenic fields determines the outcome of field cancerization. This model may explain how a field cancerization is initiated at cellular and molecular levels. Cancer-like epigenetic and genetic alterations contribute to clonal maintenance, expansion and evolution of TSCs [10-15]. In this chapter, I am going to review the recent progress in TSC research and discuss its implication in field cancerization.

3.2. Tumor Stem Cells and Tumor Development

3.2.1. Tumor Developing Stages and Tumor Malignancy

A tumor can develop from a cell with abnormal cycling. Abnormal but controllable cell proliferation may give rise to benign tumors; whereas uncontrollable cell proliferation may result in malignant tumors. The malignancy of a tumor may be determined by the capacity of proliferation, invasiveness/metastasis and tumor vasculogenesis of tumor cells [11,16]. Although benign tumors are usually limited in cell proliferation and not invasive, some of them may transform to malignant tumors or cancers upon carcinogenic stimulations. A developing cancer may have a lengthy, reversible premalignant stage before they progress to the malignant status [11,17].

Although there are a variety of histopathological changes for each type of tumors, most tumors regardless of tissue origin may exhibit three types of typical pathological changes in general: a) benign or proliferative lesions; b) premalignant lesions; and c) malignant lesions. Benign proliferative lesions mainly exhibit as hyperplasia, metaplasia or low grade dysplasia; precancerous or premalignant lesions as high grade dysplasia or carcinoma in situ (CIS); and cancerous or malignant lesions as invasive carcinoma. Accordingly, these lesions manifest clinically as benign proliferation, precancer and cancer [11,15]. While proliferative lesions and precancerous lesions are usually reversible, invasive lesions may be irreversible [18]. For an established malignant tumor, these types of changes may have occurred hierarchically. Therefore, benign proliferative lesion reflects the tumor-initiating stage, which may progress to the stages of precancer and invasive cancer, depending on environmental cues [11,15] (figure 1).

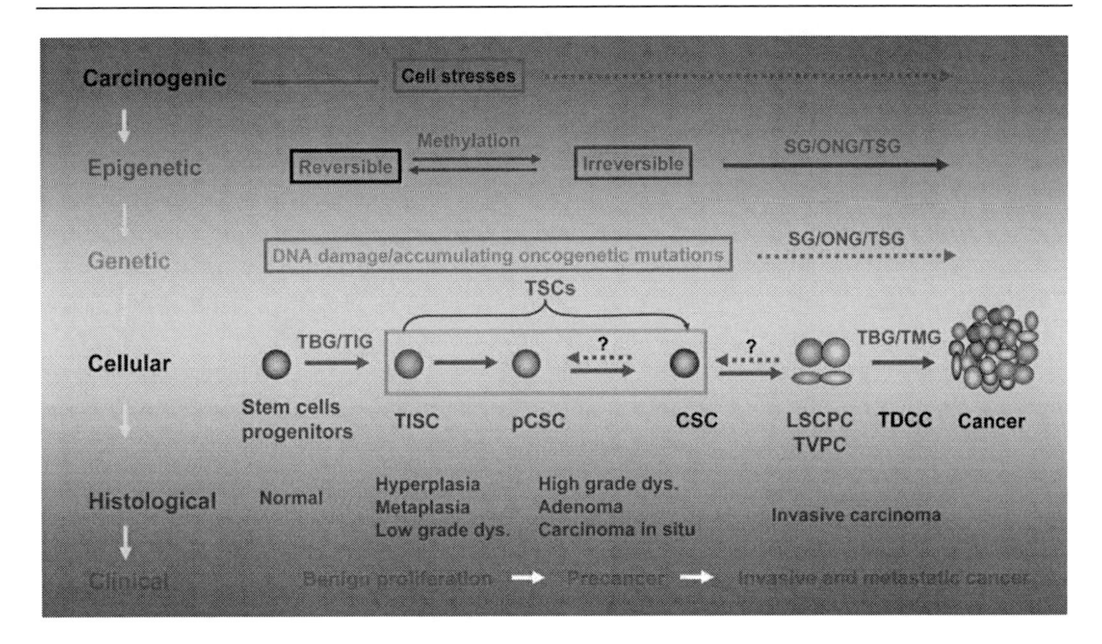

Abbreviations in the figure: TSC: tumor stem cell; TISC: tumor-initiating stem cell; pCSC: precancerous stem cell; CSC: cancer stem cell, TVPC: tumor vasculogenic progenitor cell; LSCPC: lineage-specific cancer progenitor/propagating cells; TDCC: terminal differentiated cancer cell; TBG: tumor-barrier gene; TIG: tumor-initiating gene; TMG: tumor-maintaining gene; SG: stability gene; ONG: oncogene; TSG: tumor suppressor gene; dys.: dysplasia. The figure is adopted from *Drug Discovery Today: Disease Models, 2009* [15] with modifications.

Figure 3.1. Tumor initiation, progression and establishment: molecular, cellular, histopathological and clinical manifestations. Genotoxic agents and/or cellular stresses induce DNA damage in stem/progenitor cells. The fates of DNA damaged cells depend on the activation status of TBGs and TIGs. The insulted cells that are not recovered from DNA damage are epigenetically altered and susceptible to oncogenetic mutations of SGs, ONGs and/or TSGs. The cells accumulated with epigenetic and oncogenetic alterations can develop into TSCs, including subpopulations of TISC, pCSC, and CSC. TISCs can hierarchically develop into pCSCs and then CSCs. The progenies of CSCs, called LSCPCs, have strong capacity to propagate cancers. Both pCSCs and CSCs have the potential to differentiate into TVPCs, mediating tumor vasculogenesis. Each subpopulation of TSCs can mediate corresponding histopathological and clinical changes, such as benign proliferation mediated by TISCs, precancer by pCSCs and invasive cancers by CSCs. An established cancer is comprised of a variety of tumor cells, including TISCs, pCSCs, CSCs, LSCPCs and TDCCs. Throughout the process of tumor development, TBG activation may override TMGs to suppress tumor development.

Tumor is highly heterogeneous, consisting of phenotypically and functionally different tumor cells, including parenchymal tumor cells, tumor vasculogenic progenitor cells (TVPCs) and stromal cells serving as tumor niches [11,16,19]. The parenchymal tumor cells may consist of subsets of TSCs, lineage-specific tumor progenitor or propagating cells (LSCPCs), and terminal differentiated cancer cells (TDCCs). Therefore, a tumor can be considered as a quasi-organ. Like normal organs in which tissue components are continuously replenished by tissue adult stem cells, tumor components may be replenished by stem-like tumor cells, i.e., TSCs [11]. The TSCs have been considered to be essential for a tumor development despite of controversies [20-25]. Whether TSCs can progress to pCSCs or CSCs may determine the degree of the malignancy of a tumor, which mainly depends on the outcome of interactions between TSCs and tumorigenic niches [11,15,19,26,27].

3.2.2. Roles of Tumor Stem Cell in Tumor Development

Increasing data have revealed that tumor development is mediated by TSCs [10-15,21]. Since developmental stages of tumor (benign proliferation, precancer and invasive cancer) show different pathological changes, and these changes may be mediated by developing TSCs at corresponding stages. Therefore, TSCs can be classified, based on their contribution to each stage of tumor development, as the developing stages of tumor-initiating stem cells (TISCs), pCSCs and CSCs; in other word, benign proliferation, precancer and invasive cancer can be mediated, respectively, by TISCs, pCSCs and CSCs (figure 1 and 3).

As a quai-organ, tumor is likely to mimic bone marrow, in which rare numbers of hematopoietic stem cells (HSCs) are the source for the maintenance of the supply of blood components [11,14]. HSCs can produce large numbers of blood cells every day; but they never exceed the threshold required for maintenance of blood homeostasis physiologically. However, no homeostatic balance in cancers could be established between TSCs and their progenies. TSCs may constantly give rise to various types of tumor cells as long as the tumorigenic niche is existed. TSCs themselves might also expand or be enriched in a vicious tumorigenic environment, for example, after anti-cancer therapy with chemical agents and/or X-ray irradiation [28-31]. Therefore, unlike the HSC pool, which is stable in bone marrow, TSC pool is not stable in cancers, and the frequency of TSCs in cancers may determine the rate of tumor growth.

Theoretically, benign proliferation is mediated only by TISCs; precancers by pCSCs; invasive cancers by CSCs. However, malignant tumors may contain all stages of developing TSCs, including TISCs, pCSCs and CSCs. Since TSCs are only a small population within tumors, substantial increase of tumor volume might be mediated by their progenies, i.e., LSCPCs and TDCCs. Therefore, rare number of TISCs, pCSCs and CSCs are existed in benign proliferative lesions, precancerous lesions and malignant lesions, respectively; their progenies constitute major population in respective lesions. Generally, TISCs may give rise to relatively well-differentiated but hyperplastic cells, pCSCs to less differentiated atypical cells; and CSCs to LSCPCs and TDCCs. However, the later stages of lesion always contain earlier stages of lesion. In the malignant tumors, the proliferative, precancerous and cancerous lesions may coexist and contain all stages of developing TSCs, including TISCs, pCSCs and CSCs. The co-existence of TISCs, pCSCs and CSCs in malignant tumors might be the cause of field cancerization [1-3]. The hypothesis is being verified in our laboratory.

3.2.3. New Dimension of Tumor Stem Cell Model

Because tumors are composed of phenotypically and functionally heterogeneous cells, two models, the stochastic and hierarchy models, attempted to explain how the heterogenicity arises [11,12,14,21]. The stochastic model claims that all tumor cells have initiating activity and thus can reconstitute a tumor of origin. These heterogeneous tumor cells are biologically and functionally equivalent, but their behavior varies with the influences of intrinsic and extrinsic factors and is therefore both variable and unpredictable. In contrast, hierarchy model argues that the heterogeneous tumors are biologically and functionally distinct and only a rare or small population of cells, which are capable of developing into tumor cells with differing phenotypes and biological behavior, can initiate and drive the growth of a tumor. This population has been called as CSCs [11-14,21].

Currently, most of cancer chemotherapy modes target both normal and tumor cells, because under the stochastic model, anti-cancer drugs cannot be produced without damaging normal cells. As a result many healthy cells are killed during anti-cancer chemotherapy, leading to devastating outcomes [11,32]. Therefore, it is critical for cancer therapy to specifically and effectively target tumor cells which are responsible for tumor malignancy [11]. The CSC theory has been proposed as a novel model to reach the goal [13,29,32-34].

The concept of the CSC is not novel but remains to be defined more precisely. This concept arises from the observations that only a small subset of stem-like human cancer cells can form a new tumor of origin when transplanted into non-obese diabetes/severe combined immunodeficiency disease (NOD/Scid) [35,36]. The clonal nature of these cells implicated in various types of malignancies led to the postulation of CSCs in the past by several laboratories [12,37-40]. However, CSCs were not experimentally documented for human hematopoietic cancer such as acute myelogenous leukemia (AML) until 1994 [35] and for human solid cancers such as breast cancer until 2003 [36]. Till now, whether the CSC theory truly reflects the mechanisms underlying tumor development remains highly controversial [10,11,15,16,20,25,41,42], because it is essentially derived from xenograft tumor transplantation model [35,36], with obvious limitation in accurately reflecting the physiological state of a developing tumor [10,11,15].

It is considered that CSCs are a rare population that can reconstitute a new tumor with similar composition and phenotype to the tumor of origin [11-14]. The CSCs are capable of self-renewal and have the pluripotency or multipotency of differentiation. They can give rise to "daughter" cells that are either self-renewed or variably differentiated [11,14]. The CSCs appear to be hierarchically developed from primitive precursors [10,43-45] and the rate of their cycling may determine the degree of tumor growth. Thus far, CSCs have been identified in almost all types of cancer, including the hematopoietic [35,46,47] and non-hematopoietic cancers [36,48-52]. However, the identity of these CSCs is highly variable between tumors, individuals, experimental models and even laboratories, provoking the dispute on CSC theory [11,20-22,24,25,41,53].

The CSC theory is essentially built on the blocks from xenotransplantation models of human cancers, in which a rare or small population of perspectively isolated human cancer cells with a given phenotype can reconstitute a tumor of origin in NOD/Scid mice [11,14]. The advantage of the model is that self-renewal capability of cancer cells can be reliably tested by serial transplantations; and the disadvantage is that the xenogenic hosts may offer a hostile or incompatible environment to human cancer cells, resulting in false negative or positive results [41,42,53]. A number of studies that have challenged the current CSC model might be related to the limitation of tumor xenotransplantation models [20,22,25,41,42,47,53]. In most instances, tumor cells are obtained using selection of, and enrichment for, cells with prospectively identified cell surface markers and tested in NOD/SCID mice that might offer a hostile or incompatible microenvironment for human tumor cells [36,43,46,47]. In addition, the perspective enrichment for CSCs may also underestimate or overestimate the number of CSCs and neglect their precursors and progenies. The perspectively isolated cancer cells may contain subpopulations of TSCs, such as TISCs and pCSCs, and LSCPCs, the progenies of CSCs, which cannot be distinguished by the xenotransplantation models [10,11,16,43,45,54,55]. The TISCs, pCSCs and probably

LSCPCs, might also be able to develop into tumors in SCID mice [10,20,44,56]. To circumvent the problems, we need to establish and characterize TSC lines, including TISCs, pCSCs and CSCs, which can recapitulate developing stages of tumors in appropriate models [11].

Increasing data have indicated that TSCs are existed in benign proliferations, precancers and cancers [10,11,14,16,44,57]. Recently we have identified a new type of cancer cells from murine lymphoma [58], which is called pCSCs, because they exhibit stem-like property and have the potential of both benign and malignant differentiation [10,16]. The existence of pCSCs has also been demonstrated in human acute lymphoblast leukemia (ALL) [45], human breast pre-neoplasia [59] as well as murine mammary carcinoma [55]. In addition, Stem-like cells were also isolated from benign tumor [44] and benign proliferative lesion such as hyperplastic cervix uteri [57]. Based on these findings, we have proposed an innovative TSC model (figures 1 and 3): tumor development is mediated by tumor stem cells (TSCs), which may develop from TISCs → pCSCs → CSCs → LSCPCs → terminal differentiated cancer cells (TDCCs), a cellular process unifying molecular (epigenetic and genetic), histopathological and clinical manifestations of tumor [11,15,60,61]. With this model, we may explain all aspects of tumorm development in clinicopathology, directing the divscovery and developments of cancer biomarkers, tumor vaccines as well as novel, safe and cost-effecitive anti-caner drugs.

3.3. Development of Tumor Stem Cells

3.3.1. Features of Normal Stem Cells

Stem cells are characterized as the cells that can differentiate into all or multiple cell types of an organism; and the capacity of differentiation can be maintained for lifetime through self-renewal [11,62]. In other words, they have the capacity of self-renewal and plural or multiple potencies of differentiation. Therefore, stem cells play a crucial role in all aspects of biology from the development of early embryos to the repair and maintenance of adult tissues.

In the mammals, there exist at least two types of stem cells: embryonic stem cells (ESCs) and adult tissue-specific stem cells (ATSCs). ESCs are the cells that are derived from the inner cell mass of an early stage embryo, called as blastocyst. They are pluripotent in differentiation, because they can give rise during the development to cells of all three primary germ layers, including ectoderm, endoderm and mesoderm [63]. A number of transcription factors are required for the maintenance of the pluripotency, such as Oct4, Rex1, Sox2, Nanog, Klf4 and TDGF1 [63-65]. Interestingly these factors have also been frequently detected in various types of cancer [66-70].

Unlike ESCs, ATSCs that reside in either fetal or adult tissues are multipotent in differentiation and only can differentiate into tissue-specific cell types, such as HSCs in the bone marrow (BM) and blood, neural stem cells in the brain, hepatic stem cells in the liver, and GSCs in the testis and ovary [71-75]. The ATSCs maintain a continuous supply for tissue repair throughout adult life through a mechanism of self-renewal. However, the origin of ATSCs is highly controversial, because increased data have revealed that ATSCs may be derived from bone marrow (BM) [76-82]. Whether ATSCs that are derived from BM are common or a special case of transdifferentiation [83-85] remain elusive. It is likely that some ATSCs might possess to some extent the nature of ESCs. For examples, the transcriptional profiling of neural stem cells is similar to that of ESCs [86], GSCs appear to have pluripotency of differentiation similarly to ESCs, in addition to generation of germs and eggs, [73,87].

Self-renewal is a specialized terminology for the division and proliferation of stem cells, which distinguishes from non-stem cells. When a stem cell divides into two "daughter" cells, one of them may be self-renewed and other may be differentiated or undergo apoptosis [11,88,89].

A self-renewed but not differentiated stem cell always retains the property of its parent cell. Telomere maintenance may be related to the self-renewal [90,91]. The immediately differentiated cells are called progenitor cells, which may also have oligo-potency of differentiation. Fox example, multipotent progenitors (MPP) in bone marrow (BM) can differentiate into various types of blood cells [92-94], but with self-renewal capability being greatly reduced. Thus, self-renewal is a critical feature of stem cells that distinguishes from progenitor cells or non-stem cells.

Under physiological conditions, stem cells maintain a small but stable and highly efficient pool in tissues (figure 2). For example, the HSC pool comprises only about 0.01% of marrow cells, but supplies more than 1×10^9 blood cells of various types per day [14,71,95]. To maintain homeostasis of the stem cell pool, the self-renewal of stem cells is strictly regulated by stem cell niches [88,89,96-100]. Usually, stem cells are divided asymmetrically. The asymmetric cell division produces two daughter cells: one self-renewed daughter stem cell remains the same as parent cells with slow cycling but to adapt to the needs for maintaining the stem cell pool, while the other may differentiate into progenitor cells [89]. The differentiated progenies further differentiate into lineage-restricted progenitor cells with accelerated cell cycling to meet the need for maintaining tissue homeostasis, such as common myeloid (CMP) and lymphoid progenitors (CLP) in the hematopoietic system, which can differentiate into myeloid and lymphoid blood cells, respectively [71,92-94]. With the hierarchical differentiation, stem cells gradually lose their capability of self-renewal. While the stem cell pool is reduced, stem cells may divide symmetrically into two "daughter" cells with the same self-renewal capability as parent cells to restore the reduced stem cell pool. If the stem cells lose the capability of self-renewal, the stem cell pool will be withered, leading to the diseased status (figure 2).

The fate of stem cells is determined by environmental cues referred to as the stem cell niche, which consists of stromal or accessory cells, cytokines and developmental growth factors [71,98,101,102]. Osteoblasts and endothelial cells appear to be most important accessory cells that constitute the framework of stem cell niches [96-98,101,103]. Physiologically, the balance between self-renewal and differentiation of stem cells is strictly regulated by the stem cell niche [96,101]. The property of self-renewal of stem cells is also called "stemness", which is controlled by a number of "stemness" genes, some of which have not yet been defined [86,104-107].

Interestingly, the genes that regulate self-renewal of ATSCs are also oncogenic, and can be detected in various types of cancer cells. The best studied is *Bmi-1*, an oncogene encoding a polycomb group transcription factor that is required for self-renewal of normal stem cells as well as CSCs [108-110]. However, ATSCs such as HSCs do not express ESC genes, such as *Oct4, Rex1*, *Sox2* and *TDGF1* [10].

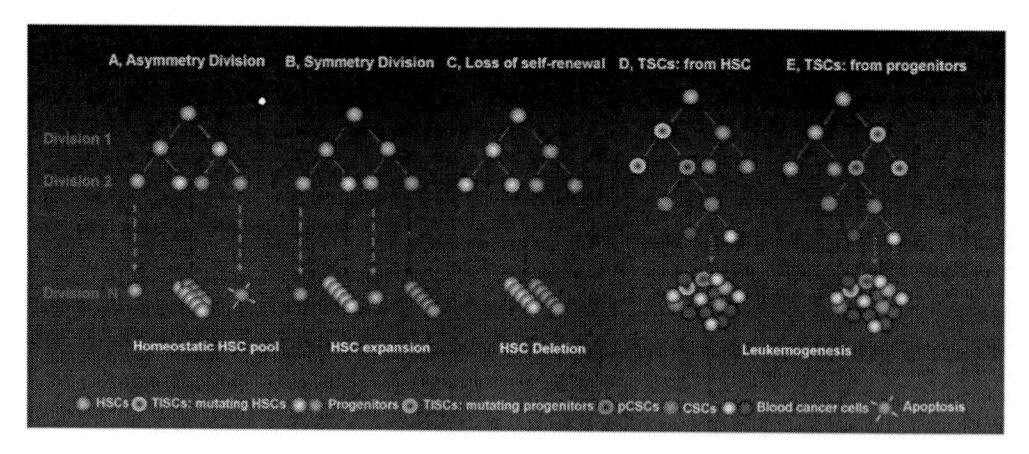

Abbreviations in the figure: HSC: hematopoietic stem cell; TSC: tumor stem cell; TISC: tumor-initiating stem cell; pCSC: precancerous stem cell; CSC: cancer stem cell. The figure is adopted from *J. Cell. Mol. Med., 2008* [11] with modifications.

Figure 3.2. Stem cell self-renewal and tumor stem cell development in blood cancers. The property of stem cell self-renewal warrants stem cells to provide all lineages required for replenishment of tissues during lifetime. Normally, self-renewing hematopoietic stem cells (HSCs) maintain their homeostasis via the mechanisms of asymmetry and symmetry division. In the physiological status, HSC pool is strictly regulated by stem cell niches in the bone marrow, in which HSCs are asymmetrically divided into two "daughter" cells to maintain the size of HSC pool: one is self-renewed, i.e., with the same property of parental cells, and the other is differentiated into progenitor cells (A). Under the pathophysiological conditions, HSC pool may be reduced because of the loss of HSCs. To recover the size of stem cell pool, HSCs divide symmetrically to generate two self-renewed "daughter" cells, i.e., with the same property of parental cells (B). However, if HSCs lose the capability of self-renewal, HSC pool will be withered, leading to hematopoietic diseases (C). In leukemogenesis, blood tumor stem cells (TSCs) or leukemic stem cells (LSCs) may be derived from mutated HSCs (D) or progenitors (E). Regardless of the origin of TSCs, HSCs and progenitors, which are insulted by genotoxic agent may develop into TSCs through the hierarchical developing stages of TISCs, pCSCs and CSCs/LSCs (refer to figure1).

3.3.2. Origin of Tumor Stem Cells

While TSCs are considered as the origin of cancer [11,12]; the origin of TSCs has not been clearly elucidated. Based on literatures, TSCs can be developed from the insulted ATSCs, progenitors, or aberrant fusion cells between the somatic and BM-derived cells [14,111-113]. With the discovery of inducible pluripotent stem (iPS) cells [65,114,115], it is conceived that TSCs might also be derived from the somatic cells with ESC genes being subverted or activated atavistically.

ATSCs are a major source of TSCs [11,116,117], because several evidences support the hypothesis. First, leukemic stem cells (LSCs) in acute myeloid leukemia (AML) are exclusively $CD34^{+}CD38^{-}$, similarly to the phenotype of normal HSCs [14,43]; second, it has been directly demonstrated that intestinal crypt stem cells (ISCs) are the source of intestinal neoplasia [51,52,118-120]. Activation of aberrant wingless (Wnt) signaling in these cells, e.g., deletion of adenomatous polyposis coli (*APC*) gene, disruption of phosphatase and tensin homolog (*PTEN*), or mutation of β-catenin (*CTNNB1*) gene, caused transformation of ISCs within days, leading to intestinal neoplasia within weeks [51,52,121]; finally, murine pCSC and CSC lines established in our laboratory exhibit a stem-like phenotype with lineage (Lin) markers being negative [10,11,36], suggesting that they are likely derived from normal stem cells. However, no stable human TSC lines have been established so far either from hematopoietic or non-hematopoietic tumors [11,53,122,123]. Traditional tumor cell lines may contain a small population of TSCs, but they are not a "real" TSC line, because Lin^+ cells are usually dominant and more likely a population of LSCPCs [124-126].

Another source of TSCs may be derived from transformed progenitor or somatic cells [112,113]. For example, granulocyte-macrophage progenitors of chronic myeloid leukemia (CML) may dedifferentiate into LSCs in blast crisis of CML [112]. Induction of pluripotent stem (iPS) cells from somatic cells by defined factors, including *Oct4*, *Sox2, c-Myc, Klf4, Nanog,* and *LIN28* [65,114,115] indirectly support the hypothesis that TSCs can be developed from progenitor cells or even from differentiated somatic cells.

Finally, cell fusion might provide additional source for TSCs. during development and tissue repair the fusion of genetic and cytoplasmic materials between cells of different origins is an important physiological process [113]. The fusion of stem cells with cells that have undergone a set of mutational events related to cancer development could be important for TSC development. Such fused cells should incorporate the characteristics of stem cell with aneuploidy chromosome [113]. For examples, *Helicobacter* infection-induced gastric epithelial CSCs appeared to be derived from BM HSCs or progenitors [127]. Whether this is caused by cell fusion or transdifferentiation needs to be elucidated further. However, it has been reported that the fusion of BM-derived cells with transformed cells may not necessarily lead to tumorigenesis [119].

3.3.3. Subpopulations of Tumor Stem Cells

3.3.3.1. The Potential of Classifying TSCs into TISCs, pCSCs and CSCs

TSC is a broad term, including all the stem-like cells that play pathogenic roles in throughout the tumor development, such as TISCs, pCSCs, and CSCs in the stage of benign proliferation, precancer and cancer, respectively. It has been difficult to define the subpopulations of TSCs based on their phenotypes; this may be related to the hierarchical development of TSCs in nature. No distinct phenotypic demarcations between TISCs, pCSCs and CSCs can be defined so far [11,14]. However, the functional heterogenicity of murine TSC lines paralleling to histopathological heterogenicity strongly indicates that TSC subpopulations indeed exist [10,11,16]. Based on their tumorigenicity in the syngeneic immunocompetent (IC) and SCID mice, TSCs can be divided into subpopulations of TISCs, pCSCs and CSCs [11,15] (Table 1). TISCs can not generate tumors in both IC and SCID mice; pCSCs can develop into tumors in SCID but not in IC mice; and CSCs can reconstitute tumors in both SCID and IC mice. The cellular process of TISC → pCSC → CSC may reflect corresponding clinical and histopathological processes of a cancer (figure 1): TISCs/benign proliferation/hyperplasia and low grade dysplasia → pCSCs/precancer/high grade dysplasia and carcinoma in situ (CIS) → CSCs/invasive cancer/invasive and metastatic carcinoma

[10,11,15,17,40,121,128-132]. In fact, proliferative lesions and precancerous lesions, regardless of tissue types, may be reversible or regressed in clinic.

The terminology between CSC, TIC and TSC has been used interchangeably, since reviving the CSC theory [11,50,133]; these three have been referred at present to as the same type of human tumor cells, in most literatures, which can reconstitute tumors of origin in NOD/Scid mice after transplantation [13,35,36,50,57,134-137]. This has caused confusion in TSC research, because the term of CSCs is not a comprehensive description of TSCs [11,15,54].

Table 1. Comparison between normal stem cells, tumor stem cells and differentiated cancer cells

	Self-renewal	Multipotency of differentiation		Expansion	Reversible Epigenetic aberration	DICD	Drug- and radiation-resistance	PL2L proteins	Reconstitute Neoplasm in	
		benign	Malig-nant						SCID mice	IC mice
NSC	+	+++	-	n.a.	n.a.	+/-?	n.a.	-	n.a.	n.a
TISC	+	+	+	-/+	+	+++	+	-/++	-/+	-
pCSC	+	+	+	-/+	+	+++	+	+++	+	-
CSC	+	-?	+	+	-	+/-	+	++	+++	+++
LSCPC	+/-	-	+/-	+++	-	+/-?	+/-	++	++	+
TDCC	n.a.	n.a.	n.a.	+	-	-	-	-	+/-	-

Abbreviations: NSC: normal stem cells; TISC: tumor-initiating stem cell; pCSC: precancerous stem cell; CSC: cancer stem cell; LSCPC: lineage-specific stem cell; TDCC: Terminal differentiated cancer cell; n.a., not applicable; DICD: differentiation-induced cell death; SCID mice: severe-combined immunodeficient mice; IC mice: immunocompetent mice.

TSCs are developed hierarchically in nature and thus are heterogeneous in function and phenotype. At the earliest stages of TSC development, TSCs, such as those isolated from benign proliferative lesion (TISCs) and benign neoplasm [benign (b) TSCs (bTSCs)] or precancerous lesion (pCSCs), might not necessarily develop into malignant tumors in their natural hosts or in the transplanted SCID recipients except for pCSCs. These TSCs (TISCs and pCSCs) are different from those (CSCs) that can form malignant tumors in both IC and SCID mice [11,16,44,45,55,57,129]. Therefore, it is important to divide the TSCs at least into three subpopulations, based on their clinicopathological characteristics. Such kind of classification will also facilitate more precise dissection of molecular events involved in TSC development. Overall, classification of TSCs as TISCs, pCSCs and CSCs will promote translational cancer medicine, leading to novel cost-effective strategies for cancer therapy.

3.3.3.2. Tumor-Initiating Stem Cells (TISCs)

TISC is the synonyms of tumor-initiating cells (TIC), which were used to refer to the TSCs mediating benign proliferative lesions (hyperplasia and low grade dysplasia) [11,15,138,139], such as TSCs isolated from cervical hyperplasia [57] or benign tumors [44], with the biological behavior differing from pCSCs and CSCs [11,15]. As the name suggested, TISCs are stem-like tumor-initiating cells (TICs), serving as the progenitors of pCSCs and CSCs [11,15].

TISCs can be derived from epigenetically and/or genetically aberrant stem cells, progenitor cells or somatic cells. The progenitor and somatic cells can acquire the property of stem cells during transformation [11,15]. These cells may mediate abnormal proliferation of tissue cells, exhibiting as hyperplasia or low-grade atypical hyperplasia. Their differentiated progenies resulted from asymmetric self-renewal may be morphologically hyperplastic but not malignant.

Although the existence of TISCs has not been directly proved, accumulating *in vitro* and *in vivo* data have suggested that TISCs are present in benign proliferative lesions [9,54,57,115,140]. For examples, clonogenic cells, one of properties of TSCs, were detected in hyperplastic endometrium [57]; mouse and human mesenchymal stem cells (MSCs) were susceptible to spontaneous transformation in long-term culture [140-145]; mammary progenitor cells underwent epigenetic changes upon genotoxic stimulations, demonstrating a cancer-like methylome [9]; TSCs have been identified in the benign pituitary adenomas [44]; and induction of iPS cells in human somatic cells with defined factors suggests that these cells have the potential to serve as TISCs [114,115]. These observations likely reflect the events that occur earlier than what happen in precancerous lesions. Therefore, authentic "TICs" should have the characteristics of TISCs. In the natural process of tumor development, benign proliferative lesions represent a tumor-initiation stage.

The fates TISCs may determine the outcomes of tumor-initiation. It is conceivable that TISCs could either progress to pCSCs or bTSCs, regress to quiescent status, undergo differentiation-induced cell death (DICD), or be eliminated by immune system. However, most TISCs are supposed to be quiescent, reversible, susceptible to DICD, or eliminated by immune surveillance, and thus unable to progress to pCSCs.

3.3.3.3. Precancerous Stem Cells (pCSCs)

pCSCs are supposed to be derived from TISCs, which may mediate precancerous lesions during tumor development, such as high grade dysplasia and CIS [10,11,15,16,45,55]. The differentiated progenies of pCSCs resulted from asymmetric self-renewal are highly atypical in morphology but have limited capacity of proliferation.

Recently, several pCSC clones have been established from murine lymphoma [10,11]. Through characterization of the lines, we have functionally defined the pCSCs as the tumor cells having the potential of both benign and malignant differentiation, depending on environmental cues [10,11,15,16]. Murine pCSCs can be distinguished from CSCs by transplantation assay with syngeneic IC mice and SCID mice. The pCSCs can develop into tumors in SCID mice but not in the syngeneic IC mice and lethally irradiated BM reconstituted (BMR) mice [11]. They can benignly differentiate into various types of tissue cells in BMR mice or blastocyst chimera (BLC) mice [10]. The benign differentiation of pCSCs in BLC mice suggests that embryonic environmental cues may play a potential and important role in reprogramming pCSCs into normal cells [146-148]. In contrast, CSCs may reconstitute malignant tumors in both SCID and IC mice (unpublished data). Although the mechanisms underlying the development of pCSCs in these model mice are not yet clear, these models provide a useful tool to explore how the interactions between pCSCs and immune system as well as microenvironments determine the fates of a pCSC.

Although the formation of tumors in the SCID mice transplanted with pCSCs may not necessarily prove the progression of pCSCs to CSCs, the facts that pCSC-derived tumor cells have altered phenotypes and karyotypes compared to their parent cells strongly suggest that some pCSCs might have developed into CSCs [10,11,16]. Further experiments are warranted to validate the hypothesis.

In addition to benign differentiation, pCSCs may undergo differentiation-induced cell death (DICD) upon stimulation by growth factors or cytokines [10]. Moreover, pCSCs lines uniquely and stably express *PIWIL2* transcripts [10,11], which might be associated with expression of Piwil2 variants, called piwil2-like (PL2L) proteins ([15] and unpublished data). Interestingly, ESC genes, such as *OCT-4*, *SOX-2, REX-1* and *TDGF1*, were ambiguously expressed in pCSCs [10,11,15]. Knockdown of *PIWIL2* in human tumor cell lines resulted down-regulation of the ESC genes, suggesting a relationship between *PIWIL2* and ESC genes (unpublished observation).

Taken together, pCSCs have the features of both normal stem cells and CSCs (table 3-1). Regardless of their origin, multiple genetic alterations reflect that the pCSCs have undergone multi-steps oncogenic mutations [10,149], and probably malignant biological behaviors have already been programmed in the pCSCs [55].

3.3.3.4. Cancer Stem Cells (CSCs)

CSCs are referred to as the stem-like tumor cells that mediate the development of invasive and metastatic cancers. They are the progenies of TISCs and pCSCs (figure 1). Tumor malignancy is associated with many factors, including uncontrollable cell division, invasiveness, metastasis, drug-resistance, and tumor neovascularization. CSCs can carry out these "missions" through the following paths:

a) *Aggressive self-renewal:* If TISCs and pCSCs mediate controllable benign proliferations and precancerous lesions through asymmetric self-renewal to maintain a stable TISC or pCSC pool; Some CSCs tend to mediate invasive cancerous lesions through symmetric self-renewal to expand the CSCs, leading to sustained tumor growth. This may explain why the percentage of CSCs in cancers varies dramatically (<0.01% to > 25%) [21,42,53,133]. Certainly, the ratio between symmetric and asymmetric self-renewal of CSCs might determine the rate of tumor growth.
b) *Generation of malignant offspring or LSCPCs:* While the division of tumor cells derived from TSICs and pCSCs is self-limited, the division rate of tumor cells derived from CSCs is uncontrollable. In most instances, the frequency of CSCs is extremely low (< 0.1%). Thus, the differentiated progenies of CSCs may inherit the malign programs of CSCs, exhibiting as aggravated uncontrollable replication and enhanced capability to evade the checkpoint of differentiation-induced cell death (DICD), leading to uncontrollable tumor growth. Some of the differentiated progenies, such as LPCSCs, might retain some CSC-like property to form tumors in SICD mice [20,41], which are defective in both innate and adaptive immunity [42,53,122]. However, these cells are susposed to be susceptible radiohterapy and chemotherapy.
c) *Invasiveness and metastasis:* CSCs also exhibited stronger capacity of invasiveness and metastasis [150-155], compared to pCSCs ([10,11] and unpublished observation). The aggressive implementation, in addition to their intrinsic migratory capacity, is supposed to be associated with their capability to evade immunosurveillance [156-158]. The notion is supported by the fact that CSCs but not pCSCs can form tumors in syngeneic IC mice ([10,11,159] and unpublished data).

d) *Tumor neovascularization:* Tumor neovascularization mediated by tumor angiogenesis and tumor vasculogenesis is critical for sustained tumor growth [11,160-164]. Like pCSCs [11,16], CSCs not only can produce angiogenic factors to promote tumor angiogenesis [165-167], but also serve as tumor vasculogenic progenitor cells (TVPCs) to support tumor vasculogenesis [16,168-171]. Especially, tumor neovascularization is a prerequisite for the establishment of metastatic tumors. A CSC that has metastatic capability but without tumor vasculogenic capacity is unable to seed and grow up in the distant "soil".
e) *Resistance to chemotherapy and radiotherapy:* Cancer recurrence after chemotherapy or radiotherapy is associated with CSCs that are resistant to the therapies [28-30,172-175]. While anti-cancer drugs or radiation can kill bulk TDCCs, these therapies are inefficient for CSCs. The mechanisms underlying the resistance to anti-cancer therapies are not yet clear but might be related to the following factors: i) CSCs are relatively quiescent compared to their progenies such as LSCPCs, and are not sensitive to anti-cancer therapies which target cycling cells; ii) CSCs, like normal stem cells, might constitutively express multiple drug resistance (MDR) transporters, which may protect the CSCs from drug toxicity [30]; and iii) dividing CSCs might be highly susceptible to mutagenesis in the therapeutic environment and thus become resistant to therapeutic drugs [176,177]; iv) The survival and proliferation of CSCs are regulated by multiple signaling pathways [178,179]; blocking one pathway might cause compensational adaption of CSCs to other survival pathways [176].

3.3.4. Lineage-Specific Cancer Progenitor/Propagating Cells (LSCPS) and Their Contribution to Tumor Growth

Based on current literatures, LSCPCs are supposed to be the differentiated progenies of CSCs. While CSCs express little or no lineage markers, LSCPCs clearly express differentiated lineage markers. However, the LSCPCs retain the malignant properties of CSCs except for the reduced potency of differentiation. Theoretically each CSC generates two daughter cells for each division. Like normal stem cells, CSCs may divide symmetrically or asymmetrically in a particular niche [11,89]. In malignant cancers, asymmetric division of CSCs appears to be dominant. Recently it is has been demonstrated that CSC division in lung cancers were mainly asymmetric [126]. While one daughter cell retains an old (parent) copy of DNA to maintain the property of CSCs, other cell containing newly synthesized DNA with some alterations differentiates into lineage-positive cell [126,180]. Compared to CSCs, the lineage-expressing progenies might acquire the strengthened capacity of proliferation to promote tumor growth. This kind of daughter cells might be the putative LSCPCs and may explain why some lineage-positive cells with unexpected high frequency in tumors clearly exhibited CSC activity in some SCID mouse models, that is, propagating human tumors in SICD mice or murine tumors in syngeneic mice [20,42,53,122].

Studies on diverse human cancers have indicated that only rare numbers of cancer cells (0.1–0.0001%) can form tumors in non-obese diabetic/severe combined immunodeficiency (NOD/SCID) mice. However, the frequency has been considered to be underestimated, when more tumorigenic cancer cells, most of which expressed lineage markers, were identified in the more immunocompromised or natural killer (NK) cell-depleted NOD/SCID mice [42,122]. The observations have caused heated debate on the concept of CSCs [21,41,53].

A number of studies using lineage-positive or differentiated human or mouse cancer cells have demonstrated that these cells, like lineage-negative cancer cells [10,11,36,47,123], can also form tumors in NOD/SCID or syngeneic mice. These cells have been considered as either lineage-positive CSCs or non-stem-like cancer propagating cells, challenging the current concept of CSCs [20,41,42,53,122,181]. The controversy may be related to the currently inaccurate definition of CSC, which is largely based on the tumorigenic capacity of the transplanted cancer cells in NOD/SCID mice [53]. While CSCs are causal "perpetrators" of tumorigenesis, their differentiated progenies could be "executors" of sustained tumor growth. Obviously, some lineage-positive cancer cells, including the hematopoietic and non-hematopoietic, could form tumors in the NK cell-depleted NOD/SCID mice, but rarely in NOD/SCID mice [20,41,42,122]. These cells are likely the same as LSCPCs we have described in this chapter (unpublished data), which can proliferate and differentiate into terminal differentiated cancer cells (TDCC), but below the hierarchy of CSCs. This concept needs to be verified further.

An important issue is whether LSCPCs or even TDCCs could be reprogrammed into stem-like status, i.e., CSC status. It is possible that TDCCs could be reverted to LSCPCs or CSCs, because it has been shown that non-stem-like cancer cells can be reverted to stem-like cancer cells because of increased genetic instability [182], although more rigorous experiments need to be done.

3.3.5. Roles and Significance of TISC, pCSCs, CSCs and LSCPCs in the Lengthy Process of Tumor Development

To understand how a tumor is developed, the best way is to link clinicopathological features of tumors with cellular and molecular changes of TSCs (figures 1, 3 and 4). Clinicopathologically, a hematopoietic or solid epithelial tumor is developed from a lengthy process from benign proliferative lesion, precancer to cancer, which may be mediated by TISCs, pCSCs and CSCs, respectively, accompanied by epigenetic and genetic evolution in the TSCs (figures 1 and 3) [11,15].

In the benign proliferative or hyperplastic lesions, TISCs may differentiate into epithelial cells with low grade transformation and abnormal but relatively limited proliferation, compared to what observed in the precancers and cancers; the damage range depends on frequency of TISCs. The differentiated progenies of TISCs are supposed to be susceptible to DICD and/or immunosurveillance. Thus, hyperplastic epithelial lesions are essentially regressed except for rare cases that progress to precancers. In the benign proliferative lesions, pCSCs and CSCs may not exist. In addition, TISCs may develop into bTSCs, mediating development of benign tumors.

The pCSCs that are considered to be developed from TISCs can either differentiate into non-malignant (tumor) cells or progress to CSCs, depending on environmental cues [10,11,15,17,18,129]. The differentiated progenies of pCSCs may exhibit as precancerous lesions in histopathology, such as high grade epithelial dysplasia, atypical epithelial lesions or carcinoma in situ (CIS), in which CSCs are not existed theoretically. Whether the precancerous lesions progress to malignant lesions depends on the fates of pCSCs within the lesions [10,11,15,17,18,129]. Increasing data suggest that malignant behavior has already been programmed in pCSCs [10,11,16,18,55], such as the capacity of tumor vasculogenesis, one of critical factors for tumor malignancy [16] and the potency to progress to uncontrollable CSCs [10]. When these programs are activated, precancer may progress to invasive and metastatic cancers. While all detached tumor cells might migrate to distant tissues, only can TSCs form various stages of neoplastic lesions in destiny, as observed in field cancerization.

Once pCSCs are developed into CSCs, they may dominantly exhibit malignant properties: uncontrollable growth of their differentiated daughter cells such as LSCPCs, active metastasis, and strong neovascularization. The LSCPCs are essentially malignant and distinct from the differentiated progenies of TISCs and pCSCs. They may retain some properties of CSCs because of increased epigenetic and genetic instability [183,184]. LSCPCs might represent predominant clones responsible for tumor mass expansion.

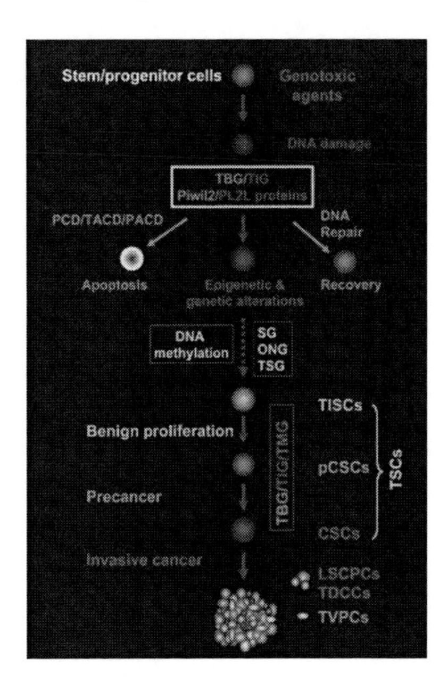

Abbreviations in the figure: TSC: tumor stem cell; TISC: tumor-initiating stem cell; pCSC: precancerous stem cell; CSC: cancer stem cell, TVPC: tumor vasculogenic progenitor cell; LSCPC: lineage-specific cancer progenitor/propagating cells; TDCC: terminal differentiated cancer cell; TBG: tumor-barrier gene; TIG: tumor-initiating gene; TMG: tumor-maintaining gene; SG: stability gene; ONG: oncogene; TSG: tumor suppressor gene; PL2L: piwil2-like; PCD: programmed cell death; TACD: transformation-associated cell death; PACD: proliferation-associated cell death. The figure is adopted from *Drug Discovery Today: Disease Models, 2009* [15] with modifications.

Figure 3.3. The potential roles of cancer-causing genes and cancer-contributing genes in tumor stem cell development. In responding to genotoxic agents, stem/progenitor cells can initiate intrinsic protective mechanisms from carcinogenesis. Among them, DNA damage response (DDR) pathways are immediately activated, which lead to either DNA repair or immediate programmed cell death (PCD) to eliminate DNA-damaged cells. Meanwhile, cancer-causing genes (CCSGs) may be activated to serve as a tumor-barrier gene (TBG) or tumor-initiating gene (TIG). TBG such as Piwil2 can induce proliferation- or transformation-associated cell death (PACD/TACD). However, Piwil2-like (PL2L) genes may serve as TIGs to antagonize TBGs. In cooperation with cancer-contributing genes (CCTGs), TIG may initiate the development of DNA damaged cells into TSCs, which are hierarchically developed via the stages of TISCs, pCSCs and CSCs. After initiation of TSC development, TIGs may serve as tumor-maintaining genes (TMG) to support TSC progression. Usually, TBGs are shut down in developing TSCs; but they can override the roles of CCTGs, such as SGs, ONGs and TSGs. Thus, it is likely that activation of TBGs in developing TSCs may effectively suppress tumor malignancy, such as uncontrollable proliferation, metastasis and tumor vasculogenesis.

The LSCPCs may further differentiate into TDCCs, which are susceptible to apoptosis in hypoxia, as observed in big tumor mass.

Taken together, while TISCs, pCSCs, CSCs and LSCPCs may perform their own duties at the corresponding stages of tumor development, they, of course, also coexist in an established malignant tumor, exhibiting a variety of histopathological changes [138,139]. The TISCs and pCSCs in the malignant cancers can also migrate to the distant areas from primary cancer, where they mediate field cancerization.

3.4. Phenotype of Tumor Stem Cells

3.4.1. Putative Phenotypes of TISCs, pCSCs and CSCs

Theoretically, functional subpopulations of TSC could be identified easily based on their phenotypes. Unfortunately, the hierarchical development of TSCs has made it difficult to phenotypically discriminate their subpopulations [11,185]. Currently, a number of TSC markers have been proposed in the name of CSCs, such as CD44, CD133 (prominin-1), CD90 and aldehyde dehydrogenase-1 (ALDH1), as well as some complementary markers, such as CD24 [36,43,50,127,137,185-187]. However, none of them are widely distributed in various types of TSCs except for CD44 [11]. The great phenotypic variation between the so called CSCs may be related to the possibility that most CSCs were characterized using the markers that identify normal ATSCs [35,50,133,137,188]. It is expected to identify and define a common phenotype of all TSCs, regardless of their tissue origin, although it is difficult so far. Increasing data have suggested the possibility to distinguish TSC subpopulations based on the clinicopathological status of tumorigenesis.

Tumorigenesis denotes a lengthy process from tumor initiation, progression to establishment of a malignant tumor. Existing clinicopathological data have suggested that the formation of a malignant tumor may undergo the stages of abnormal benign proliferation or tumor initiation, precancer and cancer, which might be mediated by TISCs, pCSCs and CSCs, respectively [11,15,17,18,54,129,138,139].

At the tumor initiation stage, some proliferative lesions, such as hyperplasia and metaplasia, probably mediated by TISCs, in breast and cervix uteri contain transforming cells expressing a germline stem cell (GSC) protein Piwil2 [138,139], the gene of which is usually silenced in normal adult somatic and stem cells, but ectopically expressed in various types of tumor [10,11,15,189,190]. Piwil2 may regulate embryonic stem cell (ESC) gene expression in tumor cells (unpublished observation). Because tumor initiation is associated with embryonic stem cell (ESC) gene expression [10,11,54], it is postulated that TISC phenotype might be associated with the expression of Piwil2 and Piwil2-regulated proteins (PRPs) such as the products of embryonic stem cell (ESC) genes [54]. Verification of Piwil2 and PRP expression in TISCs might lead to accurately delineating their phenotype.

Like TISCs, little is known about the phenotype of human pCSCs. However, pCSC activity has been demonstrated in human BRCA1 mutated CD49f^{+}EpCAM^{-} (epithelial cellular adhesion molecule) population in breast precancerous lesions [59] and CD133^{+} and Lgr5^{+} population in mouse colon pre-neoplasia [51,52,191]. Recently, we have established mouse pCSC clones from lymphoma, which are Lin^{-}CD44^{+}CD24^{-} ([10] and unpublished observation), distinct from a CSC clone (326T), which is also derived from lymphoma but with a phenotype of $Lin^{-/lo}CD44^{+}CD24^{+}$. The level of CD44 on CSCs was relatively lower than that on pCSCs (unpublished data). This observation suggests that the adhesion molecule CD44, a transmembrane receptor that is overexpressed in most of the primary cancers and associated with tumor progression [192-195], is ubiquitously expressed on pCSCs and CSCs.

The phenotype of CSCs has been explored mainly through xenotransplantation models of human tumors. As stated above, a number of markers have been considered as CSC markers [36,43,50,127,137,185-187]. In NOD/SCID mice, $CD44^{+}CD24^{-/low}ESA^{-}$(epithelial specific antigen) breast tumor cells could reconstitute the mammary tumors of origin [35,36]. Interestingly, the same activity was also observed in $CD44^{+}CD24^{+}ESA^{+}$ population of pancreatic cancer [49]. The results suggest that either both CD24 and ESA are not reliable markers for CSCs or these opposite phenotypes reflect two distinct populations, such as CSCs versus their progenies LSCPCs.

The differential levels of lineage-specific markers are thought to be a demarcation between CSCs and LSCPCs. While a CSC clone is expressing no or weak lineage markers and can differentiate into various types of LSCPCs, a given LSCPC clone may express high level of lineage markers, having less potency of differentiation but stronger capability to proliferate, forming neoplasia. This notion is supported by successful isolation of CSCs from established tumor cell lines, such as glioma cell lines [124,180]. Glioma CSCs that expressed neural stem cell-related genes were capable of self-renewal, generating tumor spheres in a factor-dependent manner but also differentiating into astrocytes and oligodendrocytes [180].

3.4.2. Means to Resolve the Dispute on CSC Concept Caused by Confusing Phenotypes

In human acute lymphoblast leukemia (ALL), $CD38^{-}CD133^{+}CD19^{-}$ cells might serve as CSCs in NOD/SCID mouse models and differentiate into $CD19^{+}$ leukemic cells [47,123]. However, both $CD19^{-}$ and $CD19^{+}$ lymphoblasts are able to propagate leukemia in natural killer (NK) cell-depleted NOD/SCID or NOD/SCID gamma (NSG) mice after intrafemoral injection [53,122], leading to heated debate whether $CD19^{+}$ leukemic cells are real CSCs [53]. Based on our experience on murine pCSC research, we would rather consider the lineage-positive (herein $CD19^{+}$) cancer propagating cells as LSCPCs rather than CSCs.

To ultimately resolve the phenotype of TSC subpopulation, establishment of human CSC lines are a prerequisite. However, the efforts to establish such kinds of cell lines have been failed. Although most of lineage-negative human tumor cells can form sphere *in vitro* in a factor-dependent manner, they will inevitably die from long-term culture [11,47,53]. Traditional tumor cell lines usually are dominant with lineage-positive cells and only contain a small population of lineage-negative cells [124,125,196]. However, most lines are transplantable, due to a small subpopulation of stem-like cells that is enriched in a side population (SP), expressing a high level of CD44 [124,125,197]. The SP expresses ATP-Binding Cassette (ABC) transporter Bcrp1 or ABCG2 [198] and has stem-like activity [124,125,199]. However, some ABCG2-negative cells also possess stem-like activity, seemingly to be more primitive in development than $ABCG2^{+}$ cells [11,125]. This may be true because the pCSC clones established in our laboratory do not express ABCG2 [10], contrasting to a CSC clone (326T) (unpublished data). Whether ABCG2 expression is a maker that distinguishes pCSCs from CSCs remains to be elucidated [11,125].

Recently, we have successfully established several stable clones of murine hematopoietic pCSC (HpCSC), mesenchymal pCSC (MpCSC) and hematopoietic CSC (hCSC) lines, which are lineage (Lin)$^-$CD44$^+$CD24$^-$ (HpCSC and MpCSC) or Lin$^{-/+}$CD44$^+$CD24$^+$ ([10,11] and unpublished data). However, a small population of Lin$^+$ cells (< 1 %) could also be detected in these lines, opposing to classical tumor cell lines, in which Lin$^+$ cells are predominant and Lin$^-$ cells are less than 1% in general (unpublished data). *In vivo*, these lines can differentiate into multi-Lin$^+$ cells ([10,11] and unpublished observations). For example, both HpCSCs and hCSCs can differentiate at least into myeloid (CD11b$^+$) and lymphoid (CD19$^+$) cells ([10,11] and unpublished observation). These Lin$^+$ cells can form tumors but with the reduced capacity compared to Lin$^-$ cells (unpublished observation). Therefore, through the study of TSC lines we can delineate phenotypes of TISCs, pCSCs and CSCs as well as precisely dissect the cellular and molecular events of tumor development.

3.4.3. Significance of c-kit and Sca-1 Expression in CSC Differentiation

CD117 (c-kit) and Sca-1 (stem cell antigen-1), which are expressed in normal HSCs [200-202], have been frequently identified in various types of progressing cancers [203-205]. These cells might be considered as TSCs. However, little or no c-kit and Sca-1 are expressed in pCSC and CSC lines ([10] and unpublished data). Interestingly, both c-kit and Sca-1 were up-regulated in some pCSC- or CSC-derived Lin$^+$ cells ([10] and unpublished data), consistently with clinical observations on human cancers [203-205]. It has been demonstrated that Sca-1 expression in stem/progenitor cells is associated with their factor-dependent lineage differentiation [206]. We have observed that c-kit expression is correlated with CD3 expression in the cultured CSC subclones (unpublished data). Thus, it is possible that c-kit and/or Sca-1 expression is a signal of CSC differentiation into LSCPCs, which are supposed to be responsible for amplification of tumor volume, as discussed above. This hypothesis is worth to be explored.

3.5. Mechanisms Underlying Tumor Stem Cell Development

3.5.1. Initiation and Progression of Tumor Stem Cells

Extensive investigations have revealed that human tumorigenesis is a complex, multistep process often requiring concordant expression of a number of oncogenes [111,178,207,208], although these steps might be checked by the mechanism of immune surveillance [11,157]. It is recognized that a cancer initially arises from the cells that fail to repair damaged DNA, leading to aberrant activity of stability genes (SGs), oncogens (ONG) and/or tumor suppressor genes (TSGs) [178,183,209]. Especially, the aberrant activity of SGs that may cause abnormal chromatin remodeling, disturbed cell replication and chromosomal instability might play critical roles in the induction of genetic mutations of ONGs and/or TSGs

[178,183]. Stem cells, progenitor cells and/or proliferating somatic cells are likely the targets accumulating the oncogenetic mutations [11,15].

Regardless of the origin of TSCs, the initial step of carcinogenesis may start from abnormal epigenetic changes of SGs, ONGs and/or TSGs of the affected cells (either stem cells or progenitor cells), which are insulted by cellular stresses or carcinogens [15,117,210]. The disturbance of SGs may affect chromatin remodeling, DNA rearrangement and cell cycling, resulting genetic mutation and/or deletion of ONGs and TSGs, accompanied by cell transformation.

These insulted cells can be transformed into TISCs, if they escape from anti-tumor-barriers, i.e., DNA repair and programmed cell death, the mechanisms responding to DNA damage to eliminate abnormal cells [211-213]. The TISCs may mediate proliferative lesions exhibiting as hyperplasia or benign neoplasm in histology. *In vitro* studies revealed that exposure of normal mammary stem/progenitor cells to estrogen led to a cancer-like methylome [9], suggesting that aberrant methylation of cancer genes is an earlier event than oncogenetic mutation during TSC development.

Theoretically, TISCs can develop into pCSCs and then CSCs which mediate premalignant and malignant lesions, respectively. The precancerous lesions exhibit as atypical dysplasia and carcinoma in situ in histopathology; whereas the malignant lesions exhibit as invasive carcinoma. The identification of pCSCs in tumors supports the notion that pCSCs are a precursor of CSC [10,11,45,55]. More and more evidences have supported the presence of pCSCs in human and animal tumors [10,11,19,45,55,59,120,191,214], although the existence of the precursors of pCSCs, i.e., TISCs, needs to be verified further. However, isolation of TSCs or bTSCs from benign tumors has implicated the existence of TISCs [44]. Thus, we think that TISCs represent a real tumor initiator, which may progress to pCSCs and CSCs [11,15].

Additional epigenetic and/or genetic alterations may drive pCSC progression to CSCs [11,15]. The novel concept is supported by a recent report that preleukemic cells in human twins with TEL-AML1 fusion proteins were driven to LSC or hematopoietic CSCs by an additional mutational hit [45].

Another study of mouse mammary carcinoma has suggested that tumor malignancy is already programmed in pCSCs [55]. Additional but random multiple deletions and translocations of chromosome occurred when pCSCs developed into tumors in SCID mice [10], probably associated with the activation of malignant program in pCSCs, including the program promoting pCSC differentiation into TVPCs [16].

Moreover, we have observed that aberrant DNA methylation was reversible in precancerous lesions but not in malignant lesion of human colorectal tumors after treatment with nonsteroidal anti-inflammatory drugs [18].

These observations suggest that additional epigenetic and/or genetic alterations are required when pCSCs progress to CSCs. The reversibility of cancer gene methylation might be a useful marker to distinguish pCSCs from CSCs.

Taken together, carcinogens-insulted stem/progenitor cells may develop into TISCs through epigenetic alterations, subsequently into pCSCs and CSCs through additionally both epigenetic and oncogenetic changes. As a result, the histology of the involved tissues will be changed accordingly [15,17,129,138,139,215] (figures 1 and 3).

3.5.2. "Atavistic" Activation of Embryonic Stem Cell Genes and Germline Stem Cell Genes in Tumor Stem Cells

Embryonic induction of oncogenesis has been observed decades ago [216]. Through investigation of bulk tumor cells, activation of embryonic stem cell (ESC) genes is a generalized phenomenon observed in malignant tumors, especially in histologically poorly differentiated tumors [54,217]. The histologically poorly differentiated tumors show more frequent overexpression of ESC genes than well-differentiated tumors, such as *Nanog, Oct4, Sox2 and c-Myc*, and repressed expression of Polycomb-regulated genes [217]. The histologically poorly differentiated tumors are usually more potent in differentiation than well differentiated tumors, because such kind of tumors contains more TSCs [196].

Increasing data have suggested that ESC gene activation is an early or initiating event of TSC development, which may be resulted from oxidative stress or DNA damage [10,11,15,54,218]. Abnormal expression of ESC genes in TSCs is likely associated with the lack of CpG island methylation of promoters, a phenomenon observed in both normal and malignant embryonic cells. This appears to be mediated by the formation of a promoter chromatin pattern particularly for ESC gene expression in TSCs. The notion is deduced from the fact that adult cancers often show aberrant promoter CpG island hypermethylation and transcriptional silencing of TSGs and pro-differentiation factors, as observed in both normal and malignant embryonic cells, which generally lack the hypermethylation of DNA [54,219]. In normal ESCs, ESC genes might be held in a "transcription-ready" state mediated by a "bivalent" promoter chromatin pattern consisting of the repressive marker, histone H3 methylated at Lys27 (H3K27), and the active marker, methylated H3K4 [219]. In the embryonic carcinoma cells, additional two repressive markers, dimethylated H3K9 and trimethylated H3K9, participate in hypermethylation of DNA. The "tetravalent" promoter chromatin pattern was also observed in adult cancers [219], suggesting a critical role in initiating TSC development. In pCSCs, a number of ESC genes such as *Poufl/Otc4, TDGF1, Zfp42/REX1and SOX2* were ambiguously expressed [10,11]. Thus, it is interesting to look at the promoter chromatin pattern of the ESC genes in TISCs, pCSCs and CSCs.

In addition to ESC genes, we have also found that pCSCs constitutively and stably expressed germline stem cell (GSC) gene *PIWIL2*; which is silenced in adult stem and somatic cells except in the GSCs of testis [10,11,15]. Importantly, Piwil2 can be detected in proliferative, precancerous and cancerous lesions of various types of cancer, such as breast and cervical carcinomas [138,139,220], strongly suggesting an important role in TSC development.

3.5.3. *PIWIL2*, a Potential Cancer-Causing Gene for Tumor Stem Cell Development

The Piwil2 is a member of PIWI/AGO protein family [190,221], which has PIWI and PAZ domain (PPD) and is exclusively expressed in the GSCs of testis [222,223]. The PAZ domain can bind siRNA [224], whereas the function of PIWI domain is not clear yet [225]. Piwi protein is essential for stem cell self-renewal in *drosophila* [221] and gametogenesis in various organisms [222,226]. Recently Piwil2 were found to bind a novel class of RNA called piwi-interacting RNA (piRNA) or repeat-associated small interfering RNAs (rasiRNAs) in mammal testis [227-232]. It may silence the selfish genetic elements, such as retrotransposons through a mechanism of methylation, in the GSCs of testis [228,232,233]. Since Piwi protein is required for stem cell self-renewal in diverse organisms and its somatic expression modulates the number of GSCs and the rate of their division [234], dysregulated Piwi protein expression appears to be associated with tumorigenesis [10,189,235]. However, the mechanisms underlying Piwil2 regulating tumor development is essentially unknown.

Argonaute (Ago) proteins that contain the same PAZ and PIWI domain as Piwi proteins are required either for the formation of RNA-induced silencing complex (RISC) for post-transcriptional silencing of mRNA [236-238] or RNA-induced initiation of transcriptional silencing (RITS) protein complex for heterochromatin formation and silencing of centromeres [239,240]. Thus, it is possible that the ectopic expression of Piwil2 in adult somatic or stem/progenitor cells might interfere with normal RNAi machinery, disturbing chromatin remodeling [241] and leading to tumorigenesis [236].

Constitutive expression of Piwil2 transcripts in pCSCs has suggested that Piwil2 might be an important gene that regulates pCSC development [10,11,15]. Normally, Piwil2 is expressed in GSCs in the testis of mammal, but silenced in adult tissues [11,189,190]. However, Piwil2 transcripts and proteins have been widely detected in various types of tumors and tumor cell lines of human and mouse, such as of brain, lung, skin, breast, cervix and blood [138,139,189,220]. In pCSCs, suppression of Piwil2 transcripts by siRNA enhanced expansion of pCSCs and up-regulated expression of *Bcl-2* and *Stat-3*, but not *Bcl-XL* [10]. However, ectopic expression of Piwil2 in normal BM-derived stem/progenitor cells induced cell proliferation and transformation followed by apoptosis [10], which is referred as to transformation-associated cell death (TACD).

While increasing data have suggested that *PIWIL2* is an important cancer gene in tumor development, it is not appreciated by the definition of ONGs, TSGs and SGs [178,242]. Based on their functions, cancer genes can be categorized into cancer-causing gene (CCSG) and cancer-contributing gene (CCTG) [178] (Figure 3). However, most of the cancer genes that are identified so far and involved in cancer development are CCTGs rather than CCSGs. No CCSG has been identified so far [178]. While the CCTGs, including ONGs, TSGs and SGs, are redundant and required as well for the control of normal cell growth and survival pathways; CCSGs are considered to be silent in normal adult somatic and stem cells and indispensable by CCTGs for natural process of tumor initiation and progression [178]. Identification of CCSGs, delineation of its causal role in TSC development or the pathways through which CCSGs act, and exploitation of the benefits of CCSG for patients with regard to diagnostic biomarker, tumor vaccines, and new anti-cancer drugs are major challenges currently we are facing [178]. *PIWIL2* is a potential CCSG, because it is not redundant in tumor development [10,11,15,138,139,189,220].

3.5.4. Tumor-Barrier Genes (TBG) and Tumor-Initiating Genes (TIGs) in Tumor Stem Cell Development

As discussed above, a CCSG should be silent in normal adult somatic and stem cells, but can be activated throughout the process of tumor initiation, progression and commitment without tissue restriction. Like CCTG family, which is classified into SG, ONG and TSG, CCSG family may also be classified at least into tumor-barrier gene (TBG) and tumor-initiating gene (TIG), based on their functions [15,243]. Loss of the function of TBGs and activation of TIGs may initiate TSC development through cooperation with CCSGs (Fig. 3). The products of such kind of genes have the potential to be used as common targets for detection, prognosis and intervention of cancers [11,15,178].

Through the studies of pCSCs, we have found that GSC protein Piwil2 and its variants Piwil2-like (PL2L) proteins, such as PL2L60, might play opposite roles in tumor development (unpublished data). Both *PIWIL2* and *PL2L60* are silenced in normal adult somatic and stem cells ([10,11,189,190] and unpublished data). However, *PIWIL2* was transiently activated to promote DNA repair in responding to DNA damages induced by genotoxic agents (unpublished data). Ectopic expression of Piwil2 in bone marrow (BM) derived stem/progenitor cells induced transformation- or proliferation-associated cell death (TACD or PACD) [10,11], whereas PL2L60 proteins that were constitutively expressed in pCSCs could promote pCSC expansion *in vitro* ([10,11] and unpublished data). Moreover, Piwil2 was mainly detected in the apoptosing cells of human primary breast cancer, whereas PL2L60 was widely detected in proliferating tumor cells of primary tumors as well as in various types of human and mouse tumor cell lines (unpublished data). The Piwil2 or Piwil2 transcripts previously detected in various types of tumors using polyclonal antibody to Piwil2 or primers common for *PIWIL2* and *PL2L* genes *de facto* mainly represent PL2L60 proteins or *PL2L60* gene ([10,11,15,138,139,189,220] and unpublished data). Failure to detect Piwil2 transcripts in bladder cancers was probably associated with the fact that the primers used for RT-PCR are specific for whole length of *PIWIL2* (within first six exon of *PIWIL2*) rather than *PL2L* genes ([244] and unpublished data). Increasing data have suggested that Piwil2 and/or PL2L proteins expression is associated with atavistic activation (reprograming) of ESC genes in TISCs [10,11,15,54]. While Piwil2 and PL2L transcripts were detected in long-term cultured primary fibroblast cell lines (unpublished data), a number of ESC genes were also activated in the cultured primary cells with a similar profile to tumor cell lines [245]. Both *PIWIL2* and ESC genes activation are probably caused by cellular stresses or favorable environmental cues during cultivation. Based on these observations, we consider that CCSGs are the "atavistic" genes, which are normally expressed in GSCs and/or ESCs, but not in adult somatic and stem cells except for the GSCs of testis [15,190].

Therefore, a TBG, unlike TSGs which are usually active in normal adult somatic and stem cells, must be silenced or dormant in the same cells, but can be activated rapidly and transiently as early as upon DNA damages caused by carcinogens; the activated TBGs are able to eliminate DNA-damaged cells, probably through promoting DNA repair and/or programmed cell death (PCD), regardless of the activation status of SGs, ONGs and/or TSGs. Should the function of TBGs be defective during tumor initiation, the DNA repair- or PCD-aborted cells are likely to evade protective mechanisms exerted by DNA-damage response (DDR) [213] and evolve into TISCs in collaboration with SGs, ONGs and/or TSGs. Although TBGs are usually inactive in malignant tumor cells; they may be activated to inhibit tumorigenesis in a favorable environmental cue.

A TIG, as the name suggested, should be able to antagonize the functions of TBG. While TIGs, like TBGs, are expressed little or not at all in normal adult tissue cells, they can be activated to antagonize TBGs in the tumorigenic environment [15]. TIGs can be the loss-of-function or gain-of-opposite function variants of TBGs, such as Piwil2 versus PL2L proteins (unpublished data).

Epigenetic disruption such as hypomethylation in TIGs might be a primary cause for TSC initiation. Especially, these changes might endow the non-stem progenitor cells some properties of stem cells at the stage of tumor initiation to promote the susceptibility of the involved cells to oncogenetic mutations of SGs, ONGs and/or TSGs. Reverted expression of ESC genes in adult stem/progenitor cells might signify the activation of TIGs. For example, *OCT4B* is activated under stress conditions to prevent cell apoptosis [246]. This may explain why *OCT4* transcripts were detected in peripheral blood mononuclear cells [68,247]. Indeed, *OCT4* is not required for somatic/adult stem cell self-renewal [248,249], suggesting that *OCT4* expression in somatic stem cells might also serve as a TIG, conducive to TSC development.

3.5.5. Other Molecular Pathways Contributing to Tumor Stem Cell Development

Since TSCs have the capacity of self-renewal similarly to normal adult and embryonic stem cells, the molecules that regulate the self-renewal of normal stem cells are also applied to TSCs, such as Notch, Wnt and hedgehog signaling pathways [11,54,179,250-252]. In addition, several proteins that are active during embryo development have been shown to induce self-renewal in adult cells, such as Oct4 and Bmi-1 [68,71,253-255].

The proteins involved in self-renewal of embryonic and adult stem cells appear to be subverted and/or activated aberrantly to allow the TSCs to maintain self-renewal capacity [252]. Among these, the polycomb protein group (PcG) gene *Bmi-1* appears to play a critical role for the self-renewal of stem cells and TSCs [106,107,256-258]. The PcG genes that are a transcriptional repressor have an essential role in embryogenesis, regulation of cell cycle, and lymphopoiesis.

The increased expression of *Bmi-1* promotes HSC self-renewal, probably through enhancing symmetrical cell division of HSCs and mediating a higher probability of inheritance of stemness through cell division. Loss-of-function analyses revealed that among the PcG genes, absence of *Bmi-1* is preferentially linked with a profound defect in HSC self-renewal. Since the molecules identified so far contributing to cancer development are also required for normal stem cell development [37,259], they are not unique for TSC development.

By comparison of self-renewal-related genes between the pCSCs and BM stem cells [10], we found that while the pCSCs expressed an elevated level of *Bmi-1* and *Stat-3*, which are required for tumorigenesis of CSCs [104,258,260,261], Piwil2 was uniquely expressed in the pCSCs but not in BM stem/progenitor cells [10]. The results suggest that the activity of adult stem cell genes may be enhanced in TSCs, but is not as unique as the Piwil2 activity for TSC development. In addition, the pCSCs also expressed a number of ESC genes such as *Poufl/Otc4, TDGF1, Zfp42/REX1and SOX2*, but these genes were expressed not as stable as *Piwil2* [10,11]. In fact, the Piwil2 transcripts detected in the murine pCSCs [10] *de facto* represent *PL2L* genes, which probably play an important role for the maintenance of pCSC self-renewal (unpublished data). In this sense, *PL2L* genes might serve as tumor-maintaining gene (TMG).

3.6. Roles of Tumor Stem Cells in Field Cancerization

3.6.1. Histopathology Underlying Field Cancerization

Cancerization or carcinogenesis is a process of transformation of a cell from normal to cancerous status. Clinically, cancerization exhibits as the stages of benign proliferation, precancer and malignant cancer in the involved tissues or organs [138,139].

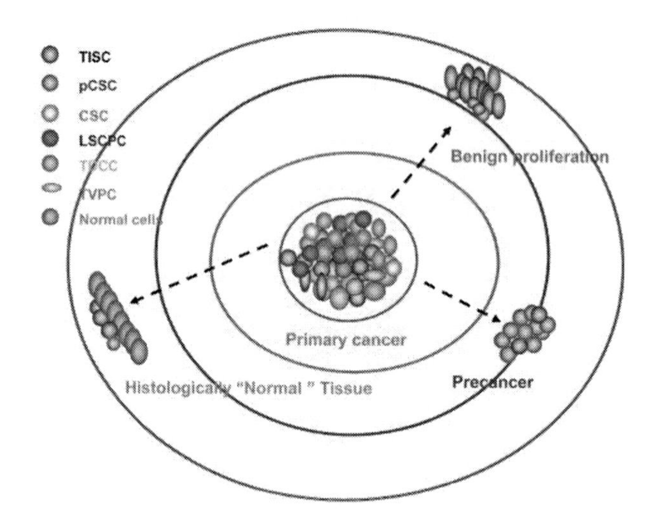

Abbreviations in the figure: TISC: tumor-initiating stem cell; pCSC: precancerous stem cell; CSC: cancer stem cell, TVPC: tumor vasculogenic progenitor cell; LSCPC: lineage-specific cancer progenitor/propagating cells; TDCC: terminal differentiated cancer cell. The figure is adopted from *Drug Discovery Today: Disease Models*, 2009 [15] with modifications.

Figure 3.4. The roles of tumor stem cells in field cancerization. Tumor stem cells (TSCs) can mediate field cancerization. Primary cancers contain the subpopulations of TSCs, including TISCs, pCSCS and CSCs. In some circumstances, TSCs can migrate out off primary cancers to distant areas where provides a niche for TSC colonization. The interaction between TSC subpopulations and niches determines the outcome of field cancerization. Accordingly, TSC niches can also be considered as benign niche, precancerous niche, and cancerous niche, where the benign proliferation, precancer, and cancer may be identified, respectively. In histologically "normal" areas, "field effects" of cancerization can be detected at epigenetic and genetic levels, suggesting that TSCs are dormant in these areas.

Histologically, as discussed above, benign proliferative lesions exhibit as hyperplasia, metaplasia and/or low grade dysplasia; precancerous lesions as high grade dysplasia and carcinoma in situ (CIS); and malignant lesions as invasive carcinomas, which are supposed to be mediated by TISCs, pCSCs and CSCs, respectively [11,15,17,138,139] (figures 1, 3 and 4). The coexistence of TISCs, pCSCs and CSCs in malignant tumors might the cause of field cancerization [1-3] (Figure 4). Increasing data have suggested that "field cancerization" is a generalized phenomenon of cancers [1-4,6] and was even observed within a primary cancer [5,138,139]. The heterogeneous lesions within or surrounding malignant tumors may be related to differential geographical microenvironments within or surrounding tumors where the status of TISCs, pCSCs and CSCs are maintained, respectively. In the invasive primary caners, not only premalignant lesions but also histologically normal appearing tissue islands could be observed [138,139]. The heterogenously histological lesions within a primary cancer suggest that a primary cancer is mediated by various stages of developing TSCs rather than clonally synchronized CSCs alone, that is, TISCs, pCSCs and CSCs likely coexist in primary cancers, providing the basis of heterogenously histological changes of a tumor (figure 4).

Field cancerization away from primary cancers is characterized by occult precancerous lesions [1-3], suggesting that TISCs and pCSCs are main mediators of field cancerization. The origin of these early TSCs are not yet clear. There might be two potential sources of TISCs and pCSCs: i) the TISCs and pCSCs might migrate from primary cancers in which TISCs and pCSCs are likely coexisted [5,138,139]; and ii) Field cancerization might occur simultaneously with the initiation of primary cancers but TISCs and/or pCSCs in the multicentric fields do not progress to CSCs as occurred in the site of primary cancers because of differential microenvironments [5] (figure 3-4). Regardless of the origin of TSCs, field cancerization provides a critical source of cancer recurrence.

3.6.2. Niche Effects on Field Cancerization

The status of field cancerization is determined by the stages of developing TSCs and stromal cells in the “seedbeds” or niches. It is likely that a favorable “seedbed” or niche is required for TSCs to colonize successfully [262,263]. Recent studies have suggested that TSCs, in contrast to normal stem cells, can actively migrate out of normal stem cell niches and disseminate among “normal” tissue cells, which provide a favorable “seedbed” for the TSCs. For examples, in premalignant human gastric intestinal tissue, normal Lgr5$^+$ intestinal stem cells were strictly located at the bottom of crypts, but precancerous Lgr5$^+$ cells (pCSCs) were distributed randomly in multiple foci at the luminal surface where provides a breeding ground for the “bad” seeds [191]. In addition, dysfunction of stem cell niches may also induce oncogenesis. Normally, mesenchymal subsets, such as endothelial cells and osteolineages, constitute stem cell niches in bone, modulating hematopoiesis [96,98,100,103,264,265]. Deletion of *Sbds* in mouse osteoprogenitors induced bone marrow dysfunction with myelodysplasia, suggesting that disruption of stem cell niche can result in secondary neoplastic disease [19]. Therefore, the TSCs in field cancerization foci might come from primary cancers or originate from the dysfunction of stem cell niches. Especially, the dysfunctioned niches or bad “seedbeds” provides a critical microenvironment for clonal evolution of TISCs to pCSCs and CSCs [5,11,15,18,61,266-270].

The phenomenon of field cancerization also suggests that the interaction between TSCs and niches determines the outcome of “field effects” of cancerization. According to histological features observed in field cancerization [138,139], TSC niches may be classified as occult niche, benign (proliferation) niche, precancerous niche, and cancerous niche. The occult TSC niche may host TSCs in a dormant state, exhibiting as the histologically “normal” appearing tissues, but can be detected at epigenetic and genetic levels [3,4,8] (figure 3-4). The size of TSC niches may determine the scope of involved tissues, which appears not to be affected by macro-environment of primary cancers but by the quality of stromal cells in the niches [19,138]. In the precancerous lesions of gastrointestinal tissue, Lgr5$^+$ intestinal stem cells or epithelial cells always show a sharp transition between $Lgr5^+$ cells and the negative cells [19], indicating that the precancerous lessions are strictly regulated by precancerous niches. Accordingly, the pCSCs and pCSC-derived progenies are strictly regulated by the niches and would not progress to CSCs, if malignant niches remain absent surrounding the precancerous lesions (figure 3-4).

3.6.3. Piwil2 is a Potential Biomarker for Field Cancerization

Field cancerization is an important phenomenon associated with cancer recurrence and metastasis [2-4]. The epigenetic and/or genetic alterations in the "normal" appearing tissues are often the risk factors of cancerization [271,272], and thus this change in the normal tissues distant from primary cancers could be a cause of tumor recurrence and metastasis [8]. Especially, chemotherapy and radiation therapy may incur progressive recurrence and metastasis of the occult precancerous lesions. Detection and resecting precancerous lesions surrounding primary cancers before treatment can effectively prevent the recurrence or metastasis of the field precancers. However, the field cancerization is usually occult, exhibiting as proliferative or precancerous lesions under microscope. In some circumstances, some foci of field cancerization may only exhibit as histologically normal appearing tissues, though with cancer-like epigenetic and genetic changes [7,8]. Thus, these occult lesions could not be detected with microscopy. Although some gene-specific field effects could be detected at molecular levels based on their cancer-like methylome [3,4,8,9], the application of the methods to detection of occult field cancerization are still limited, because these genes, with individual variations, are unlikely detected in all types of cancers. Recently, we have found that Piwil2 is expressed in the histologically normal appearing epithelium adjacent to cancerous lesions of breast and cervical uteri, regardless of tumor types [138,139]. This may be related to the "field effect" of cancerization [7]. Since *PIWIL2* or *PL2L* genes are expressed in various types of tumors [10,11,138,139,189,220], they could be a potential biomarker for detection of occult field precancerous lesions.

3.6.4. Therapeutic Approaches to Field Cancerization

Because field cancerization is a generalized phenomenon of cancers, as discussed above, eradication of occult field precancerous lesions is critical for preventing cancer recurrence and metastasis. However, it is difficult to completely remove occult precancerous lesions by surgery, even though some of them can be detected before surgery. Adjuvant therapy such as chemotherapy and radiotherapy might incur progression, accelerate the recurrence and promote metastasis of occult precancerous lesions, because both therapies themselves are genotoxic and may elicit the progression of TISC and pCSC to CSCs [11,29,30]. To prevent cancer recurrence and metastasis caused by field precancerous lesions, immunotherapy is of choice as adjuvant therapy. Recently, we have found that pCSCs are highly immunogenic in IC mice. Immunization of the mice with live pCSCs induced effective anti-tumor immunity. The immunized mice could reject challenging tumor cells unrelated to live pCSCs ([159] and unpublished data). The results suggest that pCSCs contain common tumor-specific antigens (CTSAs), and can be eliminated by appropriate immunotherapeutic modes through targeting of the antigens. Identification of such kind of antigens will lead to develop novel tumor vaccines for cancer immunotherapy. Therefore, immunotherapy through targeting of TSCs is of choice to prevent cancer recurrence and metastasis or eliminate field cancerization.

Conclusion

Field cancerization is a generalized phenomenon of cancers. It appears to be closely associated with cancer recurrence and metastasis. Accumulating data have suggested that the field cancerization is mediated by TSCs. TSCs undergo developmental stages of TISC, pCSC and CSC, which mediates proliferative, precancerous and cancerous lesions, respectively. In addition to the signaling pathways common for normal stem cells, TSC development may be initiated by "atavistic" expression of GSC gene *PIWIL2* and ESC genes in adult stem/progenitor cells. Among them, *PIWIL2* may play as a TBG, whereas its variants *PL2L* genes may plays as a TIG. *PIWIL2* is belonged to cancer-causing gene (CCSG) family, which is silenced in normal adult stem/progenitor cells and distinct from cancer-contributing genes (CCTGs) including SGs, ONGs and TSGs, which are expressed in normal adult stem/progenitor cells as well. Elimination of occult field precancerous lesions may cost-effectively prevent the recurrence and metastasis of cancers. Through targeting of TSCs, we may develop novel tumor vaccines to prevent cancer recurrence and metastasis caused by field cancerization.

References

[1] Danely P. Slaughter HWSWS. "Field cancerization" In oral stratified squamous epithelium. Clinical implications of multicentric origin. *Cancer* 1953, 6:963-968.

[2] Dakubo GD, Jakupciak JP, Birch-Machin MA, Parr RL. Clinical implications and utility of field cancerization. *Cancer Cell Int.* 2007, 7:2.

[3] Braakhuis BJM, Tabor MP, Kummer JA, Leemans CR, Brakenhoff RH. A genetic explanation of slaughter's concept of field cancerization: Evidence and clinical implications. *Cancer Res.* 2003, 63:1727-1730.

[4] Shen L, Kondo Y, Rosner GL, Xiao L, Hernandez NS, Vilaythong J, Houlihan PS, Krouse RS, Prasad AR, Einspahr JG, Buckmeier J, Alberts DS, Hamilton SR, Issa JP. Mgmt promoter methylation and field defect in sporadic colorectal cancer. *J. Natl. Cancer Inst.* 2005, 97:1330-1338.

[5] Rhiner C, Moreno E. Super competition as a possible mechanism to pioneer precancerous fields. *Carcinogenesis* 2009, 30:723-728.

[6] Chai H, Brown RE. Field effect in cancer-an update. *Ann. Clin. Lab. Sci.* 2009, 39:331-337.

[7] Giovannucci E, Ogino S. DNA methylation, field effects, and colorectal cancer. *J. Natl. Cancer Inst.* 2005, 97:1317-1319.

[8] Yan PS, Venkataramu C, Ibrahim A, Liu JC, Shen RZ, Diaz NM, Centeno B, Weber F, Leu YW, Shapiro CL, Eng C, Yeatman TJ, Huang TH. Mapping geographic zones of

cancer risk with epigenetic biomarkers in normal breast tissue. *Clin. Cancer Res.* 2006, 12:6626-6636.

[9] Cheng ASL, Culhane AC, Chan MWY, Venkataramu CR, Ehrich M, Nasir A, Rodriguez BAT, Liu J, Yan PS, Quackenbush J, Nephew KP, Yeatman TJ, Huang THM. Epithelial progeny of estrogen-exposed breast progenitor cells display a cancer-like methylome. *Cancer Res.* 2008, 68:1786-1796.

[10] Chen L, Shen R, Ye Y, Pu XA, Liu X, Duan W, Wen J, Zimmerer J, Wang Y, Liu Y, Lasky LC, Heerema NA, Perrotti D, Ozato K, Kuramochi-Miyagawa S, Nakano T, Yates AJ, Carson Iii WE, Lin H, Barsky SH, Gao JX. Precancerous stem cells have the potential for both benign and malignant differentiation. *PLoS ONE* 2007, 2:e293.

[11] Gao JX. Cancer stem cells: The lessons from precancerous stem cells. *J. Cell Mol. Med.* 2008, 12:67-96.

[12] Reya T, Morrison SJ, Clarke MF, Weissman IL. Stem cells, cancer, and cancer stem cells. *Nature* 2001, 414:105-111.

[13] Clarke MF, Dick JE, Dirks PB, Eaves CJ, Jamieson CH, Jones DL, Visvader J, Weissman IL, Wahl GM. Cancer stem cells--perspectives on current status and future directions: Aacr workshop on cancer stem cells. *Cancer Res.* 2006, 66:9339-9344.

[14] Dick JE. Stem cell concepts renew cancer research. *Blood* 2008, 112:4793-4807.

[15] Gao J-X, Zhou Q. Epigenetic progenitors in tumor initiation and development. *Drug Discovery Today: Disease Models* 2009, 6:5-12.

[16] Shen R, Ye Y, Chen L, Yan Q, Barsky SH, Gao JX. Precancerous stem cells can serve as tumor vasculogenic progenitors. *PLoS ONE* 2008, 3:e1652.

[17] Berman JJ, Albores-Saavedra J, Bostwick D, Delellis R, Eble J, Hamilton SR, Hruban RH, Mutter GL, Page D, Rohan T, Travis W, Henson DE. Precancer: A conceptual working definition -- results of a consensus conference. *Cancer Detect. Prev.* 2006, 30:387-394.

[18] Shen R, Tao L, Xu Y, Chang S, Brocklyn JV, Gao JX. Reversibility of aberrant global DNA and estrogen receptor-a gene methylation distinguishes the colorectal precancer from cancer. *Int. J. Clin. Exp. Pathol.* 2009, 2:21-33.

[19] Raaijmakers MHGP, Mukherjee S, Guo S, Zhang S, Kobayashi T, Schoonmaker JA, Ebert BL, Al-Shahrour F, Hasserjian RP, Scadden EO, Aung Z, Matza M, Merkenschlager M, Lin C, Rommens JM, Scadden DT. Bone progenitor dysfunction induces myelodysplasia and secondary leukaemia. *Nature* advance online publication.

[20] Kelly PN, Dakic A, Adams JM, Nutt SL, Strasser A. Tumor growth need not be driven by rare cancer stem cells. *Science* 2007, 317:337.

[21] Dick JE. Looking ahead in cancer stem cell research. *Nat. Biotech.* 2009, 27:44-46.

[22] Eaves CJ. Cancer stem cells: Here, there, everywhere? *Nature* 2008, 456:581-582.

[23] Cancer stem cells are everywhere. *Nat. Med.* 2009, 15:23-23.

[24] Jordan CT. Cancer stem cells: Controversial or just misunderstood? *Cell Stem. Cell* 2009, 4:203-205.

[25] Gupta PB, Chaffer CL, Weinberg RA. Cancer stem cells: Mirage or reality? *Nat. Med.* 2009, 15:1010-1012.

[26] Lin H-JL, Zuo T, Lin C-H, Kuo CT, Liyanarachchi S, Sun S, Shen R, Deatherage DE, Potter D, Asamoto L, Lin S, Yan PS, Cheng A-L, Ostrowski MC, Huang THM. Breast cancer-associated fibroblasts confer akt1-mediated epigenetic silencing of cystatin m in epithelial cells. *Cancer Res.* 2008, 68:10257-10266.

[27] Zhao H, Peehl DM. Tumor-promoting phenotype of cd90hi prostate cancer-associated fibroblasts. *Prostate* 2009, 69:991-1000.

[28] Bao S, Wu Q, McLendon RE, Hao Y, Shi Q, Hjelmeland AB, Dewhirst MW, Bigner DD, Rich JN. Glioma stem cells promote radioresistance by preferential activation of the DNA damage response. *Nature* 2006, 444:756-760.

[29] Diehn M, Clarke MF. Cancer stem cells and radiotherapy: New insights into tumor radioresistance. *J. Natl. Cancer Inst.* 2006, 98:1755-1757.

[30] Donnenberg VS, Donnenberg AD. Multiple drug resistance in cancer revisited: The cancer stem cell hypothesis. *J. Clin. Pharmacol.* 2005, 45:872-877.

[31] Huang EH, Heidt DG, Li CW, Simeone DM. Cancer stem cells: A new paradigm for understanding tumor progression and therapeutic resistance. *Surgery* 2007, 141:415-419.

[32] Dean M. Cancer stem cells: Redefining the paradigm of cancer treatment strategies. *Mol. Interv.* 2006, 6:140-148.

[33] Klonisch T, Wiechec E, Hombach-Klonisch S, Ande SR, Wesselborg S, Schulze-Osthoff K, Los M. Cancer stem cell markers in common cancers - therapeutic implications. *Trends in Molecular Medicine* 2008, 14:450-460.

[34] Sell S. Cancer stem cells and differentiation therapy. *Tumour Biol.* 2006, 27:59-70.

[35] Lapidot T, Sirard C, Vormoor J, Murdoch B, Hoang T, Caceres-Cortes J, Minden M, Paterson B, Caligiuri MA, Dick JE. A cell initiating human acute myeloid leukaemia after transplantation into scid mice. *Nature* 1994, 367:645-648.

[36] Al-Hajj M, Wicha MS, Benito-Hernandez A, Morrison SJ, Clarke MF. Prospective identification of tumorigenic breast cancer cells. *Proc. Natl. Acad. Sci. USA* 2003, 100:3983-3988.

[37] Warner JK, Wang JC, Hope KJ, Jin L, Dick JE. Concepts of human leukemic development. *Oncogene* 2004, 23:7164-7177.

[38] Al-Hajj M, Clarke MF. Self-renewal and solid tumor stem cells. *Oncogene* 2004, 23:7274-7282.

[39] Barsky SH, Grossman DA, Ho J, Holmes EC. The multifocality of bronchioloalveolar lung carcinoma: Evidence and implications of a multiclonal origin. *Mod. Pathol.* 1994, 7:633-640.

[40] Sternlicht M, Mirell C, Safarians S, Barsky SH. A novel strategy for the investigation of clonality in precancerous disease states and early stages of tumor progression. *Biochem. Biophys. Res. Commun.* 1994, 199:511-518.

[41] Adams JM, Strasser A. Is tumor growth sustained by rare cancer stem cells or dominant clones? *Cancer Res.* 2008, 68:4018-4021.

[42] Quintana E, Shackleton M, Sabel MS, Fullen DR, Johnson TM, Morrison SJ. Efficient tumour formation by single human melanoma cells. *Nature* 2008, 456:593-598.

[43] Bonnet D, Dick JE. Human acute myeloid leukemia is organized as a hierarchy that originates from a primitive hematopoietic cell. *Nat. Med.* 1997, 3:730-737.

[44] Xu Q, Yuan X, Tunici P, Liu G, Fan X, Xu M, Hu J, Hwang JY, Farkas DL, Black KL, Yu JS. Isolation of tumour stem-like cells from benign tumours. *Br. J. Cancer* 2009, 101:303-311.

[45] Hong D, Gupta R, Ancliff P, Atzberger A, Brown J, Soneji S, Green J, Colman S, Piacibello W, Buckle V, Tsuzuki S, Greaves M, Enver T. Initiating and cancer-

propagating cells in tel-aml1-associated childhood leukemia. *Science* 2008, 319:336-339.

[46] Castor A, Nilsson L, Astrand-Grundstrom I, Buitenhuis M, Ramirez C, Anderson K, Strombeck B, Garwicz S, Bekassy AN, Schmiegelow K, Lausen B, Hokland P, Lehmann S, Juliusson G, Johansson B, Jacobsen SEW. Distinct patterns of hematopoietic stem cell involvement in acute lymphoblastic leukemia. *Nat. Med.* 2005, 11:630-637.

[47] Cox CV, Diamanti P, Evely RS, Kearns PR, Blair A. Expression of cd133 on leukemia-initiating cells in childhood all. *Blood* 2009, 113:3287-3296.

[48] Dalerba P, Dylla SJ, Park IK, Liu R, Wang X, Cho RW, Hoey T, Gurney A, Huang EH, Simeone DM, Shelton AA, Parmiani G, Castelli C, Clarke MF. Phenotypic characterization of human colorectal cancer stem cells. *Proc. Natl. Acad. Sci. USA* 2007, 104:10158-10163.

[49] Li C, Heidt DG, Dalerba P, Burant CF, Zhang L, Adsay V, Wicha M, Clarke MF, Simeone DM. Identification of pancreatic cancer stem cells. *Cancer Res.* 2007, 67:1030-1037.

[50] Singh SK, Hawkins C, Clarke ID, Squire JA, Bayani J, Hide T, Henkelman RM, Cusimano MD, Dirks PB. Identification of human brain tumour initiating cells. *Nature* 2004, 432:396-401.

[51] Zhu L, Gibson P, Currle DS, Tong Y, Richardson RJ, Bayazitov IT, Poppleton H, Zakharenko S, Ellison DW, Gilbertson RJ. Prominin 1 marks intestinal stem cells that are susceptible to neoplastic transformation. *Nature* 2009, 457:603-607.

[52] Barker N, Ridgway RA, van Es JH, van de Wetering M, Begthel H, van den Born M, Danenberg E, Clarke AR, Sansom OJ, Clevers H. Crypt stem cells as the cells-of-origin of intestinal cancer. *Nature* 2009, 457:608-611.

[53] Heidenreich O, Vormoor J. Malignant stem cells in childhood all: The debate continues! *Blood* 2009, 113:4476-4477.

[54] Werbowetski-Ogilvie TE, Bhatia M. Pluripotent human stem cell lines: What we can learn about cancer initiation. *Trends in Molecular Medicine* 2008, 14:323-332.

[55] Damonte P, Hodgson JG, Chen J, Young L, Cardiff R, Borowsky A. Mammary carcinoma behavior is programmed in the precancer stem cell. *Breast Cancer Research* 2008, 10:R50.

[56] Michor F. Cml blast crisis arises from progenitors. *Stem. Cells* 2007.

[57] Hubbard SA, Friel AM, Kumar B, Zhang L, Rueda BR, Gargett CE. Evidence for cancer stem cells in human endometrial carcinoma. *Cancer Res.* 2009, 69:8241-8248.

[58] Gao JX, Liu X, Wen J, Zhang H, Durbin J, Liu Y, Zheng P. Differentiation of monocytic cell clones into cd8alpha(+) dendritic cells (dc) suggests that monocytes can be direct precursors for both cd8alpha(+) and cd8alpha(-) dc in the mouse. *J. Immunol.* 2003, 170:5927-5935.

[59] Lim E, Vaillant F, Wu D, Forrest NC, Pal B, Hart AH, Asselin-Labat M-L, Gyorki DE, Ward T, Partanen A, Feleppa F, Huschtscha LI, Thorne HJ, Fox SB, Yan M, French JD, Brown MA, Smyth GK, Visvader JE, Lindeman GJ. Aberrant luminal progenitors as the candidate target population for basal tumor development in brca1 mutation carriers. *Nat. Med.* 2009, 15:907-913.

[60] Gao JX, Zhou Q. Epigenetic progenitors in tumor initiation and development. *Drug Discovery Today: Disease Models* 2009, 5:In press.

[61] Shackleton M, Quintana E, Fearon ER, Morrison SJ. Heterogeneity in cancer: Cancer stem cells versus clonal evolution. *Cell* 2009, 138:822-829.
[62] Orkin SH, Zon LI. Hematopoiesis: An evolving paradigm for stem cell biology. *Cell* 2008, 132:631-644.
[63] Koestenbauer S, Zech NH, Juch H, Vanderzwalmen P, Schoonjans L, Dohr G. Embryonic stem cells: Similarities and differences between human and murine embryonic stem cells. *Am. J. Reprod. Immunol.* 2006, 55:169-180.
[64] Chambers I, Colby D, Robertson M, Nichols J, Lee S, Tweedie S, Smith A. Functional expression cloning of nanog, a pluripotency sustaining factor in embryonic stem cells. *Cell* 2003, 113:643-655.
[65] Takahashi K, Yamanaka S. Induction of pluripotent stem cells from mouse embryonic and adult fibroblast cultures by defined factors. *Cell* 2006, 126:663-676.
[66] Xing PX, Hu XF, Pietersz GA, Hosick HL, McKenzie IF. Cripto: A novel target for antibody-based cancer immunotherapy. *Cancer Res.* 2004, 64:4018-4023.
[67] Monk M, Holding C. Human embryonic genes re-expressed in cancer cells. *Oncogene* 2001, 20:8085-8091.
[68] Tai MH, Chang CC, Kiupel M, Webster JD, Olson LK, Trosko JE. Oct4 expression in adult human stem cells: Evidence in support of the stem cell theory of carcinogenesis. *Carcinogenesis* 2005, 26:495-502.
[69] Raman JD, Mongan NP, Liu L, Tickoo SK, Nanus DM, Scherr DS, Gudas LJ. Decreased expression of the human stem cell marker, rex-1 (zfp-42), in renal cell carcinoma. *Carcinogenesis* 2006, 27:499-507.
[70] Dong C, Wilhelm D, Koopman P. Sox genes and cancer. *Cytogenet Genome Res.* 2004, 105:442-447.
[71] Kondo M, Wagers AJ, Manz MG, Prohaska SS, Scherer DC, Beilhack GF, Shizuru JA, Weissman IL. Biology of hematopoietic stem cells and progenitors: Implications for clinical application. *Annu. Rev. Immunol.* 2003, 21:759-806.
[72] Johnson J, Canning J, Kaneko T, Pru JK, Tilly JL. Germline stem cells and follicular renewal in the postnatal mammalian ovary. *Nature* 2004, 428:145-150.
[73] Kanatsu-Shinohara M, Inoue K, Lee J, Yoshimoto M, Ogonuki N, Miki H, Baba S, Kato T, Kazuki Y, Toyokuni S, Toyoshima M, Niwa O, Oshimura M, Heike T, Nakahata T, Ishino F, Ogura A, Shinohara T. Generation of pluripotent stem cells from neonatal mouse testis. *Cell* 2004, 119:1001-1012.
[74] Amariglio N, Hirshberg A, Scheithauer BW, Cohen Y, Loewenthal R, Trakhtenbrot L, Paz N, Koren-Michowitz M, Waldman D, Leider-Trejo L, Toren A, Constantini S, Rechavi G. Donor-derived brain tumor following neural stem cell transplantation in an ataxia telangiectasia patient. *PLoS Med.* 2009, 6:e29.
[75] Thorgeirsson SS. Hepatic stem cells in liver regeneration. *FASEB J.* 1996, 10:1249-1256.
[76] Lagasse E, Connors H, Al-Dhalimy M, Reitsma M, Dohse M, Osborne L, Wang X, Finegold M, Weissman IL, Grompe M. Purified hematopoietic stem cells can differentiate into hepatocytes in vivo. *Nat. Med.* 2000, 6:1229-1234.
[77] Petersen BE, Bowen WC, Patrene KD, Mars WM, Sullivan AK, Murase N, Boggs SS, Greenberger JS, Goff JP. Bone marrow as a potential source of hepatic oval cells. *Science* 1999, 284:1168-1170.

[78] Theise ND, Badve S, Saxena R, Henegariu O, Sell S, Crawford JM, Krause DS. Derivation of hepatocytes from bone marrow cells in mice after radiation-induced myeloablation. *Hepatology* 2000, 31:235-240.

[79] Zhan YT, Wang Y, Wei L, Liu B, Chen HS, Cong X, Fei R. Differentiation of rat bone marrow stem cells in liver after partial hepatectomy. *World J. Gastroenterol.* 2006, 12:5051-5054.

[80] Brazelton TR, Rossi FM, Keshet GI, Blau HM. From marrow to brain: Expression of neuronal phenotypes in adult mice. *Science* 2000, 290:1775-1779.

[81] Mezey E, Chandross KJ, Harta G, Maki RA, McKercher SR. Turning blood into brain: Cells bearing neuronal antigens generated in vivo from bone marrow. *Science* 2000, 290:1779-1782.

[82] Zhao LR, Duan WM, Reyes M, Keene CD, Verfaillie CM, Low WC. Human bone marrow stem cells exhibit neural phenotypes and ameliorate neurological deficits after grafting into the ischemic brain of rats. *Exp. Neurol.* 2002, 174:11-20.

[83] Orkin SH. Stem cell alchemy. *Nat. Med.* 2000, 6:1212-1213.

[84] Shen CN, Slack JM, Tosh D. Molecular basis of transdifferentiation of pancreas to liver. *Nat. Cell Biol.* 2000, 2:879-887.

[85] Orlic D. Bm stem cells and cardiac repair: Where do we stand in 2004? *Cytotherapy* 2005, 7:3-15.

[86] Ramalho-Santos M, Yoon S, Matsuzaki Y, Mulligan RC, Melton DA. "Stemness": Transcriptional profiling of embryonic and adult stem cells. *Science* 2002, 298:597-600.

[87] Conrad S, Renninger M, Hennenlotter Jr, Wiesner T, Just L, Bonin M, Aicher W, BÃ¼hring H-Jr, Mattheus U, Mack A, Wagner H-J, Minger S, Matzkies M, Reppel M, Hescheler Jr, Sievert K-D, Stenzl A, Skutella T. Generation of pluripotent stem cells from adult human testis. *Nature* 2008, 456:344-349.

[88] Oguro H, Iwama A. Life and death in hematopoietic stem cells. *Curr. Opin. Immunol.* 2007, 19:503-509.

[89] Lin H. Cell biology of stem cells: An enigma of asymmetry and self-renewal. *J. Cell Biol.* 2008, 180:257-260.

[90] Harrington L. Does the reservoir for self-renewal stem from the ends? *Oncogene* 2004, 23:7283-7289.

[91] Morrison SJ, Prowse KR, Ho P, Weissman IL. Telomerase activity in hematopoietic cells is associated with self-renewal potential. *Immunity* 1996, 5:207-216.

[92] Spangrude GJ, Heimfeld S, Weissman IL. Purification and characterization of mouse hematopoietic stem cells. *Science* 1988, 241:58-62.

[93] Akashi K, Traver D, Miyamoto T, Weissman IL. A clonogenic common myeloid progenitor that gives rise to all myeloid lineages. *Nature* 2000, 404:193-197.

[94] Adolfsson J, Mansson R, Buza-Vidas N, Hultquist A, Liuba K, Jensen CT, Bryder D, Yang L, Borge OJ, Thoren LA, Anderson K, Sitnicka E, Sasaki Y, Sigvardsson M, Jacobsen SE. Identification of flt3+ lympho-myeloid stem cells lacking erythro-megakaryocytic potential a revised road map for adult blood lineage commitment. *Cell* 2005, 121:295-306.

[95] Morrison SJ, Uchida N, Weissman IL. The biology of hematopoietic stem cells. *Annu. Rev. Cell Dev. Biol.* 1995, 11:35-71.

[96] Yin T, Li L. The stem cell niches in bone. *J. Clin. Invest.* 2006, 116:1195-1201.

[97] Martinez-Agosto JA, Mikkola HK, Hartenstein V, Banerjee U. The hematopoietic stem cell and its niche: A comparative view. *Genes Dev.* 2007, 21:3044-3060.
[98] Li L, Xie T. Stem cell niche: Structure and function. *Annu. Rev. Cell Dev. Biol.* 2005, 21:605-631.
[99] Hirao A, Arai F, Suda T. Regulation of cell cycle in hematopoietic stem cells by the niche. *Cell Cycle* 2004, 3.
[100] Arai F, Suda T. Maintenance of quiescent hematopoietic stem cells in the osteoblastic niche. *Ann. N. Y. Acad. Sci.* 2007, 1106:41-53.
[101] Moore KA, Lemischka IR. Stem cells and their niches. *Science* 2006, 311:1880-1885.
[102] Zhang J, Niu C, Ye L, Huang H, He X, Tong WG, Ross J, Haug J, Johnson T, Feng JQ, Harris S, Wiedemann LM, Mishina Y, Li L. Identification of the haematopoietic stem cell niche and control of the niche size. *Nature* 2003, 425:836-841.
[103] Yang YX, Miao ZC, Zhang HJ, Wang Y, Gao JX, Feng MF. Establishment and characterization of a human telomerase catalytic subunit-transduced fetal bone marrow-derived osteoblastic cell line. *Differentiation* 2007, 75:24-34.
[104] Constantinescu S. Stemness, fusion and renewal of hematopoietic and embryonic stem cells. *J. Cell Mol. Med.* 2003, 7:103-112.
[105] Ivanova NB, Dimos JT, Schaniel C, Hackney JA, Moore KA, Lemischka IR. A stem cell molecular signature. *Science* 2002, 298:601-604.
[106] Iwama A, Oguro H, Negishi M, Kato Y, Morita Y, Tsukui H, Ema H, Kamijo T, Katoh-Fukui Y, Koseki H, van Lohuizen M, Nakauchi H. Enhanced self-renewal of hematopoietic stem cells mediated by the polycomb gene product bmi-1. *Immunity* 2004, 21:843-851.
[107] Park IK, Qian D, Kiel M, Becker MW, Pihalja M, Weissman IL, Morrison SJ, Clarke MF. Bmi-1 is required for maintenance of adult self-renewing haematopoietic stem cells. *Nature* 2003, 423:302-305.
[108] Clarke MF, Fuller M. Stem cells and cancer: Two faces of eve. *Cell* 2006, 124:1111-1115.
[109] Nowak K, Kerl K, Fehr D, Kramps C, Gessner C, Killmer K, Samans B, Berwanger B, Christiansen H, Lutz W. Bmi1 is a target gene of e2f-1 and is strongly expressed in primary neuroblastomas. *Nucleic Acids Res.* 2006, 34:1745-1754.
[110] Park IK, Morrison SJ, Clarke MF. Bmi1, stem cells, and senescence regulation. *J. Clin. Invest.* 2004, 113:175-179.
[111] Fearon ER, Vogelstein B. A genetic model for colorectal tumorigenesis. *Cell* 1990, 61:759-767.
[112] Jamieson CH, Ailles LE, Dylla SJ, Muijtjens M, Jones C, Zehnder JL, Gotlib J, Li K, Manz MG, Keating A, Sawyers CL, Weissman IL. Granulocyte-macrophage progenitors as candidate leukemic stem cells in blast-crisis cml. *N. Engl. J. Med.* 2004, 351:657-667.
[113] Bjerkvig R, Tysnes BB, Aboody KS, Najbauer J, Terzis AJA. The origin of the cancer stem cell: Current controversies and new insights. *Nat. Rev. Cancer* 2005, 5:899-904.
[114] Takahashi K, Tanabe K, Ohnuki M, Narita M, Ichisaka T, Tomoda K, Yamanaka S. Induction of pluripotent stem cells from adult human fibroblasts by defined factors. *Cell* 2007, 131:861-872.

[115] Yu J, Vodyanik MA, Smuga-Otto K, Antosiewicz-Bourget J, Frane JL, Tian S, Nie J, Jonsdottir GA, Ruotti V, Stewart R, Slukvin II, Thomson JA. Induced pluripotent stem cell lines derived from human somatic cells. *Science* 2007, 318:1917-1920.

[116] Gao JX, Zhou Q. Epigenetic progenitors in tumor initiation and development. *Drug Discovery Today: Disease Models* In Press, Corrected Proof.

[117] Feinberg AP, Ohlsson R, Henikoff S. The epigenetic progenitor origin of human cancer. *Nat. Rev. Genet.* 2006, 7:21-33.

[118] Lobachevsky PN, Radford IR. Intestinal crypt properties fit a model that incorporates replicative ageing and deep and proximate stem cells. *Cell Prolif* 2006, 39:379-402.

[119] Rizvi AZ, Swain JR, Davies PS, Bailey AS, Decker AD, Willenbring H, Grompe M, Fleming WH, Wong MH. Bone marrow-derived cells fuse with normal and transformed intestinal stem cells. *Proc. Natl. Acad. Sci. USA* 2006, 103:6321-6325.

[120] Barker N, van Es JH, Kuipers J, Kujala P, van den Born M, Cozijnsen M, Haegebarth A, Korving J, Begthel H, Peters PJ, Clevers H. Identification of stem cells in small intestine and colon by marker gene lgr5. *Nature* 2007, 449:1003-1007.

[121] He XC, Yin T, Grindley JC, Tian Q, Sato T, Tao WA, Dirisina R, Porter-Westpfahl KS, Hembree M, Johnson T, Wiedemann LM, Barrett TA, Hood L, Wu H, Li L. Pten-deficient intestinal stem cells initiate intestinal polyposis. *Nat. Genet.* 2007, 39:189-198.

[122] le Viseur C, Hotfilder M, Bomken S, Wilson K, Röttgers S, Schrauder A, Rosemann A, Irving J, Stam RW, Shultz LD, Harbott J, Jürgens H, Schrappe M, Pieters R, Vormoor J. In childhood acute lymphoblastic leukemia, blasts at different stages of immunophenotypic maturation have stem cell properties. *Cancer Cell* 2008, 14:47-58.

[123] Cox CV, Evely RS, Oakhill A, Pamphilon DH, Goulden NJ, Blair A. Characterization of acute lymphoblastic leukemia progenitor cells. *Blood* 2004, 104:2919-2925.

[124] Kondo T, Setoguchi T, Taga T. Persistence of a small subpopulation of cancer stem-like cells in the c6 glioma cell line. *Proc. Natl. Acad. Sci. USA* 2004, 101:781-786.

[125] Patrawala L, Calhoun T, Schneider-Broussard R, Zhou J, Claypool K, Tang DG. Side population is enriched in tumorigenic, stem-like cancer cells, whereas abcg2+ and abcg2- cancer cells are similarly tumorigenic. *Cancer Res.* 2005, 65:6207-6219.

[126] Pine SR, Ryan BdM, Varticovski L, Robles AI, Harris CC. Microenvironmental modulation of asymmetric cell division in human lung cancer cells. *Proceedings of the National Academy of Sciences* 107:2195-2200.

[127] Houghton J, Stoicov C, Nomura S, Rogers AB, Carlson J, Li H, Cai X, Fox JG, Goldenring JR, Wang TC. Gastric cancer originating from bone marrow-derived cells. *Science* 2004, 306:1568-1571.

[128] Bond JH. Colon polyps and cancer. *Endoscopy* 2003, 35:27-35.

[129] Cardiff RD, Anver MR, Boivin GP, Bosenberg MW, Maronpot RR, Molinolo AA, Nikitin AY, Rehg JE, Thomas GV, Russell RG, Ward JM. Precancer in mice: Animal models used to understand, prevent, and treat human precancers. *Toxicol. Pathol.* 2006, 34:699-707.

[130] Maglione JE, Moghanaki D, Young LJ, Manner CK, Ellies LG, Joseph SO, Nicholson B, Cardiff RD, MacLeod CL. Transgenic polyoma middle-t mice model premalignant mammary disease. *Cancer Res.* 2001, 61:8298-8305.

[131] Namba R, Maglione JE, Davis RR, Baron CA, Liu S, Carmack CE, Young LJ, Borowsky AD, Cardiff RD, Gregg JP. Heterogeneity of mammary lesions represent molecular differences. *BMC Cancer* 2006, 6:275.

[132] Wistuba, II. Genetics of preneoplasia: Lessons from lung cancer. *Curr Mol Med* 2007, 7:3-14.

[133] O'Brien CA, Pollett A, Gallinger S, Dick JE. A human colon cancer cell capable of initiating tumour growth in immunodeficient mice. *Nature* 2007, 445:106-110.

[134] Bussolati B, Bruno S, Grange C, Ferrando U, Camussi G. Identification of a tumor-initiating stem cell population in human renal carcinomas. *FASEB J.* 2008, 22:3696-3705.

[135] Friedman S, Lu M, Schultz A, Thomas D, Lin R-Y. Cd133⁺ anaplastic thyroid cancer cells initiate tumors in immunodeficient mice and are regulated by thyrotropin. *PLoS ONE* 2009, 4:e5395.

[136] Ji Q, Hao X, Zhang M, Tang W, Yang M, Li L, Xiang D, DeSano JT, Bommer GT, Fan D, Fearon ER, Lawrence TS, Xu L. Microrna mir-34 inhibits human pancreatic cancer tumor-initiating cells. *PLoS ONE* 2009, 4:e6816.

[137] Ricci-Vitiani L, Lombardi DG, Pilozzi E, Biffoni M, Todaro M, Peschle C, De Maria R. Identification and expansion of human colon-cancer-initiating cells. *Nature* 2007, 445:111-115.

[138] He G, Chen L, Ye Y, Xiao Y, Hua K, Jarjoura D, Nakano T, Barsky SH, Shen R, Gao JX. Piwil2 expressed in various stages of cervical neoplasia is a potential complementary marker for p16ink4a. *Am. J. Transl. Res.* 2010, 2:14.

[139] Liu JS, R.; Gang, H.; Chen, L.;Yin, Y.; Hua, K.; Jarjoura, D.; Nakano, T.; Ramesh, GK; Shapiro, CL.;Barsky, SH.; Gao, JX. Piwil2 is expressed in various stages of breast cancers and has the potential to be used as a novel biomarker. *Int. J. Clin. Exp. Pathol.* 2010, 3:10.

[140] Rosland GV, Svendsen A, Torsvik A, Sobala E, McCormack E, Immervoll H, Mysliwietz J, Tonn J-C, Goldbrunner R, Lonning PE, Bjerkvig R, Schichor C. Long-term cultures of bone marrow-derived human mesenchymal stem cells frequently undergo spontaneous malignant transformation. *Cancer Res.* 2009, 69:5331-5339.

[141] Miura M, Miura Y, Padilla-Nash HM, Molinolo AA, Fu B, Patel V, Seo BM, Sonoyama W, Zheng JJ, Baker CC, Chen W, Ried T, Shi S. Accumulated chromosomal instability in murine bone marrow mesenchymal stem cells leads to malignant transformation. *Stem Cells* 2006, 24:1095-1103.

[142] Rubio D, Garcia-Castro J, Martin MC, de la Fuente R, Cigudosa JC, Lloyd AC, Bernad A. Spontaneous human adult stem cell transformation. *Cancer Res.* 2005, 65:3035-3039.

[143] Tolar J, Nauta AJ, Osborn MJ, Panoskaltsis Mortari A, McElmurry RT, Bell S, Xia L, Zhou N, Riddle M, Schroeder TM, Westendorf JJ, McIvor RS, Hogendoorn PC, Szuhai K, Oseth L, Hirsch B, Yant SR, Kay MA, Peister A, Prockop DJ, Fibbe WE, Blazar BR. Sarcoma derived from cultured mesenchymal stem cells. *Stem. Cells* 2007, 25:371-379.

[144] Wang Y, Huso DI, Harrington J, Kellner J, Jeong DK, Turney J, McNiece IK. Outgrowth of a transformed cell population derived from normal human bm mesenchymal stem cell culture. *Cytotherapy* 2005, 7:509-519.

[145] Rubio D, Garcia S, Paz MF, De la Cueva T, Lopez-Fernandez LA, Lloyd AC, Garcia-Castro J, Bernad A. Molecular characterization of spontaneous mesenchymal stem cell transformation. *PLoS ONE* 2008, 3:e1398.

[146] Blelloch RH, Hochedlinger K, Yamada Y, Brennan C, Kim M, Mintz B, Chin L, Jaenisch R. Nuclear cloning of embryonal carcinoma cells. *Proceedings of the National Academy of Sciences of the United States of America* 2004, 101:13985-13990.

[147] Durr M, Harder F, Merkel A, Bug G, Henschler R, Muller AM. Chimaerism and erythroid marker expression after microinjection of human acute myeloid leukaemia cells into murine blastocysts. *Oncogene* 2003, 22:9185-9191.

[148] Geiger H, Sick S, Bonifer C, Muller AM. Globin gene expression is reprogrammed in chimeras generated by injecting adult hematopoietic stem cells into mouse blastocysts. *Cell* 1998, 93:1055-1065.

[149] Shipitsin M, Campbell LL, Argani P, Weremowicz S, Bloushtain-Qimron N, Yao J, Nikolskaya T, Serebryiskaya T, Beroukhim R, Hu M, Halushka MK, Sukumar S, Parker LM, Anderson KS, Harris LN, Garber JE, Richardson AL, Schnitt SJ, Nikolsky Y, Gelman RS, Polyak K. Molecular definition of breast tumor heterogeneity. *Cancer Cell* 2007, 11:259-273.

[150] Allan AL, Vantyghem SA, Tuck AB, Chambers AF. Tumor dormancy and cancer stem cells: Implications for the biology and treatment of breast cancer metastasis. *Breast Dis.* 2006, 26:87-98.

[151] Sheridan C, Kishimoto H, Fuchs RK, Mehrotra S, Bhat-Nakshatri P, Turner CH, Goulet R, Jr., Badve S, Nakshatri H. Cd44+/cd24- breast cancer cells exhibit enhanced invasive properties: An early step necessary for metastasis. *Breast Cancer Res.* 2006, 8:R59.

[152] Shmelkov SV, Butler JM, Hooper AT, Hormigo A, Kushner J, Milde T, St Clair R, Baljevic M, White I, Jin DK, Chadburn A, Murphy AJ, Valenzuela DM, Gale NW, Thurston G, Yancopoulos GD, D'Angelica M, Kemeny N, Lyden D, Rafii S. Cd133 expression is not restricted to stem cells, and both cd133+ and cd133- metastatic colon cancer cells initiate tumors. *J. Clin. Invest.* 2008, 118:2111-2120.

[153] Townson JL, Chambers AF. Dormancy of solitary metastatic cells. *Cell Cycle* 2006, 5:1744-1750.

[154] Wicha MS. Cancer stem cells and metastasis: Lethal seeds. *Clin. Cancer Res.* 2006, 12:5606-5607.

[155] Yu S-c, Bian X-w. Enrichment of cancer stem cells based on heterogeneity of invasiveness. *Stem Cell Reviews and Reports* 2009, 5:66-71.

[156] Aguirre-Ghiso JA. Models, mechanisms and clinical evidence for cancer dormancy. *Nat. Rev. Cancer* 2007, 7:834-846.

[157] Dunn GP, Old LJ, Schreiber RD. The three es of cancer immunoediting. *Annu Rev Immunol* 2004, 22:329-360.

[158] Thomas L. On immunosurveillance in human cancer. *Yale J. Biol. Med.* 1982, 55:329-333.

[159] Gao J-X, Chen L, Yan Q, Waldman J, Ye Y, Barsky SH, Shen R. Immunoprevention of cancer through targeting of precancerous stem cells. *FASEB J.* 2008, 22:1077.1024-.

[160] Bergers G, Benjamin LE. Tumorigenesis and the angiogenic switch. *Nat. Rev. Cancer* 2003, 3:401-410.

[161] Carmeliet P, Jain RK. Angiogenesis in cancer and other diseases. *Nature* 2000, 407:249-257.
[162] Folkman J. Tumor angiogenesis: Therapeutic implications. *N. Engl. J. Med.* 1971, 285:1182-1186.
[163] Kim M-Y, Oskarsson T, Acharyya S, Nguyen DX, Zhang XHF, Norton L, Massagué J. Tumor self-seeding by circulating cancer cells. *Cell* 2009, 139:1315-1326.
[164] Furuya M, Nishiyama M, Kasuya Y, Kimura S, Ishikura H. Pathophysiology of tumor neovascularization. *Vasc. Health Risk Manag.* 2005, 1:277-290.
[165] Bao S, Wu Q, Sathornsumetee S, Hao Y, Li Z, Hjelmeland AB, Shi Q, McLendon RE, Bigner DD, Rich JN. Stem cell-like glioma cells promote tumor angiogenesis through vascular endothelial growth factor. *Cancer Res.* 2006, 66:7843-7848.
[166] Furstenberger G, von Moos R, Lucas R, Thurlimann B, Senn HJ, Hamacher J, Boneberg EM. Circulating endothelial cells and angiogenic serum factors during neoadjuvant chemotherapy of primary breast cancer. *Br. J. Cancer* 2006, 94:524-531.
[167] Zhang L, Yang N, Park JW, Katsaros D, Fracchioli S, Cao G, O'Brien-Jenkins A, Randall TC, Rubin SC, Coukos G. Tumor-derived vascular endothelial growth factor up-regulates angiopoietin-2 in host endothelium and destabilizes host vasculature, supporting angiogenesis in ovarian cancer. *Cancer Res.* 2003, 63:3403-3412.
[168] Hilbe W, Dirnhofer S, Oberwasserlechner F, Schmid T, Gunsilius E, Hilbe G, Woll E, Kahler CM. Cd133 positive endothelial progenitor cells contribute to the tumour vasculature in non-small cell lung cancer. *J. Clin. Pathol.* 2004, 57:965-969.
[169] Ayesha BA, Han-Hsuan F, Jennie H, Irene V, Liora M, Carlos Cano M, Jessica O, Dan-Arin S, Gil M. Stem-like ovarian cancer cells can serve as tumor vascular progenitors. *Stem Cells* 2009, 9999:N/A.
[170] Bussolati B, Grange C, Sapino A, Camussi G. Endothelial cell differentiation of human breast tumor stem/progenitor cells. *J. Cell Mol. Med.* 2008.
[171] Folkins C, Shaked Y, Man S, Tang T, Lee CR, Zhu Z, Hoffman RM, Kerbel RS. Glioma tumor stem-like cells promote tumor angiogenesis and vasculogenesis via vascular endothelial growth factor and stromal-derived factor 1. *Cancer Res.* 2009, 69:7243-7251.
[172] Phillips TM, McBride WH, Pajonk F. The response of cd24-/low/cd44+ breast cancer-initiating cells to radiation. *J. Natl. Cancer Inst.* 2006, 98:1777-1785.
[173] Tanei T, Morimoto K, Shimazu K, Kim SJ, Tanji Y, Taguchi T, Tamaki Y, Noguchi S. Association of breast cancer stem cells identified by aldehyde dehydrogenase 1 expression with resistance to sequential paclitaxel and epirubicin-based chemotherapy for breast cancers. *Clin. Cancer Res.* 2009, 15:4234-4241.
[174] Kavalerchik E, Goff D, Jamieson CHM. Chronic myeloid leukemia stem cells. *J. Clin. Oncol.* 2008, 26:2911-2915.
[175] Lou H, Dean M. Targeted therapy for cancer stem cells: The patched pathway and abc transporters. *Oncogene* 2007, 26:1357-1360.
[176] Rudin CM, Hann CL, Laterra J, Yauch RL, Callahan CA, Fu L, Holcomb T, Stinson J, Gould SE, Coleman B, LoRusso PM, Von Hoff DD, de Sauvage FJ, Low JA. Treatment of medulloblastoma with hedgehog pathway inhibitor gdc-0449. *N. Engl. J. Med.* 2009, NEJMoa0902903.
[177] Von Hoff DD, LoRusso PM, Rudin CM, Reddy JC, Yauch RL, Tibes R, Weiss GJ, Borad MJ, Hann CL, Brahmer JR, Mackey HM, Lum BL, Darbonne WC, Marsters JC,

Jr., de Sauvage FJ, Low JA. Inhibition of the hedgehog pathway in advanced basal-cell carcinoma. *N. Engl. J. Med.* 2009, NEJMoa0905360.

[178] Vogelstein B, Kinzler KW. Cancer genes and the pathways they control. *Nat. Med.* 2004, 10:789-799.

[179] Campbell C, Risueno RM, Salati S, Guezguez B, Bhatia M. Signal control of hematopoietic stem cell fate: Wnt, notch, and hedgehog as the usual suspects. *Curr. Opin. Hematol.* 2008, 15:319-325.

[180] Zhou Z-h, Ping Y-f, Yu S-c, Yi L, Yao X-h, Chen J-h, Cui Y-h, Bian X-w. A novel approach to the identification and enrichment of cancer stem cells from a cultured human glioma cell line. *Cancer Letters* 2009, 281:92-99.

[181] Yamazaki J, Mizukami T, Takizawa K, Kuramitsu M, Momose H, Masumi A, Ami Y, Hasegawa H, Hall WW, Tsujimoto H, Hamaguchi I, Yamaguchi K. Identification of cancer stem cells in a tax-transgenic (tax-tg) mouse model of adult t-cell leukemia/lymphoma. *Blood* 2009, 114:2709-2720.

[182] Liang Y, Zhong Z, Huang Y, Deng W, Cao J, Tsao G, Liu Q, Pei D, Kang T, Zeng Y-X. Stem-like cancer cells are inducible by increasing genomic instability in cancer cells. *Journal of Biological Chemistry* 285:4931-4940.

[183] Charames GS, Bapat B. Genomic instability and cancer. *Curr. Mol. Med.* 2003, 3:589-596.

[184] Isaacs JT, Wake N, Coffey DS, Sandberg AA. Genetic instability coupled to clonal selection as a mechanism for tumor progression in the dunning r-3327 rat prostatic adenocarcinoma system. *Cancer Res.* 1982, 42:2353-2371.

[185] Hubbard S, Gargett C. A cancer stem cell origin for human endometrial carcinoma? *Reproduction* REP-09-0411.

[186] Zhang YQ, Kritzik M, Sarvetnick N. Identification and expansion of pancreatic stem/progenitor cells. *J. Cell Mol. Med.* 2005, 9:331-344.

[187] Ginestier C, Hur MH, Charafe-Jauffret E, Monville F, Dutcher J, Brown M, Jacquemier J, Viens P, Kleer CG, Liu S, Schott A, Hayes D, Birnbaum D, Wicha MS, Dontu G. Aldh1 is a marker of normal and malignant human mammary stem cells and a predictor of poor clinical outcome. *Cell Stem. Cell* 2007, 1:555-567.

[188] Collins AT, Berry PA, Hyde C, Stower MJ, Maitland NJ. Prospective identification of tumorigenic prostate cancer stem cells. *Cancer Res.* 2005, 65:10946-10951.

[189] Lee JH, Schutte D, Wulf G, Fuzesi L, Radzun HJ, Schweyer S, Engel W, Nayernia K. Stem-cell protein piwil2 is widely expressed in tumors and inhibits apoptosis through activation of stat3/bcl-xl pathway. *Hum. Mol. Genet.* 2006, 15:201-211.

[190] Sasaki T, Shiohama A, Minoshima S, Shimizu N. Identification of eight members of the argonaute family in the human genome small star, filled. *Genomics* 2003, 82:323-330.

[191] Becker L, Huang Q, Mashimo H. Immunostaining of lgr5, an intestinal stem cell marker, in normal and premalignant human gastrointestinal tissue. *ScientificWorldJournal* 2008, 8:1168-1176.

[192] Adamia S, Maxwell CA, Pilarski LM. Hyaluronan and hyaluronan synthases: Potential therapeutic targets in cancer. *Curr Drug Targets Cardiovasc Haematol Disord* 2005, 5:3-14.

[193] Nair KS, Naidoo R, Chetty R. Expression of cell adhesion molecules in oesophageal carcinoma and its prognostic value. *J. Clin. Pathol.* 2005, 58:343-351.

[194] Agnantis NJ, Goussia AC, Batistatou A, Stefanou D. Tumor markers in cancer patients. An update of their prognostic significance. Part ii. *In Vivo* 2004, 18:481-488.

[195] Nagano O, Saya H. Mechanism and biological significance of cd44 cleavage. *Cancer Sci.* 2004, 95:930-935.

[196] Yu S-c, Ping Y-f, Yi L, Zhou Z-h, Chen J-h, Yao X-h, Gao L, Wang JM, Bian X-w. Isolation and characterization of cancer stem cells from a human glioblastoma cell line u87. *Cancer Letters* 2008, 265:124-134.

[197] Hirschmann-Jax C, Foster AE, Wulf GG, Nuchtern JG, Jax TW, Gobel U, Goodell MA, Brenner MK. A distinct "Side population" Of cells with high drug efflux capacity in human tumor cells. *Proc. Natl. Acad. Sci. USA* 2004, 101:14228-14233.

[198] Zhou S, Schuetz JD, Bunting KD, Colapietro AM, Sampath J, Morris JJ, Lagutina I, Grosveld GC, Osawa M, Nakauchi H, Sorrentino BP. The abc transporter bcrp1/abcg2 is expressed in a wide variety of stem cells and is a molecular determinant of the side-population phenotype. *Nat. Med.* 2001, 7:1028-1034.

[199] Szotek PP, Pieretti-Vanmarcke R, Masiakos PT, Dinulescu DM, Connolly D, Foster R, Dombkowski D, Preffer F, Maclaughlin DT, Donahoe PK. Ovarian cancer side population defines cells with stem cell-like characteristics and mullerian inhibiting substance responsiveness. *Proc. Natl. Acad. Sci. USA* 2006, 103:11154-11159.

[200] Yang L, Bryder D, Adolfsson J, Nygren J, Mansson R, Sigvardsson M, Jacobsen SE. Identification of lin(-)sca1(+)kit(+)cd34(+)flt3- short-term hematopoietic stem cells capable of rapidly reconstituting and rescuing myeloablated transplant recipients. *Blood* 2005, 105:2717-2723.

[201] Osawa M, Nakamura K, Nishi N, Takahasi N, Tokuomoto Y, Inoue H, Nakauchi H. In vivo self-renewal of c-kit+ sca-1+ lin(low/-) hemopoietic stem cells. *J. Immunol.* 1996, 156:3207-3214.

[202] Wong SH, Lowes KN, Bertoncello I, Cook MJ, Simmons PJ, Kornberg AJ, Kapsa RM. Evaluation of sca-1 and c-kit as selective markers for muscle remodelling by non-hemopoietic bone marrow cells. *Stem. Cells* 2007, 25:1364-1374.

[203] Potti A, Ganti AK, Tuchman SA, Sholes K, Langness E, Koka V, Koch M. Her-2/neu and cd117 (c-kit) overexpression in patients with pesticide exposure and extensive stage small cell lung carcinoma (essclc). *J. Carcinog.* 2005, 4:8.

[204] Demetri GD. Targeting c-kit mutations in solid tumors: Scientific rationale and novel therapeutic options. *Semin. Oncol.* 2001, 28:19-26.

[205] Xin L, Lawson DA, Witte ON. The sca-1 cell surface marker enriches for a prostate-regenerating cell subpopulation that can initiate prostate tumorigenesis. *Proc. Natl. Acad. Sci. USA* 2005, 102:6942-6947.

[206] Chang HH, Hemberg M, Barahona M, Ingber DE, Huang S. Transcriptome-wide noise controls lineage choice in mammalian progenitor cells. *Nature* 2008, 453:544-547.

[207] Hanahan D, Weinberg RA. The hallmarks of cancer. *Cell* 2000, 100:57-70.

[208] Tahara E. Genetic pathways of two types of gastric cancer. *IARC Sci. Publ.* 2004, 327-349.

[209] Bartek J, Bartkova J, Lukas J. DNA damage signalling guards against activated oncogenes and tumour progression. *Oncogene* 26:7773-7779.

[210] Widschwendter M, Fiegl H, Egle D, Mueller-Holzner E, Spizzo G, Marth C, Weisenberger DJ, Campan M, Young J, Jacobs I, Laird PW. Epigenetic stem cell signature in cancer. *Nat. Genet.* 2007, 39:157-158.

[211] Bartkova J, Horejsi Z, Koed K, Kramer A, Tort F, Zieger K, Guldberg P, Sehested M, Nesland JM, Lukas C, Orntoft T, Lukas J, Bartek J. DNA damage response as a candidate anti-cancer barrier in early human tumorigenesis. *Nature* 2005, 434:864-870.

[212] Bartek J, Lukas J, Bartkova J. DNA damage response as an anti-cancer barrier: Damage threshold and the concept of 'conditional haploinsufficiency'. *Cell Cycle* 2007, 6:2344-2347.

[213] Harper JW, Elledge SJ. The DNA damage response: Ten years after. *Molecular Cell* 2007, 28:739-745.

[214] Mullighan CG, Phillips LA, Su X, Ma J, Miller CB, Shurtleff SA, Downing JR. Genomic analysis of the clonal origins of relapsed acute lymphoblastic leukemia. *Science* 2008, 322:1377-1380.

[215] Kanai Y, Hirohashi S. Alterations of DNA methylation associated with abnormalities of DNA methyltransferases in human cancers during transition from a precancerous to a malignant state. *Carcinogenesis* 2007, 28:2434-2442.

[216] James AW, Joseph MVDW, Helmuth G. Role of embryonic induction in benign transformation of neuroblastomas. *Cancer* 1967, 20:1335-1342.

[217] Ben-Porath I, Thomson MW, Carey VJ, Ge R, Bell GW, Regev A, Weinberg RA. An embryonic stem cell-like gene expression signature in poorly differentiated aggressive human tumors. *Nat. Genet.* 2008, 40:499-507.

[218] James E T. From adult stem cells to cancer stem cells. *Annals of the New York Academy of Sciences* 2006, 1089:36-58.

[219] Ohm JE, McGarvey KM, Yu X, Cheng L, Schuebel KE, Cope L, Mohammad HP, Chen W, Daniel VC, Yu W, Berman DM, Jenuwein T, Pruitt K, Sharkis SJ, Watkins DN, Herman JG, Baylin SB. A stem cell-like chromatin pattern may predispose tumor suppressor genes to DNA hypermethylation and heritable silencing. *Nat. Genet.* 2007, 39:237-242.

[220] Feng DQ, Peng C, Li CR, Zhou Y, Li M, Ling B, Wei HM, Tian ZG. Identification and characterization of cancer stem-like cells from primary carcinoma of the cervix uteri. *Oncol. Rep.* 2009, 22:1129-1134.

[221] Cox DN, Chao A, Baker J, Chang L, Qiao D, Lin H. A novel class of evolutionarily conserved genes defined by piwi are essential for stem cell self-renewal. *Genes. Dev.* 1998, 12:3715-3727.

[222] Kuramochi-Miyagawa S, Kimura T, Ijiri TW, Isobe T, Asada N, Fujita Y, Ikawa M, Iwai N, Okabe M, Deng W, Lin H, Matsuda Y, Nakano T. Mili, a mammalian member of piwi family gene, is essential for spermatogenesis. *Development* 2004, 131:839-849.

[223] Kuramochi-Miyagawa S, Kimura T, Yomogida K, Kuroiwa A, Tadokoro Y, Fujita Y, Sato M, Matsuda Y, Nakano T. Two mouse piwi-related genes: Miwi and mili. *Mech. Dev.* 2001, 108:121-133.

[224] Song JJ, Liu J, Tolia NH, Schneiderman J, Smith SK, Martienssen RA, Hannon GJ, Joshua-Tor L. The crystal structure of the argonaute2 paz domain reveals an rna binding motif in rnai effector complexes. *Nat. Struct. Biol.* 2003, 10:1026-1032.

[225] Cerutti L, Mian N, Bateman A. Domains in gene silencing and cell differentiation proteins: The novel paz domain and redefinition of the piwi domain. *Trends Biochem. Sci.* 2000, 25:481-482.

[226] Lee JH, Engel W, Nayernia K. Stem cell protein piwil2 modulates expression of murine spermatogonial stem cell expressed genes. *Mol. Reprod. Dev.* 2006, 73:173-179.

[227] Aravin A, Gaidatzis D, Pfeffer S, Lagos-Quintana M, Landgraf P, Iovino N, Morris P, Brownstein MJ, Kuramochi-Miyagawa S, Nakano T, Chien M, Russo JJ, Ju J, Sheridan R, Sander C, Zavolan M, Tuschl T. A novel class of small rnas bind to mili protein in mouse testes. *Nature* 2006, 442:203-207.

[228] Aravin AA, Sachidanandam R, Girard A, Fejes-Toth K, Hannon GJ. Developmentally regulated pirna clusters implicate mili in transposon control. *Science* 2007, 316:744-747.

[229] Grivna ST, Beyret E, Wang Z, Lin H. A novel class of small rnas in mouse spermatogenic cells. *Genes. Dev.* 2006, 20:1709-1714.

[230] Grivna ST, Pyhtila B, Lin H. Miwi associates with translational machinery and piwi-interacting rnas (pirnas) in regulating spermatogenesis. *Proc. Natl. Acad. Sci. USA* 2006, 103:13415-13420.

[231] Lau NC, Seto AG, Kim J, Kuramochi-Miyagawa S, Nakano T, Bartel DP, Kingston RE. Characterization of the pirna complex from rat testes. *Science* 2006, 313:363-367.

[232] Saito K, Nishida KM, Mori T, Kawamura Y, Miyoshi K, Nagami T, Siomi H, Siomi MC. Specific association of piwi with rasirnas derived from retrotransposon and heterochromatic regions in the drosophila genome. *Genes. Dev.* 2006, 20:2214-2222.

[233] Brennecke J, Aravin AA, Stark A, Dus M, Kellis M, Sachidanandam R, Hannon GJ. Discrete small rna-generating loci as master regulators of transposon activity in drosophila. *Cell* 2007, 128:1089-1103.

[234] Cox DN, Chao A, Lin H. Piwi encodes a nucleoplasmic factor whose activity modulates the number and division rate of germline stem cells. *Development* 2000, 127:503-514.

[235] Qiao D, Zeeman AM, Deng W, Looijenga LH, Lin H. Molecular characterization of hiwi, a human member of the piwi gene family whose overexpression is correlated to seminomas. *Oncogene* 2002, 21:3988-3999.

[236] Carmell MA, Xuan Z, Zhang MQ, Hannon GJ. The argonaute family: Tentacles that reach into rnai, developmental control, stem cell maintenance, and tumorigenesis. *Genes. Dev.* 2002, 16:2733-2742.

[237] Liu J, Carmell MA, Rivas FV, Marsden CG, Thomson JM, Song JJ, Hammond SM, Joshua-Tor L, Hannon GJ. Argonaute2 is the catalytic engine of mammalian rnai. *Science* 2004, 305:1437-1441.

[238] Preall JB, Sontheimer EJ. Rnai: Risc gets loaded. *Cell* 2005, 123:543-545.

[239] Ekwall K. The rits complex--a direct link between small rna and heterochromatin. *Molecular Cell* 2004, 13:304-305.

[240] Buhler M, Verdel A, Moazed D. Tethering rits to a nascent transcript initiates rnai- and heterochromatin-dependent gene silencing. *Cell* 2006, 125:873-886.

[241] Jaronczyk K, Carmichael JB, Hobman TC. Exploring the functions of rna interference pathway proteins: Some functions are more riscy than others? *Biochem. J.* 2005, 387:561-571.

[242] Stratton MR, Campbell PJ, Futreal PA. The cancer genome. *Nature* 2009, 458:719-724.

[243] Mader RM. Disease models in cancer. *Drug Discovery Today: Disease Models* 2009, 6:1-3.

[244] Nikpour P, Forouzandeh-Moghaddam M, Ziaee SA-M, Dokun OY, Schulz WA, Mowla SJ. Absence of piwil2 (hili) expression in human bladder cancer cell lines and tissues. *Cancer Epidemiology* In Press, Corrected Proof.

[245] Mongan NP, Martin KM, Gudas LJ. The putative human stem cell marker, rex-1 (zfp42): Structural classification and expression in normal human epithelial and carcinoma cell cultures. *Mol. Carcinog.* 2006, 45:887-900.

[246] Wang X, Zhao Y, Xiao Z, Chen B, Wei Z, Wang B, Zhang J, Han J, Gao Y, Li L, Zhao H, Zhao W, Lin H, Dai J. Alternative translation of oct4 by an internal ribosome entry site and its novel function in stress response. *Stem Cells* 2009, 27:1265-1275.

[247] Kotoula V, Papamichos SI, Lambropoulos AF. Revisiting oct4 expression in peripheral blood mononuclear cells. *Stem Cells* 2008, 26:290-291.

[248] Berg JS, Goodell MA. An argument against a role for oct4 in somatic stem cells. *Cell Stem Cell* 2007, 1:359-360.

[249] Lengner CJ, Camargo FD, Hochedlinger K, Welstead GG, Zaidi S, Gokhale S, Scholer HR, Tomilin A, Jaenisch R. Oct4 expression is not required for mouse somatic stem cell self-renewal. *Cell Stem. Cell* 2007, 1:403-415.

[250] Duncan AW, Rattis FM, DiMascio LN, Congdon KL, Pazianos G, Zhao C, Yoon K, Cook JM, Willert K, Gaiano N, Reya T. Integration of notch and wnt signaling in hematopoietic stem cell maintenance. *Nat. Immunol.* 2005, 6:314-322.

[251] Liu S, Dontu G, Wicha MS. Mammary stem cells, self-renewal pathways, and carcinogenesis. *Breast Cancer Res.* 2005, 7:86-95.

[252] Dreesen O, Brivanlou A. Signaling pathways in cancer and embryonic stem cells. *Stem Cell Reviews and Reports* 2007, 3:7-17.

[253] Devine SM, Lazarus HM, Emerson SG. Clinical application of hematopoietic progenitor cell expansion: Current status and future prospects. *Bone Marrow Transplant* 2003, 31:241-252.

[254] Campbell PA, Perez-Iratxeta C, Andrade-Navarro MA, Rudnicki MA. Oct4 targets regulatory nodes to modulate stem cell function. *PLoS ONE* 2007, 2:e553.

[255] Kim JB, Sebastiano V, Wu G, Araúzo-Bravo MJ, Sasse P, Gentile L, Ko K, Ruau D, Ehrich M, van den Boom D, Meyer J, Hübner K, Bernemann C, Ortmeier C, Zenke M, Fleischmann BK, Zaehres H, Schöler HR. Oct4-induced pluripotency in adult neural stem cells. *Cell* 2009, 136:411-419.

[256] Dick JE. Stem cells: Self-renewal writ in blood. *Nature* 2003, 423:231-233.

[257] Lessard J, Sauvageau G. Bmi-1 determines the proliferative capacity of normal and leukaemic stem cells. *Nature* 2003, 423:255-260.

[258] Raaphorst FM. Self-renewal of hematopoietic and leukemic stem cells: A central role for the polycomb-group gene bmi-1. *Trends Immunol.* 2003, 24:522-524.

[259] Passegue E, Jamieson CH, Ailles LE, Weissman IL. Normal and leukemic hematopoiesis: Are leukemias a stem cell disorder or a reacquisition of stem cell characteristics? *Proc. Natl. Acad. Sci. USA* 2003, 100 Suppl 1:11842-11849.

[260] Chiarle R, Simmons WJ, Cai H, Dhall G, Zamo A, Raz R, Karras JG, Levy DE, Inghirami G. Stat3 is required for alk-mediated lymphomagenesis and provides a possible therapeutic target. *Nat. Med.* 2005, 11:623-629.

[261] Yu H, Jove R. The stats of cancer--new molecular targets come of age. *Nat. Rev. Cancer* 2004, 4:97-105.

[262] Dingli D, Michor F, Antal T, Pacheco JM. The emergence of tumor metastases. *Cancer Biol. Ther.* 2007, 6:383-390.

[263] Li L, Neaves WB. Normal stem cells and cancer stem cells: The niche matters. *Cancer Res.* 2006, 66:4553-4557.

[264] Arai F, Hirao A, Suda T. Regulation of hematopoiesis and its interaction with stem cell niches. *Int. J. Hematol.* 2005, 82:371-376.

[265] Jones DL, Wagers AJ. No place like home: Anatomy and function of the stem cell niche. *Nat. Rev. Mol. Cell Biol.* 2008, 9:11-21.

[266] Baylin SB, Herman JG, Graff JR, Vertino PM, Issa JP. Alterations in DNA methylation: A fundamental aspect of neoplasia. *Adv. Cancer Res.* 1998, 72:141-196.

[267] Lichtenstein A. Carcinogenesis: Evolution of concepts. *Biochemistry (Moscow)* 2009, 74:353-361.

[268] Nowell PC. The clonal evolution of tumor cell populations. *Science* 1976, 194:23-28.

[269] Salk JJ, Salipante SJ, Risques RA, Crispin DA, Li L, Bronner MP, Brentnall TA, Rabinovitch PS, Horwitz MS, Loeb LA. Clonal expansions in ulcerative colitis identify patients with neoplasia. *Proceedings of the National Academy of Sciences* 2009, 106:20871-20876.

[270] Armengol G, Capella G, Farre L, Peinado MA, Miro R, Caballin MR. Genetic evolution in the metastatic progression of human pancreatic cancer studied by cgh. *Lab. Invest.* 2001, 81:1703-1707.

[271] Maekita T, Nakazawa K, Mihara M, Nakajima T, Yanaoka K, Iguchi M, Arii K, Kaneda A, Tsukamoto T, Tatematsu M, Tamura G, Saito D, Sugimura T, Ichinose M, Ushijima T. High levels of aberrant DNA methylation in helicobacter pylori-infected gastric mucosae and its possible association with gastric cancer risk. *Clin. Cancer Res.* 2006, 12:989-995.

[272] Lewis CM, Cler LR, Bu DW, Zochbauer-Muller S, Milchgrub S, Naftalis EZ, Leitch AM, Minna JD, Euhus DM. Promoter hypermethylation in benign breast epithelium in relation to predicted breast cancer risk. *Clin. Cancer Res.* 2005, 11:166-172.

Part II - Epedemiological Aspects of Field Cancerization

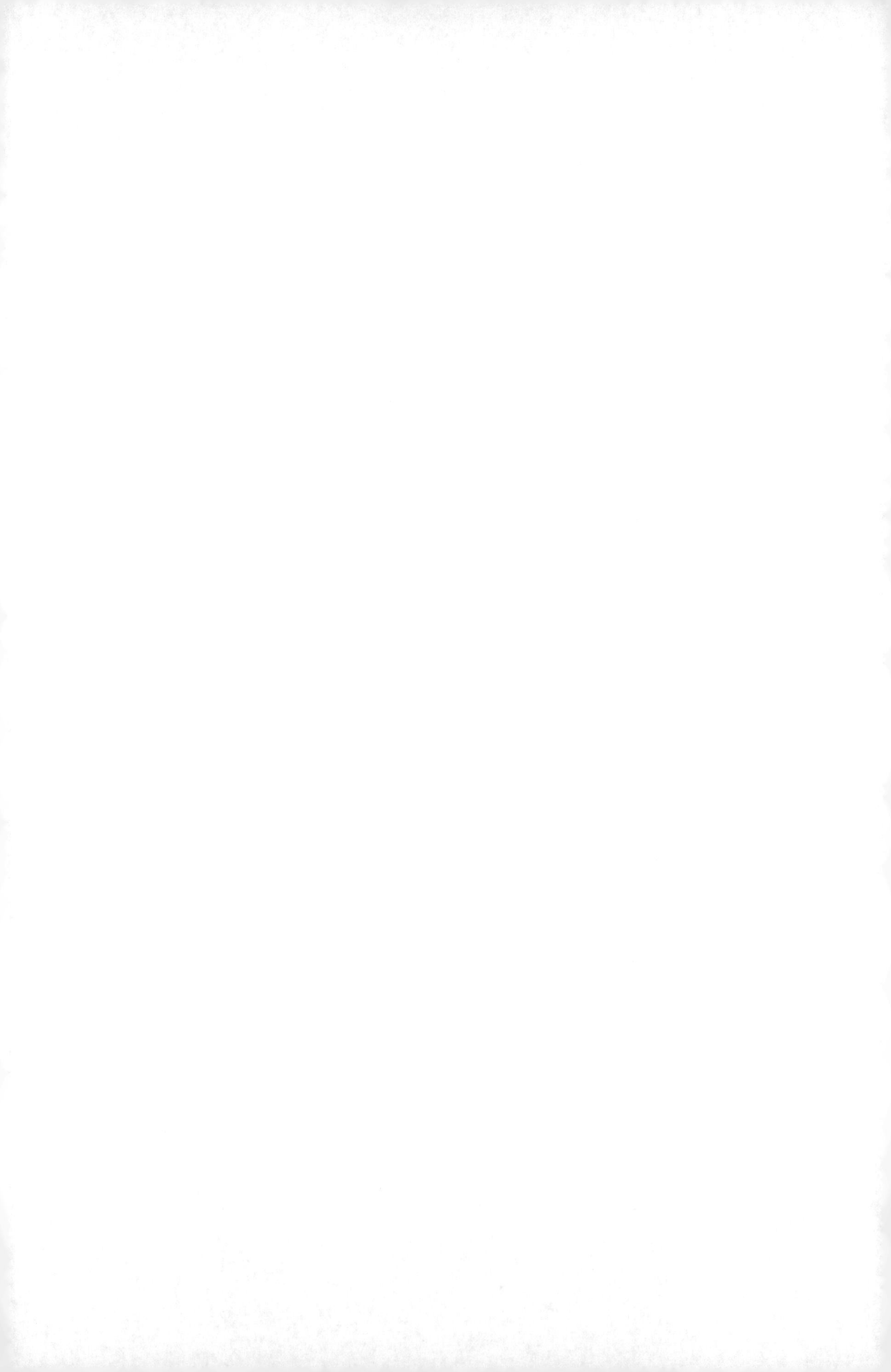

In: Field Cancerization: Basic Science and Clinical Applications ISBN 978-1-61761-006-6
Editor: Gabriel D. Dakubo

Chapter 4

Epidemiology of Synchronous and Metachronous Type Multiple Primary Neoplasms

Sevil Kılçıksız and Beste M. Atasoy

Abstract

Multiple primary neoplasms (MPNs) comprise synchronous or metachronous tumors. They arise after diagnosis of the first primary tumor, and are commonly reported with an incidence of 0.7% to 11.7% of all cancer patients. By appropriate statistical methods, these tumors are shown to occur more frequently than expected, and therefore, may provide a model for generating and testing hypotheses on mechanisms of carcinogenesis. Some studies suggest that men are more frequent than women to develop both synchronous and metachronous tumors. Despite the controversial reports about the age of onset for MPNs, the consensus is that the mean age of developing MPNs at first diagnosis is high, such that many patients with MPNs are over 50 years. However, the risk of developing multiple cancers after the first primary for cancers like those of the thyroid increases for patients younger than 40 years of age. The mean age at diagnosis for synchronous and metachronous tumors do not differ significantly. Generally, the same organ or systems are involved. For instant MPN of the respiratory, gastrointestinal, and genitourinary systems are common. Most of the studies look for the association between MPNs and a specific system or organ such as the gastrointestinal, breast, head and neck, thyroid or brain. On the other hand, there are different definitions for MPNs and also the discrepancy in classifications and coding for reporting make comparisons difficult. Hence, in order to interpret the discordance and decrease the bias on this issue, it is highly recommended for researchers to use the international rules in their national registries.

4.1. Introduction

Multiple primary neoplasms (MPNs) are tumors that either occur concomitantly with the primary tumor (synchronous) or later, after diagnosis of the first primary tumor (metachronous). They represent ~0.7% to 11.7% of all cancer cases in the literature [1-5]. Improved survival rates and long-term remissions of cancer patients, mostly due to early diagnosis and modern radiotherapy/chemotherapy, allow more patients with neoplastic disease to survive long enough to develop metachronous tumors and also contribute to detection of synchronous occult tumors which were formerly undetected [2,6-8].

4.2. Incidence of Multiple Primary Neoplasms

The pattern of cancer incidence is very different between countries and therefore, each study is very valuable in enlightening us on both the incidence and etiology of MPNs. However, there are currently different definitions for MPNs, and the divergence in classifications and topographic coding used for reporting of these tumors make comparisons difficult [3,6,9]. The formation of tumor registries based on the rules of the International Association of Cancer Registries (IACR) and International Agency for Research on Cancer (IARC), has greatly aided in the diagnosis and analysis of multiple primary cancer patients [10-16]. For this reason, establishment of national registry systems respecting these international cancer registry rules in different countries may reduce the discordance and decrease the bias on this issue. Therefore, it is recommended for investigators to use these rules in their national registries. The rules for the diagnosis of MPNs according to ICD-O-3 were as follows:

1. the recognition of the existence of $\geq$ 2 primary cancers does not depend on time,
2. a primary cancer is one that originates in a primary site or tissue, and is not an extension, a recurrence, or metastasis,
3. only one tumor shall be recognized as arising in an organ or a pair of organs or a tissue. Multifocal tumors-that is, discrete masses apparently not in the continuity with other primary cancers originating in the same primary site or tissue, for example bladder-are counted as a single cancer,
4. the previous rule does not apply in 2 circumstances: systemic (or multicentric) cancers potentially involving many different organs are only counted once in any individual (e.g., Kaposi's sarcoma and tumors of the hematopoietic system); and neoplasm of different morphology should be regarded as multiple cancers even if they are diagnosed simultaneously in the same site [11,17].

Commonly, the metachronous tumors are defined as those that are diagnosed after an interval of > 6 months. Park et al found 39 (0.7%) metachronous colorectal cancer in their series of 5,447 patients [18]. The mean time interval between sequential metachronous cancers was 39 months ranging from 6 to 215 months. In this series, however, 13 (33.3%) patients were diagnosed with metachronous cancer after 5 years. In another study, the mean time interval between index and metachronous cancer was 44.4 ± 30.8 months [19]. In a study related to multiple primary neoplasm in patients with gastric cancer, the authors reported that 87% of patients were diagnosed with a second neoplasm within the first two years and considerating metachronous cases, the average interval was 20± 14 months [20].

Multiple primary neoplasms may give signs of the complex etiology of human cancer, and might offer a model for generating and testing hypotheses on mechanisms of carcinogenesis [1-5]. For example, "field cancerization", which is the term used to describe the multicentric pathogenic process in which carcinogenesis occurs in different organs subjected to the same carcinogens, has a higher probability of being associated with the development of synchronous tumors than metachronous tumors [3,6,7,15,21]. In a Japanese study, 36.5% of MPNs were reported to be in the same organ [22]. The studies from Turkey addressed a propensity of synchronous tumors occurrence in the same organ system (40% of synchronous vs. 21% of metachronous [6] and 75.8% of synchronous vs. 24.2% of metachronous [19], respectively). Long-term exposure to carcinogens as seen in excess tobacco and alcohol use may also be an ideal biologic model to demonstrate the effects of lifestyle-hypothesis of field cancerization on carcinogenesis beyond genetics. Patients with head and neck cancer (HNC) have a risk of developing multifocal primary epithelial tumors in the upper respiratory or digestive tracts (URDT) [7, 23-26]. In a retrospective study from Germany, a total of 649 patients with HNC were evaluated and 77 patients (11.8%) developed a second cancer either synchronous (18.2%) or metachronous (76.6%), whereas the incidence of second cancer inside the head and neck region was 7.5% [23]. The risk of developing lung cancer in addition to HNC is approximately 7% within 15 years after the diagnosis of the primary cancer [24]. In another study, investigation by bronchoscopy in patients with primary oral squamous cell carcinoma (SCC) revealed synchronous pulmonary carcinomas in 2% of all cases [25]. Some investigators identified lip-oral cavity and pharynx-esophagus combinations, which were formerly reported as significant associations, attributed to tobacco and alcohol consumption [7,26]. Moreover, gene mutations, genetic susceptibility and also genetic instability may influence the development of MPNs [27-30].

4.3. Family History, Gender and Age as Risk Factors for Development of Multiple Primary Neoplasms

Family history: The other related issue in the development of MPNs is the role of family history. The risk of a second primary cancer is expressed as the standardized incidence ratio (SIR). By using SIR calculated from site-, sex- and age-specific rates for all offspring, Dong et al found that the family history was one of the major risk factors for occurrence of MPNs in the colon (SIR = 59.1), skin (SIR = 48.2) and female breast (SIR = 7.9) in the Swedish Family-Cancer Database [3]. In this study, the corresponding SIRs in patients without family history were reported as 13.8, 10.5 and 5.2 at the three sites respectively. The authors also suggested that the high risk of second cancer in their series would be consistent with a polygenic model of carcinogenesis [3,28].

Gender: According to gender, some studies suggest that more men than women are observed in both synchronous and metachronous groups [5,7].

In an Italian study, which was comprised of eleven Italian population-based cancer registries, 240,111 patients were followed for 544,438 person-years during which 8,766-second primary cancers were found. Restricting the analysis to metachronous cancers, there were 6,974 second primary cancers diagnosed among 198,303 patients [5]. In this study there was no difference in gender representation.

On the contrary, in another study it was reported that 56.7% of cancer patients with two primaries were men, and men comprised about two thirds of the cases in the synchronous and metachronous groups [7]. The authors argued that the difference might be due to the higher consumption of tobacco and alcohol in males, or the screening effect of occult prostatic cancers.

Age: Age of onset is another consideration for MPNs, and the reports are controversial. Most of the earlier studies of MPNs did not include patients with MPNs who were older than those with a single primary malignant neoplasm. Later review indicated the potential of older cancer patients being at a high risk of developing second primaries [9]. In most reports, the mean ages of MPNs at first diagnosis are higher in the West than those in the East. In general, more than 75% of patients with MPNs are over 50 years [6-9,31]. In their descriptive cohort Crocetti et al reported that for metachronous cancers, the SIR pattern significantly differed between the age groups with consistent excess risks in subjects younger than 65 years in comparison with older people [5].

Similarly, in the Swedish Family-Cancer Database, the incidence of second primary was higher when the age at diagnosis of the first primary was less than 40 years [3]. On the other hand, in another study, more than 80% of all MPNs were equal to or older than 50 years, and synchronous and metachronous groups did not show a significant difference in mean ages [19].

The impact of age on the development of cancer in different organs such as breast, thyroid, head and neck, and, colorectal are reported [18, 32-35]. In a breast cancer study comprised of 45,229 surgically treated non-metastatic breast cancer patients, there was an increased in synchronous and metachronous contralateral breast cancer incidence in young patients [32]. In this study, the SIR of metachronous contralateral breast cancer was 11.4 (95% CI 8.6-14.8) in patients younger than 35 years, and this number decreased to 1.5 (95% CI 1.4-1.7) in women equal or older than 60 years. In another study, synchronous breast cancers were found more common in older patients, whereas metachronous breast cancer was much more common in younger subjects [33].

Ronckers et al studied both the risk of thyroid cancer after an earlier primary cancer, and the risk of developing multiple primaries after an earlier thyroid cancer in a Surveillance Epidemiology and End Results (SEER) cancer registries program (1973-2000) [34]. The patients less than 40 years of age at diagnosis of thyroid cancer had a 39% increased risk of a second cancer, whereas for older patients the risk was elevated 6%. Friedrich et al reported that oral and maxillofacial (OMF) cancer patients who developed second cancers were younger than the patients who had OMF, solely [35]. Park et al reported that the average age of metachronous colorectal cancer patients was 53 years, which is a much younger age than 58 years that was the average age of sporadic colorectal cancer patients [18].

4.4. Tissues Distribution of Multiple Primary Neoplasms

Expanded topographic evaluation shows that most of the malignancies with MPNs involve the genitourinary, respiratory and gastrointestinal systems [2,9,20,36]. It was reported in the study from Connecticut Tumor Registry that the most frequent simultaneous tumors were cancers of the colon, rectum, prostate, lung, breast, and bladder [37]. In the case series of multiple primary cancers of the Tuscany Tumor Registry (1985-1991), bladder, prostate, and renal cell carcinoma were significantly higher in synchronous tumors [5]. Flannery et al reported that genitourinary system rose to the first place when the main topographic groups were condensed [37]. Yet, carcinoma of the prostate is a frequent incidental finding at autopsy of elderly men, hence, it is argued whether or not men with prostate cancer and MPNs are 'true cases' [9]. Furthermore, slow-growing silent tumors are more frequent in patients with prostate, bladder, or renal cell cancers, which are most frequently diagnosed during ascertainment of another cancer [4,5,7,26]. Skin is also reported as the most frequent location, and the higher occurrence of skin tumors was related to climatic factors and exposure to ultraviolet radiation [19]. The most frequent site-association with respect to different topographic groups was reported for genitourinary systems, and the rate was higher in the synchronous than in the metachronous groups [19]. All these findings might be due to field cancerization in the epithelium, the alternative theory of a common clonal origin where the second tumor is clonally related to an index tumor, or to screening effect [1,20,38-40].

Most of the studies have examined the association of MPNs and a specific system/region or organ such as the gastrointestinal system, breast, head and neck, thyroid and brain [36, 41-47, 55-58]. In a study from Taiwan, the authors analyzed 2,109 gastric cancer patients treated between 1987 and 2002 and they found 99 MPNs (4.7%) [41]. These investigators found that about 78% of second cancers was discovered within the first 5 years, whereas 34% of the synchronous tumors were discovered within 1 year after the onset of gastric cancer. In this study, in males, prostate cancer was the most common (19.5%) followed by cancers of the colon (18.2%) and liver (14.3%), while in females, colon cancer was the most common (31.9%) followed by breast and cervix cancers (22.7%). Cheng et al also analyzed the characteristics of MPNs of the gastrointestinal system in their study [42]. Among 129 patients, there were 43 synchronous and 86 metachronous cancers, and 120 (93.02%) had two primary cancers and 9 (6.98%) had three primary cancers. The major sites of MPNs of gastrointestinal system were large intestine, stomach, and liver. Reproductive tract cancers, especially cervical, ovarian, bladder, and prostate cancers were the most commonly associated non-gastrointestinal cancers, followed by cancer of the lung and breasts. Eom et al reviewed 4,593 gastric cancer patients diagnosed between 1999 and 2005 [36]. The synchronous or metachronous cancer incidence was 3.4%, and the most common other primary cancer was colorectal cancer (20.1%), followed by lung cancer and liver cancer. An Italian analysis was based on a total of 4286 gastrointestinal cancer patients comprised of 1742 patients with colorectal carcinoma, 1418 patients with gastric cancer, 91 patients with malignant tumor of the small bowel, 867 patients with pancreatic cancer and 68 with hepatocellular carcinoma [43]. Eleven cases of synchronous tumors and 170 metachronous tumors were found in 151 patients, and seven patients had multiple second primary tumors. Female genital tract tumors (37 cases), hematopoietic system tumors (34 cases), breast tumors

(29 cases), and cutaneous tumors (20 cases) were the most frequently observed. The authors reported an elevated incidence of second tumors in patients with small bowel neoplasms (19.8%) than in patients with other tumors of the gastrointestinal tract.

A number of investigators have examined the incidence of MPNs following primary breast cancer diagnosis [33, 44-46]. The increase in breast cancer incidence rates, improvements in prognosis and the estimated survival expectancy may have changed the potential risk for the development of second cancers in this population. Breast cancer patients have an increased risk for second cancers of the contralateral breast, endometrium, ovary, esophagus, stomach, colon, lung, skin, bone, connective tissue, thyroid gland and hematopoietic system (leukemia) [33, 44-46]. The incidence of synchronous breast cancer has been reported to be up to 2% in most series [33,45,46]. The relative risk of developing a metachronous breast cancer is estimated to be in the range of 1.4 to 4.5 times the risk in the normal population [45]. The 10-year incidence for development of a metachronous contralateral breast cancer is as high as 6.4-9%, with yearly hazard function (annual incidence rates for each event) of 0.75% per year of follow-up [46]. According data from Sweden, the incidence of synchronous and metachronous breast cancer in a 30-year period of follow up was approximately 29% and 69%, respectively [33]. The correlation between long-term Tamoxifen usage for breast cancer treatment and the development of endometrial carcinoma has been attributed to its estrogen agonist properties [47]. There is also 1.3 - 2 fold increase in the risk of endometrial carcinoma in Tamoxifen users in Western countries [48,49]. In a Japanese series, the risk of uterine cancer among breast cancer patients diagnosed at ages 50 - 74 was 3.4 times higher than the general population [50]. The British Tamoxifen Second Cancer Study Group reported that there is an increase in the relative risk for developing various types of uterine carcinomas and sarcomas, and this risk correlates with the duration of Tamoxifen treatment [51]. The relative risk of endometrial carcinoma according to total dose of Tamoxifen exposure was 1.00 in patients with breast cancer who underwent an annual pelvic examination and cytologic and/or histologic screening of the cervix and endometrium.

An increased risk of developing ovarian cancer is described in breast cancer patients that may be due to shared reproductive risk factors, inherited susceptibility (*BRCA* mutations) or iatrogenic effects [19,44,50,53]. In a study of hospital-based cancer registry, the most frequent association in the metachronous group was detected between breast and ovary [19]. This finding was supported with the hypothesis that the same types of carcinogens like hormones and oncogenes may have the responsibility for the development of neoplasms in topographic associations, such as breast/breast and endometrium/ovary [44,50,53].

Patients who develop a primary cancer of the upper respiratory or digestive tracts (URDT) frequently develop a synchronous or metachronous bronchial carcinoma [54,55]. In a single center prospective study, 60 patients (55 men) in remission following treatment of non-metastatic HNC (the buccal cavity, pharynx and larynx) were examined. In this study, a high prevalence (6.7%) of bronchial carcinoma in index URDT patients was detected [54]. Van der Haring et al reviewed the incidence of second primary tumors after treatment of a first primary in 917 HNC (oral or oropharyngeal squamous cell carcinomas) [55]. They reported 149 (16%) metachronous tumor development in a 2.6 years median follow-up time. Most of these secondary tumors were diagnosed in the URDT (44%) and lung (23%). They found the 5-year and 10-year cumulative incidences were 13% (S.E. 1.2) and 21% (S.E. 1.7), respectively.

Omur et al reviewed in their series of 1680 differentiated thyroid carcinoma patients followed over twenty years [56]. A total of 45second primary tumors, 15 synchronous tumors and 30 metachronous tumors, were found. The most common second primary was URDT tumors in synchronous group, whereas a variety of tumors were noted in the metachronous group.

Inskip et al investigated multiple primary neoplasms involving cancer of the brain and central nervous system (CNS) using data from SEER registries program (1973-1998) [57]. They reported that among patients who were diagnosed first with cancer of the brain or CNS, statistically significant excesses were observed for cancers of bone (SIR = 14.4), soft tissue (SIR = 4.6), brain and CNS (SIR = 5.9), salivary gland (SIR = 5.1), and thyroid gland (SIR = 2.7) in addition to acute myelocytic leukemia (SIR = 4.1) and melanoma of the skin (SIR = 1.7). In childhood CNS tumours, the excess risk of new malignancies was markedly greater than in adulthood patients with similar diagnosis. In reverse associations, significant excesses of cancer of the brain and CNS were observed only after diagnoses of acute lymphocytic leukemia (SIR = 7.4) and cancer of the testis (SIR = 1.8) or the thyroid gland (SIR = 1.7). They concluded that cancer treatment appears to have been the major factor underlying most of the positive associations between brain cancer and primary cancers of other types, with a probable lesser contribution from shared genetic susceptibility.

Conclusion

This chapter provides some insights into the incidence of synchronous and metachronous tumors. A sophisticated analysis of MPNs requires a large, well-defined population under observation for at least 10 years. Therefore, the formation in population based tumor registries, efficient surveillance and, increasing the number of studies from different geographical regions may greatly aid in identifying multiple primary cancer patients and elucidating important tumoral associations.

References

[1] Tachimori, Y. Cancer screening in patients with cancer. *Jpn J. Clin. Oncol.* 2002; 32:118-9.

[2] Artac, M; Bozcuk, H; Ozdogan, M, et al. Different clinical features of primary and secondary tumors in patients with multiple malignancies. *Tumori* 2005; 91:317-20.

[3] Dong, C; Hemminki, K. Second primary neoplasms in 633,964 cancer patients in Sweden, 1958-1996. *Int. J. Cancer* 2001; 93:155-61.

[4] Van Westreenen, HL; Westerterp, M; Jager, PL, et al. Synchronous primary neoplasms detected on 18F-FDG PET in staging of patients with esophageal cancer. *J. Nucl. Med.* 2005; 46:1321-5.

[5] Crocetti, E; Arniani, S; Buiatti, E. Synchronous and metachronous diagnosis of multiple primary cancers. *Tumori* 1998; 84:9-13.

[6] Aydiner, A; Karadeniz, A; Uygun, K, et al. Multiple primary neoplasm at a single institution: Differences between synchronous and metachronous neoplasms. *Am. J. Clin. Oncol.* 2000; 23:364-70.
[7] Kaneko, S; Yamaguchi, N. Epidemiological analysis of site relationships of synchronous and metachronous multiple primary cancers in the National Cancer Center, Japan, 1962-1996. *Jpn J. Clin. Oncol.* 1996; 29:96-105.
[8] Engin K. Cancers in multiple primary sites. *Int. Surg.* 1994; 79:33-7.
[9] Demandante, CG; Troyer, DA; Miles, TP. Multiple primary malignant neoplasm: case report and a comprehensive review of the literature. *Am. J. Clin. Oncol.* 2003; 26:79-83.
[10] Schoenberg, BS; Myers, MH. Statistical methods for studying multiple primary malignant neoplasms. *Cancer* 1977; 40:1892-8.
[11] International Rules for Multiple Primary Cancers (ICD-O Third Edition), Internal Report No. 2004/ 02. Lyon (France), IARC, 2004.
[12] Giles, GG; Thursfield, V. Cancer Statistics: Everything you wanted to know about the cancer registry data but were too afraid to ask. *ANZ J. Surg.* 2004; 74:931-4.
[13] Merrill, RM; Capocaccia, R; Feuer, EJ, et al. Cancer prevalence estimates based on tumour registry data in the Surveillance, Epidemiology and End results (SEER) Program. *Int. J. Epidemiol.* 2000; 29:197-207.
[14] Fidaner, C; Eser, SY; Parkin, DM. Incidence in Izmir in 1993-1994: first results from Izmir Cancer Registry. *Eur. J. Cancer* 2001; 37:83-92.
[15] Buiatti, E; Crocetti, E; Gafa, L, et al. Agreement estimate among three Italian cancer registries in the coding of multiple primary cancers. *Tumori* 1996; 82:533-8.
[16] Crocetti, E; Lecker, S; Buiatti. E, et al. Problems related to the coding of multiple primary cancers. *Eur. J. Cancer* 1996; 32A:1366-70.
[17] Fritz, A; Percy, C; Jack, A, et al, editors. International Classification of Diseases for Oncology (ICD-O-3). Geneva (Switzerland); WHO; 2000.
[18] Park, IJ; Yu, CS; Kim, HC, et al. Metachronous colorectal cancer. *Colorectal Dis.* 2006; 8:323-7.
[19] Kilciksiz, S; Gokce, T; Baloglu, A, et al. Characteristics of synchronous- and metachronous-type multiple primary neoplasms: A study of hospital-based cancer registry in Turkey. *Clin. Genitourinary Cancer* 2007; 5:438-45.
[20] Muela Molinero, A; Jorquera Plaza, F; Ribas Arino, T, et al. Multiple malignant primary neoplasms in patients with gastric neoplasms in the health district of Leon. *Rev. Esp. Enferm. Dig.* 2006; 98:907-16.
[21] Carey, TE. Field cancerization: are multiple primary cancers monoclonal or polyclonal? *Ann. Med.* 1996; 28:183-8.
[22] Ueno, M; Muto, T; Oya, M, et al. Multiple primary cancer: an experience at the Cancer Instute Hospital with special reference to colorectal cancer. *Int. J. Clin. Oncol.* 2003; 8:162- 7.
[23] Friedrich RE. Primary and second primary cancer in 649 patients with malignancies of the maxillofacial region. *Anticancer Res.* 2007; 27:1805-18.
[24] Deleyiannis , FW; Thomas, DB. Risk of lung cancer among patients with head and neck cancer. *Otolaryngol. Head Neck Surg.* 1997; 116:630-6.
[25] Kesting, MR; Robitzky, L; Al-Benna, S, et al. Bronchoscopy screening in primary oral squamous cell carcinoma: a 10-year experience. *Br. J. Oral. Maxillofacial Surg.* 2009; 47:279-83.

[26] Kagei, K; Hosokawa, M; Shirato, H, et al. Efficacy of Intense Screening and treatment for synchronous second primary cancers in patients with esophageal cancer. *Jpn J. Clin. Oncol.* 2002; 32:120-7.
[27] Koutsopoulos, AV; Dambaki, KI; Datseris, G, et al. A novel combination of multiple primary carcinomas: urinary bladder transitional cell carcinoma, prostate adenocarcinoma and small cell lung carcinoma – report of a case and review of the literature. *World J. Surg. Oncol.* 2005; 3:51.
[28] Dong, C; Hemminki, K. Multiple primary cancers of the colon, breast and skin (melanoma) as models for polygenic cancers. *Jpn J. Clin. Oncol.* 2001; 31:349-51.
[29] Hemminki, K; Boffett, P. Multiple primary cancers as clues to environmental and heritable causes of cancer and mechanisms of carcinogenesis. *IARC Sci. Publ.* 2004; 157:289-97.
[30] Miki, Y; Swensen, J; Schattuck-Eidens, D, et al. A strong candidate for the breast and ovarian cancer susceptibility gene BRCA 1. *Science* 1994; 266:66-71.
[31] Crocetti, E; Buiatti, E; Falini, P. Multiple Primary Cancers in Italy. Italian Multiple Primary Cancer Working Group. *Eur. J. Cancer* 2001; 37:2449-56.
[32] Schaapveld, M; Visser, O; Louwman, WJ, et al. The impact of adjuvant therapy on contralateral breast cancer risk and the prognostic significance of contralateral breast cancer: a population based study in the Netherlands. *Breast Cancer Res. Treat.* 2008; 110:189-97.
[33] Hartman, M; Czene, K; Reilly, M, et al. Incidence and prognosis of synchronous and metachronous bilateral breast cancer. *J. Clin. Oncol.* 2007; 25:4210-6.
[34] Ronckers, CM; McCarron, P; Ron, E. Thyroid cancer and multiple primary tumors in the SEER cancer registries. *Int. J. Cancer* 2005; 117:281-8.
[35] Friedrich RE. Primary and second primary cancer in 649 patients with malignancies of the maxillofacial region. *Anticancer Res.* 2007; 27:1805-18.
[36] Eom, BW; Lee, HJ; Yoo, MW, et al. Synchronous and metachronous cancers in patients with gastric cancer. *J. Surg. Oncol.* 2008; 98:106-10.
[37] Flannery, JT; Boice, JD Jr; Devesa, SS, et al. Cancer registration in Connecticut and the study of multiple primary cancers, 1935-82. *Natl. Cancer Inst. Monogr.* 1985; 68:13-24.
[38] Wang, X; Wang, M; MacLennan, GT, et al. Evidence for common clonal origin of multifocal lung cancers. *J. Natl. Cancer Inst.* 2009; 101:560-70.
[39] Palou, J; Rodriguez-Rubio, F; Huguet, J, et al. Multivariate analysis of clinical paramets of synchronous primary superficial bladder cancer and upper urinary tract tumor. *J. Urol.* 2005; 174:859-61.
[40] Bedi, GC; Westra, WH; Gabrielson, E, et al. Multiple head and neck tumors: evidence for a common clonal origin. *Cancer Res.* 1996; 56:2484-7.
[41] Wu, CW; Lo, SS; Chen, JH, et al. Multiple primary cancers in patients with gastric cancer. Hepatogastroenterology 2006; 53:463-7.
[42] Cheng, HY; Chu, CH; Chang, WH, et al. Clinical analysis of multiple primary malignancies in the digestive system: a hospital-based study. *World J. Gastroenterol.* 2005; 11:4215-9.
[43] Minni, F; Casadei, R; Marrano, N, et al. Second tumours in patients with malignant neoplasms of the digestive apparatus. A retrospective study on 2406 cases. *Ann. Ital. Chir.* 2005; 76:467-72. [Article in Italian]

[44] Evans, HS; Lewis, CM; Robinson, D, et al. Incidence of multiple primary cancers in a cohort of women diagnosed with breast cancer in Southeast England. *Br. J. Cancer* 2001; 84:35-40.

[45] Polednak, AP. Bilateral synchronous breast cancer: A population-base study of characteristics, method of detection and survival. *Surgery* 2003; 133:383-389.

[46] Broet, P; de la Rochefordiere, A; Scholl, SM, et al. Contralateral breast cancer: annual incidence and risk parameters. *J. Clin. Oncol.* 1995; 13:1578-83.

[47] Volk, N; Pompe-Kirn, V. Second primary cancers in breast cancer patients in Slovenia. *Cancer Causes Control* 1997; 8:764-770.

[48] Neven, P; Vergote, I. Controversies regarding tamoxifen and uterine carcinoma. *Curr. Opin. Obstet. Gynecol.* 1998; 10:9-14.

[49] Benson, JR; Pitsinis, V. Update on clinical role of tamoxifen. *Curr. Opin. Obstet. Gynecol.* 2003; 15:13-23.

[50] Tanaka, H; Tsukuma, H; Koyama, H, et al. Second primary cancers following breast cancer in the Japanese female population. *Jpn J. Cancer Res.* 2001; 92:1-8.

[51] Swerdlow, AJ; Jones, MA. Tamoxifen treatment for breast cancer and risk of endometrial cancer: A case-control study. *J. Natl. Cancer Inst.* 2005; 97:375-84.

[52] Katase, K; Sugiyama, Y; Hasumi, K, et al. The incidence of subsequent endometrial carcinoma with tamoxifen use in patients with primary breast carcinoma. *Cancer* 1998; 82:1698-703.

[53] Miki, Y; Swensen. J; Schattuck-Eidens. D, et al. A strong candidate for the breast and ovarian cancer susceptibility gene BRCA-1. *Science* 1994; 266:66-71.

[54] Bertrand, D; Righini, C; Ferretti, G, et al. Early diagnosis of bronchial carcinoma after head and neck cancer. *Rev. Mal. Respir.* 2008; 25:559-68. [Article in French]

[55] Van der Haring, IS; Schaapveld, MS; Roodenburg, JL, et al. Second primary tumours after a squamous cell carcinoma of the oral cavity or oropharynx using the cumulative incidence method. *Int. J. Oral. Maxillofac. Surg.* 2009; 38:332-8.

[56] Omur, O; Ozcan, Z; Yazici, B, et al. Multiple primary tumors in differentiated thyroid carcinoma and relationship to thyroid cancer outcome. *Endocr. J.* 2008; 55:365-72.

[57] Inskip, PD. Multiple primary tumors involving cancer of the brain and central nervous system as the first or subsequent cancer. *Cancer* 2003; 98:562-7.

In: Field Cancerization: Basic Science and Clinical Applications ISBN 978-1-61761-006-6
Editor: Gabriel D. Dakubo

Chapter 5

Field Cancerization in Derivatives of the Embryonic Foregut: An Observation Based on Epidemiological Patterns

Donald E. Henson, Jorge Albores-Saavedra, Arnold M. Schwartz and Kristen Batich

5.1. Introduction

Carcinogenic fields have been described for a number of anatomic sites [1-4] These fields are characterized by: 1) a common anatomic or regional continuity, 2) a common embryologic origin, and 3) common exposure to putative carcinogens. A well-known example is the occurrence of synchronous and metachronous carcinomas in the lung and head and neck; anatomic sites that are continuous, share a common embryology from the anterior foregut, and are exposed to a common carcinogen, namely cigarette smoke.

Previous work, based largely on epidemiological patterns, has indicated that the extrahepatic biliary system including the gallbladder and pancreas shares in a field of carcinogenesis [5].

The extrahepatic biliary system, liver, and pancreas are anatomically continuous and share a common embryological origin from the mid foregut. Nothing is known, however, about carcinogenic agents, although gallbladder cancer has often been associated with the presence of gallstones [6].

In this chapter we consider the field changes in the extrahepatic biliary system and describe novel ways based on epidemiology to test for a field. These epidemiological methods can be used for less common cancers and may further substantiate clinical observations on common cancers.

In this chapter we initially consider: 1) the embryology and anatomy of the extrahepatic biliary system 2) clinicopathological observations that suggest a field phenomenon, and 3) the carcinogenic field based on descriptive epidemiology.

5.2. Data Source

Data were obtained from the Surveillance, Epidemiology, and End Results (SEER) Program at the National Cancer Institute for the years 1973 through 2006 [7]. Initiated in 1973, SEER has collected demographic, anatomic, histologic, extent of disease, mortality, and limited treatment information on cancer patients in the US. Currently, SEER collects information on 26% of the population that includes four states and large regional metropolitan areas.

5.3. Histopathologic Codes

In SEER, the histopathlogic types of neoplasia are coded from the pathology reports according to the *International Classification of Disease for Oncology* (ICD-O) published by the World Health Organization (1992). Data are not available for benign tumors. Specific codes are also available for anatomic sites.

5.4. Data Analysis

Incidence trends and age specific incidence rates (2000 US standard population) were calculated using SEER*Stat (6.1.4) and expressed as number of cases per 100,000 persons per year [7]. Data were obtained from SEER Registries 9 and 13, which contains data from 1973-2006. Registry 9 contains 81,936 cases of pancreatic cancer, 10,001 of gallbladder cancer, 6,286 cancers of the extrahepatic biliary system, and 3,507 cases of the ampulla of Vater. Registry 13, which contains data from 1992 to 2006, was used to calculate age specific incidence rates.

All racial/ethnic groups were included. Only invasive cancers that had histological confirmation were selected. Cases identified through death certificates were excluded. Age-specific incidence rates, calculated for 5-year intervals, were plotted on linear as well as on logarithmic scales. Age frequency density plots were constructed on linear scales as previously described [5].

5.5. Embryological Development

The anatomic derivatives of the foregut (i.e., liver, gallbladder, extrahepatic bile ducts, ampulla of Vater, and pancreas) have a common and complex embryonic ancestry [8]. Along with the liver, the gallbladder and bile duct progenitors develop from primitive endodermal cells located in the mid-embryonic foregut.

By the fourth week of fetal life a ventral-medial outgrowth buds from the endoderm, near the junction of the foregut and yolk sac, opposite the dorsal pancreatic bud. Pushing into the splanchnic mesenchyme, this outgrowth will eventually become the hepatic diverticulum.

The cranial part differentiates into the liver and intrahepatic bile ducts, while the caudal part branches to form the gallbladder and cystic duct. A small bud, the ventral pancreas, which eventually becomes part of the head of the pancreas, arises from the hepatic diverticulum near its origin from the foregut. The original hepatic diverticulum then elongates to form the common bile duct.

As the stomach rotates, causing torsion on the duodenum, the hepatic diverticulum comes to lie dorsal to the duodenum and the small ventral pancreas comes around to fuse with the larger dorsal pancreas, which is now ventral because of torsion, to form the head and uncinate process.

The dorsal bud forms the remainder of the pancreas. As a result of fusion, the ventral pancreatic duct becomes the proximal segment of the main pancreatic duct (duct of Wirsung), which, because of its origin from the hepatic diverticulum, usually opens into the duodenum through the terminal part of the common bile duct creating in many cases the ampulla of Vater. By the eighth week of fetal development, a lumen has been established throughout most of the biliary tract.

5.6. Anatomy of the Extrahepatic Biliary System

The extrahepatic biliary system consists of the left and right hepatic ducts, common hepatic duct, gallbladder, cystic duct, and common bile duct. The extrahepatic system conducts bile from the liver to the small intestine to facilitate digestion [6].

The right and left hepatic ducts emerge from the liver and almost immediately join to form the common hepatic duct. The gallbladder connects to the common hepatic duct via the cystic duct to form the common bile duct, which descends behind the duodenum and traverses the head of the pancreas where it joins the main pancreatic duct. This junction forms the pancreatic-biliary ampulla (ampulla of Vater) and duodenal papilla or papilla of Vater. It must be noted that there are many anatomic variations in the extrahepatic system and a true pancreatic-biliary ampulla is not always present. The common hepatic duct varies from 0.8 to 5.2 cm in length, the cystic duct from 0.4 to 6.5 cm, the common bile duct from 1.5 to 9.0 cm, and the pancreatic-biliary ampulla 0.1 to 1.2 cm when present.

5.6.1. Histology

The extrahepatic biliary system is lined by a single layer of tall columnar epithelium, often referred to as biliary type epithelium. The larger pancreatic ducts are lined by columnar epithelial cells. However, as the pancreatic and common bile ducts approach the duodenal papilla, their lining epithelium becomes papillary and often projects towards the lumen of the duodenum. These papillary projections reflect the progressive transition from the relatively flat epithelium of the distal ducts to the intestinal type epithelium that covers the duodenal papilla.

5.7. Clinical Pathological Observations Indicating a Field Effect

Published clinical pathological observations have suggested a carcinogenic field in the extrahepatic system, similar to the field in upper aerodigestive tract. The co-occurrence of carcinomas of the pancreas, extrahepatic bile ducts, and ampulla of Vater, and the coexistence of ampullary neoplasms with pancreatic intraepithelial neoplasia has been reported [9-13]. Adenomas and adenocarcinomas of the ampulla have been associated with intraepithelial neoplasia of the pancreatic ducts [12] In one case, 3 synchronous carcinomas were found in the common bile duct, papilla of Vater, and main pancreatic duct that were similar by histology, immunohistochemistry, and flow cytometry [9]. Although small in number, these reports suggest the existence of a carcinogenic field effect since the bile duct, ampulla of Vater and pancreatic ducts are anatomically continuous. However, because cancers arising in these areas tend to be diagnosed late and are followed by relatively short survival times, the opportunity for primary metachronous carcinomas to develop over time is limited.

The conclusions of these case reports can be extended by evaluating the observed/expected (O/E) ratios of second primary cancers found in the SEER Program. Of 6,561 cases of gallbladder cancer, there were 14 cases with second primary cancers occurring in the extrahepatic bile ducts. While only 14 cases, this was highly significant ($p<.05$) since the O/E ratio was 10.86. There were 12 cases with second primary tumors occurring in the ampulla of Vater. Again, this was highly significant, with an O/E ratio of 13.52. In addition, gallbladder cancer was associated with 19 cases of pancreatic cancer, which was also significant ($p<.05$) with an O/E ratio of 2.86. The significance arises because these cancers are relatively uncommon, except for pancreas, and survival is very short which reduces the opportunity for second primary cancers to develop in the same field.

5.8. Epidemiology

The number of cases and the median and mean age at time of diagnosis for each cancer site is shown in table 5-1. Our analysis was limited to cases less than 85 years of age since all patients more than 85 years at diagnosis were assigned by SEER to a single category 85+ and not stratified by 5-year age intervals.

Table 5.1. Number of cases and mean age of diagnosis

Anatomic Site	Total No. Cases	No. Cases <85 Years	Mean Age at Diagnosis*
Ampulla	6,079	5,388	67.2
EHBD**	9,810	8,419	68.2
Gallbladder	14,968	12,888	68.7
Pancreas	127,586	112,830	67.6

*Mean age only for patients < 85 years of age.
**Extrahepatic bile duct.

5.8.1. Age Specific Incidence Rates

The age specific incidence rates of all cancers arising in the gallbladder, extrahepatic bile ducts, ampulla, and pancreas from 1973 through 2006 were calculated at 5-year intervals to age 85+ (Figure 5-1). Pancreatic cancer is clearly the most common and its age specific rate rises rapidly in all age groups.

It is often more informative, however, to explore age specific incidence rates by logarithmic plots since these plots often reveal information that is not always obvious on linear plots. Our results showed a potential common pathogenesis of carcinomas arising in the pancreas, gallbladder, EHBD, and ampulla of Vater. As background to the log-log plots (figure 5-2), Armitage and Doll in 1954 demonstrated that the age specific incidence rates of certain epithelial cancers have a linear slope when plotted against the age of diagnosis on logarithmic scales [14,15].

This logarithmic transformation of population data confirmed a theoretical equation relating the sequential development of carcinoma to a series of molecular changes and cellular events, and thereby supporting the multistage process of carcinogenesis with a continuous increase in cancer rate as a function of age [16]. Many investigators have since exploited logarithmically scaled plots to investigate both the rates and origins of human cancer [17-19].

These log-log plots represent a mathematic transformation that provides insight into tumor development and comparisons among tumor populations. Similar graphical patterns imply that similar tumors arising in different organs or tissues represent a single population with similar mechanisms of transformation or a similar carcinogenic process.

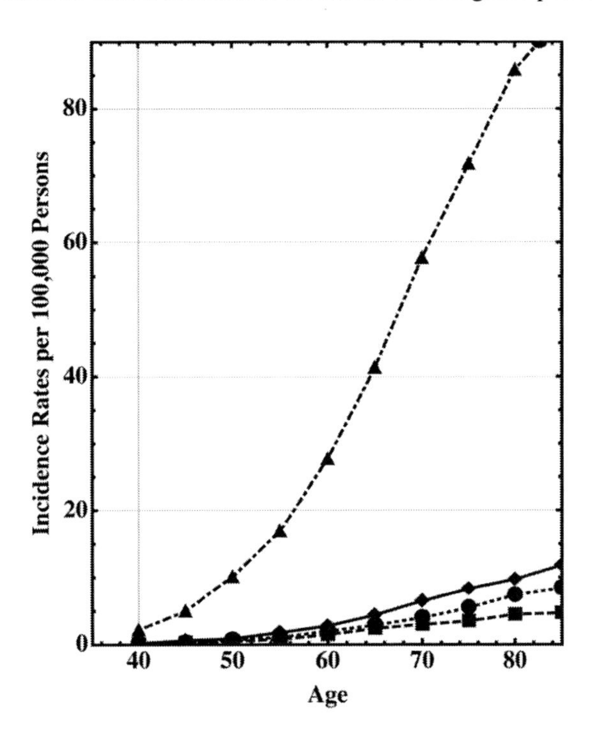

Figure 5.1. Linear plot of age specific rates for cancers of the pancreas (▲), gallbladder (♦), extrahepatic bile duct (●), and ampulla of Vater (■), SEER, 1973-2006,

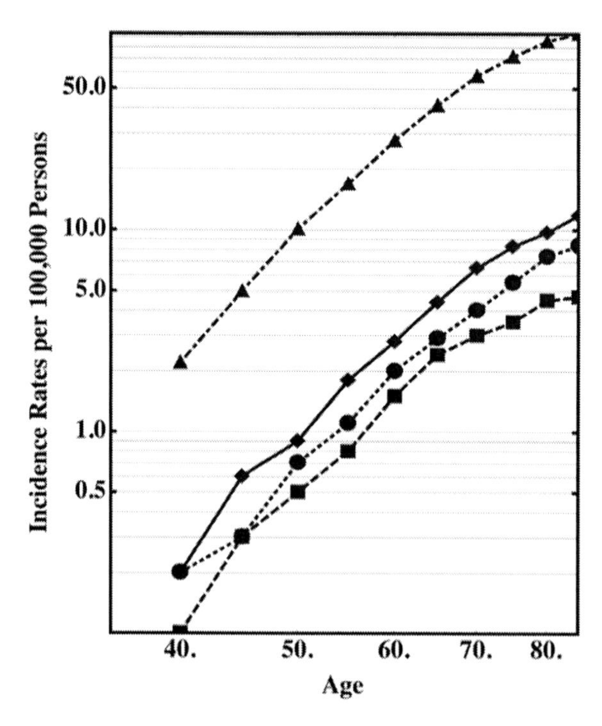

Figure 5.2. Log-log plot of age specific rates for cancers of the pancreas (▲), gallbladder (♦), extrahepatic bile duct (●), and ampulla of Vater (■), SEER, 1973-2006.

The age specific rates were graphically analyzed on a logarithmic scale and plotted as the log age specific rate versus the log age at diagnosis (figure 5-2).

The log-log plot revealed nearly parallel linear rate patterns for the four anatomic sites. On a log-log plot, parallel rate patterns indicate that age specific incidence rates are increasing by the same exponential rate. Therefore, parallel rate patterns indicate that the percentage change of each rate is similar even though the rates among the four tumors differ significantly in absolute incidence.

Because on a log-log plot, a straight line indicates that tumor incidence increases at a constant exponential rate, the parallel lines, therefore, are indicative of a single cohort population among the tumors in the four anatomic sites that differ only in absolute incidence. The implication of a single cohort population suggests that the rate of development of cancer is the same in the four sites even though the incidence rates are remarkably different.

5.8.2. Age Frequency Density

The age frequency density plots for carcinomas of the gallbladder, extrahepatic bile ducts, ampulla, and pancreas are shown in figure 5-3. Even though the incidence rates varied significantly for all four anatomic sites, the frequency density plots were isomorphic with a peak age at 71 years and median age of 72 years.

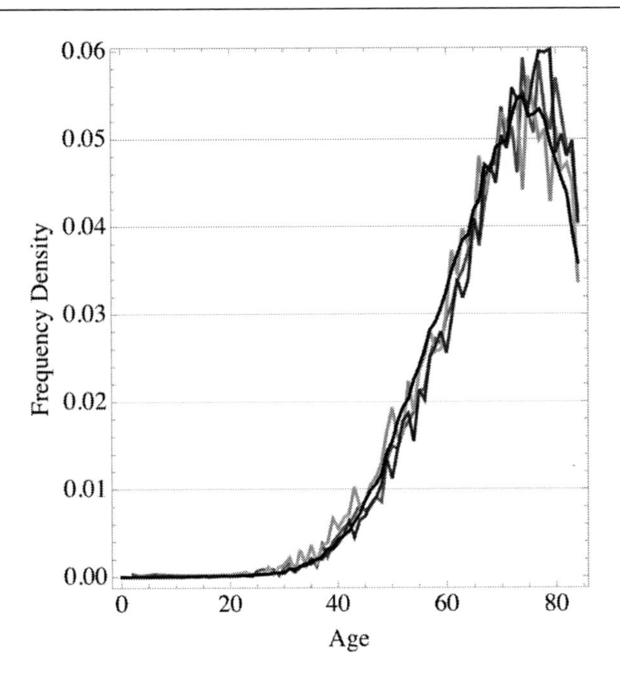

Figure 5.3. Age frequency density plot showing four isomorphic patterns one for pancreas, gallbladder, extrahepatic bile duct, and ampulla of Vater, SEER 1973-2006.

5.9. Molecular Evidence

In many anatomic sites, field effects are characterized by similar pathologic and related molecular changes [20]. It is, however, difficult to show molecular fields in the extrahepatic biliary system because: 1) investigators usually do not compare the molecular changes arising in all anatomic divisions, 2) the relatively short survival eliminates the opportunity for second primary cancers to develop, and 3) there are variations in existing molecular results. Published data shows wide variation in the molecular changes in cancers arising in the extrahepatic biliary system. For extrahepatic bile duct carcinoma, for example, the reported rates of K-*ras* mutation have ranged from 0% to 100% and for gallbladder carcinoma the rate has ranged from 5% to 57% [21,22].

Conclusion

A carcinogenic field effect may be proposed based on the concatenation of embryologic development, histopathologic findings, epidemiologic evidence, and molecular biologic support. The mucosa or epithelium at risk for the field effect must have a similar or overlapping embryologic development whose differentiation involves shared histogenesis despite the separation in anatomic location or disparate organ development. The histopathologic findings demonstrate that field carcinomas have similar or analogous mucosae, similar patterns of progressive epithelial dysplasia or carcinoma-in-situ, similar histologic types of carcinomas, and similar biologic behavior and patterns of tumor dissemination. The epidemiologic evidence must show that the field carcinomas have similar age-related density plots, similar patterns of logarithmically transformed age-adjusted incidence plots, and second primary cancers within the field whose observed incidence markedly exceeds the expected incidence in sporadic cases. It is helpful, but may not be determined, that the etiology of the field carcinogenesis be identical. The carcinogenic field effect is strengthened by the molecular biology support demonstrating similar or overlapping carcinogenic pathways among the field carcinomas. These shared molecular biologic signals may include identical activation of oncogenes, loss or inactivation of tumor suppressor genes, and other cellular events or molecular changes. The accumulated evidence from these scientific disciplines adds proof to the proposed carcinogenic field effect, and, suggests areas for research, from one discipline to another, to increase the accumulated evidence supporting a field effect for carcinogenesis.

A carcinogenic field seems to exist in the extrahepatic biliary system and pancreas based on similar descriptive epidemiology patterns. These tissues, in addition, satisfy other conditions for a field, they are anatomically continuous and share a common embryologic origin. Epidemiologically, tumors arising in these sites have similar age specific incidence rates and isomorphous age frequency density plots. From this, we propose that the carcinogenic mechanism of cancer arising in the extrahepatic biliary ductal system including the pancreas is similar in all of its anatomic divisions [5]. To account for the variation in the incidence rate of cancer in each site, we have suggested that the rate is a function of the relative surface area of the ducts in these sites [5].

Assuming that a common carcinogenic mechanism exists in the extrahepatic biliary system, then the phenotypic variations seen morphologically in cancers arising in these sites most likely occur after initiation of carcinogenesis. While the gallbladder and extrahepatic bile ducts are lined by biliary epithelium, the pancreas by pancreatic epithelium, and the ampulla in part by intestinal epithelium, tumors arising in this area can exhibit divergent histological patterns. Because there are different patterns, these phenotypic variations must be laid down following the initiation of carcinogenesis; otherwise the log-log plots would vary for each pattern. Evidence for this conclusion is seen in pancreatic cancer. Adenosquamous carcinomas of the pancreas have KRAS2, DPC4, and TP53 molecular changes that are similar to conventional ductal adenocarcinomas of the pancreas [23].

The use of descriptive epidemiology to reveal field effects, especially in unusual sites, is now possible because of the SEER Program, which serves as a population based national cancer registry. SEER has recorded more than 5 million cases of cancer covering all demographic segments of the US. In unpublished studies, we have shown that epidemiological patterns of lung and laryngeal cancers are similar, which is consistent with clinical observations. Laryngeal cancer is relatively rare, but its occurrence is usually associated with lung cancer and is attributable to smoking.

It was difficult to prove that molecular fields exist in the extrahepatic system since no systematic efforts have been made to identify common molecular alterations. There are several reasons for this: 1) investigators usually study only a single site and rarely compare molecular changes arising in all anatomic divisions of the extrahepatic system; 2) variations in racial/ethnic populations and geography; 3) the relatively short survival of most patients precludes the development of subsequent second primary tumors, and 4) variation in different assay techniques.

In summary, these data based primarily on descriptive epidemiology suggest that carcinomas that develop in the anatomic derivatives of the embryonic foregut are likely to be pathogenically related, since they share a common field of carcinogenesis. This implies, therefore, that the potential for carcinogenesis is similar in each of the four anatomic sites, even though the incidence rates vary greatly. We have hypothesized that the divergent rates in each site can be explained by the differences in the area of the ductal surface epithelium within each site. Most cancers arise in the pancreas because the ductal system has the largest surface area since it ramifies and often branches through the pancreas, while the ampulla of Vater has the least surface area of all four anatomic sites. Descriptive epidemiology offers a novel method to uncover new fields or to confirm existing fields discovered through clinical observations.

References

[1] Willis RA. The Pathology of Tumours. 4th Edition, 1967, pp107-126, Butterworths, London.

[2] Slaughter DL, Southwick HW, Smejkal W. "Field cancerization" in oral squamous epithelium: clinical implications of multicentric origin. *Cancer* 1953;6:963-968.

[3] Monique GCT, van Oijen MG, Slootweg PJ. Oral field cancerization: carcinogen-induced independent events or micrometastatic deposits? *Cancer Epidemiol. Biomarkers Prev.* 2000;9:249-256.

[4] Strong MS, Incze J, Vaughan CW. Field carcerization in the aerodigestive tract—its etiology, manifestation, and significance. *J. Otolaryngol.* 1984;13:1-6.

[5] Henson DE, Schwartz AM, Nsouli H, Albores-Saavedra J. Carcinomas of the pancreas, gallbladder, extrahepatic bile ducts, and ampulla of Vater share a field for carcinogenesis. *Arch. Pathol. Lab. Med.* 2009;133:67-71.

[6] Albores-Saavedra J, Henson DE, Klimstra DS. *Tumors of the Gallbladder, Extrahepatic Bile Ducts, and Ampulla of Vater*. Atlas of Tumor Pathology, Third Series, Armed Forces Institute of Pathology, 2000, Washington DC.

[7] Surveillance, Epidemiology, and End Results (SEER) Program (www.seer.cancer.gov) SEER*Stat Database: Incidence - SEER 17 Regs Limited-Use, Nov 2006 Sub (1973-2004 varying) - Linked To County Attributes - Total U.S., 1969-2006 Counties, National Cancer Institute, DCCPS, Surveillance Research Program, Cancer Statistics Branch, released April 2009, based on the November 2006 submission.

[8] Slack JMW. Developmental biology of the pancreas. *Development* 1995;121:1569-1580.

[9] Nishihara K, Tsuneyoshi M, Shimura H, Yasunami Y. Three synchronous carcinomas of the papilla of Vater, common bile duct and pancreas. *Pathol. Int.* 1994;44:325-332.

[10] Fava M, Foradori G, Cruz F, Guzman S. Papillomatosis of the common bile duct associated with ampullary carcinoma. *Am. J. Roentgenol.* 1991;156:405-406.

[11] 11.Nordback IH, Hruban RH, Cameron JL. Second primary lesions in the biliary tree after successful resection of ampullary carcinoma. *Surgery* 1992;112:111-115.

[12] Agoff SN, Crispin DA, Bronner MP, Dail DH, Hawes SE, Haggitt RC. Neoplasms of the ampulla of Vater with concurrent pancreatic intraductal neoplasia: a histological and molecular study. *Mod. Pathol.* 2001;14:139-146.

[13] Liu TH, Chen J, Zeng XJ. Histogenesis of pancreatic head and ampullary region carcinoma. *Chin. Med. J.* (Engl) 1983;96:167-174.

[14] Armitage, P. and Doll, R. The age distribution of cancer and a multi-stage theory of carcinogenesis. 1954. *Int. J. Epidemiol.* 2004;33:1174-1179.

[15] Armitage, P. and Doll, R. A two-stage theory of carcinogenesis in relation to the age distribution of human cancer. *Br. J. Cancer* 1957;11:161-169.

[16] Knudson AG. Two genetic hits (more or less) to cancer. *Nature* 2001;1:157-162.

[17] Pierce DA, Mendelsohn ML. A model for radiation-related cancer suggested by atomic bomb survivor data. *Radiat Res.* 1999;152:642-654.

[18] Kaldor JM, Day NE. Mathematical models in cancer epidemiology. In: Cancer Epidemiology and Prevention, 2nd Edition, JF Schottenfeld and J Fraumeni, editors, pp.127-137, Oxford University Press, 1996, NY.

[19] Moolgavkar SH. Carcinogenesis models: an overview. *Basic Life Sci.* 1991;58:387-396, Discussion 396-399.

[20] Wang X, Wang M, Maclennan GT, Abdul-Karim FW, Eble JN, Jones TD, et al. Evidence for common clonal origin of multifocal lung cancers. *J. Natl. Cancer Inst.* 2009;101:560-570.

[21] Rashid A, Cellular and molecular biology of biliary tract cancers. *Surg. Oncol. Clin. N.* Am 11:2002:995-1009.

[22] Rashid A, Ueki T, Gao YG, Houlihan PS, Wallace C, Wang BS, Shen MC, Deng J, Hsing AW. K-ras mutation, p53 overexpression, and microsatellite instability in biliary tract cancers: a population based study in China. *Clin. Cancer Res.* 2002;8:3156-3163.

[23] Brody JR, Costantino CL, Potoczek M, Cozzitorto J, McCue P, Yeo CJ, Hruban RH, Witkiewicz AK. Adenosquamous carcinoma of the pancreas harbors KRAS2, DPC4, and TP53 molecular alterations similar to pancreatic ductal adenocarcinoma. *Mod. Pathol.* 2009;22:651-659.

Part III – Clincal and Molecular Aspects of Field Cancerization in Specific Tissues

In: Field Cancerization: Basic Science and Clinical Applications ISBN 978-1-61761-006-6
Editor: Gabriel D. Dakubo

Chapter 6

Field Cancerization and Oral Leukoplakia

Liviu Feller and Johan Lemmer

Abstract

There is evidence that several clinical, histological and cytogenetic factors are associated with greater risk of carcinomatous transformation of oral leukoplakia: older age, anatomical site (floor of mouth, ventrolateral surface of the tongue, maxillary retromolar and adjoining soft palate), size larger than 5mm, erythroleukoplakia, high-grade epithelial dysplasia, DNA aneuploidy, and loss of heterozygosity of certain defined chromosomal loci. Paradoxically, idiopathic leukoplakia possesses a greater risk of malignant transformation than tobacco related leukoplakia. There is convincing evidence that while either oral leukoplakia or oral squamous cell carcinoma can arise *de novo*, in the great majority of cases these lesions develop at single or at multiple sites within fields of epithelial precancerous cells. Leukoplakias may remain in a steady state or may progress to carcinoma.

There is a series of molecular, genetic and histopathological events or processes whereby oral epithelium which is in every respect normal, at certain sites develops clones of transformed cells which by replicative clonal expansion become fields of genetically transformed, or ultimately of precancerous cells. Transformation of keratinocytes to precancerous cells depends on the number of mutagenic events rather than on the sequence in which they occur.

6.1. Introduction

Leukoplakia is the most common potentially malignant lesion of the oral cavity. It can be idiopathic or associated with tobacco or areca nut use. Oral leukoplakia is a term for a white plaque that cannot be characterised clinically or microscopically as any other specific pathological entity, and cannot be associated with any aetiologic agent other than tobacco or areca nut use [1,2]. A definitive diagnosis of oral leukoplakia must be established by exclusion of other entities on clinical (Table 7-1) or histopathological grounds [1,2].

There is evidence that several clinical, histological and cytogenetic factors are associated with greater risk of carcinomatous transformation of oral leukoplakia: older age, anatomical site (floor of mouth, ventrolateral surface of the tongue, maxillary retromolar and adjoining soft palate), size larger than 5 mm, erythroleukoplakia, high-grade epithelial dysplasia, DNA aneuploidy, and loss of heterozygosity of certain defined chromosomal loci. Paradoxically, idiopathic leukoplakia possesses a greater risk of malignant transformation than tobacco related leukoplakia.

While either oral leukoplakia or oral squamous cell carcinoma (SCC) can arise *de novo*, in the great majority of cases these lesions develop at single or at multiple sites within fields of epithelial precancerous cells. Leukoplakias may remain in a steady state or may progress to carcinoma.

Biopsy is mandatory not only to distinguish leukoplakia from other specific pathological entities, but also to determine whether or not there is epithelial dysplasia [3]. Some oral leukoplakias develop within fields of clinically and histopathologically normal, but genetically altered keratinocytes termed fields of precancerization.

There is a series of molecular, genetic and histopathological events or processes whereby oral epithelium that is in every respect normal, at certain sites develops clones of transformed cells which by replicative clonal expansion become fields of genetically transformed, and ultimately of precancerous cells. Transformation of keratinocytes to precancerous cells depends on the number of mutagenic events rather than on the sequence in which they occur. Such a field of genetically altered or 'precancerized' keratinocytes in the oral cavity can be contiguous with or discrete from other such precancerized fields which may or may not show epithelial dysplasia. A field of genetically altered keratinocytes may display a normal microscopic appearance but may nevertheless be sufficiently cytogenetically altered to constitute a field of precancerization and thus to present a risk of malignant change [4-11].

Table 6.1. Clinical differential diagnosis of oral leukoplakia

- Tobacco-associated white lesions (stomatitis nicotina, tobacco pouch keratosis)
- Leukoedema
- Candida-associated white lesions (chronic hyperplastic candidosis, pseudomembranous candidosis)
- Oral hairy leukoplakia
- Oral lichen planus
- Oral discoid lupus erythematosus
- Oral white sponge naevus
- Linea alba
- Habitual cheek, lip and tongue biting
- Frictional keratosis
- Chemical burn (e.g aspirin)
- Non-ulcerative squamous cell carcinoma
- Verrucous carcinoma.

6.2. Clinical and Clinical Statistical Aspects of Oral Leukoplakia

6.2.1. Clinical Features

Oral leukoplakias are classified into two main types according to their clinical appearances. Homogeneous leukoplakias are uniformly white plaques that can vary in size from a few millimeters to several centimeters, and have relatively flat surfaces that exhibit irregular shallow fissures (Figure 6-1A).

Non-homogeneous leukoplakias are either mixed white and red plaques called erythroleukoplakia, or are nodular or verrucous showing wrinkled or corrugated surfaces (Figure 6-1B) [1,2,12,13]. Non-homogeneous leukoplakia has a greater risk of carcinomatous transformation than homogeneous leukoplakia [14,15], the greatest risk being associated with the erythroplakic component (Figure 6-2). However, most leukoplakias remain stable or will regress [15-17]. Oral leukoplakia in any of its forms can be single, multiple or diffusely widespread [15,18].

The eryrthoplakic component of oral erythroleukoplakia is identical to erythroplakia *per se,* a velvety red plaque that carries the greatest risk of carcinomatous transformation of all oral precancerous lesions. More than 50% of all cases of clinical erythroplakia prove to be SCCs on biopsy [19].

Proliferative verrucous leukoplakia, considered by some to be a distinct entity, is characterised by multiple lesions that affect different oral mucosal sites. Proliferative verrucous leukoplakia usually runs an aggressive course, is not strongly associated with tobacco use, is persistent, irreversible and progressive. Usually it cannot be recognized in its initial stages because it presents identically to an isolated leukoplakia, and therefore the diagnosis is often made late in the course of the disease [20-23].

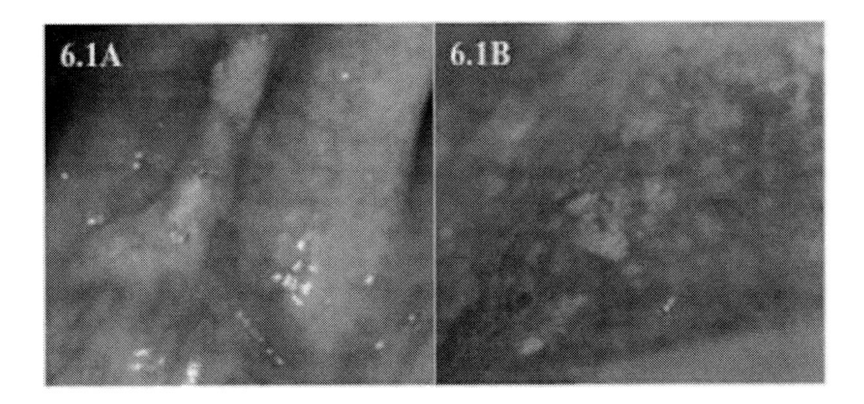

Figure 6.1. Multiple leukoplakic lesions in a 72 years white male: smoked 20 cigarettes per day for 55 years. Two discrete homogeneous leukoplakic lesions on the sublingual frenulum (Figure 6.1A) and erythroleukoplakia (speckled leukoplakia) at the junction of the hard and soft palate (Figure 6.1B): clear evidence of a wide field of precancerization. On biopsy the palatal lesion proved to have become carcinomatous.

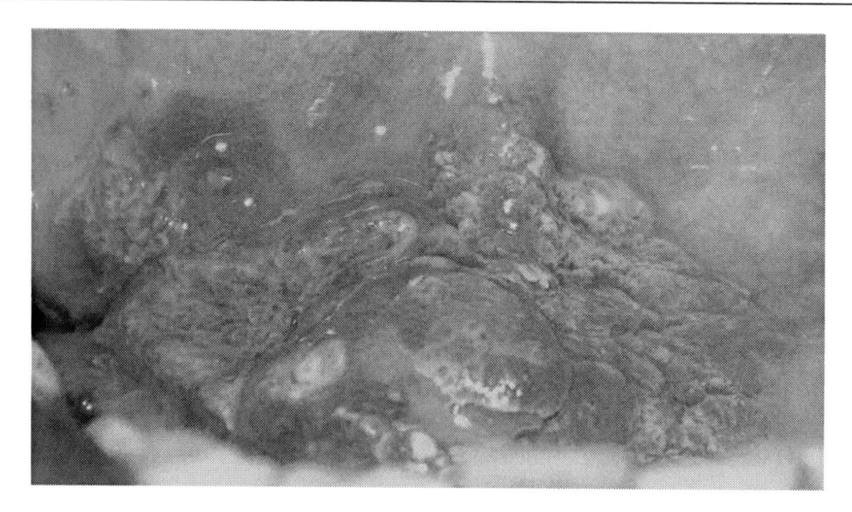

Figure 6.2. Erythroleukoplakia of floor of the mouth in a 55-year old black male who smoked 15 cigarettes per day for 40 years. On biopsy it proved to be squamous cell carcinoma.

The potentially malignant nature of oral leukoplakia, in particular that of erythroleukoplakia and of proliferative verrucous leukoplakia, and the multifocality of the latter support the notion that they arise within fields of oral epithelium containing genetically altered transformed keratinocytes. In one study, 63% of subjects with proliferative verrucous leukoplakia developed oral SCC, and 53% of these subjects continued to develop additional verrucous carcinomas or SCCs at different oral anatomical sites [21].

6.2.2. Clinical Aspects of Oral Leukoplakia Related to its Malignant Potential

The risk of carcinomatous transformation of oral leukoplakia is generally unpredictable but overall is relatively low [14,18]. The reported rate of carcinomatous transformation of oral leukoplakia varies from study to study ranging from less than 1% to about 20-25% [13,15]. This is undoubtedly owing to significant differences between the studies with respect to methodology and case selection (gender, age, race, social factors, habits, etc), as well as to whether or not the leukoplakia had previously been treated, and very importantly whether the study sample is or is not drawn from a hospital population [12,13].

Non-homogeneous leukoplakia carries a greater risk of progression to carcinoma (20-25%) than homogeneous leukoplakia (0.6%-5%) [13,15], but the overall risk of carcinomatous transformation of oral leukoplakia is less than 2% per year if the estimate is to be believed [15]. If proliferative verrucous leukoplakia is regarded as a distinct entity, almost all cases progress to verrucous carcinoma, or ultimately to SCC [22,24]. Since the erythroplakic part of non-homogeneous leukoplakia to all intents and purposes is identical to erythroplakia, it is noteworthy that the rate of transformation of the latter to carcinoma ranges from 14% to 50% [19].

It has long been believed that a higher risk of carcinomatous transformation attaches to larger leukoplakias (arbitrarily more than 5mm in size) and to leukoplakias at high-risk sites which are floor of the mouth, ventrolateral surface of the tongue and maxillary retromolar/soft palate complex [13,15,25,26]. Oral leukoplakia at high-risk sites as defined above exhibits epithelial dysplasia and undergoes carcinomatous transformation more frequently than does leukoplakia elsewhere in the mouth. However, the increased malignant potential of oral leukoplakia at high-risk sites is not directly related to degree of dysplasia, as dysplastic leukoplakia at high-risk sites is more likely to undergo carcinomatous transformation than comparably dysplastic leukoplakia at other oral sites [26].

6.2.3. The Natural Course of Oral Leukoplakia

In populations with high frequencies of tobacco related oral leukoplakia, as in Southeast Asia, where heavy smoking, reverse smoking and the use of smokeless tobacco are very common, most SCC arise from oral leukoplakia. In European and North American populations, for example, who use less tobacco and where reverse smoking or the use of smokeless tobacco are much less common, many oral SCC arise *de novo* from apparently normal oral mucosa [14]. Many such '*de novo*' SCC nevertheless exhibit tell-tale signs of leukoplakic origins [13]; and about one third arise in close proximity to leukoplakias [2].

There is evidence that oral SCC that arises from pre-existing leukoplakia behaves less aggressively and has a better prognosis than oral SCC that arises *de novo* [14,19]; and the frequency of carcinomatous transformation, unexpectedly, is higher in idiopathic than in tobacco-associated oral leukoplakias [13,18]. If carcinomatous transformation of oral leukoplakia occurs, the rate of transformation is highly variable, ranging unpredictably from a few months to many years [2].

Between 70% and 90% of oral leukoplakias are associated with tobacco smoking, and most tobacco-associated oral leukoplakias regress or resolve following cessation of smoking [14]. Cigarette, pipe and cigar smoking are all risk factors for oral leukoplakia and there is a clear relationship between the frequency and the duration of smoking, and the prevalence of oral leukoplakia [2,27]; but tobacco smoking is a poor predictor of carcinomatous transformation of oral leukoplakia [25]. By definition, the aetiology of idiopathic oral leukoplakia is at present unknown [14].

It appears that the risk of carcinomatous transformation of dysplastic oral leukoplakia is questionably influenced by treatment [28]. The estimated rate of recurrance of surgically treated oral leukoplakia may be as high as 30% [29]; and SCC occurs at 12% of sites of surgically excised leukoplakia [17]. These facts are consistent with the view that many oral leukoplakias develop in a field of precancerization of the oral mucosa that is populated by transformed keratinocytes.

In the light of avalaible evidence it is safe to conclude that some cases of oral leukoplakia, despite treatment, are destined to recur or to progress to cancer [29]; but neither clinical, nor histological, nor molecular methods are yet available confidently to identify these cases.

6.3. Epidemiology

As mentioned earlier, the documented epidemiological data regarding oral leukoplakia are highly variable owing to great differences in factors such as selection criteria and methods of data collection among others, and the reported results are at best an approximation. Where people often practise the habits of tobacco chewing (smokeless tobacco), or of areca nut chewing, the prevalence of oral leukoplakia is greater than where smoking of tobacco is the most common practice [14].

The association between race and oral leukoplakia is not reported in many studies. In a South African study, 86% of subjects with oral leukoplakia were whites, 9% were blacks and 5% were Asians, in spite of the fact that the vast majority of the South African population is black. These results are difficult to explain. It is possible that fewer blacks have oral leukoplakia, but it is equally possible that black people often seek medical attention later in the course of their disease, so that at the time of presentation the leukoplakia has already become carcinomatous [30], and thus would not be included in the statistics for leukoplakia.

Estimates of the global prevalence of oral leukoplakia range from 0.5% to 3.46% [31]; about 10% of all cases of oral leukoplakias are idiopathic and the rest are associated with tobacco use [14,15]; and about 70% of subjects with oral leukoplakias are males. Oral leukoplakia is seldom detected before middle-age and the prevalence increases with age [2]. In populations in which women use tobacco as much as men, the gender prevalence of oral leukoplakia is equal. Approximately 25% of oral leukoplakias affect the buccal mucosa, 20% the lower gingiva, 10% the tongue, 10% the floor of the mouth and the remainder affect other oral sites [15]. Between 0.7% and 2.9%, of oral leukoplakias are estimated to undergo carcinomatous transformation and these malignantly transformed leukoplakias represent between 17% and 35% of oral SCC, the remaining number of carcinomata arising *de novo* [31].

6.4. Histopathological Aspects Related to Malignant Potential of Oral Leukoplakia

The presence of dysplasia is an important marker of the malignant potential of oral leukoplakia [13,16,26] and it is probable that the dysplastic features are a reflection of the genomic and molecular alterations occurring in the field of keratinocytes in which the dysplasia arose [32].

The reported frequency of epithelial dysplasia in oral leukoplakias ranges from 5% to 25% of all cases [2]; and it is more prevalent in non-homogeneous than in homogeneous leukoplakias [13]. The risk of carcinomatous transformation of an individual leukoplakic lesion is proportional to the grade of dysplasia, and indeed is twice as great for lesions with moderate and severe dysplasia as for lesions with mild dysplasia or simple epithelial hyperplasia [13,16,18,33]. In this regard it must be remembered that the grading of epithelial dysplasia is highly subjective with low reproducibility [7,19,28], and that microscopical diagnosis of an incisional biopsy specimen does not reflect the nature of the entire lesion, which in different parts may display different grades of epithelial dysplasia [28,34].

However some dysplastic oral leukoplakias remain clinically and/or histologically stable or even regress, while some leukoplakias which do not exhibit epithelial dysplasia at the time of biopsy, may progress to carcinoma. [13,18,33]. In one study of the pattern of progression of dysplastic oral leukoplakias and oral erythroplakias to carcinoma, 36% of the carcinomata developed directly from the leukoplakias or erythroplakias, 49% developed contiguous to the precancerous lesions and 15% at remote oral sites [25], thus suggesting the probable existence of fields of precancerization.

It is thus evident that while dysplasia, particurlarly high-grade dysplasia, is asociated with carcinomatous transformation of oral leukoplakia, dysplasia cannot confidently be used as a predictor of progression to cancer [3,16]. However, in spite of the predictive shortcomings outlined above, epithelial dysplasia remains an important guide to clinical management of oral leukoplakia, and has been found overall to be a significant indicator of possible future malignant change [13,32].

6.5. Oral Leukoplakias and Oral Precancerous Fields

6.5.1. General Characteristics of Precancerized Fields in the Oral Cavity

There is strong evidence that most, if not all, SCC of the oral cavity develop within fields of genetically altered keratinocytes [10]. It is not entirely clear whether the initial genetic lesions in keratinocytes populating a field of precancerization in normal looking oral epithelium are caused by a single genetic event or by multiple events; whether the field of precancerization comprises a population of monoclonal cells originating from one transformed cell that undergoes clonal expansion and consequently spreads laterally; or whether many keratinocytes acquire identical or different genetic lesions concurrently and subsequently evolve into a number of homologous monoclones, or polyclones [35]. Regardless of the yet-uncertain fine details of the process, the evolution in the oral mucosa of a field of genetically altered keratinocytes is a distinct biopathological process in the continuum of epithelial carcinogenesis [9].

It would appear that oral SCC is a monoclonal lesion arising from a progenitor cell in the basal cell layer of the oral epithelium. The cell acquires one or more genetic alterations and evolves into an expanding clone that may be clinically inapparent, may manifest as leukoplakia or may undergo clonal divergences consequent to additional genetic events, and eventually progresses to SCC [36,37].

On the other hand, it is conceivable that oral leukoplakia that remains stable or even regresses may have had an aetiology that did not bring about genetic alterations, and that produces a field of benign cells that would not subsequently progress to carcinoma. Leukoplakia arising from a precancerous field of cells cannot be distinguished clinically from leukoplakia arising from a benign field; and even after long-term observation a distinction may not be possible since leukoplakia of either origin can remain stable without either progressing or regressing. It is possible that only the molecular profile of the keratinocytes of a stable leukoplakia will allow the identification of its true nature.

It is possible that ectodermal cells destined to become oral keratinocytes may have undergone genetic and/or epigenetic changes during organogenesis. The altered ectodermal stem cells then differentiate into oral epithelium constituting a field of initially transformed keratinocytes [35,36]. Additional post-developmental genomic lesions may culminate in the evolution of a clone or clones of precancerous cells that undergo clonal expansion [Figure 6-3].

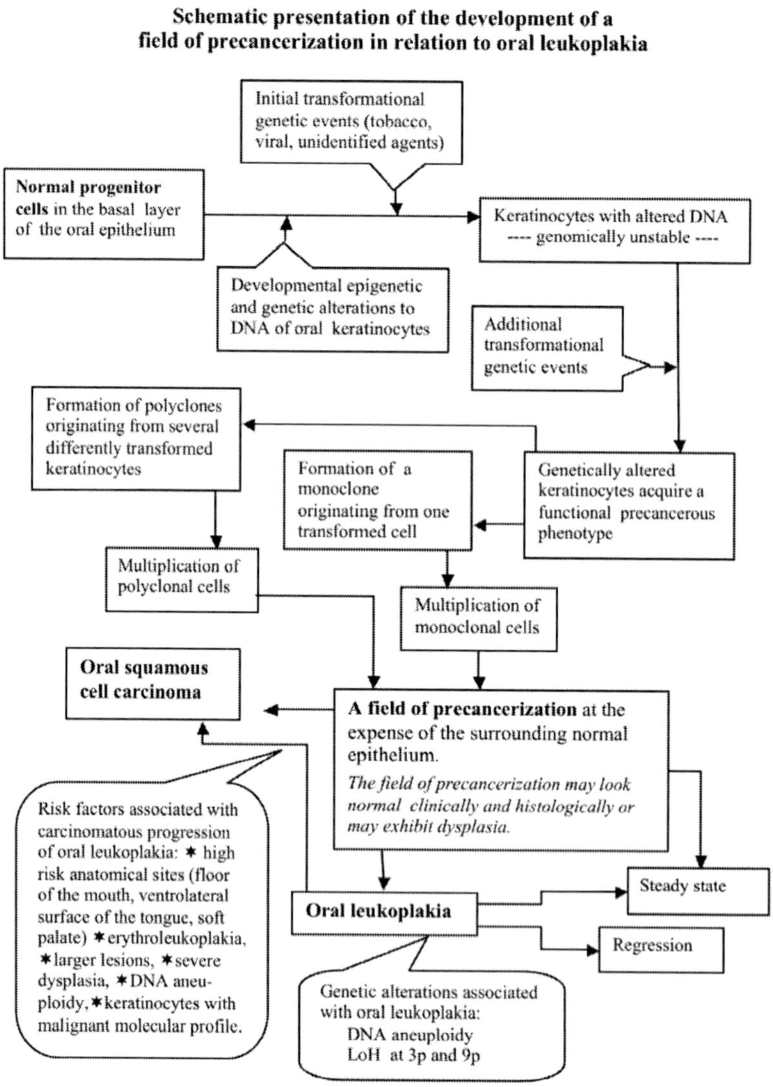

Schematic presentation of the development of a field of precancerization in relation to oral leukoplakia

Initial transformational genetic events (tobacco, viral, unidentified agents)

Normal progenitor cells in the basal layer of the oral epithelium

Keratinocytes with altered DNA ---- genomically unstable ----

Developmental epigenetic and genetic alterations to DNA of oral keratinocytes

Additional transformational genetic events

Formation of polyclones originating from several differently transformed keratinocytes

Formation of a monoclone originating from one transformed cell

Genetically altered keratinocytes acquire a functional precancerous phenotype

Multiplication of polyclonal cells

Multiplication of monoclonal cells

Oral squamous cell carcinoma

A field of precancerization at the expense of the surrounding normal epithelium.

The field of precancerization may look normal clinically and histologically or may exhibit dysplasia.

Risk factors associated with carcinomatous progression of oral leukoplakia: ✱ high risk anatomical sites (floor of the mouth, ventrolateral surface of the tongue, soft palate) ✱erythroleukoplakia, ✱larger lesions, ✱severe dysplasia, ✱DNA aneuploidy,✱keratinocytes with malignant molecular profile.

Oral leukoplakia

Steady state

Regression

Genetic alterations associated with oral leukoplakia: DNA aneuploidy LoH at 3p and 9p

Figure 6.3. Schematic presentation of the development of a field of precancerization in relation to oral leukoplakia.

6.5.2. The Evolution of a Field of Precancerized Cells in the Oral Cavity

A precancerized field constitutes a large pool of genetically altered keratinocytes at different stages of transformation [38]. It is estimated that 3 to 12 sequential genetic mutations are necessary for a cell to undergo malignant transformation. The number is an imponderable, but is determined by the inherent resistance of the cell to transformation [36,38]. This is a function of the efficiency of the cellular DNA repair mechanisms, of the number of signal transduction pathways that must be dysregulated for a cell to be transformed, and of the critical number of genetic lesions that will confer a selective growth advantage and enhanced fitness (competitive advantage) upon the transformed cells [36,38].

The initial genetic events leading to cell transformation are not well characterized, and not all the molecular changes associated with the formation of a field of precancerization in normal looking oral epithelium are known [36]. In oral epithelium, the initial transformational events probably occur in amplifying cells in the progenitor compartment of the basal and/or parabasal layers. These amplifying cells constantly divide to produce new cells that maintain the integrity and the proliferative capacity of the basal and parabasal cell layers, then enter the maturation sequence and gradually rise through the epithelial cell layers to the desquamating surface [39].

Precancer and cancer of the oral epithelium are not uncommon. Malignant transformation of a normal cell requires the occurrence of several singular genetic events, but the estimated spontaneous mutation rate (random DNA damage) in a normal cell during its life-span is not sufficient to account for the complex genetic lesions in a cancerous cell [38,40]. It has therefore been proposed that an early event in carcinogenesis is the evolution of a transformed cell that expresses a 'mutator phenotype'. This mutator phenotype is characterised by functional alterations in those genes responsible for maintaining the genomic stability of normal cells. A cell with a mutator phenotype enters a cascade of mutations at a rate above that of accumulated spontaneous mutations [40] with a consequent quantum jump in the number of the genetic lesions, leading to the clonal expansion of the altered cell population, and to clonal divergences [41]. This drives the genetic evolution of the transformed cells towards cancerization [40].

With time, as the mutagenic events accumulate with subsequent loss of effectiveness of cellular repair mechanisms, genetically altered keratinocytes can acquire a functional malignant phenotype [36,38,42]. These changes may occur in a field of clinically normal-looking oral epithelium, so if leukoplakia or SCC becomes clinically apparent, it represents only the 'tip of the iceberg'. The vast majority of the genetically altered cells are still at precancerous stages of transformation, are clinically, and frequently also microscopically indistinguishable from normal cells, but they have many genetic alterations in common with cancer cells, with the potential to become cancer cells [36].

Thus, the development of an oral keratinocyte having a complete set of genomic alterations of a malignant phenotype is preceded by the evolution of a multitude of either polyclonal or monoclonal altered cells [7,9,10,38], creating an expanding field of precancerous keratinocytes at the expense of the surrounding normal epithelium [36] (Figure 6-3). The keratinocytes in this field will share similar genetic changes if the altered cell population is clonally related by descent from a monoclone; but the genetic changes in the keratinocytes will be dissimilar if the field of cells has a polyclonal origin [43,44].

Although the cell population in a monoclone arises from a single cell, the molecular profiles of the monoclonal cells are not necessarily identical because repeated spontaneous or induced mutations may have different genetic effects on different cells in the field. On the other hand, polyclonal cells within a field may acquire some similar genetic alterations by exposure to identical micro-environments and to secondary transforming agents. It is probable that the initial genetic alterations in the molecularly atypical keratinocytes in the field confer upon them a competitive growth advantage in relation to the normal neighbouring keratinocytes. The altered keratinocytes in the field are fitter, have increased metabolic activity and proliferation rates, and it is suggested that these altered cells can trigger apoptosis of normal neighbouring keratinocytes and may even remove the detritus of the dead cells. This process favours the expansion of the precancerized field [36].

6.5.3. A Model of Oral Epithelial Carcinogenesis

Carcinomatous transformation of normal keratinocytes is the outcome of a sufficient number of genetic alterations rather than the sequence in which such alterations occur. Although there appear to be patterns of sequential genetic alterations in the carcinogenesis of oral epithelial lesions, and although genetic lesions found in precancerous stages appear to be associated with initiating early transformational events, while genetic changes seen in frank carcinoma may be the consequence of late events [45,46], the varying sequential order of the events is probably concealed by the complex process of carcinogenesis [41,47,48].

It is not surprising that within either oral leukoplakia or within oral SCC there is marked molecular variety in the form of cytogenetically related sub-clones and of cytogenetically unrelated sub-clones. The related sub-clones probably reflect clonal divergence and the unrelated sub-clones reflect polyclones arising independently. When a monoclone undergoes clonal expansion, the initial genetic alteration that affects the progenitor cell of the clone will necessarily be present in all cells of that clone and its sub-clones. Additional genetic events can lead to increasingly divergent cytogenetic profiles of cells in successive generations of sub-clones [42].

There are no reliable molecular or genetic predictors of carcinomatous transformation for oral leukoplakia. Carcinomatous transformation of oral leukoplakia may or may not occur irrespective of the detection of molecular markers usually related to early or late genetic events associated with cancer [3,49].

6.5.4. Limitations of Certain Existing Studies of Molecular Predictors of Carcinomatous Transformation of Potentially Malignant Oral Lesions

From an oral medical perspective it is difficult to interpret the results of many studies that aim to evaluate the association between specific molecular markers and carcinomatous transformation of potentially malignant lesions. Many studies do not distinguish lesions of different anatomical regions of the upper aerodigestive mucosae, and therefore it is not possible to extract the information specifically relevant to the oral mucosa. Since the natural courses of potentially malignant epithelial lesions of the oral mucosa, and of the larynx for example, are different, and may be induced by different spectra of aetiological factors [37], the results of such 'portmanteau' studies have limited value in relation to the oral medical field.

Many studies also do not specify the potentially malignant entities investigated. In the mouth there are several distinct potentially malignant lesions including leukoplakia, each being characterized by its own distinct clinical features and natural courses, though having some common histological features such as epithelial hyperplasia and dysplasia. In many of the studies, the inclusion criteria for lesions to be categorized as potentially malignant are based on these very histopathological features of epithelial hyperplasia and dysplasia, without giving the specific diagnosis of the lesion. As certain reactive inflammatory lesions and benign tumours of the oral mucosa may also show the histopathological features of epithelial hyperplasia and low-grade dysplasia [13], such lesions may well have been included in some of the studies of malignant transformation of supposedly potentially malignant lesions, thus skewing the results.

6.5.5. Molecular Markers Associated with Oral Leukoplakia and its Carcinomatous Transformation

Regardless of inherited predispositions and suspected aetiological factors, genetic changes associated with the development of both oral leukoplakia and oral SCC include alterations in the p53 protein tumour-suppressor gene (PT 53), dysregulation of the mechanism controlling the G1 transition to the S phase of the cell cycle at the G1 checkpoint, activation of proto-oncogenes, inactivation of several tumour-suppressor genes as a result of loss of heterozygosity (LoH) [3,49,50], alteration of mitochondrial DNA [51], and aberration of DNA content [52].

Alterations in PT53 and subsequent dysfunction of p53 protein are observed in apparently normal, in potentially malignant, and in carcinomatous oral epithelia [53-55]; are associated with dysregulation of the cell cycle, of DNA replication and repair, and of apoptosis [41]; and are observed in about 53% of subjects with SCC of the head and neck (oral, pharyngeal and laryngeal). There is a considerable heterogeneity of PT53 alterations in SCC of the head and neck. Specific molecular changes are associated with different clinical courses of the disease, and not all alterations in PT53 give rise to dysfunctional p53 protein [53]. Alterations in PT53 are considered to be an initial genetic event in the continuum of oral carcinomatous transformation, inducing genomic instability, and are present in apparently normal epithelium in the precancerized field before the appearance of oral leukoplakia or SCC [9,40].

Loss of chromosomal regions that contain tumour-suppressor genes are associated with genomic instability [40]. Loss of heterozygosity (LoH) within chromosomal regions with candidate tumour-suppressor genes that may be associated with carcinomatous transformation occurs frequently in oral leukoplakia [46,56]. Increasing LoH in cells of the epithelium of the upper aerodigestive tract correlates with the progression of histopathological changes from hyperplasia through increasing grades of dysplasia to carcinoma *in situ,* and ultimately to invasive carcinoma. Apparently normal keratinocytes adjacent to the precancerous or cancerous lesions, and keratinocytes of these lesions have similar genetic alterations in common [5]. Oral and oropharyngeal dysplastic epithelial lesions with high rates of proliferation manifested by a high proportion of Ki-67 positive cells have a greater frequency of LoH than epithelial lesions with low proliferative rates [7].

In the oral keratinocytes, LOH at the chromosome arms 3p and 9p is associated with progression of potentially malignant lesions, including oral leukoplakia, to carcinoma [5,25,46,56,57]. In one study of keratinocytes of oral leukoplakia [56] 45% of subjects had LOH at 3p14 and 36% at 9p21. Thirty-seven percent (37%) of these subjects with LOH at 3p14 and at 9p21 progressed to SCC as compared to only 6% of subjects without LOH at either of these chromosomes [56]. In another study of unspecified oral precancerous epithelial lesions [46] the keratinocytes that carried LOH limited to 3p and/or 9p had a 3.8-fold increase of carcinomatous transformation of the lesions compared to precancerous lesions without LOH at either 3p or at 9p. Those precancerous lesions, which carry LOH at 3p and/or at 9p and additional losses at any of chromosomes 4q, 8p, 11q and 17p, had a 33-fold increased risk compared to lesions that retain these chromosomal arms intact, and they progressed to carcinoma significantly more rapidly than precancerous lesions with LOH only at 3p and/or at 9p. However, the time of progression to carcinoma differed greatly and randomly between lesions [46,58].

A question still to be answered is this: what are the genetic events preceding the progressive transformation of keratinocytes in which LOH as outlined above cannot be demonstrated, to carcinomatous cells?

The chromosomes of keratinocytes of dysplastic leukoplakia of the floor of the mouth, the ventrolateral surface of the tongue and of the maxillary retromolar/soft palate complex (high-risk anatomical sites) more frequently exhibit LOH compared to the chromosomes of keratinocytes of leukoplakia from low-risk regions of the mouth [26]. For oral leukoplakia with epithelial dysplasia, the risk of malignant transformation is much greater (84%) for those lesions manifesting aneuploidy than for those (3%) with normal (diploid) DNA content [52]. Moreover subjects with oral SCC evolving from aneuploid dysplastic leukoplakia have a lower rate of survival than subjects with oral SCC arising from diploid dysplastic leukoplakia. Surgical removal of aneuploid dysplastic oral leukoplakia with clear margins, as evidenced by histopathological examination, does not improve the prognosis [59]. Therefore DNA aneuploidy may be a reliable predictor of progression of dysplastic leukoplakia to carcinoma and an indicator of poor prognosis [26,50,52,59]. Both numerical and structural clonal chromosomal aberrations may be present in fields of apparently normal epithelium of the upper aerodigestive tract of elderly people [60].

Ha et al. (2002) found alterations in the mitochondrial DNA (mtDNA) in about 37% of premalignant lesions of the oral cavity, oropharynx and larynx. Although this figure is very much lower than the 84% risk of malignant transformation of cells manifesting aneuploidy, as these alterations in mtDNA occur early in the continuum of carcinogenesis and increase in number with the increasing severity of the epithelial dysplasia, alterations in mtDNA may serve as a supporting indicator of carcinomatous transformation [51].

Although epithelial premalignancy and SCC are clearly the result of an accumulation of genetic alterations in keratinocytes [61], genomic alterations in the cells of the connective tissue stroma underlying the epithelium may also play an important rôle in carcinomatous transformation [62,63]. Genomic changes in stromal fibroblasts with expression of aberrant mediators may dysregulate the relationship of the connective tissue to the overlying keratinocytes which have previously undergone initiation of transformation, contributing to the formation of a field of precancerization and to the induction or promotion of epithelial carcinogenesis [62,64].

6.5.6. Field of Precancerization and the Course of Oral Leukoplakia

The existence of a field of precancerization may explain the course of oral leukoplakia (Figure 6-3). Firstly, transformed keratinocytes in an oral field of precancerization may give rise to multiple synchronous and/or metachronous precancerous oral leukoplakias. These multiple lesions may be clonally related if they arise from sub-clones of a clone developed from a single cell, but not if they arose from the independent cloning of several cells. Secondly, additional genetic alterations to the precancerous keratinocytes of the oral leukoplakia may lead to the evolution of a malignant clone, thus explaining why some early oral SCC are embedded within leukoplakias while other oral SCC are contiguous to leukoplakias.

Lastly, the concept of a field of precancerization may explain the recurrence at the same site of leukoplakia with the identical molecular profile to that of an apparently successfully surgically excised leukoplakia, or the development of more than one leukoplakia of similar or dissimilar DNA molecular profiles depending upon whether the lesions developed from precancerous cells left behind at surgery or from related or unrelated clones adjacent to the excision.

However, the concept of field cancerization cannot easily explain the mechanisms of regression or resolution of some oral leukoplakias. As not all oral leukoplakias are potentially malignant, and as only some are committed to a malignant pathway, those leukoplakias that are not precancerous may resolve when the aetiological factor, whatever it might be, is withdrawn. Regarding regression of those leukoplakias that show high-grade epithelial dysplasia and that have undergone genetic alterations associated with early events in carcinogenesis, it is possible that the acquired genetic profile could have rendered the dysplastic cells inferior, rather than superior in their growth capacity, resulting in their replacement by, rather than in their replacing the surrounding cells.

What factors influence the rapidity of malignant transformation of a precancerous leukoplakia is unknown. The rate of the progression to cancer of different lesions that are already committed to the pathway to cancerization may unpredictably vary from 6 months to 8 years [46,58].

Conclusion

Leukoplakia is the most common potentially malignant lesion of the oral cavity. It can develop at single or multiple sites within fields of precancerous epithelial cells. Older age, high risk anatomical sites, larger lesions, erythroleukoplakia, high grade epithelial dysplasia, DNA aneuploidy and LoH at certain defined chromosomal loci are associated with greater risk of carcinomatous transformation of oral leukoplakia.

Carcinomatous transformation of oral leukoplakia may or may not occur irrespective of the detection of molecular markers related to early or late genetic events associated with cancer. The question still to be answered is: what are the genetic events associated with the progressive transformation of keratinocytes in which LOH or aneuploidy cannot be demonstrated, in carcinomatous cells?

References

[1] Warnakulasuriya S, Johnson NW, van der Waal I. Nomenclature and classification of potentially malignant disorders of the oral mucosa. *J. Oral. Pathol. Med.* 2007; 36: 575-580.

[2] Neville RW, Damm DD, Allen CM, Buquot JE. *Oral and maxillofacial pathology.* 3rd Edition. China, Saunders Elsevier; 2009, Chapter 10: pg 388-397.

[3] Warnakulasuriya S. Histological grading of oral epithelial dysplasia: revisted. *J. Pathol.* 2001; 194:294-297.
[4] Thomson PJ. Field change and oral cancer: new evidence for widespread carcinogenesis? *Int. J. Oral. Maxillofac. Surg.* 2002; 31:262-266.
[5] Califano J, van der Riet P, Westra W, Nawroz H, Clayman G, Piantadosi S, Corio R, Lee D, Greenberg B, Koch W, Sidransky D. Genetic progression model for head and neck cancer: implications for field cancerization. *Cancer Res.* 1996; 56:2488-2492.
[6] Tabor MP, Brakenhoff RH, van Houten VMM, Alain Kummer J, Snel MHJ, Snijders PJF, Snow GB, Leemans CR, Braakhuis BJM. Persistence of genetically altered fields in head and neck cancer patients: biological and clinical implications. *Clin. Cancer Res.* 2001; 7:1523-1532.
[7] Tabor MP, Braakhuis BJM, van der Wal JE, van Diest PJ, Leemans CR, Brakenhoff RH, Kummer JA. Comparative molecular and histological grading of epithelial dysplasia of the oral cavity and the oropharynx. *J. Pathol.* 2003; 199:354-360.
[8] Tabor MP, Brakenhoff RH, Ruijter-Schippers HJ, Kummer JA, Leemans CR, Braakhuis BJM. Genetically altered fields as origin of locally recurrent head and neck cancer: A retrospective study. *Clin. Cancer Res.* 2004; 10:3607-3613.
[9] Braakhuis BJM, Tabor MP, Kummer JA, Leemans CR, Brakenhoff RH. A genetic explanation of Slaughter's concept of field cancerization: evidence and clinical implications. *Cancer Res.* 2003; 63:1727-1730.
[10] Braakhuis BJM, Brakenhoff RH, Leemans CR. Second field tumours: A new opportunity for cancer prevention? *Oncologist* 2005; 10:493-500.
[11] Ha PK, Califano JA. The molecular biology of mucosal field cancerization of the head and neck. *Crit. Rev. Oral. Biol. Med.* 2003; 14:363-369.
[12] Lodi G, Sardella A, Bez C, Demarosi F, Carrassi A. Interventions for treating oral leukoplakia. Cochrane database of systematic reviews 2006, Issue 4. Art No.: CD001829. DOI:10.1002/14651858.CD001829.pub3.
[13] Reibel J. Prognosis of oral pre-malignant lesions: significance of clinical histopathological, and molecular biological characteristics. *Crit. Rev. Oral. BIol. Med.* 2003; 14:47-62.
[14] Suarez P, Batsakis JG, El-Naggar AK. Leukoplakia: Still a gallimaufry or is progress being made? A review. *Adv. Anat. Pathol.* 1998; 5:137-155.
[15] Napier SS, Speight PM. Natural history of potentially malignant oral lesions and conditions: an overview of the literature. *J. Oral. Pathol. Med.* 2008; 37:1-10.
[16] Scully C, Sudbø J, Speight PM. Progress in determining the malignant potential of oral lesions. *J. Oral. Pathol. Med.* 2003; 32:251-256.
[17] Holmstrup P, Vedtofte P, Reibel J, Stolze K. Long-term treatment outcome or oral premalignant lesions. *Oral. Oncol.* 2006; 42:461-474.
[18] van der Waal I, Axéll T. Oral leukoplakia: a proposal for uniform reporting. *Oral. Oncol.* 2002; 38:521-526.
[19] Reichart PA, Philipsen HP. Oral erythroplakia – a review. *Oral. Oncol.* 2005; 41:551-561.
[20] Feller L, Wood NH, Raubenheimer EJ. Proliferative verrucous leukoplakia and field cancerization: Report of a case. *J. Int. Acad. Periodontol.* 2006; 8:67-70.
[21] Bagan JV, Murillo J, Poveda R, Gavalda C, Jimenez Y, Scully C. Proliferative verrucous leukoplakia: unusual locations of oral squamous cell carcinomas, and field

cancerization as shown by the appearance of multiple OSCCs. *Oral. Oncol.* 2004; 40:440-443.

[22] Silverman S Jr, Gorsky M. Proliferative verrucous leukoplakia. A follow-up study of 54 cases. *Oral. Surg. Oral. Med. Oral. Pathol. Oral. Radiol. Endod.* 1997; 84:154-157.

[23] Cabay RJ, Morton TH Jr, Epstein JB. Proliferative verrucous leukoplakia and its progression to oral carcinoma: a review of the literature. *J. Oral. Pathol. Med.* 2007; 36:255-261.

[24] Zakrzewska JM, Lopes V, Speight P, Hopper C. Proliferative verrucous leukoplakia. A report of ten cases. *Oral. Surg. Oral. Med. Oral. Pathol. Oral. Radiol. Endod.* 1996; 82:396-401.

[25] Partridge M, Pateromichelakis S, Phillips E, Emilion GG, A'Hern RP, Langdon JD. A case control study confirms that microsatellite assay can identify patients at risk of developing oral squamous cell carcinoma within a field of cancerization. *Cancer Res.* 2000; 60:3893-3898.

[26] Zhang L, Cheung KJ Jr, Lam WL, Cheng X, Poh C, Priddy R, Epstein J, Le ND, Rosin MP. Increased genetic damage in oral leukoplakia from high risk sites. Potential impact on staging and clinical management. *Cancer* 2001; 91:2148-2155.

[27] Dietrich T, Reichart PA, Scheifele C. Clinical risk factors of oral leukoplakia in a representative sample of the US population. *Oral. Oncol.* 2004; 40:158-163.

[28] Lumerman H, Freedman P, Kerpel S. Oral epithelial dysplasia and the development of invasive squamous cell carcinoma. *Oral. Surg. Oral. Med. Oral. Pathol. Oral. Radiol. Endod.* 1995; 79:321-329.

[29] Lodi G, Porter S. Management of potentially malignant disorders: evidence and critique. *J. Oral. Pathol. Med.* 2008; 37:63-69.

[30] Feller L, Altini M, Slabbert H. Pre-malignant lesions of the oral mucosa in a South African sample – a clinicopathological study. *J. Dent. Assoc. S. Afr.* 1991; 46:261-265.

[31] Petti S. Pooled estimate of world leukoplakia prevalence: a systematic review. *Oral. Oncol.* 2003; 39:770-780.

[32] Warnakulasuriya S, Reibel J, Bouqout J, Dabelsteen. Oral epithelial dysplasia classification systems: predictive value, utility, weaknesses and scope for improvement. *J. Oral. Pathol. Med.* 2008; 37:127-133.

[33] Silverman S Jr, Gorsky M, Lozada F. Oral leukoplakic and malignant transformation. A follow up study of 257 patients. *Cancer* 1984; 53:563-568.

[34] Holmstrup P, Vedtofte P, Reibel J, Stolze K. Oral premalignant lesions: is a biopsy reliable? *J. Oral. Pathol. Med.* 2007; 36:262-266.

[35] Dakubo GD, Jakupciak JP, Birch-Machin MA, Parr RL. Clinical implications and utility of field cancerization. *Cancer Cell Int.* 2007; 7:2.

[36] Rhiner C, Moreno E. Super competition as a possible mechanism to pioneer pre-cancerous fields. *Carcinogenesis* 2009; 30:723-728.

[37] Mao L, El-Naggar AK, Papadimitrakopoulou V, Shin DM, Shin HC, Fan Y, Zhou X, Clayman G, Lee JJ, Lee JS, Hittelman WN, Lippman SM, Hong WK. Phenotype and genotype of advanced premalignant head and neck lesions after chemopreventive therapy. *J. Natl. Cancer Instit.* 1998; 90: 1545-1551.

[38] Lichtenstein AV. On evolutionary origin of cancer. *Cancer Cell Int.* 2005; 5:5.

[39] Nanci A. *Ten Cate's Oral Histology. Development, structure and function.* 7th Edition. Missouri: Mosby Elsevier; 2008, Chapter 12: pg 319-357.

[40] Loeb LA. A mutator phenotype in cancer. *Cancer Res.* 2001; 61:3230-3239.
[41] Mandard AM, Hainaut P, Hollstein M. Genetic steps in the development of squamous cell carcinoma of the esophagus. *Mutat Res.* 2000; 462:335-342.
[42] Jin C, Jin Y, Wennerberg J, Åkervall J, Dictor M, Mertens F. Karyotypic heterogeneity and clonal evolution in squamous cell carcinomas of the head and neck. *Cancer genet. Cytogenet.* 2002; 132:85-96.
[43] Jang SJ, Chiba I, Hirai A, Hong WK, Mao L. Multiple oral squamous epithelial lesions: are they genetically related? *Oncogene* 2001; 20:2235-2242.
[44] van Oijen MGCT, Slootweg PJ. Oral field cancerization: carcinogen-induced independent events or micrometastatic deposits? *Cancer Epidemiol, Biomarkers Prev.* 2000; 9:249-256.
[45] Kim MM, Califano JA. Molecular pathology of head-and-neck cancer. *Int. J. Cancer* 2004; 112:545-553.
[46] Rosin MP, Cheng X, Poh C, Lam WL, Huang Y, Lovas J, Berean K, Epstein JB, Priddy R, Le ND, Zhang L. Use of allelic loss to predict malignant risk for low-grade oral epithelial dysplasia. *Clin. Cancer Res.* 2000; 6:357-362.
[47] Garnis C, Buys TP, Lam WL. Genetic alteration and gene expression modulation during cancer progression. *Mol. Cancer* 2004; 3:9.
[48] Grizzi F, Di Ieva A, Russo C, Frezza EE, Cobos E, Muzzio PC, Chiriva-Internati M. Cancer initiation and progression: an unsimplifiable complexity. *Theor Biol. Med. Model.* 2006; 3:37.
[49] Warnakulasuriya S. Lack of molecular markers to predict malignant potential of oral precancer. *J. Pathol.* 2000; 190:407-409.
[50] Greenspan D, Jordan RCK. The white lesion that kills – Aneuploid dysplastic oral leukoplakia. *N. Eng. J. Med.* 2004; 350:1382-1384
[51] Ha PK, Tong BC, Westra WH, Sanchez-Cespedes M, Parrella P, Zahurak M, Sidransky D, Califano JA. Mitochondrail C-tract alteration in premalignant lesions of the head and neck: a marker for progression and clonal proliferation. *Clin. Cancer Res.* 2002; 8:2260-2265.
[52] Sudbø J, Kildal W, Risberg B, Koppang HS, Danielsen HE, Reith A. DNA content as a prognostic marker in patients with oral leukoplakia. *N. Engl. J. Med.* 2001; 344:1270-1278.
[53] Poeta ML, Manola J, Goldwasser MA, Forastiere A, Benoit N, Califano JA, Ridge JA, Goodwin J, Kenady D, Saunders J, Westra W, Sidransky D, Koch WM. TP53 mutations and survival in squamous cell carcinoma of the head and neck. *N. Engl. J. Med.* 2007; 357:2552-2561.
[54] Jin YT, Myers J, Tsai ST, Goepfert H, Batsakis JG, El-Naggar AK. Genetic alterations in oral squamous cell carcinoma of young adults. *Oral. Oncol.* 1999; 35:251-256.
[55] Santos-García A, Abad-Hernández MM, Fonseca-Sánchez E, Cruz Hernández JJ, Bullón-Sopelana A. Proteic expression of p53 and cellular proliferation in oral leukoplakias. *Med. Oral. Patol. Oral. Cir. Bucal.* 2005; 10:1-8.
[56] Mao L, Lee JS, Fan YH, Ro JY, Batsakis JG, Lippman S, Hittleman W, Hong WK. Frequent microsatellite alterations at chromosome 9p21 and 3p14 in oral premaligant lesions and their value in cancer risk assessment. *Nat. Med.* 1996; 2:682-685.
[57] Lee JJ, Hong WK, Hittelman WN, Mao L, Lotan R, Shin DM, Benner SE, Xu XC, Lee JS, Papadimitrakopoulou VM, Geyer C, Perez C, Martin JW, El-Naggar AK, Lippman

SM. Predicting cancer development in oral leukoplakia: Ten years of translational research. *Clin. Cancer Res.* 2000; 6:1702-1710.

[58] Zhang L, Williams M, Poh CF, Laronde D, Epstein JB, Durham S, Nakamura H, Berean K, Hovan A, Le ND, Hislop G, Priddy R,. Hay J, Lam WL, Rosin MP. Toluidine blue staining identifies high-risk primary oral premalignant lesions with poor outcome. *Cancer Res.* 2005; 65:8017-8021.

[59] Sudbø J, Lippman SM, Lee JJ, Mao L, Kildal W, Sudbø A, Sagen S, Bryne M, El-Naggar A, Risberg B, Evensen JF, Reith A. The influence of resection and aneuploidy on mortality in oral leukoplakia. *N. Engl. J. Med.* 2004; 350:1405-1413.

[60] Jin C, Jin Y, Wennerberg J, Åkervall J, Grenthe B, Mandahl N, Heim S, Mitelman F, Mertens F. Clonal chromosome aberrations accumulate with age in upper aerodigestive tract mucosa. *Mutat Res.* 1997; 374:63-72.

[61] Zhang L, Rosin MP. Loss of heterozygosity: a potential tool in management of oral premalignant lesion? *J. Oral. Pathol. Med.* 2001; 30:513-520.

[62] Weber F, Xu Y, Zhang L, Patocs A, Shen L, Platzer P, Eng C. Microenvironmental genomic alterations and clinicopathological behaviour in head and neck squamous cell carcinoma. *JAMA* 2007; 297:187-195.

[63] Baker SG, Kramer BS. Paradoxes in carcinogenesis: New opportunities for research directions. *BMC Cancer*; 2007; 7:151.

[64] Hong WK, Sporn MB. Recent advances in chemoprevention of cancer. *Science* 1997; 278:1073-1077.

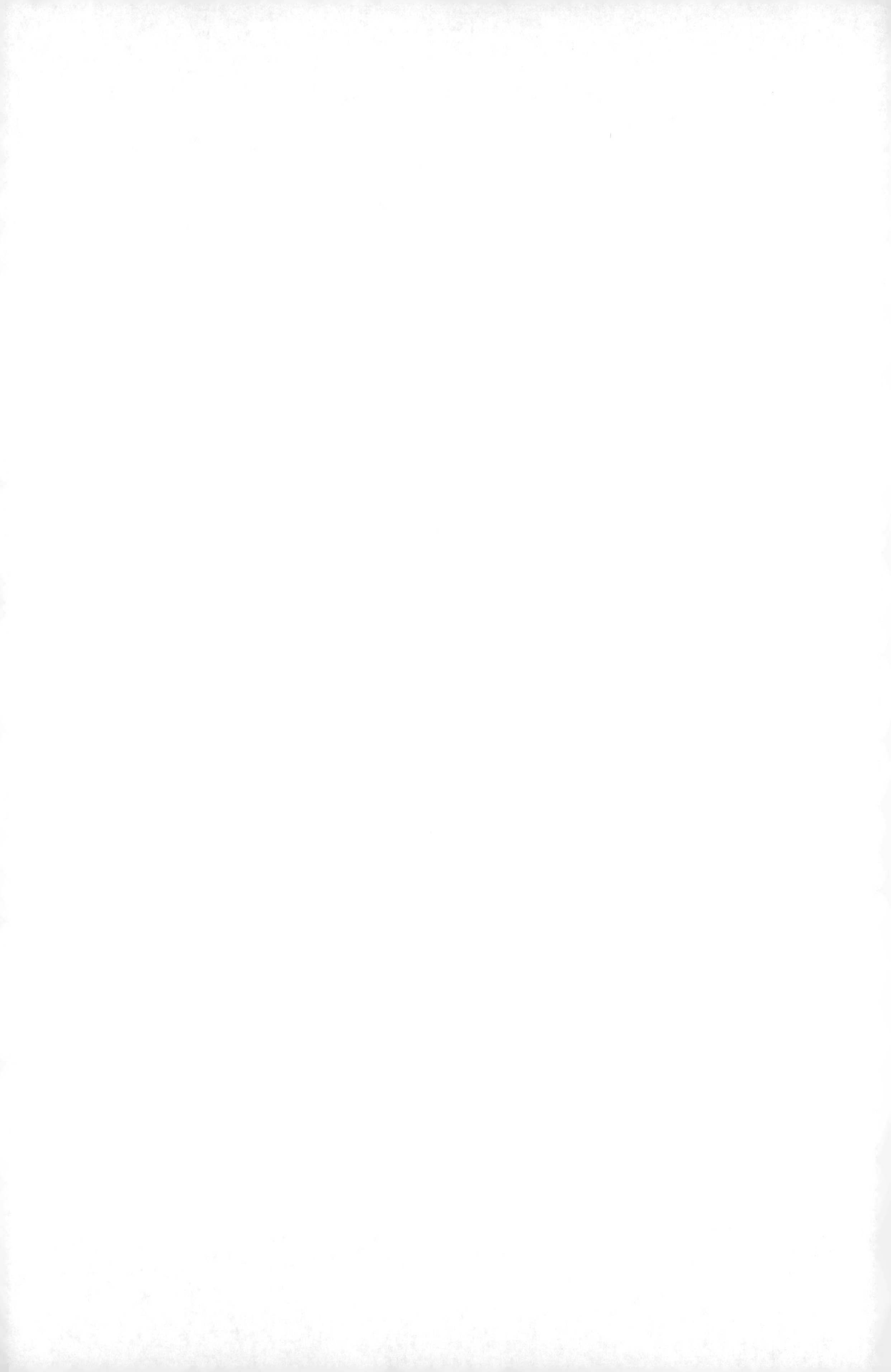

In: Field Cancerization: Basic Science and Clinical Applications ISBN 978-1-61761-006-6
Editor: Gabriel D. Dakubo

Chapter 7

Field Cancerization in Head and Neck Squamous Cell Carcinoma with Focus on Second Primary Tumors

Rostam D. Farhadieh

7.1. Introduction

Head and Neck Squamous Cell Carcinoma (HNSCC) remains a serious public health problem. Head and Neck Squamous Cell Carcinoma represents 5-10% of all newly diagnosed malignancies in Western Europe and the United States [1]. Laryngeal cancer is the most common HNSCC [1,2]. In the United States an estimated 37, 000 new cases and 12,000 expected deaths are recorded [3] each year. It has a worldwide incidence of 500, 000 cases per year [4]. The etiological risk factors in developing HNSCC clearly rest with tobacco and alcohol consumption [5]. The role of tobacco has been particularly reinforced by anatomical localization of tumors to the oral cavity of tobacco chewers and evidence of correlation of disease prevalence with the level of consumption of alcohol and tobacco [6,7] in combination.

Despite relatively early diagnosis and anatomical access for immediate surveillance, overall survival remains poor [8,9,10]. This overall dismal survival outcome from the disease has changed little in the past twenty years, the chief reason being loco-regional recurrent disease [11,12]. Approximately half the patients present with relatively advanced local disease with a 5 year expected survival rate of 10 to 40% [13]. In all, about 10% of patients with HNSCC develop regional recurrences while 10-15% present with distant metastasis, the main contributing factors to such low overall survival rate [12]. Surgery, radiotherapy (RT) and a combination of both are the mainstay of modern therapies. More recently evidence in support of chemo-induction and post operative synchronous chemotherapy has enhanced therapeutic outcomes [14,15].

The extent of disease is grouped into clinical staging in TNM prognostic classification stratifications. Histologically, the tumors are classified as well, moderate to well and undifferentiated in accordance with the degree of keratin formation and the maturity of the cancer cells. Large primary tumor size [16,17], presence of lymph node metastasis [18,19], positive margins after surgical excision [20,21] and perineural invasion [22] have been established as reliable clinical indicators of a poor outcome. The presence of extracapsular spread in the cervical lymph nodes remains the most significant prognostic indicator of survival, loco-regional recurrence and distant metastasis in patients suffering from HNSCC [23,24,25,26].

Briefly, RT continues to form one of the main pillars of treatment of HNSCCs. Ionizing radiation, which includes X-Rays and Gamma Rays, is considered carcinogenic. This same biological ability to break DNA strands, cause mutations, chromosomal aberrations and cell damage is utilized in external beam RT [27]. In the head and neck area however, this adverse carcinogenic effect has not been as clear [28,29,30,31]. The possibility of localized radiotherapy leading to the formation of Second Primary Tumors (SPTs), either regional or remote, has been weighed against the possible benefit of regional RT preventing at least a number of pre-neoplastic epithelial islands of the upper aero-digestive tract (UADT) from progressing to frankly invasive foci of SPTs [32]. Currently the literature indicates contradictory evidence in this regard. Evidence from several studies lends support to the assumption that RT leads to increased SPT incidence [28,29,30,33]. Other reports indicate that there is either a reduction or no significant difference in reported subsequent SPTs [32,34].

7.2. Biological Model

Since the discovery of p53, a dizzying number of other proteins and proportionately larger number of studies have sought to establish molecular progression theory of malignancies as fact. This ever exponentially expanding body of literature has demonstrated with some success, landmark steps in malignant transformation of normal mucosa to malignant tissue. The relevance of these investigations are not only in the inherent value of solving the riddle but with manifest improvement of clinical care and discarding of the current gross staging which although still relevant is outdated and in fact shown to be not overwhelmingly reliable. Groome et al showed that none of the staging systems currently used for HNSCC can account for a poultry 30% of variation in survival. In other words, the vast majority of survival variations are not accounted for by the current scheme [35,36]. This offers the prospect of significant improvement of the current understanding and clinical grouping of patients. Although, a complete review of the subject is out of the scope of this chapter salient features will be highlighted below before moving onto the next logical subject of predicting field changes and SPTs in HNSCC.

7.3. Neoplastic Progression Model

Original theory of multistep progression of neoplastic transformation was proposed for colon cancer a generation ago [37]. Since then, much like evolution, another biological model based on gains and losses of traits amongst organized collection of cells, species has become more or less accepted as the basic premise of carcinogenesis. This painful task of piecing this jigsaw together has proved elusive, although in recent years the advent of whole genome profiling through rapidly developing microarray and proteomic techniques have substantially added to the toolbox. It is now possible to analyze the expressions of hundreds or even thousands of genes at the same time in single samples. This allows development of molecular signatures, which in fact is a map that allows seeing the wood from the trees. These signatures can be used to determine aggression, risk of local disease failure, lymphatic as well as distant metastases in patients who would otherwise be classified in the same T, N, M staging. HNSCC progresses through well defined histopathologic stages that run parallel to genetic aberrations. Microsatellite analyses have identified several chromosomal areas that are thought to be rich with tumor suppressor genes [38,39,40]. Chromosomal loss at 9p, 3p, and 17p are considered early transforming events whilst *TP53* mutations and loss at 13q, 18q and 8p are considered late events [41,42,43,44]. There are some dated but excellent reviews on this subject [45,46,47].

7.4. Preneoplastic Clustering

The threat of malignant transformation and relative differing degrees of dysplasia of leukoplakia and erythroplakia are well known. These premalignant conditions have suffered some genetic changes, which has rendered their morphological and gross appearance abnormal [48,49,50]. This has led to the perspective that a screening tool should be possible not only for these premalignant lesions but to herald the prospect of future malignancies. Multiplex Ligation-Dependent Probe Amplification (MLPA) [51,52] technique was used for microsatellite analysis of oral exfoliated cells [53] and DNA ploidy status [51,54,55]. More recent application of microarray techniques has yielded some interesting results. It has demonstrated a closer relationship between genetic expression profiles of frankly malignant and premalignant lesions than the latter with control mucosal tissues [56].

7.5. Second Primary Tumors

Second Primary Tumors (SPTs) have a reported widely varied incidence of 5-30% following successful treatment of the index tumor (Table 7-1), and are considered an important negative prognostic marker [31, 57, 58, 59, 60, 61, 62, 63, 64, 65, 66, 67, 68, 69, 70, 71, 72, 73, 74]. The original definition of SPTs published by Warren and Gates in 1932 is still applied by most clinicians [75,76,77]. Slaughter's concept of "field of cancerization" or "condemned mucosa" has long been accepted as a coherent explanation of this phenomenon [78]. It has been postulated that repeated assault on the mucosa, by carcinogens results in the mucosal tissues developing multiple, independent neoplastic foci, separated by geography and time. It is now broadly accepted that the exposure of the upper aero-digestive tract (UADT), including lung and esophageal tissues, to tobacco and alcohol, is the main contributing environmental risk factor for the development of SPTs and index tumors alike. Currently there is no method of confidently predicting which of the patients will go on to develop SPTs.

Table 7.1. Patient series examining the incidence of Second Primary Tumors

Author	Patients (N)	Index Site	Time Delay To SPT (Yrs)	Incidence of SPTs		Site of SPTs							
						HNSCC-SPTs		Lung-SPTs		Esophagus-SPTs		Remote-SPTs	
				No	%	No	%	No	%	No	%	No	%
Berg[57]	1651	HNSCC	-	167	10.1	30	1.8	39	2.4	11	0.7	-	-
Boice[58]	4139	Larynx	1-4	541	13.1	40	1.0	178	4.3	19	0.5	139	3.4
Brown[59]	1600	HNSCC	5	61	3.8	16	1	18	1.1	-	-	17	1.1
Cohn[60]	267	Larynx	-	44	17	16	6.0	10	3.7	12	4.5	10	3.7
De Viri[61]	1660	Larynx	5.5	84	5	5	0.3	25	1.5	4	0.2	52	3.1
DeVries[62]	748	Larynx	4	104	14	9	1.2	64	8.6	0	0	31	4.1
Gluckman[63]	5337	HNSCC	-	548	11.2	246	5.0	181	3.7	120	2.5	-	-
Haughey[64]	3706	HNSCC	-	475	12.8	246	6.6	106	2.9	17	0.5	159	4.3
Larson[65]	875	HNSCC	1.5	207	23.7	126	14.4	54	6.2	13	1.5	-	-
Leon[66]	1074	Larynx	-	169	15.7	48	4.5	66	6.1	13	1.2	39	3.9
Lin[67]	662	Larynx	-	51	7.7	6	0.9	31	4.7	2	0.3	-	-
Lundgren[68]	295	Larynx	6.3	32	10.8	10	3.4	12	4.1	2	0.7	-	-
Masaki[69]	3162	HNSCC	-	182	5.8	66	2.1	34	1.1	-	-	18	0.6
McDonald[70]	235	Larynx	4	50	21	9	3.8	22	9.4	-	-	16	6.8
Miyahara[31]	1389	Larynx	0-23	138	9.95	43	3.1	23	1.7	3	0.2	68	4.9
Olsen[71]	3847	HNSCC	1-4	368	9.6	16	0.4	131	3.4	-	-	100	2.6
Tsou[72]	1477	HNSCC	1.9	108	7.3	63	4.2	5	0.3	14	0.9	39	2.6
Vaamonde[73]	636	HNSCC	-	48	7.5	34	5.3	7	1.1	4	0.6	3	0.5
Wagenfeld[74]	740	Larynx	-	48	6.5	16	48	25	52	-	-	-	-
Farhadieh	987	Larynx	3.5	143	14.5	83	8.4	56	5.7	4	0.41	65	6.6

The group of patients who develop SPTs would most likely benefit from closer follow up surveillance, and the development of more aggressive or novel approaches to therapeutic algorithms. Biological models of the gradual accumulation of genetic alterations form the current understanding of neoplastic transformation from normal to malignant cells. More recently, attempts have been made to explain the biological origins of SPTs [49,79]. It would be of great clinical and therapeutic significance if predictive biological marker(s) in the index tumor could, with some level of reproducible certainty, herald the development of SPTs.

Diagnosis of Second Primary Tumors (SPTs) was based on standard criteria [80]:

- Each lesion is distinct and separated by normal tissue,
- The possibility of metastasis is excluded,
- Histological documentation of each malignancy at the time of diagnosis,
- Any tumor identified within 6 months of diagnosis of the index tumor was designated Synchronous and those occurring beyond 6 months as Metachronous,
- Lung lesions were designated SPTs only if solitary and histologically distinct from the index tumor.

Alternative theories have since been put forward which suggest that malignant cells from the index tumor may migrate in one of two ways to the SPT site. A clone of the cells may migrate through the tissues, saliva, or lymphatics to form a metastasis diagnosed as an SPT. Another theory suggests that from a field of clonally identical premalignant cells, an independent processes may occur resulting in two different tumors, the so called Second Field Tumors (SFTs) [49,75,79,81,82].

7.6. Genetic Changes in Head and Neck Squamous Cell Carcinoma

7.6.1. Role of Tumor Suppressor Genes and Abnormal Expression of Oncogenes

Recent advances in molecular biology have gone some way to unraveling the complex nature of acquired genetic abnormalities in neoplastic transformation of cells. Simplistically these include functional groups of proteins responsible for growth of the cell, regulation of growth rate, cohesion of cell mass, and migration as well as repair of cellular damage. In HNSCC, slowly the body of evidence is accumulating to indicate potential correlations of some of these genetic changes with morphologic and ultimately clinical behavior [45,82,83,84]. This transformation process includes inactivation of tumor suppressor genes such as p16, p21, and p53, as well as the activation of oncogenes, including c-Myc and c-Abl [46]. Dysregulation of the G1/S point in the cell cycle, owing to mutations in oncogenes or tumor suppressor genes, is the most common point of cellular dysregulation in neoplastic transformation [85]. Cyclins are the major regulators of the cell cycle. Cyclin D1 and p16ARF have already been established as independent prognostic factors of disease-free and overall survival in HNSCC. The p53 protein plays a pivotal role in genomic stability, cell differentiation, cell cycle arrest, DNA repair and apoptosis [86]. Dysfunction of this gene at any of the vulnerable points of regulation, promotion, suppression, protein expression, degradation and function remains the most common abnormality detected in human cancers, and is a relatively early change in the development of HNSCCs [87]. Human analogue of Murine Double Minute protein (MDM-2) forms a negative autoregulatory loop with p53, but is also involved in the modulation of many other signals of cell proliferation as well as apoptosis including pRB, E2F1, INK4A, p21 and p19ARF [88,89,90,91,92]. Another tumor suppressor, p33ING1b, further regulates this interactive loop. The exact mechanism of action of p33ING1b is not yet clear, however it appears to stabilize and enhance intranuclear expression of the p53 protein at least in part by antagonizing MDM2 related negative regulation of p53 expression [93,94,95].

7.6.2. Cell Cycle Aberrations

The tumor suppressor gene, p53, located on the short arm of chromosome 17, encodes a 53kD protein which plays a central role in genomic stability, cell differentiation, cell cycle arrest, DNA repair, and apoptosis [96,97]. The p53 protein was identified in 1979 [98,99,100] and its gene, *TP53*, was cloned in 1983 [101]. In 1989, the p53 protein was shown to block the transformation of rat embryo fibroblasts and in 1990 [102] it was implicated in most cases of Li-Fraumeni syndrome, a rare inherited condition associated with frequent occurrence of several types of cancer in affected individuals. The *TP53* gene consists of 11 exons, the first of which is non-coding [86]. The p53 protein is made up of 393 amino acids and comprises four regions with different functions. In the N-terminus of the protein there is a transactivation domain that is important for activation of specific genes, especially the *MDM2* gene. The central part contains the DNA binding site through which the p53 protein binds to specific sites. The C-terminal contains the tetramerization domain, which allows formation of the most active conformation state of the protein. The C-terminus also contains a regulatory binding site, which can negatively regulate the central DNA binding domain thus inhibiting specific p53 binding to different promoters. The p53 protein has a very short half life of about twenty minutes, which means it is normally undetectable by immunohistochemistry in the wild type state [86]. However, due to mutations, defects in the degradation pathway or binding to other proteins, it is functionally compromised and may be detectable in an almost exclusively nuclear distribution. As an example, p53 is known to bind to certain DNA virus encoded proteins such as SV40 large T, which blocks its DNA binding activity, or adenovirus E1B (55kD) which blocks its transcriptional activity, and HPV E6 which targets it for accelerated degradation [103].

Although the upstream activation of p53 is not as well understood as its downstream activity, hypoxia, UV exposure, irradiation and DNA damage can cause its activation, most likely through phosphorylation of specific residues. Three main categories are recognized to stimulate its activation: Oncogenic stimuli through the ARF pathway [104], UV and ionizing radiation through the ATM pathway, as well as other ways such as hypoxia [105], cytokines and growth factors [106]. Once activated it functions by means of activating other genes and mobilizing protein products by non-specifically binding to DNA. This is achieved through the C-terminus, which as pointed out earlier, blocks the central specific DNA sites. This process is reversed through phosphorylation or acetylation of the C-terminus, thus enabling specific DNA binding and hence activation by the p53 protein. The p53 protein is regulated by rapid degradation and export from the nucleus as detailed below. The Nuclear Export Signals (NES) are within the C-terminus and once in tetramer conformation they are inaccessible by exportins [43,107].

The p53 gene is functionally impaired through deletion or mutation in nearly half of human cancers [108]. Although in the remaining human cancers it may retain wild type status, its function can be inhibited by its primary cellular inhibitor, the murine double minute 2 (MDM-2, HDM-2 in humans). MDM-2 was first discovered as the product of an oncogene found over-expressed by amplification in a spontaneously transformed mouse cell line [109]. Over expression of MDM-2 due to amplification of its gene was first discovered in sarcomas retaining wild type p53 [110]. This observation has since been observed in several other cancers [111]. Dysfunction of the *TP53* gene due to mutation is the most common abnormality detected in human cancers [112]. In most studies of HNSCC, however, p53 expression alone has not been consistently correlated with prognosis [113,114,115,116].

Most *TP53* alterations are mutations. These mutations may take the form of point mutations, deletions, or insertions. Most of the mutations are missense point mutations, which tend to concentrate within exons 5-8, spanning the evolutionary conserved region of the protein. Many of these mutations alter the p53 wild type conformation and yield stabilised proteins, which are detectable by immunohistochemistry. Moreover studies suggest that after mutation on one *TP53* allele, the remaining wild type allele is deleted, consequently, the mutant phenotype is the only one expressed [117,118]. Mutations of *TP53* are found in approximately 60% of HNSCCs. The reported mutation rates however, are widely disparate, ranging from 30-70% [119,120,121,122,123,124]. This frequency has been correlated with the level of alcohol and tobacco exposure. The frequency of mutations in smokers was twice that of non-smokers [124]. These are predominantly in the codons 238-248, which constitute a mutation hotspot region [125]. One recent study suggests that the mutation rate may be found to be even higher when all 11 exons of the *TP53* are sequenced [126]. The pattern of this mutation is consistent with tobacco related carcinogenesis, the most prevalent being G:C>A:T transitions and G:C>T:A tranversions. Furthermore it has been noted that p53 frameshift mutations occur more frequently in HNSCC (16%) than in other cancers in which this rate is around 9%[127].

Successive genetic alterations are responsible for the development of HNSCCs. p53 alterations are an early step in HNSCC pathogenesis, being detected in premalignant lesions [83]. Indeed evidence of suprabasal expression has been highly predictive of malignant transformation [128]. Furthermore, the presence of the full length p53 in the index tumour and nodal metastatic tissue were concordant confirming that the early mutations were preserved [129]. In relation to SPTs and the postulations of SFT changes, analysis of DNA extracted from morphologically normal tissue taken a distance of 0.5 cm from the margins demonstrated identical mutations in 3 of 8 samples, in support of clonal field changes in at least a proportion of SPTs [50,87,130]. This is even more relevant as clinical treatment is based on the clearance of the margins from disease. In an interesting report, Brennan and colleagues evaluated the presence/absence of mutant p53 in the surgically and morphologically cleared surgical margins and demonstrated that 13 patients had positive p53 mutations in the morphologically normal surgical margins. Moreover, among these patients, 38% had recurred locally whereas none of the 12 patients with negative mutation status in the margins had local recurrence [131]. This has been further confirmed in other reports [132,133].

Attempts to correlate the expression of wild type or mutant p53 in HNSCC with clinico-pathologic parameters have given contradictory findings. A number of studies have shown that *TP53* mutations are associated with an increased risk of locoregional recurrence and poor overall outcome [134,135,136,137]. Other reports describe over-expression of mutated p53 protein correlating with increased tumour recurrence, increased local control, decreased disease-free survival, and poorer overall survival [138,139,140]. However, equally there are many studies to suggest that *TP53* mutations or protein over-expression do not correlate with clinical outcome in patients with HNSCC [141,142,143,144]. Although the prognostic value of p53 expression is controversial on the whole, the case concerning *TP53* mutations is more convincing [137,145,146]. In a critical review of the evidence, Oh and Mao [147] concluded that although tumors with p53 over-expression tend to be more aggressive, the majority of studies have not been shown to demonstrate a statistically significant correlation with disease progression. However, they highlighted the report by Shin and colleagues, that using stringent criteria, patients with increased p53 expression had a poorer survival [148]. There has been further support for this view in two other reports, where p53 over-expression was defined strictly only when >75% of tumour cells stained positively for p53 expression [149,150]. Furthermore, accumulation of p53, as is the case for the mutant protein leads to the production by the patient of anti-p53 antibodies, which have been found in up to 17-19% of patients [122,151]. This is of vital importance as the absence of these antibodies is associated with a significantly increased risk of recurrence and poor overall survival. In fact the overall survival at 2 years was 63% when patients did not have anti-p53 antibodies compared to 29% where anti-p53 antibodies were present [152]. Interestingly the strongest correlation between p53 expression and clinical outcome is ascribed to an anatomical subset of HNSCCs in the larynx [153]. It has been claimed that the different survival rates for pharyngeal and laryngeal cancers (< 30% vs. 60% 5 year survival) is chiefly related to the difference in *TP53* mutational status, and actual mutations related to the increased carcinogenecity in the pharynx where alcohol is a more significant aetiological factor [154].

Cyclins are the major regulators of the cell cycle. Cyclin A1 is a highly tissue specific alternative CDK2 associated A-type cyclin [155,156,157]. It has been found to play an important role in neoplasia by encouraging G1/S cellular transition and thus promoting cellular proliferation [158]. Cyclin A1 is also a known downstream target of p53. It has been further implicated in a recent study demonstrating a direct relationship between forced cyclinA1 and wild type p53 expression in HNSCC cell lines [159]. The exact mechanism of action of cyclin A1 in neoplastic transformation is not clear. Cyclin A1 is present throughout the cell cycle and reaches its maximum expression during G2/M phase [160]. Its expression has been correlated directly to increased survival in myeloid leukemias and inversely with Multi-Drug-Resistant (MDR) relapse [161]. Cyclin A1/CDK2 interaction encourages cellular progression from G1 into the S phase, most likely through release of E2F from E2F/retinoblastoma protein (pRb) complex [160,161]. Other recent investigations have shown variable expression of cyclin A1 in testicular, cervical, endometrial, non-small cell lung, and breast cancers. In prostate cancer cell lines, Vascular Endothelial Growth Factor (VEGF) expression has been correlated with cyclin A1 expression. There is also some contradictory evidence in support of its role in cellular apoptosis [162,163].

MDM-2 has been shown to be a negative regulator of p53 mediated transactivation [164]. Together, they form an autoregulatory feedback loop [93]. Upon activation, p53 transcribes the *MDM-2* gene and in turn MDM-2 protein inhibits p53 activity through several means:

i. MDM-2 binds to the p53 transactivation domain in the N-terminus and inhibits its transcriptional activity [164,165];
ii. MDM-2 exports p53 out of the nucleus, promoting its degradation and rendering it inaccessible to its target genes [166]; the process is achieved through specific nuclear proteins called exportins;
iii. MDM-2 also promotes proteasome-mediated degradation of p53, functioning as an E3 ubiquitin ligase [167].

MDM-2 itself can be bound by p14ARF protein forming a complex with p53/MDM-2 that is retained in the nucleus. Furthermore it can also target MDM-2 for degradation causing release of p53 and return to function [168,169]. Dysfunction of *TP53* gene owing to mutations is the most common abnormality detected in human cancers [112]. In most studies of HNSCC however, p53 expression alone has not consistently been correlated with prognosis [113,114,115,116].

7.6.3. Role of p53 in Predicting Development of Second Primary Tumors

Until recently it was thought that development of SPTs represented progression of multiple separate genetically altered mucosal foci [75]. However, evidence from genetic studies including p53 mutation status, suggests that at least a proportion of these SPTs arise from residual portions of a single contiguous preneoplastic field after the complete gross resection of the index tumor. This proportion of SPTs have been termed Second Field Tumors (SFTs) to indicate their common genetic origin [81,130]. Indeed in an interesting report, Brennan and colleagues analyzed p53 mutation status in surgically and morphologically cleared surgical margins of patients with oral squamous cell carcinoma (OSCC) and demonstrated 13 patients had positive p53 mutation at the morphologically normal surgical margins. Moreover, among these patients 38% had recurred locally whereas none of the 12 patients with negative mutation status in the margins had local recurrence [131]. Observed widespread early neoplastic transformation underpinning future SPT formation with identical microsatellite changes in areas of dysplasia and synchronous OSCC in the same patients lend support to this theory [170].

A report from MD Anderson compared the results of survival as well as time to SPT and rate of SPT occurrence in 69 patients with HNSCC. In this series, patients with positive expression of p53 protein through DO7 immunohistochemistry were correlated with SPT diagnosis ($p=0.47$) as well as shorter time to SPT ($p=0.035$) [148].

More recently, we analyzed the SPT predictive measure of mutant p53, MDM-2 and Cyclin A1 protein in primary laryngeal SCC in 106 patients [171,172]. Tumor samples from 106 patients included in the study were used for immunohistochemical analysis. During the median follow up 41.0 ± 36.4 months, 4 patients died of unrelated causes, 42 died of HNSCC related causes and 60 patients were still alive. The latter patient group had a median survival of 75.8 ± 52.2 months (14-205). Protein expression was noted in a nuclear distribution within the tumor fields and was considered positive in 83/106 (78.3%) and 25/106 (23.6%) cases for cyclin A1 and mut-p53 expression respectively. There was a significant correlation between mut-p53 and cyclin A1 expression (Spearman's correlation coefficient=0.301, $p=0.002$).

MDM-2 protein expression was noted in a nuclear distribution within the tumor fields and was considered positive in 51/106 (48.1%) of cases.

Concurrent local and nodal recurrence also showed a significant inverse correlation with mut-p53 expression (p=0.038, p=0.029 Fisher's test). There were however, no other significant correlations between expression of any of the markers (mut-p53 and cyclin A1) and clinico-pathologic parameters or occurrence of SPTs.

Interestingly, Cyclin A1 is a known downstream target of p53. A recent investigation in HNSCCs demonstrated a 45% promoter hypermethylation of the cyclin A1 gene in twenty primary HNSCC tissue samples as well as in multiple cell lines, suggesting that cyclin A1 translation would be down-regulated. A further statistically significant inverse correlation between cyclin A1 promoter hypermethylation and p53 mutational status was demonstrated in a sample of thirty-nine primary HNSCC tissue samples. Eleven of nineteen patients with wild type p53 status showed cyclin A1 promoter hypermethylation compared to only four of twenty patients with a p53 mutation. This study concluded that a selective pressure against cyclin A1 expression exists when p53 is of wild-type status [1,159]. In our larger series (n=106) we were able to confirm this relationship between expression of mut-p53 and cyclin A1 proteins. However, we were unable to demonstrate any correlation with clinico-pathologic status including disease-free and overall survival or correlation with SPT occurrence during follow up.

7.7. Epidermal Growth Factor Receptor Expression in Head and Neck Squamous Cell Carcinomas

7.7.1. Potential Role of Epidermal Growth Factor Receptor Pathway

Dysregulation of the Epidermal Growth Factor Receptor (EGFR) is one of the best studied and most significant transmembrane cellular signalling systems leading to activation of intracellular signalling pathways in turn leading to inhibition of apoptosis, cellular proliferation, and angiogenesis [173]. Elevated levels of EGFR expression and abnormal function have been reported in many malignancies including HNSCC [174,175]. Adjuvant clinical application of EGFR inhibitors has recently been shown to improve survival and response to radiotherapy [176].

Epidermal Growth Factor Receptor (EGFR), so called type 1 Tyrosine Kinase (TK) receptor, was first purified in 1980, some 15 years after isolation of its ligand EGF [62,177]. Epidermal growth factor receptor is a 170kD glycoprotein with an encoding gene located on chromosome 7p12. It belongs to the ErbB receptor family (Her-1[EGFR], Her-2/*neu*, Her-3, Her-4). These receptors are composed of an extracellular N-terminal ligand binding domain, a hydrophobic transmembrane segment and an intracellular C-terminal tyrosine kinase domain, which also contains multiple phosphorylation sites involved in regulating TK activity. Once EGF or TGF-a, the natural ligands of the receptor bind with EGFR, it undergoes a conformational change. This promotes homodimerization with other EGFR molecules or heterodimerization with other Her family members, in particular with Her-2. This dimerization results in subsequent autoactivation of the tyrosine kinase from the intracellular domain of the receptor. The activated receptor is then able to recruit and activate several downstream signalling cascades including Ras/RAF/MEK/ERK, phosphtidilinositol-3 kinase (PI3K)-Akt, Stat and phospholipase C gamma pathways [178]. This process leads to further intracellular activation and induction of cellular proliferation, angiogenesis, inhibition of apoptosis as well as increased metastatic potential [179]. In HNSCCs, EGFR activation has been shown to result in activation of Src, which ultimately promotes invasion of cells [180]. Furthermore, EGFR translocates to the nucleus, where it acts as a transcription activator. It has been shown to activate the transcription of inducible nitric oxide (iNO) synthase by interacting with Stat 3 within the nucleus [181]. In a study of patients with oropharyngeal cancer, those with higher nuclear immunohistochemical EGFR expression had a higher local recurrence rate and lower disease free survival [182].

Epidermal growth factor receptor is over-expressed in many solid tumors of epithelial origin. In normal cells EGFR expression ranges from 40,000-100,000 receptors per cell, whilst in HNSCCs, EGFR is over-expressed in up to 80-90% of cases, and this is often associated with over expression of its natural ligand [183,184]. The magnitude of increase is 1.7 fold (P=0.005) and 1.9 fold (P=0.006) for receptor and ligand respectively [175]. The pathological end results of EGFR in HNSCC are achieved through at least four major mechanisms:

i. Over expression of EGFR ligands and establishment of autocrine/paracrine loops,
ii. Mutational activation of EGFR,
iii. Amplification of EGFR
iv. Transactivation by other receptor and non receptor TKs

Activating mutations of EGFR are an uncommon event in HNSCCs. A recent study showed that only 7.3% somatic mutations occurred in the gene in 41 tumor samples [185]. The amplification of EGFR gene does not appear to be a frequent event in HNSCCs and has only been demonstrated in 15% of tumors [186]. Mutational truncation of the extracellular domain, EGFR vIII, occurs infrequently in HNSCC and is more common in high-grade gliomas and non-small lung cancers. EGFR vIII results from the deletion of exons 2 to 7 and results in a constitutively activated intracellular kinase domain [187].

Epidermal growth factor receptor over-expression has been shown to be an independent prognostic indicator in patients with HNSCC. A study of 140 patients with laryngeal SCC showed that 5 year survival rate was 81% for patients with negative EGFR expression, whilst it was only 25% for those expressing EGFR (P<0.0001) [188]. This observation has since been corroborated by others [189]. In relation to radiotherapy (RT), employed as a vital tool in treatment of HNSCCs, another phase III study showed that EGFR expression, present in 148/155 patients, was an independent prognosticator of overall survival (P=0.006), disease-free survival (P=0.003) and locoregional recurrence (P=0.002) but not distant metastasis (P=0.5)[190]. There is more convincing evidence for radioresistance in the presence of high EGFR expression both in the clinical setting as well as in preclinical experiments performed using xenograft models [191,192,193]. This fact is highlighted by increased RT efficacy in conjunction with cetuximab, an anti-EGFR antibody [194]. The most significant of these studies involved a phase III trial of 424 patients with locally advanced HNSCC treated with RT alone or RT in conjunction with cetuximab. This trial showed a clear significant increase in the local control time period (24.4 months vs. 14.9 months; P=0.005), survival (49 months vs. 29.3 months; P=0.03) as well as tumour control and Overall Survival (OS) at 2 and 3 years. The most striking gains were made in patients with oropharyngeal cancers. Moreover, the grade 3-4 RT toxicities were not different [176].

Although not completely clear yet, part of the biological premise for this clinical phenomenon of radioresistance in the presence of EGFR over-expression may be found in its actual activation by ionising radiation and increased phosphorylation levels of downstream signalling pathways that are vital for cell survival; these include the Raf-1, MAPK, and Akt pathways [195,196]. Finally, in HNSCCs, EGFR derangement and over expression appears to be a relatively early process in neoplasia involving the field change concept. Elevated levels of EGFR have been demonstrated in morphologically normal margins as well as in dysplastic oral mucosal lesions [197].

7.7.2. Role of Epidermal Growth Factor Receptor in Development of Second Primary Tumors

Elevated levels of EGFR have been demonstrated in morphologically normal margins as well as dysplastic oral mucosal lesions [197]. More recently cyclo-oxygenase-2 (COX-2) enzyme, over-expressed in many premalignant and malignant human cancers including HNSCC has been targeted along with EGFR for chemoprevention in HNSCC cell lines as well as nude mice [198,199]. The results have demonstrated HNSCC cell line G1 cell cycle arrest [199] as well as reduced Vascular Endothelial Growth Factor (VEGF) expression and capillary angiogenesis arrest [198]. These results have clear implication in preventing SPT foci development.

We analyzed the predictive correlation of EGFR protein expression in 106 primary laryngeal SCC and subsequent SPT diagnosis. EGFR protein distribution was purely cytoplasmic.

It was considered positive in 82/106 (77.4%) and intensely positive in 53/106 (50.0%) cases [172]. In this cohort, 21/106 patients (19.8%) developed SPTs during the follow up period. There was a significant correlation between incidence of new primaries and both positive EGFR (p=0.003) as well as intensely positive EGFR expression (p=0.01). No correlation was noted between MDM-2 expression and incidence of new primaries. A univariate and multivariate analysis of both positive (p=0.02 and p=0.02) as well as intensely positive (p=0.03 and p=0.03) EGFR protein marker expression was correlated with diagnosis of second primary tumors respectively.

7.8. Future Directions

The advent of microarray studies has led to a revolutionary large amount of data being presented and fitted into patterns of correlation. Undoubtedly prediction of SPTs through analysis of patterns of protein expression aberrations in the index tumour will yield better clinical outcomes and more focused follow-up protocols.

References

[1] Pisani P, Bray F, Parkin DM (2002) Estimates of the world-wide prevalence of cancer for 25 sites in the adult population. *International Journal of Cancer* 97: 72-81.

[2] Jemal A, Thomas A, Murray T, Thun M (2002) Cancer statistics. *Cancer J. Clin.* 52: 23-47.

[3] Ries L, Eisner M, Kosary C (2003) SEER cancer statistics review, 1975-2000. National Cancer institute: Online http://seer.cancer,gov/csr/1975_2000.

[4] Parkin DM, Laara E, CS Muir (1988) Estimates of the worldwide frequecy of sixteen major cancers in 1980. *Int. J. Cancer* 41: 184-197.

[5] Tuyns AJ, Esteve J, Raymond L, Berrino F, Benhamou E, et al. (1988) Cancer of the larynx/pharynx, tobacco and alcohol: IARC internationla case control study in Turin and Varese (Italy), Zaragoza and Navarra (Spain), Geneva (Switzerland) and Calvados (France). *Int. J. Cancer* 41: 483-491.

[6] Ahrendt SA, Chow JT, Yang SC, Wu L, Zhang MJ, et al. (2000) Alcohol consumption and cigarette smoking increase in frequency of p53 mutation in non small cell lung cancer. *Cancer Research* 60: 3155-3159.

[7] Balaram P, Sridhar SB, Overgaard J (2001) TP53 mutation is related to to poor prognosis after radiotherapy, but not surgery, in squamous cell carcinoma fo the head and neck. *Radiother Oncol.* 59: 179-185.

[8] Porceddu SV, Campbell B, Rischin D, Corry J, Weih L, et al. (2004) Postoperative chemoradiotherapy for high-risk head-and-neck squamous cell carcinoma. *Int. J. Radiat. Oncol. Biol. Phys.* 60: 365-373.

[9] Temam S, Koka V, Mamelle G, Julieron M, Carmantrant R, et al. (2005) Treatment of the N0 neck during salvage surgery after radiotherapy of head and neck squamous cell carcinoma. *Head and Neck* 27: 653-658.

[10] Leemans CR, Tiwari R, Nauta JJ, van der Wall I, Snow G (1994) Recurrence at the primary site in the head and neck cancer and the significance of neck lymph node metastases as a prognostic factor. *Cancer* 73: 187-190.

[11] Leemans CR, Tiwari R, Nauta JJ, van der Waal I, Snow GB (1994) Recurrence at the primary site in head and neck cancer and the significance of neck lymph node metastases as a prognostic factor. *Cancer* 73: 187-190.

[12] Leemans CR, Tiwari R, Nauta JJ, van der Waal I, Snow GB (1993) Regional lymph node involvement and its significance in the development of distant metastases in head and neck carcinoma. *Cancer* 71: 452-456.

[13] Goldberg H, Lockwood S, Wyatt S, Crossett L (1994) Trends and differentials in mortality from cancers of the oral cavity and pharynx in the United States 1973-1987. *Cancer* 74: 565-572.

[14] Bernier J, Domenge C, Ozsahin M, Matuszewska K, Lefèbvre JL, et al. (2004) Postoperative irradiation with or without concomitant chemotherapy for locally advanced head and neck head and neck cancer. *N. Engl. J. Med.* 350: 1945-1952.

[15] Cooper JS, Pajak TF, Forastiere AA, Jacobs J, Campbell BH, et al. (2004) Postoperative current radiotherapy and chemotherapy for high risk squamous cell carcinoma of the head and neck. *N. Engl. J. Med.* 350: 1937-1944.

[16] Tytor M, Olofsson J (1992) Prognostic factors in oral cavity carcinomas. *Acta Otolaryngol. Supp*. 492: 75-78.
[17] Eiband J, Elias E, Suter C, Gray W, E D (1989) Prognostic factors in squmous cell carcinoma of larynx. *Am. J. Surg*. 158: 314-317.
[18] Nogouchi M, Kido Y, Kubota H, Kinjo H, Kohama G (1999) Prognostic factors and relative risk for survival in N1-3 oral squamous cell carcinoma: a multivariate analysis using Cox's hazard model. *Br. J. Oral. Maxillofac. Surg.* 37: 433-437.
[19] Shingaki Z, Li J, Li Z (2002) Circulating levels of vascular endothelial growth factor in patients with oral squmous cell carcinoma *Int. J. Oral. Maxillofac. Surg.* 31: 495-498.
[20] Jacobs J, Ahmad K, Casiano R, et al (1993) Implications of positive margins *Laryngoscope* 103 (Part 1): 64-68.
[21] Sutton D, Brown J, Rogers S, Vaughan E, Woolgar J (2003) The prognostic implications of the surgical margin in oral squamous cell carcinoma. *Int. J. Oral. Maxillofac. Surg.* 32: 30-34.
[22] Rahima B, Shingaki S, Nagata M, Saito C (2004) Prognostic significance of perineural invasion in oral and orophayrngeal carcinoma. *Oral. Surg. Oral. Med. Oral. Path. Oral. Radiol. Endod.* 97: 423-431.
[23] Greenberg J, Fowler R, Gomez J, et al (2003) Extent of extracapsular spread: a critical prognosticator in oral tongue cancer. *Cancer* 97: 1464-1470.
[24] Jose J, Coatesworth A, Johnsoton C, McLennan K (2003) Cervical node metastasis in squmous cell carcinoma of the upper aerodigestive tract: the significance of extracapsular spread and soft tissue deposits. *Head and Neck* 25: 451-456.
[25] Puri SK, Fan CY, Hanna E (2003) Signifgicance of extracapsular lymph node metastases in patients with head and neck squamous cell carcinoma. *Curr. Opinn. Otolaryngol. Head Neck Surg.* 11: 119-123.
[26] Woolgar JA, Rogers S, Lowe D, Brown J, E V (2003) Cervical lymph node metastasis in oral cancer: the importance of even extracapsular spread. *Oral. Oncol.* 39: 130-137.
[27] Hall J, Angele S (1999) Radiation DNA damage and cancer. *Mol. Med. Today* 5: 157-164.
[28] Begg CB , Zhang ZF, Sun M, Herr HW, Schantz SP (1995) Methodology for evaluating the incidence of second primary cancers with application to smoking-related cancers from the surveillance, epidemiology, and end results (SEER) program. *Am. J. Epidemiol.* 142 653–665.
[29] Gao X, Fisher SG, Mohideen N, Emami B (2003) Second primary cancers in patients with laryngeal cancer: a population-based study. *Int. J. Radiat. Oncol. Biol. Phys.* 56: 427-435.
[30] Hashibe M, Ritz B, Le AD, Li G, R S, et al. (2005) Radiotherapy for oral cancer as a risk factor for second primary cancers. *Cancer Letters:* 185-195.
[31] Mihara H, Sato T, Yoshino K (1998) Radiation-induced cancers of the head and neck region. *Acta Otolaryngol. Suppl.* 553: 60-64.
[32] Rusthoven K, Chen C, Raben D, Kavanagh B (2007) USe of external beam radiotherapy is associated with reduced incidence of second primary head and neck cancer: A SEER database analysis. *Int. J. Radiat. Oncol. Biol. Phys.*: E Pub.
[33] Lawson W, Som M (1975) Seoncd primary cancer after irradiation of laryngeal cancer. *Ann. Otol.* 84: 771-775.

[34] Jones AS, Morar P, Phillips DE, Field JK, Husband D, et al. (1995) Second primary tumors in patients with head and neck squamous cell carcinoma. *Cancer* 75: 1343–1353.

[35] Groome PA SK, Boyen M, SF Hall (2001) A comparison of published head and neck stage groupings in carcinomas of the oral cavity. *Head and Neck* 23: 613-624.

[36] Groome PA SK, Boyen M, SF Hall (2002) A comparison of published head and neck stage groupings in laryngeal cancer using data from 2 countries. *J. Clin. Epidemiology* 55: 533-544.

[37] Fearon ER, Vogelstein B (1990) A genetic model for colorectal tumorigenesis. *Cell* 61: 759-767.

[38] Gupta VK, Schmidt AP, Pashia ME, Sunwoo JB, Scholnick S (1999) Multiple regions of deletion on chromosome arm 13q in head and neck squamous cell carcinoma. *Int. J. Cancer* 84: 453-457.

[39] Sunwoo JB, Bolt MS, Radford DM, Deeker C, Scholnick S (1996) Evidence of multiple tumor suppressor genes on chromosome arm 8p in supraglottic laryngeal cancer. *Genes Chromosome and Cancer* 16: 164-169.

[40] Takebayashi S, Ogawa T, Jung KY, Muallem A, Mineta H, et al. (2000) Identification of new minimally lost regions on 18q in head and neck squamous cell carcinoma. *Cancer Res.* 60: 3397-3403.

[41] Bedi GC, Westra WH, Gabrielson E, Koch W, Sidransky D (1996) Multiple head and neck tumors: evidence for a common clonal origin. *Cancer Research* 56: 2484-2487.

[42] Ishwad CS, Ferrell RE, Rossie KN, et al (1996) Loss of heterozygosity of the short arm of chromosome 3 and 9 in oral cancer. *Int. J. Cancer* 69: 1-4.

[43] Sakaguchi K, Herrera JE, Saito S, et al (1998) DNA damage activates p53 through phosphorylation-acetylation cascade. *Genes Dev* 12: 2831-2841.

[44] Roz L, Wu CL, Porter S, et al (1996) Allelic imbalance on chromosome 3p in oral dysplastic changes: an early event in oral cancer. *Cancer Res.* 56: 1228-1231.

[45] Califano J, van der Riet P, Westra W, Nawroz H, Clayman G, et al. (1996) Genetic progression model for head and neck cancer: implications for field cancerization. *Cancer Research* 56: 2488-2492.

[46] Scully C, Field JK, Tanzawa H (2000) Genetic abberations in oral or head and neck squmous cell carcinoma: clinico-pathological applications III. *Oral. Oncol.* 36: 404-413.

[47] Scully C, Field JK, Tanzawa H (2000) Genetic abberations in oral or head and neck squmous cell carcinoma: clinico-pathological applications II. *Oral. Oncol.* 36: 311-327.

[48] Schepman KP, Van Der Meij EH, Smeele LE, Van Der Waal I (1998) Malignant transformation of oral leukoplakia: A follow-up study of a hospital basd population of 166 patients with oral leukoplakia from the Netherlands. *Oral. Oncol.* 34: 270-275.

[49] Braakhuis BJM, Tabor MP, Kummer JA, Leemans CR, Brakenhoff RH (2003) A genetic explanation of Slaughter's concept of field cancerization: evidence and clinical implications. *Cancer Research* 63: 1727-1730.

[50] Tabor MP, Brakenhoff RH, Ruijter-Schippers HJ, Kummer JA, Leemans CR, et al. (2004) Genetically altered fields as origin of locally recurrent head and neck cancer: a retrospective study. *Clinical Cancer Research* 10: 3607-3613.

[51] Bremmer JF, Braakhuis B J, Brink A, Broeckaert MA, Belien JA, et al. (2008) Comparative evaluation of genetic assays to identify oral precancerous fields. *J. Oral. Pathol. Med.* 37: 599-606.

[52] Bremmer JF, Braakhuis B J, Ruijter-Schippers, et al (2005) A non invasive genetic screening test to detect oral preneoplastic lesions. *Laboratory Investigation* 85.

[53] Rosin MP, Epstein JB, Berean K, et al (1997) The use of exfoliative cell samples to map clonal genetic alterations in the oral epithelium of high risk patients. *Cancer Res.* 57: 5258-5260.

[54] Mehrotra R, Gupta A, Singh M, Ibrahim R (2006) Application of cytology and molecular biology in diagnosing premalignant or malignant oral lesions. *Mol. Cancer* 5: 11.

[55] Remmerbach TW, Weidenbach H, Pomjanski N, et al (2001) Cytologic and DNA cytometric early diagnosis of oral cancer. *Annal. Cell Pathology* 22: 211-221.

[56] Ha PK, Benoit NE, Yochem R, et al (2003) A transcriptional progression model of head and neck cancer. *Clin. Cancer Research* 9: 3058-3064.

[57] Berg J, Schottenfield D, Ritter F (1970) Incidence of multiple primary cancers III. Cancers of the respiratory and upper digestive system as multiple primary cancers. *J. Natl. Cancer Inst.* 44: 263-274.

[58] Boice JD Jr, Fraumeni JFJ (1985) Second cancer following cancer of the respiratory system in Connecticut. *Natl. Cancer Inst. Monogr.* 68: 83-98.

[59] Brown M (1978) Second primaries in cases of cancer of larynx. *J. Layngol. Otol.* 92: 991-996.

[60] Cohn AM, Peppard SB (1980) Multiple primary malignant tumous of the head and neck. *Am J Otolaryngol* 1: 411-417.

[61] Deviri E, Bartal A, Goldsher M, Eliachar I, Steinitz R, et al. (1982) Occurrence of additional primary neoplasms in patients with laryngeal carcinoma in Israel (1960-1976). *Ann. Otol. Rhinol. Laryngol.* 91: 261-265.

[62] De Vries N, Snow GB (1986) Multiple primary tumours in patients with laryngeal cancer. *J. Layngol. Otol.* 100: 915-918.

[63] Gluckman JL, Crissman JD (1983) Survival rates in 548 patients with multiple neoplasms of the upper aero-digestive tract. *Laryngosope* 93: 71-74.

[64] Haughey BH, Gates GA, Arfken CL, Harvey J (1992) Meta-Analysis of second malignant tumors in Head and neck cancer: The case for and endoscopic screening protocol. *Ann. Otol. Rhinol. Laryngol.* 101: 105-112.

[65] Larson JT, Adams GL, Fattah H (1990) Survival Statistics for multiple primaries in head and neck cancer. *Otolarngol. Head and Neck Surg* 103: 14-23.

[66] Leon X, Quer M, Diez S, Orus C, Lopez-Pousa A, et al. (1999) Second neoplasm in patients with head and neck cancer. *Head and Neck* 21: 204-210.

[67] Lin K, Patel SG, Chu PY, Matsuo JMS, Singh B, et al. (2005) Second primary malignancy of the aerodigestive tract in patients treated for cancer of the oral cavity and larynx. *Head and Neck* 27: 1042-1048.

[68] Lundgren J, Olofsson J (1986) Multiple primary malignancies in patients treated for laryngeal carcinoma. *J. Otolaryngol.* 15: 145-150.

[69] Masaki N, Hashimoto T, Ikeda H, Inoue T, Kozuka T (1987) Multiple primary malignancies in patients with head and neck cancer. *Jpn J. Clin. Oncol.* 7: 303-307.

[70] McDonald S, Haie C, Rubin P, Nelson D, Divers L (1989) Second Malignant tumors in patients with laryngeal carcinoma: diagnosis, treatment and prevention. *Int. J. Radiat. Oncol. Biol. Phys.* 17: 457-465.

[71] Olsen J (1985) Second cancer following cancer of the respiratory system in Denmark, 1943-80. *Natl. Cancer Inst. Monogr.* 68: 309-324.

[72] Tsou Y, Hua CH, Tseng HC, Lin MH, Tsai M (2007) Survival study and treatment strategy for second primary malignancies in patients with head and neck squamous cell carcinoma and nasopharyngeal carcinoma. *Acta Oto-Laryngologica* 127: 651-657.

[73] Vaamonde P, Martin C, del Rio M, LaBella T (2003) second primary malignancies in patients with cancer of the head and neck. *Otolarngol. Head and Neck Surg* 129: 65-70.

[74] Wagenfeld D.J.H., Harwood A.R., Byrce D.P., van Nostrand P., DeBoer G (1981) Second primary respiratory tract malignant neoplasms in supraglottic carcinoma. *Arch Otolaryngol* 102: 135-137.

[75] Braakhuis BJM, Tabor MP, Leemans CR, van der Waal I, Snow GB, et al. (2002) Second primary tumors and field cancerization in oral and oropharyngeal cancer: molecular techniques provide new insights and definitions. *Head and Neck* 24: 198-206.

[76] Hong WK, Lippman SM, Itri LM, Karp DD, Lee JS, et al. (1990) Prevention of second primary tumors with isotretinoin in squamous-cell carcinoma of the head and neck.[see comment]. *New England Journal of Medicine* 323: 795-801.

[77] Warren S GO (1932) Multiple primary malignant tumours. A survey of the literature and a statistical study. *AmericanJournal of Cancer* 16: 1358-1414.

[78] Slaughter DP, Southwick HW, Smejkal W (1953) Field cancerization in oral stratified squamous epithelium. *Cancer* 6: 963-968.

[79] Braakhuis BJM, Leemans CR, Brakenhoff RH (2005) Expanding fields of genetically altered cells in head and neck squamous carcinogenesis. *Seminars in Cancer Biology* 15: 113-120.

[80] Warren S, Gates O (1932) Multiple primary malignant tumours: A survey of the literature and a statistical study. *Am. J. Cancer* 15: 1348-1414.

[81] Braakhuis BJM, Brakenhoff RH, Leemans CR (2005) Second field tumors: a new opportunity for cancer prevention? *Oncologist* 10: 493-500.

[82] Braakhuis BJM, Brakenhoff RH, Leemans CR (2005) Head and neck cancer: molecular carcinogenesis. *Annals of Oncology* 16 Suppl 2: ii249-250.

[83] Boyle JO, Hakim J, Koch W, van der Riet P, Hruban RH, et al. (1993) The incidence of p53 mutations increases with progression of head and neck cancer. *Cancer Research* 53: 4477-4480.

[84] Braakhuis BJM, Leemans CR, Brakenhoff RH (2004) A genetic progression model of oral cancer: current evidence and clinical implications. Jou*rnal of Oral Pathology and Medicine* 33: 317-322.

[85] Knudson AG (2002) Cancer genetics. *American Journal of Medical Genetics* 111: 96-102.

[86] Gomez-Lazaro M, Fernandez-Gomez FJ, Jordan J (2004) p53: twenty five years understanding the mechanism of genome protection. *Journal of Physiology and Biochemistry* 60: 287-307.

[87] Tabor MP, Brakenhoff RH, van Houten VM, Kummer JA, Snel MH, et al. (2001) Persistence of genetically altered fields in head and neck cancer patients: biological and clinical implications. *Clinical Cancer Research* 7: 1523-1532.

[88] Momand J, Zambetti GP, Olson DC, George D, Levine A (1992) The mdm-2 oncogene product forms a complex with the p53 protein and inhibits p53-mediated transactivation. *Cell* 69: 1237-1245.

[89] Michael D, Oren M (2002) The p53 and MDM2 families in cancer. *Curr. Opin. Genet.* Dev 12: 53-59.

[90] Zhang Z, Wang H, Li M, Agrawal S, Chen X, et al. (2004) MDM2 as a negative regulator of p21 WAF1/CIP1, independent of p53 *J. Biol. Chem.* 279: 16000-16006.

[91] Pomerantz J, Schreiber-Agus N, NJ L (1998) The Ink4a tumour suppressor gene product, pARF19, interacts with MDM2 neutralises MDM2 inhibition of p53. *Cell* 92: 713-723.

[92] Xiao ZX, Chen J, Levine AJ, Modjtahedi N, J X, et al. (1995) Interaction between the retinoblastoma protein and the oncogene MDM2. *Nature* 375: 694-698.

[93] Wu X, Bayle JH, Olson D, Levine A (1993) The p53-MDM2 autoregulatory feedback loop. *Genes. Dev.* 7: 1126-1132.

[94] Juven T, Barak Y, Zauberman A, George DL, Oren M (1993) Wild type p53 can mediate sequence specific transactivation of an internal promoter within the MDM2 gene. *Oncogene* 8: 3411-3416.

[95] Garkasvstev I, Kazarov A, Gudkov A, Riabowol K (1996) Suppression of the novel growth inhibitor p33ING1 promotes neoplastic transformation. *Nat. Genet.* 14: 415-420.

[96] Levin AJ, J M, Finlay C (1991) The p53 tumour suppressor gene. *Nature* 351: 453-456.

[97] Lane D (1992) p53: The guardian of the genome. *Nature* 358: 15-16.

[98] Linzer DI, Levine AJ (1979) Characterisation of a 54K dalton cellular SV40 tumour antigen present in SV40 transformed cells and uninfected embryonal carcinoma cells. *Cell* 17: 43-52.

[99] Del Leo AB, Jay G, Appella E, Dubois GC, Law LW, et al. (1979) Detection of a transformation related antigen in chemically induced sarcomas and other transofrmed cells of mouse. *Proc. Natl. Acad. Sci.* 76: 2420-2424.

[100] Lane DP, Crawford LV (1979) T antigen is bound to a host protein in SV40-transformed cells. *Nature* 278: 261-263.

[101] Oren M, Levine AJ (1983) Molecular clonining of a cDNA specific for the murine p53 cellular tumour antigen. *Proc. Natl. Acad. Sci.* 80: 56-59.

[102] Finlay CA, Hinds PW, Levine AJ (1989) The p53 proto-oncogene can act as a suppressor of transformation. *Cell* 57: 1083-1093.

[103] Lane DP (1998) Killing tumour cells with viruses- a question of specificity. *Nat. Med.* 4: 1012-1013.

[104] Lowe SW, Ruley HE (1993) Stabilisation of the p53 tumour suppressor gene is induced by adenovirus E1A and accompanies apoptosis. *Genes. Dev.* 7: 535-547.

[105] Graeber TG, Osmanian C, Jacks T, et al (1996) Hypoxia mediated selection of cells with diminished apoptotic potential in solid tumours. *Nature* 379: 88-91.

[106] Canman CE, Gilmer TM, Coutts SB, Kastan MB (1995) Growth factor modulation of p53-mediated growth arrest vesrsus apoptosis. *Genes. Dev.* 9: 600-611.

[107] Anderson ME, Woelker B, Reed M, Wang P, Tegtmayer P (1997) Reciprocal interference between the sequence specific core and nonspecific C-terminal DNA binding domains of p53: implications for regulation. *Mol. Cell Biol.* 17: 6255-6264.

[108] Feki A, Irminger-Finger I (2004) Mutational spectrum of p53 mutation in primary breast and ovarian tumours. *Crit. Rev. Oncol. Hematol.* 52: 103-116.

[109] Fakharzadeh SS, Trusko SP, George DL (1991) Tumourigenic potential associated with enhanced expression of a gene that is amplified in a mouse tumour cell line. *EMBO J.* 10: 1565-1569.

[110] Oliner JD, Kinzler KW, Meltzer PS, George DL, Vogelstein B (1992) Amplification of a gene encoding p53 associated protein in human sarcomas. *Nature* 358: 80-83.

[111] Mormand J, Jung D, Wilczynski S, Niland J (1998) The MDM2 gene amplification database. *Nucliec Acids Res.* 26: 3453-3459.

[112] Hollstein M, Sindransky D, Vogelstein B, Harris C (1991) p53 mutations in human cancers. *Science* 253: 49-53.

[113] Nylander K, Scildt EB, Eriksson M, Roos G (1997) PCNA, Ki67, p53, bcl-2 and prognosis in intraoral squamous cell carcinoma of the head and neck. *Analyt Cell Pathol.* 14: 1-10.

[114] Pande P, Soni S, Kaur J, Agarwal S, Mathur M, et al. (2002) Prognostic factors in betel and tobacco related oral cancer. *Oral. Oncol.* 38: 491-499.

[115] Yuen PW, Chow V, Choy J, Lam KY, Ho WK, et al. (2001) The clinicopahtologic significance of p53 and p21 expression in the surgical management of lingual squamous cell carcinoma. *Am. J. Clin. Pathol.* 116: 240-245.

[116] Kapranos N, Stathopolous GP, Manopoulos L, Kokka E, Papadimitriou C, et al. (2001) p53, p21, p27 protein expression in head and neck cancer and their prognostic value. *Anticancer Res.* 21: 521-528.

[117] Yin XY, Smith ML, Whiteside TL, Johnson JT, Berberman RB, et al. (1993) Abnormalities in the *P53* gene in tumours and cell lines of human squamous cell carcinomas of the head and neck. *Int. J. Cancer* 54: 322-327.

[118] Kiuru A, Servomaa K, Grenman R, Pulkkinen J, Rytomma T (1997) *P53* mutations in human head and neck cancer cell lines. *Acta Otolaryngol. Supp.* 529: 237-240.

[119] Temam S, Flahault A, Perie S, Monceaux G, Coulet F, et al. (2000) p53 gene status as a predictor of tumour response to induction chemotherapy of patients with locoregioanlly advanced squamous cell carcinomas of the head and neck *J. Clin. Oncol.* 18: 385-394.

[120] Brennan CT, Boyle JO, Koch WM, Goodman SN, Hruban R H, et al. (1995) Association between cigarette smoking and mutation of the p53 gene in squamous cell carcinoma of the head and neck. *N. Engl. J. Med.* 322: 712-717.

[121] Alsner J, Sorensen SB, Overgaard J, (2001) TP53 mutation is related to porr prognosis after radiotherapy, but no surgery, in squamous cell carcinoma of the head and neck. *Radiat. Oncol.* 59: 179-185.

[122] Cabelguenne A, Blons H, de Wazier I, Carnot F, Houllier AM, et al. (2000) p53 alterations predict tumour response to neoadjuvant chemotherapy in head and neck squmaous cell cell carcinoma: a prospective series. *J. Clin. Oncol.* 18: 1465-1473.

[123] Gillison ML, Koch WM, Capone RB, Spafford M, Westra WH, et al. (2000) Evidence for a causal assoication between human papillomavirus and a subset of head and neck cancers. *J. Natl. Cancer* 92: 709-720.

[124] Ko Y, Abel J, Harth V, Brode P, Antony C, et al. (2001) Association of CYP1B1 codon 432 mutant allele in head and neck squamous cell cancer reflected by somatic mutations of p53 in tumour tissue. *Cancer Res*. 61: 4398-4404.

[125] Wallace-Brodeur RR, Lowe SW (1999) Clinical implications of p53 mutations. *Cell Mol. Life Sci.* 55: 64-75.

[126] Kropveld A, Rozemuller EH, Leppers FG, Scheidel KC, de Weger RA, et al. (1999) Sequencing analysis of RNA and DNA of exons 1 through 11 shows p53 gene alterations to be present in almost 100% of head and neck squamous cell cancers. *Laboratory Investigation* 79: 347-353.

[127] Olivier M, Eeles R, Hollstein M, Khan MA, Harris CC, et al. (2002) The IARC TP53 database: new online mutation analysis and recommendations to users. *Hum. Mutat.* 19: 607-614.

[128] Cruz IB, Snijders PJ, Meijer CJ, Braakhuis BJ, Snow GB, et al. (1998) p53 expression above the basal cell layer in oral mucosa is an early event of malignant transformation and has predictive value for developing oral squamous cell carcinoma. *Journal of Pathology* 184: 360-368.

[129] Tjebbes GW, Leppers Vd Straat F G, Tilanus M G, Hordijk G J, Slootweg P J (1999) p53 tumour suppressor gene as clonal marker in head and neck squamous cell carcinoma: p53 mutations in primary tumour and matched lymph node metastases. *Oral. Oncol.* 35: 384-389.

[130] Tabor MP, Brakenhoff RH, Ruijter-Schippers HJ, Van Der Wal JE, Snow GB, et al. (2002) Multiple head and neck tumors frequently originate from a single preneoplastic lesion. *American Journal of Pathology* 161: 1051-1060.

[131] Brennan CT, Mao L, Hruban RH, Boyle JO, Eby YJ, et al. (1995) Molecular assessment of histopathological staging in squmous cell carcinoma of the head and neck. *N. Engl. J. Med.* 332: 429-435.

[132] Ball V, Righi P, Tejada E, Radpour S, Pavelic Z, et al. (1997) Immunostaining of surgical margins as a predictor of local recurrence in squamous cell carcinoma of the oral cavity and oropharynx. *Ear Nose Throat J.* 76: 818-823.

[133] Jin X, Zhou L, Zhao A (2000) Mutants of *P53* gene presence in laryngeal carcinoma and adjacent histopathologically normal tissue. *ORL J. Otolarhingol. Rel. Spec.* 62: 140-142.

[134] Koch WM, Brennan J, Zahurak ML (1996) *P53* mutation and locoregional treatment failure in head and neck squamous cell carcinoma. *J. Natl. Cancer* 88: 1580-1586.

[135] Erber R, Conradt C, Homann N, et al (1998) *TP53* DNA contact mutation are selectively assoicated with allelic loss and have a striong impact in head and neck cancer. *Oncogene* 16: 1671-1679.

[136] Ma L, Ronai A, Riede U, Kohler G (1998) Clinical implication of screening *P53* gene mutations in head and neck squmous cell carcinomas. *J. Cancer Res. Clin. Oncol.* 124: 389-396.

[137] Mineta H, Borg A, Dictor M, Wahlberg P, Akervall J, et al. (1998) *P53* mutation, but not p53 overexpression, correlates with survival in head and neck squamous cell carcinoma *Brit. J. Cancer* 78: 1084-1090.

[138] Khademi B, Shirazi F, Vasei M, et al (2002) The expression of p53, c-erbB-1 and c-erbB-2 molecules and their correlation with prognostic markers in patients with head and neck tumours. *Cancer Letters* 184: 223-230.

[139] Vielba R, Bilbao J, Ispizua A, et al (2003) p53 and cyclin D1 as prognostic factors in squamous cell carcinoma of the larynx. *Laryngoscope* 113: 167-172.

[140] De Vicente C, Junquera Gutierrez L, Zapatero A, et al (2004) Prognostic significance of p53 expression in oral squamous cell carcinoma without neck metastases. *Head and Neck* 26: 22-30.

[141] Gapany M, Pavelic Z, Gapany S, et al (1993) Relationship between immunohitochemistry detectable p53 protein and prognostic factors in head and neck tumours. *Cancer Detect Prev.* 17: 379-383.

[142] Friedman M, Lim J, Manders E, et al (2001) Prognostic significance of Bcl-2 and p53 expression in advanced laryngeal squamous cell carcinoma of the tongue. *Head and Neck* 23: 280-285.

[143] Pukkila M, Kumpulainen E, Virtaniemi J, et al (2002) Nuclear and cytoplasmic p53 expression in pharyngeal squamous cell carcinoma: prognostic implications. *Head and Neck* 24: 784-791.

[144] Smardova J, Ksicova K, Binkova H, et al (2004) Analysis of tumour suppressor p53 status in head and neck squamous cell carcinoma *Oncol. Rep.* 11: 923-929.

[145] Bradford CR, Zhu S, Poore J, Fisher SG, Beals TF, et al. (1997) p53 mutation as a prognostic marker in advanced laryngeal carcinoma. Department of vetrens affairs laryngeal cancer cooperative study group. *Acta Otolaryngol. Head Neck Surg* 123: 605-609.

[146] Bandoh N, Hayashi T, Kishibe K, Takahara M, Imada M, et al. (2002) Prognostic value of p53 mutations, bax, and spontanous apoptosis in maxillary sinus squamous cell carcinoma. *Cancer* 94: 1968-1980.

[147] Oh Y, Mao L (1997) Biomarkers in head and neck carcinoma. *Curr. Opin. Oncol.* 9: 247-256.

[148] Shin DM, Lee JS, Lippman SM, Lee JJ, Tu ZN, et al. (1996) p53 expressions: predicting recurrence and second primary tumours in head and neck squamous cell carcinoma. *J. natl. Cancer Inst.* 88: 519-529.

[149] Jin YT, Kayser S, Kemp BL, Ordonez NG, Tucker SL, et al. (1998) The prognostic significance of biomarkers p21WAF(CIP1), PR1WAF1(CIP1), p53, and bcl-2 in laryngeal squamous cell carcinoma *Cancer* 82: 2159-2165.

[150] Caminero MJ, Nunez F, Suarez C, Ablanedo P, Riera JR, et al. (1996) Detection of p53 protein in oropharyngeal carcinoma. Prognostic implications. *Arch. Otolaryngol. Head and Neck Surg.* 122: 769-772.

[151] Bourhis J, Lubin R, Roche B, Koscienly S, Bosq J, et al. (1996) Analysis of p53 serum antibodies in patients with head and neck squamous cell cancer. *J. Natl. Cancer* 88: 1228-1233.

[152] Chow V, Yuen AP, Lam KY, Ho WK, Wei WI (2001) Prognostic siginificance of serum p53 protein and p53 antibody in patients with surgical treatment for head and neck squamous cell carcinoma. *Head and Neck* 23.

[153] Narayanna A, Vaughan AT, Gunaratne S, Kathuria S, Walter S, et al. (1998) Is p53 an independent prognostic factor in patients with laryngeal carcinoma? *Cancer* 82: 286-291.

[154] Rowley H, Roland NJ, Helliwell TR, Caslin A, Kinsella AR, et al. (1998) p53 protein expression in tumours from head and neck subsites, larynx and hypopharynx and differences in relationship to survival *Clin. Otolaryngol.* 23: 57-62.

[155] Sweeney C, Murphy M, Kubelka M, Ravnik SE, Hawkins CF, et al. (1996) A distinct cyclin A is expressed in germ cells in the mouse. *Development* 122: 53-64.
[156] Diederichs S, Baumer N, Ji P, Metzelder SK, Idos GE, et al. (2004) Identification of interaction partners and substrates of the cyclin A1-CDK2 complex. *Journal of Biological Chemistry* 279: 33727-33741.
[157] Yang R, Nakamaki T, Lubbert M, Said J, Sakashita A, et al. (1999) Cyclin A1 expression in leukemia and normal hematopoietic cells. *Blood* 93: 2067-2074.
[158] Yang R, Morosetti R, Koeffler HP (1997) Characterization of a second human cyclin A that is highly expressed in testis and in several leukemic cell lines. *Cancer Research* 57: 913-920.
[159] Tokumaru Y, Yamashita K, Osada M, Nomoto S, Sun DI, et al. (2004) Inverse correlation between cyclin A1 hypermethylation and p53 mutation in head and neck cancer identified by reversal of epigenetic silencing. *Cancer Research* 64: 5982-5987.
[160] Yang R, Muller C, Huynh V, Fung YK, Yee AS, et al. (1999) Functions of cyclin A1 in the cell cycle and its interactions with transcription factor E2F-1 and the Rb family of proteins. *Molecular and Cellular Biology* 19: 2400-2407.
[161] Nakamaki T, Hamano Y, Hisatake J, Yokoyama A, Kawakami K, et al. (2003) Elevated levels of cyclin A1 and A (A2) mRNA in acute myeloid leukaemia are associated with increased survival. *British Journal of Haematology* 123: 72-80.
[162] Wegiel B, Bjartell A, Ekberg J, Gadaleanu V, Brunhoff C, et al. (2005) A role for cyclin A1 in mediating the autocrine expression of vascular endothelial growth factor in prostate cancer. *Oncogene* 24: 6385-6393.
[163] Muller-Tidow C, Diederichs S, Schrader MG, Vogt U, Miller K, et al. (2003) Cyclin A1 is highly expressed in aggressive testicular germ cell tumors. *Cancer Letters* 190: 89-95.
[164] Mormand J, Zambetti GP, Olson DC, George D, Levine AJ (1992) The MDM2 oncogene product forms a complex with p53 protein and inhibits p53 mediated transactivation. *Cell* 69: 1237-1245.
[165] Chen J, Marechal V, Levine AJ (1993) Mapping of the p53 and MDM2 interaction domains. *Mol. Cell Biol.* 13: 4107-4114.
[166] Freedman DA, Levine AJ (1998) Nuclear export is required for degradation of endogenous p53 by MDM2 and human papilloma virus E^. *Mol. Cell Biol.* 18: 7288-7293.
[167] Haupt Y, Maya R, Kazaz M, Oren M (1997) Oncoprotein MDM2 promotes rapid degradation of p53. *Nature* 387: 296-299.
[168] Bates S, Phillips AC, Clark A, et al (1998) p14ARF links the tumour suppressor RB and p53. *Nature* 395: 124-125.
[169] Prives C (1998) Signalling to p53: breaking the MDM2-p53 circuit. *Cell* 95: 5-8.
[170] Scholes AG, Woolgar JA, Boyle MA, Brown JS, Vaughan ED, et al. (1998) Synchronous oral carcinomas: independent or common clonal origin? *Cancer Research* 58: 2003-2006.
[171] Farhadieh RD, Smee R, Rees CG, Salardini A, Jiang L, et al. (2009) Cyclin A1 Expression in Laryngeal Cancers Correlates with Diagnosis of New HNSCCs Primary. *ANZ Journal of Surgery* 79: 48-54.
[172] Farhadieh RD, Salardini A, Rees CG, Jia-Lin Yang, Russell PJ, et al. (2009) Protein Expression of Epidermal Growth Factor Receptor in Laryngeal Squamous Cell

Carcinoma Index Tumours Correlates with Diagnosis of Second Primary Tumours of the Upper Aero-Digestive Tract Annals of Surgical Oncology In Review.

[173] Jorissen RN, Walker F, Pouliot N, Garret TP, Ward CW, et al. (2003) Epidermal growth factor receptor: mechanisms of activation and signalling. *Exp. Cell Res.* 284: 31-53.

[174] Grandis J, Melhem M, Gooding W (1998) Levels of TGF-α and EGFR protein in head and neck squamous cell carcinoma and patient survival. *J. Natl. Cancer Inst.* 90: 824–832.

[175] Grandis J, Tweardy D (1993) Elevated levels of transforming growth factor α and epidermal growth factor receptor messenger RNA are early markers of carcinogenesis in head and neck cancer. *Cancer Res.* 53: 3579–3584.

[176] Bonner JA, Harari PM, Giralt J, et al (2006) Radiotherapy plus cetuximab for squmous cell carcinoma of the head and neck N. *Engl. J. Med.* 354: 567-578.

[177] Cohen S, Carpernter G, King L Jr (1980) Epidermal growth factor receptor protein kinase interactions: co-purification of receptor and epidermal growth factor enhanced phosphorylation activity. *J. Biol. Chem.* 255: 4834-4842.

[178] Grandis JR, Sok JC (2004) Signalling through the epidermal growth receptor during the development of malignancy. *Pharmacol Ther.* 102: 37-46.

[179] Roskoski R Jr (2004) The ErbB/HER receptor protein tyrosine kinases and cancer. *Biochem. Biophys. Res. Com.* 319: 1-11.

[180] Zhang Q, Thomas SM, Xi S, et al (2004) SRC family kinases mediate epidermal growth factor receptor ligand cleavage, proliferation, and invasion of head and neck cancer cells. *Cancer Research* 64: 6166-6173.

[181] Lo HW, Hsu SC, Ali-Seyed M, et al (2001) Nuclear interactionof EGFR receptor and its poteintial new role as a transcription factor. *Nat. Cell Biol.* 3: 802-808.

[182] Psyrri A, Yu Z, Weinberger P (2005) Quantitative determination of nuclear and cytoplasmic epidermal growth factor receptor expression in oropharyngeal squamous cell cancer by using automated quantitative analysis. *Clin. Cancer Res.* 11: 5856–5862.

[183] Bei R, Budillon A, Masulli L, et al (2004) Frequent overexpression of multiple ErbB receptors by head and neck squamous cell carcinoma contrasts with rare antibody immunity in patients. *J. Pathol.* 204: 317-325.

[184] Ongkeko WM, Altuna X, Weisman RA, Wang-Rodriguez J (2005) Expression of protein tyrosine kinases in head and neck squamous cell carcinomas. *Am. J. Clin. Pathol.* 124: 71-76.

[185] Lee JW, Soung YH, Kim SY, et al (2005) Somatic mutations of EGFR gene in squamous cell carcinoma of the head and neck *Clin. Cancer Res.* 11: 2879-2882.

[186] Temam S, Kawaguchi H, El-Naggar AK, et al (2007) Epidermal growth factor receptor copy number alterations correlate with poor clinical outcome in patients with head and neck squamous cell *Cancer J. Clin. Oncol* 16: 2164-2170.

[187] Zhu HJ, Iaria J, Orchard S, Walker F, Burgess AW (2003) Epidermal growth factor receptor: association of extracellular domain negatively regulates intracellular kinase activation in the absence of Ligand. *Growth Factors* 21: 15-30.

[188] Maurizi M, Almadori G, Ferrandina G (1996) Prognostic significance of epidermal growth factor receptor in laryngeal squamous cell carcinoma. *Br. J. Cancer* 74: 1253–1257.

[189] Ang KK, Andratschke NH, Milas L (2004) Epidermal growth factor receptor and response of head and neck carcinoma to therapy. *Int. J. Radiat. Oncol. Biol. Phys.* 58: 959-965.

[190] Ang KK, Berkey BA, Tu X, Zhang HZ, Katz R, et al. (2002) Impact of epidermal growth factor receptor expression on survival and pattern of relapse in patients with advanced head and neck carcinoma. *Cancer Res.* 62: 7350-7356.

[191] Milas L, Raju U, Liao Z, Ajani J (2005) Targeting molecular determinants of chemo-radioresistance. *Semin. Oncol.* 32: 578-581.

[192] Milas L, Fan Z, Andratschke NH, Ang KK (2004) Epidermal growth factor receptor and tumour response to radiation: in vivo preclinical studies *Int. J. Radiat. Oncol. Biol. Phys.* 58: 966-971.

[193] Sheridan MT, O'Dwyer T, Seymour CB (1997) Potential indicators of radiosensitivity in squamous cell carcinoma of the head and neck. *Radiat. Oncol. Invest.* 5: 180–186.

[194] Bianco C, Tortora G, Bainco R, Caputo R, Veneziani BM, et al. (2002) Enhancement of antitumour activity of ionising radiation b y combined treatment with selective epidermal growth factor receptor tyrosine kinase inhibitor ZD1839 (Iressa). *Clin. Cancer Res.* 8: 3250-3258.

[195] Yusoff P, Lao DH, Ong SH, Wong ES, Lim J, et al. (2002) Sprouty2 inhibits the Ras/MAP kinase pathway by inhibiting the activation of Raf. *J. Biol. Chem.* 277: 3195-3201.

[196] Gupta AK, McKenna WG, Weber CN, Feldman MD, Goldsmith JD, et al. (2002) Local recurrence in head and neck cancer: relationship to radiation resistance and signal transduction. *Clin. Cancer Res.* 8: 885-892.

[197] Grandis JR, Melhem MF, Barnes EL, Tweardy DJ (1996) Quantitative immunohistochemical analysis of transforming growth factor alpha and epidermal growth factor receptor in patients with squamous cell carcinoma of the head and neck. *Cancer* 78: 1284-1292.

[198] Zhang X, Chen Z, Choe MS, Lin Y, Sun SY, et al. (2005) Tumor Growth Inhibition by Simultaneously Blocking Epidermal Growth Factor Receptor and Cyclooxygenase-2 in a Xenograft Model. *Clin. Cancer Research* 11: 6261-6269.

[199] Chen Z, Zhang X, Li M, Wang Z, Wieand HS, et al. (2004) Simultaneously Targeting Epidermal Growth Factor Receptor Tyrosine Kinase and Cyclooxygenase-2, an Efficient Approach to Inhibition of Squamous Cell Carcinoma of the *Head and Neck Clin Cancer Research* 10: 5930-5939.

In: Field Cancerization: Basic Science and Clinical Applications ISBN 978-1-61761-006-6
Editor: Gabriel D. Dakubo

Chapter 8

Field Cancerization in Esophageal Epithelia Demonstrated by Telomere Shortening and Chromosomal Instability

Makoto Kammori

Abstract

Esophageal squamous cell carcinoma (ESCC) is an aggressive human malignancy with an extremely poor prognosis, possibly due to genomic instability in the tumor cells. Quantitative fluorescence in situ hybridization was used to compare chromosomal aberrations and telomere shortening in cells taken from ESCC tissue and from adjacent normal tissue. The results showed that the mean telomere length in ESCC cells was significantly less than in normal cells. Furthermore, chromosomal gains were greater in the ESCC cells. The ESCC cells also displayed several anaphase bridges, which are evidence of chromosomal instability. This chapter describes how telomere shortening and chromosomal instability are consistent with the concept of field cancerization in the esophagus.

8.1. Introduction

Esophageal squamous cell carcinoma (ESCC) is a fairly common cancer that shows striking variations in geographic distribution, reflecting exposure to specific environmental factors that are still poorly defined. Esophageal squamous cell carcinoma develops as a sequence of histopathological changes that typically involve esophagitis, atrophy, mild to severe dysplasia, carcinoma in situ, and finally, invasive cancer. Genetic changes associated with the development of ESCC include mutations of the p53 gene, disruption of cell-cycle control in G1 by several mechanisms (inactivation of *p16MTS1*, amplification of *cyclin D1*, alteration of RB), activation of oncogenes (e.g., *EGFR*, *c-MYC*) and inactivation of several tumor suppressor genes. Loss of heterozygosity on chromosome 17q25 has been linked with Howel-Evans syndrome (also known as familial keratoderma with carcinoma of the esophagus, or Tylosis), a rare autosomal dominant syndrome associated with high predisposition to ESCC. Chronic esophagitis is a frequent occurrence in populations at high risk of ESCC. These lesions often show focal accumulation of p53 protein, and in some instances, patches of cells positive for p53 gene mutation have been found in areas of esophagitis at the margins of tumors. This observation is consistent with the concept of field cancerization in the esophagus, and suggests that esophagitis may represent a promising target for early detection of ESCC [1, 2].

Telomeres are nucleoprotein complexes located at the ends of eukaryotic chromosomes, and play an important role in the maintenance of genomic integrity. Telomeres cap the ends of human chromosomes, protecting them against chromosome fusion and preventing the chromosome termini from being recognized as double-stranded DNA breaks [3-7]. Because conventional DNA replication cannot completely replicate the ends of linear chromosomes, normal somatic cells lose telomeric repeats with each cell division, both in vivo and in vitro: a phenomenon referred to as the "end-replication problem". Human telomeres thus play critical roles in the maintenance of chromosomal stability as well as in limiting the ultimate replication capacity of cells. It has been proposed that telomere shortening is an important biological factor in carcinogenesis, cell senescence, cell replication, cell immortality, and aging [8-12]. To further understand the relationship between telomere metabolism and field cancerization in ESCCs and adjacent non-neoplastic esophageal epithelium (NNEE), it is important to measure and compare the telomere lengths of these two regions [13].

We hypothesized that the very rapid cell proliferation that occurs in ESCC might accelerate the telomere loss in this region as compared with the adjacent NNEE. In this chapter, we introduce some of the techniques that have been used to test this hypothesis. First, we measured the telomere lengths of different cell types within human esophageal epithelial tissue using quantitative fluorescence in situ hybridization (Q-FISH) with peptide nucleic acid (PNA) probes for the telomere and centromere. To overcome the problem of measurements from incomplete nuclei, we based our estimates on the telomere to centromere intensity ratio (TCR). The rationale is that a similar proportion of centromere to telomere within any given slice will be the same as that in the entire cell, and that the length of the centromere is constant among individuals. Second, immunohistochemistry (IHC) was also used to determine telomerase activity, cell proliferation and basal-cell markers as well as expression of other markers including human telomerase reverse transcriptase (hTERT) protein, MIB-1 (Ki-67) and CD49f. Third, we quantified chromosomal instability by counting the frequency of anaphase bridges and comparing them between ESCC and NNEE cells [13, 14].

8.2. Results

8.2.1. Tissue Quantitative Fluorescence in Situ Hybridization (Tissue Q-FISH)

Digital images were acquired from DAPI-stained nuclei, FITC-labeled centromeres, and Cy3-labeled telomeres. We combined the three images after assigning pseudo-colors (Figures

8-1A and B) and subjected the images to computer analysis. The average TCR in ESCC was significantly lower than that in the basal cell layer, prickle cell layer, and stromal cells, respectively ($p < 0.0001$).

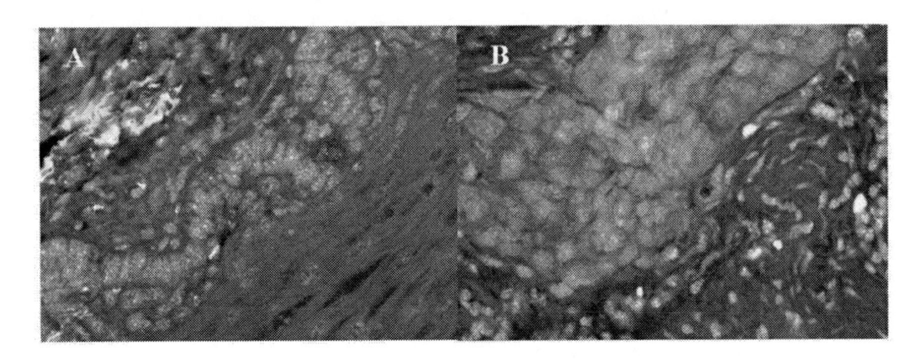

Figure 8.1. A and B. Examples of quantitative fluorescence in situ hybridization (Q-FISH) using normal and cancerous esophageal tissues and a PNA telomeric probe, a PNA centromeric probe, and DAPI counterstain. Telomere shortening is evident in the esophageal epithelium and in cancer cells. A: Tissue Q-FISH analysis of a specimen of esophageal cancer tissue. The tissue section was hybridized with a Cy3-conjugated telomeric PNA probe (red) and a FITC-conjugated centromeric PNA probe (green). The section was then counterstained with the fluorescent DNA dye DAPI (blue), and examined by normal microscopy. We used image analysis to identify nuclei and to correct for nuclear autofluorescence. An esophageal cancer tissue specimen shows reduced signal intensity from the telomeres but not the centromeres in cancer cells, as compared to stromal cells. B: Telomeric (red), centromeric (green), and nuclear counterstaining (blue) in a specimen of normal esophageal tissue shows stronger signal intensity from the telomeres in basal cells and stromal cells in the esophageal mucosa.

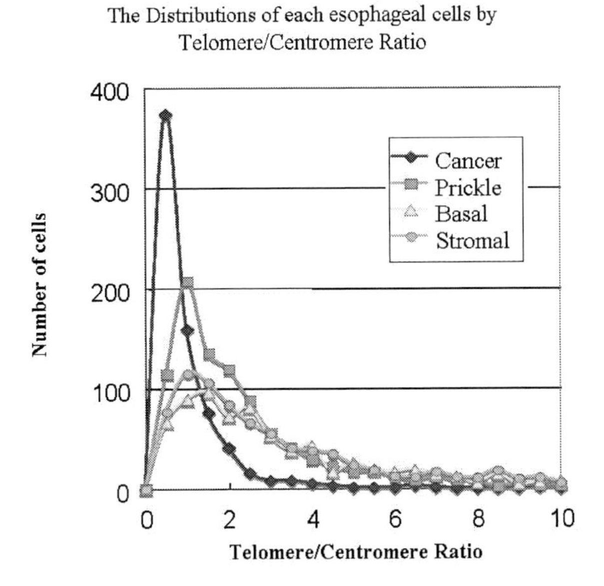

Figure 8.2. The TCR distributions of each esophageal cell type in esophageal tissue: basal, prickle, cancer, and stromal cells. The peak ratio in cancer cells is less than 1 whereas that in normal esophageal cells is greater than 1. A considerable number of non-cancerous cell types have telomeres similar in length to those of cancer cells.

We also analyzed the TCR distribution of each esophageal cell type using tissue Q-FISH. The peak percentage of TCR was less than 1 for ESCC, and greater than 1 for normal esophageal cell types. However, a considerable number of NNEE cells had telomeres similar in length to those of cancer cells (Figure 8-2).

8.2.2. Immunohistochemical Staining and in Situ Hybridization

The hTERT protein detected by IHC was strongly expressed in the nuclei and cytoplasm of almost all basal layer cells, a few of the parabasal layer cells, and almost all of the lymphocytes in the stromal layer (Figures 8-3A). The cell proliferation marker MIB-1 was strongly expressed in the nuclei of almost all the parabasal layer cells (including prickle cells) and a few basal layer cells (Figure 8-3B). CD49f, an epithelial marker, was strongly expressed in the cytoplasm of almost all basal cells (Figure 8-3C).

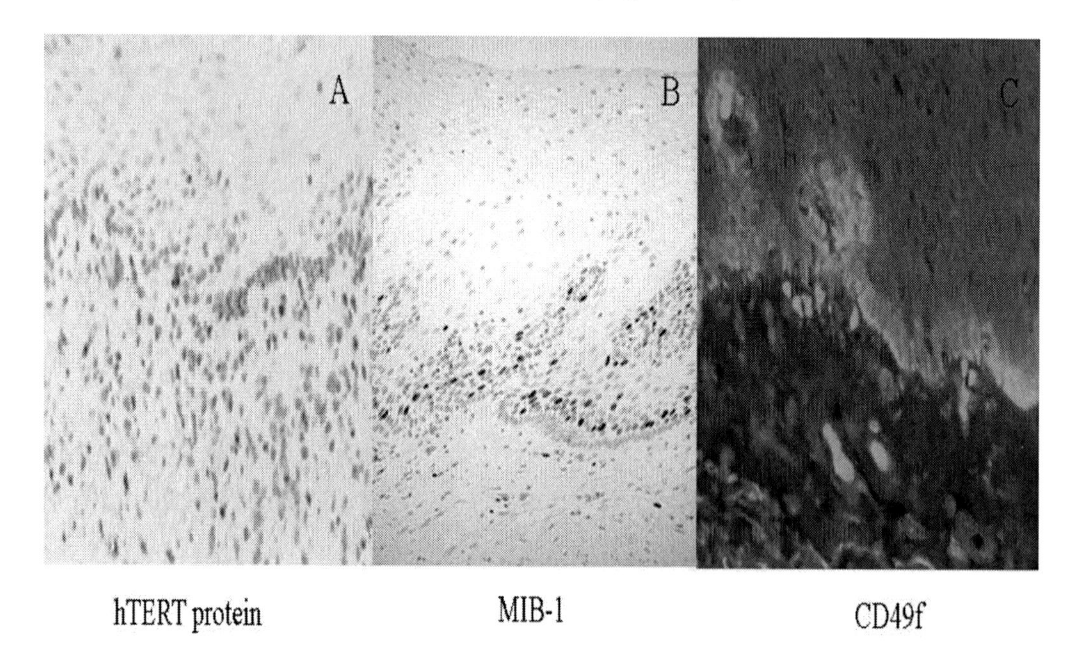

Figure 8.3. A,B and C. Immunohistochemical (IHC) staining of normal esophageal epithelium. A: IHC shows that the hTERT protein is expressed in the basal cells in normal esophageal epithelium and in lymphocytes of the normal esophageal submucosa. B: IHC shows that MIB-1, a marker of proliferating cells, is expressed in the epibasal cells, including prickle cells, of the normal esophageal epithelium. C: IHC-FISH shows that CD49f, an epithelial stem cell marker, is expressed in the basal layer cells of the normal esophageal epithelium.

8.2.3. Anaphase-Bridge Analysis

We examined the frequency of anaphase bridges in two ESCC cell lines (Figure 8-4A), two NNEE cell lines (Figure 8-4B), and tissue sections from esophageal cancer (Figure 8-4C). Although anaphase bridges were observed in both cancer and non-cancer cell lines, their frequency was significantly higher in cell lines derived from cancer and in sections of cancer tissue than in cell lines derived from NNEE (p = 0.002, p = 0.001), respectively (Figure 8-4).

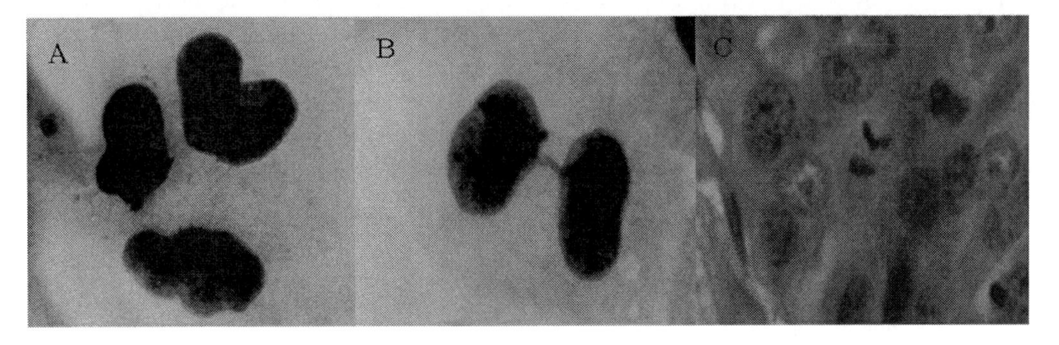

Figure 8.4. A, B and C. Anaphase bridge analysis. A: Cells line derived from ESCC. Images show a chromatin string connecting the nuclei in three adjacent cells, connecting three lobes of a nucleus, and connecting three nuclei. B: Epithelial cells of NNEE. Image shows a chromatin string connecting two lobes of a nucleus. C: H&E. staining shows an anaphase bridge in a tissue section of esophageal cancer.

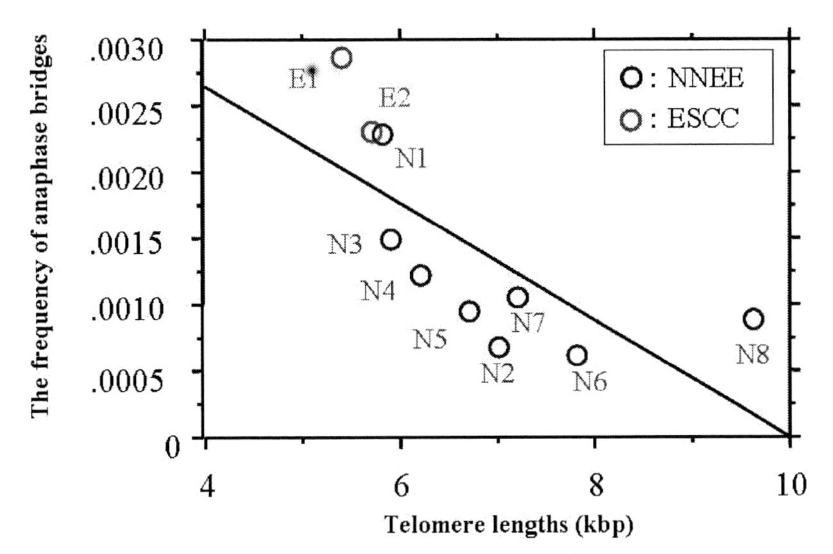

The frequency of anaphase bridges = 0 .00441 - .00044 * TRF; R^2 = .508
r=-0.696, p=0.0231

Figure 8.5. Correlation between telomere length and anaphase bridges in ESCC and NNEE cell lines. The frequency of anaphase bridges showed a significant inverse correlation with telomere length in ESCC and NNEE (p=0.0231).

8.5. Discussion

In normal esophageal mucosa, the basal layer cells have significantly longer telomeres than prickle layer cells and stromal cells. A telomerase component, hTERT, is strongly expressed in the nuclei and cytoplasm of almost all cells in the basal layer, a few cells in the parabasal layer, and almost all lymphocytes and stromal cells. Furthermore, MIB-1, a cell proliferation marker, is strongly expressed in the nuclei of almost all cells in the parabasal layer and a few cells in the basal layer. MIB-1 is present only in the nucleus during cell proliferation, and is commonly used as a measure of proliferative activity [15]. Telomerase consists of an RNA component, human telomerase RNA (hTERC), a catalytic protein subunit (hTERT), and other telomerase-associated proteins whose functions remain to be established. The expression of hTERT is largely restricted to cells with telomerase activity [15].

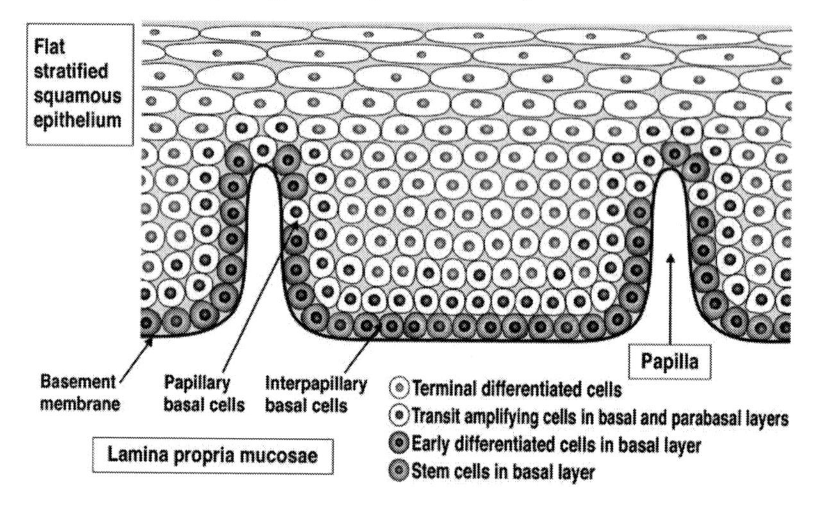

Figure 8.6. A schematic drawing of the cellular organization of human esophageal squamous epithelium. The basal layer contains stem cells, early-differentiated cells, and transit-amplifying cells. Stem cell division always gives rise to one daughter stem cell and one cell that becomes an early-differentiated cell. This early-differentiated cell divides into two cells, which are both early-differentiated cells, and these then differentiate into transit-amplifying cells in the basal layer. Thereafter, a transit-amplifying cell arises and divides into either a transit-amplifying cell or a terminally differentiated cell in the parabasal layer; these are then transferred to the upper epithelial layer.

Some stem cells express telomerase activity [16]. In this chapter, we have described that MIB-1 and hTERT are expressed in different cell layers. CD49f, a squamous epithelial cell-surface marker, was strongly expressed in the cytoplasm of almost all basal layer cells. These results suggest that squamous epithelial stem cells remain in the basal layer and have the longest telomeres of all cell types. In many invertebrate systems, stem cell division always gives rise to one daughter stem cell and one transit-amplifying cell [17]. Seery reported that esophageal epithelial stem cells remain in the basal layer while dividing into one daughter stem cell and one transit-amplifying cell [18]. Therefore, we hypothesize that the system of cellular organization in human esophageal squamous epithelium (Figure 8-6), and esophageal epithelial stem cells may exhibit several unusual properties, identification of which may facilitate future studies of esophageal carcinogenesis.

Anaphase bridges are chromatin bridges that are not resolved after anaphase [19]. They are a hallmark of telomere dysfunction and can lead to chromosomal losses, gains and rearrangements after breakage [20]. Although NNEE cell lines had anaphase bridges, their frequency was significantly lower than in ESCC cell lines, and a considerable number of anaphase bridges were observed in ESCC tissue sections. Here, the distribution of telomere fluorescence intensity for ESCC and NNEE cell lines overlapped. These results suggest that telomere shortening may be linked to a specific genetic alteration characteristic of esophageal squamous cancers.

Conclusion

We have provided evidence that esophageal epithelial stem cells remain in the basal layer of the normal esophageal epithelium. Both cancerous and normal epithelial cells occasionally have very short telomeres and anaphase bridges. Therefore, genetically unbalanced chromosomal translocations and anaphase bridges may be a result of shortened telomeres in ESCC and normal epithelial cells. The details outlined in this chapter further our understanding of the process by which telomere shortening and chromosomal instability lead to carcinogenesis and field cancerization in the esophagus.

References

[1] Mandard AM, Hainaut P, Hollstein M (2000). Genetic steps in the development of squamous cell carcinoma of the esophagus. *Mutation Res. 462,* 335-342.

[2] Tian D, Feng Z, Hanley NM, Setzer RW, Mumford JL, Demarini DM (1998). Multifocal accumulation of p53 protein in esophageal carcinoma: evidence for field cancerization. *Int. J. Cancer 78,* 568-575.

[3] Autexier C, Greider CW (1996). Telomerase and cancer: revisiting the telomere hypothesis. *Trends Biochem. Sci. 21*, 387-391.

[4] Artandi SE, Chang S, Lee SL, Alson S, Gottlieb GJ, Chin L, DePinho RA (2000). Telomere dysfunction promotes non-reciprocal translocations and epithelial cancers in mice. *Nature 406*, 641-645.

[5] Gisselesson D, Jonson T, Petersen A, Strombeck B, Dal Cin P, Hoglund M, Mitelman F, Mertens F, Mandahl N (2001). Telomere dysfunction triggers extensive DNA fragmentation and evolution of complex chromosome abnormalities in human malignant tumors. *Proc. Natl. Acad. Sci. USA 98,* 12683-12688.

[6] Blasco MA (2002). Telomerase beyond telomeres. *Nat. Rev. Cancer 2,* 627-33.

[7] Hackett JA, Greider CW (2002). Balancing instability: dual roles for telomerase and telomere dysfunction in tumorigenesis. *Oncogene 21*, 619-626.

[8] Harley CB, Villeponteau B (1995). Telomeres and telomerase in aging and cancer. *Curr. Opin. Genet. Dev. 5,* 249–55.

[9] Shay JW (1995). Aging and cancer: are telomeres and telomerase the connection? *Molecular Medical Today 1,* 378–384.

[10] de Lange T (1998). Telomeres and senescence: ending the debate. *Science 279,* 334–335.

[11] Greider CW (1998). Telomeres and senescence: the history, the experiment, the future. *Current Biology 8,* R178–181.

[12] DePinho RA (2000). The age of cancer. *Nature 408,* 248–254.

[13] Kammori M, Poon SS, Nakamura K, Izumiyama N, Ishikawa N, Kobayashi M, Naomoto Y, Takubo K (2007). Squamous cell carcinoma of the esophagus arises from a telomere-shortened epithelial field. *Int. J. Mol. Med. 20,* 793-799.

[14] Kammori M, Izumiyama N, Nakamura K, Kurabayashi R, Kashio M, Aida J, Poon SS, Kaminishi M (2006). Telomere metabolism and diagnostic demonstration of telomere measurement in the human esophagus for distinguishing benign from malignant tissue by tissue quantitative fluorescence in situ hybridization. *Oncology 71,* 430-436.

[15] Smith DL, Soria JC, Morat L, Yang Q, Sabatier L, Liu DD, Nemr RA, Rashid A, Vauthey JN (2004). Human telomerase reverse transcriptase (hTERT) and Ki-67 are better predictors of survival than established clinical indicators in patients undergoing curative hepatic resection for colorectal metastases. *Annuls of Surgical Oncology 11*, 45-51.

[16] Jaras M, Edqvist A, Rebetz J, Salford LG., Widegren B, Fan X (2006). Human short-term repopulating cells have enhanced telomerase reverse transcriptase expression. *Blood 108,* 1084-91.

[17] Watt FM, Hogan BL (2000). Out of Eden: stem cells and their niches. *Science 287*,1427-30.

[18] Seery, JP (2002). Stem cells of the esophageal epithelium. *J. Cell Sci. 115*,1783-9.

[19] Gisselsson D, Jonson T, Petersen A, Strombeck B, Dal Cin P, Hoglund M, Mitelman F, Mertens F, Mandahl N (2001). Telomere dysfunction triggers extensive DNA fragmentation and evolution of complex chromosome abnormalities in human malignant tumors. *Proc. Natl. Acad. Sci. USA 98*, 12683-8.

[20] O'Sullivan JN, Bronner MP, Brentnall TA, Finley JC, Shen WT, Emerson S, Emond MJ, Gollahon KA, Moskovitz AH, Crispin DA, Potter JD, Rabinovitch PS (2002). Chromosomal instability in ulcerative colitis is related to telomere shortening. *Nat. Genet. 32*, 280-4.

In: Field Cancerization: Basic Science and Clinical Applications ISBN 978-1-61761-006-6
Editor: Gabriel D. Dakubo

Chapter 9

Field Cancerization in Mammary Tissues

Marco Bisoffi, Christopher M. Heaphy and Jeffrey K. Griffith

Abstract

In this chapter we review published evidence for field cancerization within human mammary tissues. First, breast tissue development and morphology is revisited with a focus on the different cell types that can be affected by or contribute to field cancerization. Different definitions and possible concepts and cellular mechanisms of breast field cancerization are also presented. This is followed by a review of published molecular data including genetic, epigenetic, and expressional that is in support of mammary field cancerization. We then discuss the clinical importance of field cancerization in breast tissues as a source for biomarkers with diagnostic and prognostic potential, and its relationship to surgical margins and disease recurrence. We conclude with a future outlook of further research in breast field cancerization addressing experimental methods and the development of possible models to increase knowledge of this important field of research.

9.1. Introduction

The term "field cancerization" was originally introduced by D.P. Slaughter and colleagues as early as 1953 in the context of oral squamous cell carcinoma [3]. Field cancerization was used to describe the presence of histologically abnormal tissue surrounding cancerous lesions and was proposed to be the reason for the development of multiple primary tumors and locally recurrent cancer. The occurrence of field cancerization was then proposed for other organ systems [4,10,11], including mammary tissues, although it must be noted that the definition of the term has evolved to accommodate organ specificities and possible mechanisms. Of note, due to the tremendous progress in molecular biology and biotechnology since the 1950's, the description of field cancerization has changed from a largely histological perspective to a more refined molecular definition. This change is perhaps best reflected in the following definitions used previously in the literature; accordingly, field cancerization can denote:

> "The presence of histologically abnormal tissue surrounding cancerous lesions" as originally intended by Slaughter and colleagues in 1953 [3];
>
> Or:
>
> "The monoclonal or multiclonal displacement of normal epithelium by a genetically altered but microscopically undistinguishable homologue" as described by more recent authors [11] who used the term "hydra phenomenon of cancer".

The latter definition emphasizes the need to explain the general mechanisms of field cancerization in the context of specific organs. The occurrence of field cancerization in human mammary tissues is now an accepted phenomenon, as outlined in excellent recent reviews by D.L. Ellsworth and colleagues [12] and by G.D. Dakubo and co-workers [10], although it must be noted that to date, information on breast field cancerization remains relatively scarce compared to the literature relating to head and neck cancer. Current knowledge on mammary field cancerization will be discussed in detail in the subsequent sections of this chapter. However, before the various molecular evidences of field cancerization in mammary tissues are discussed, some general and subsequently more specific definitions of field cancerization must be considered for mammary tissues (see section 9.1.2). These definitions in turn are intricately linked to overall structure, histology, and development of human mammary tissues.

9.1.1. Developmental and Morphological Aspects of Human Mammary Tissue

To understand pathological alterations in human mammary tissues it is necessary to review mammary tissue development and histological structure. This includes a closer look at the cell types that are part of the complex structure of mammary tissue, and that can contribute to the molecular alterations defining mammary pathologies. In addition, the mammary gland is a structurally dynamic organ, varying with age, menstrual cycle and reproductive status. The dynamic changes in breast structure over time, from its embryologic inception, to pubertal growth, and onto its postmenopausal involution are characterized by highly complex cellular processes that offer multiple opportunities for initiating events related to field cancerization. For more detailed information, the reader is referred to text books and review articles covering aspects of mammary tissue development, physiology and morphology, *e.g.* [1,13,14,15,16,17].

Prenatal Development: The first visible indication of the mammary gland during prenatal development is the proliferation of paired areas of epithelial cells in the epidermis of the thoracic region. These proliferative areas then extend between the fetal axilla and inguinal region and form two indistinct ridges, termed the mammary ridges or milk lines. After some regression, two solid epithelial masses (the mammary buds) begin to grow downwards into the underlying mesenchyme. This solid core of cells continues to evaginate into the underlying mesenchyme and becomes surrounded by a more cellular zone of fibroblast-like cells within a dense collagenous mesenchyme. Solid secondary epithelial buds grow and branch off the main mammary bud, establishing the future lobed structure of the mature gland. During this period, the mesenchymal cells differentiate to form fibroblasts, smooth muscle cells, capillary endothelial cells and adipocytes: The future stroma. The epithelial cells form ductules consisting of a bilayer of cuboidal cells. The luminal layer rapidly gains the characteristics of secretory cells, while the basal layer becomes myoepithelial. This marks the establishment of the basic tubular architecture of the mammary gland, where the tubules are separated by "fat islands" within a dense fibrous stroma, and the rudimentary secretory epithelial cells have become functional. All of these prenatal cellular events are driven by maternal estrogens. After birth, the mammary glands remain at this rudimentary stage until puberty.

Puberty: The changing hormonal environment at the onset of puberty is the controlling factor for the sexually dimorphic (female *vs.* male) growth and development of the mammary gland. In the female, estrogen acts on the mesenchymal cells to stimulate further development. The gland increases in size, mainly due to the deposition of interlobular fat. The ducts extend and branch into the expanding stroma. This expansion includes epithelial cell proliferation and basement membrane remodeling, as controlled by stromal fibroblasts. By adulthood the complete ductal architecture of the gland is established. The small intralobular ducts end in epithelial buds which become the secretory alveoli. While the mammary glands remain in this mature but inactive state until pregnancy, relatively small cyclical changes induced by ovarian hormones occur during the menstrual cycle. Menstruation induces changes in both the stroma and the epithelial cells, with the latter changing morphology from cuboidal during the follicular phase to columnar during the luteal phase, which allows lumina with small secretions to develop. Importantly, there is a moderate level of cell proliferation, especially towards the end of the luteal phase. This is followed by abrupt involution and apoptosis during the last few days, before the onset of menstruation. The basement membrane (basal lamina) undergoes cyclical remodeling in concert with these cellular changes.

9.1.1.1. Structure of Adult Mammary Tissue

The developmental processes outlined above result in a branched tubulo-alveolar gland with secretory acini grouped within lobules and draining into *intra*lobular ducts, which in turn drain into *inter*lobular ducts (Figure 9-1A). The lobules are organized into 15 to 20 lobes, each of which empties into separate lactiferous sinuses and into lactiferous ducts that lead to the nipple. The stroma of the gland consists of a dense interlobular connective tissue, within which are varying amounts of adipose (fat) tissue and fibrous suspensory ligaments providing structural support.

The intralobular stroma consists of a loose cellular connective tissue with a zone of hormone sensitive fibroblasts surrounding the lobular epithelial components. The right upper panel in Figure 9-1B shows the schematic morphology of a terminal end bud within a lobule, embedded in adipose tissue and featuring its prominent cells: The epithelium consisting of non-secretory myoepithelial and secretory luminal epithelial cells, which become multilayered at the cap (body cells), separated by a basement membrane (basal lamina) from fibroblasts and adipocytes. Figure 9-1C shows a corresponding histological section through multiple ducts of a lobe at low magnification.

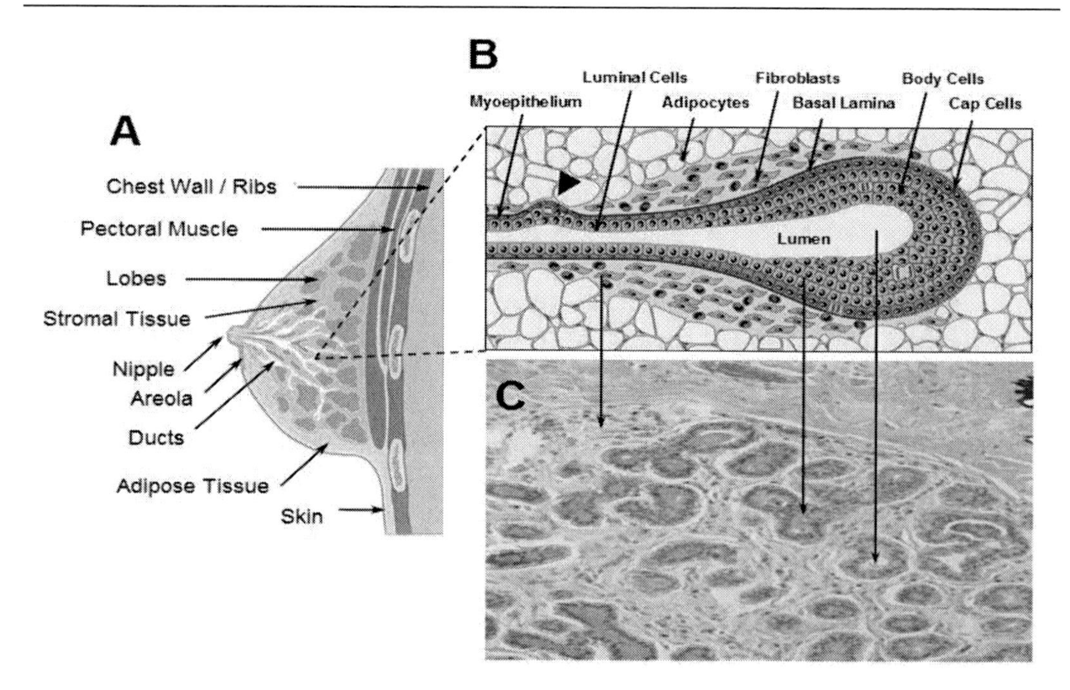

Figure 9.1. Structure of adult mammary tissue. (A) Morphology of the mammary gland consisting of ducts and lobes surrounded by stroma and adipose (fat) tissue. (B) Schematic morphology of a terminal end bud within a lobule, and its subtending ducts; different epithelial cells make up the epithelium separated by a basal lamina from fibroblasts and adipocytes. The arrow heads denote stromal macrophages/eosinophils (reproduced with permission from [1]). (C) Hematoxylin & eosin stained histological section of mammary tissue at low magnification. Arrows from left to right denote stromal area, ductal epithelium, and ductal lumen.

9.1.1.2. Pregnancy, Lactation, and Menopause

During pregnancy, the mammary gland epithelium experiences its greatest and most rapid phase of proliferation in response to a variety of hormones. During this phase, the terminal ductules branch and elongate and the epithelial cells proliferate from stem cells distributed throughout the gland. At the same time the adipose tissue and stroma of the gland progressively thin as the glandular components of the breast enlarge. The epithelial cells become cuboidal, with an extensive basal endoplasmic reticulum, basally situated nuclei, apical granules and cytoplasmic lipid droplets. The rate of milk secretion increases as the alveoli distend. Intralobular connective tissue surrounds the alveoli, the original dense connective tissue of the stroma thins to the extent that it appears as septae separating the lobules. A switch from estrogen and progesterone to prolactin control renders the secretory fully active in producing large volumes of milk, causing the alveoli to fully dilate. The dense interlobular connective tissue is reduced to a fibrous capsule surrounding the lobules. The alveolar contents are secreted by contraction of the myoepithelial cells.

After lactation ceases, epithelial cell numbers are reduced through apoptosis, the remaining cells become inactive and reduce in size and the alveoli and ducts regress back to a resting state. The stromal fibroblasts reconstruct the collagenous interlobular connective tissue and the gland becomes reinvested with adipose tissue.

The resting state is maintained in a manner similar to that of the post-pubertal gland, with the potential to re-enter the fully functional state during subsequent pregnancies. With age, the amount of elastic tissue increases, the stroma becomes more fibrous and less cellular and adipose tissue is lost. As menopause sets in, the ductal elements degenerate and dense connective tissue replaces the intralobular connective tissue.

9.1.1.3. Conclusions and Implication for Field Cancerization

It is important to note that two phenomena common to all of these events are proliferation and migration. Both are ultimately related to the malignant behavior of cancers, and may also pertain to mechanisms underlying field cancerization as described in the following sections. It is thus not surprising to find hypotheses in the literature that allude to the possibility that breast disease, including cancer, may start in the womb [18].

9.1.2. General Concepts and Definitions of Field Cancerization in Mammary Tissues

The dynamic processes outlined in section 9.1.1 offer multiple opportunities for molecular alterations to occur, even in the absence of histological change, which is the very definition of field cancerization. In addition, the glandular and rather complex structure of human mammary tissues raises a number of questions about the nature of the field, which need to be addressed before delving into the molecular details. First, it must be pointed out that "field cancerization" in human mammary tissue can be understood, and is being reported in the literature, in two ways:

i. The effect of altered epithelial cells, be they histologically cancerous or phenotypically normal yet genetically/biochemically altered, on their surrounding stroma as defined by fibroblasts, smooth muscle cells, capillary endothelial cells, and adipocytes; and
ii. The presence of altered epithelial cells throughout a tissue area, as defined in (i) above, that are seemingly independent from each other.

For the sake of clarity, these two possibilities should be separated using different terms. The effect of altered epithelial cells on the adjacent and/or further surrounding stromal cells in mammary tissues as described in (i) (see Figure 9-1 in section 9.1.1) should be viewed as one form of "reactive stroma" as described for solid tumors in general [19,20], notably prostate [21,22,23] and breast [24] cancers. Reactive stroma associated with tumors is usually discussed in the context of inflammatory processes as a reaction to the presence of tumor cells, or *vice versa* as a consequence of systemic inflammation priming the stroma to support cancer development and progression. It may also be meaningful to discriminate alterations into genetic and purely epigenetic changes. Both may lead to biochemical changes, as evidenced by RNA and protein expression, but the former is based on mutational events, while the latter can be a transient and reversible reaction to external stimuli. We generally refer to the second definition outlined above when discussing the phenomenon of field cancerization, and will thus not review here the literature describing the nature and importance of reactive stroma. In addition, we propose to define "alterations" in the context of field cancerization to reflect different cellular and molecular behavior as genetic, *i.e.* based on mutational events, as opposed to epigenetic as defined above. Finally, because we make the case that field cancerized cells may represent initiators of tumorigenesis, we tend to restrict these definitions to epithelial cells only, as solid tumors such as mammary carcinomas are epithelial in origin. However, caution must be used when applying the latter restriction, as it has been shown in breast cancer that cancerous epithelial cells are able to induce permanent karyotypic changes in the genome of adjacent stromal cells [25,26,27,28]. Some of these issues relating to the definition of field cancerization will again be approached, albeit from different points of view, in the next sections.

While it is clear that cancerous lesions are located in a field of phenotypically normal yet genetically and/or biochemically altered tissues, one fundamental and as yet unanswered question about field cancerization in solid tumors, including breast cancer, is whether the field precedes and gives rise to the tumor lesion at a location of highest genetic alteration, or whether the tumor lesion induces the field, or both, as shown in Figure 9-2A. A similar question relates to the extent and structure of the field itself: Is it uniform around the lesion, or is it comprised of multiple heterogeneous areas (patches) containing cells with different levels of genetic and/or biochemical alterations, as shown in Figure 9-2B? While these questions may seem to be of more interest to basic science, we propose in section 9.5 that the answers to these questions are of clinical importance.

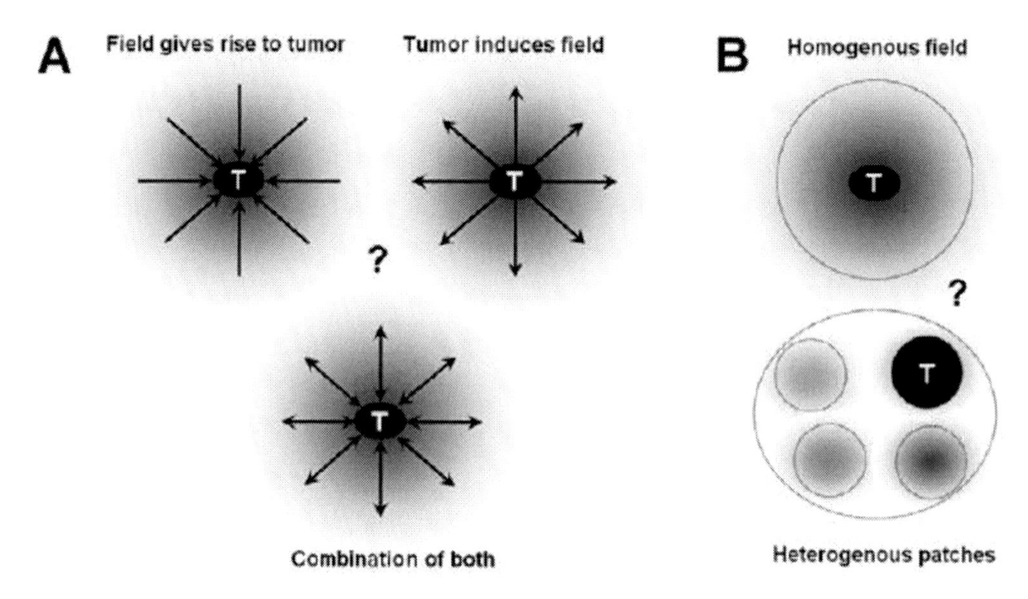

Figure 9.2. General concepts of field cancerization in mammary tissues. (A) The field (gradually shaded area), as defined by the occurrence of genetically and/or biochemically altered, yet phenotypically normal cells could precede and give rise to the tumor (T); or the tumor could induce the field; or both mechanisms could be at play. (B) The field could be uniform; or consists of heterogeneous areas (patches) of cells with different levels of genetic and/or biochemical alterations.

These questions centered on the general concepts of field cancerization are justified for human mammary tissues in the light of the relatively vast area (centimeters as opposed to millimeters) that can be affected. This distribution over relatively large distances will be confirmed at the molecular level in subsequent sections of this chapter and raises another question of general nature: How are the fields, as defined by the occurrence of genetically/biochemically altered cells and described in Figure 9-2, formed? This question partially overlaps with the previous ones but seeks a more mechanistic and cellular answer. As shown in Figure 9-3, we propose two possible major model processes that need not be exclusive of each other and could be at work simultaneously: The *stationary model* (Figure 9-3A) and the *migratory model* (Figure 9-3B). According to the *stationary model*, cells within a tissue area are continuously insulted by one or more external factors that are able to induce genetic alterations. These induced cells may gain a proliferative advantage and may divide to some extent. As a consequence, a field of cell patches with different levels of genetic and/or biochemical alteration is formed. In this model however, cells remain stationary and where the genetic/biochemical alterations are highest, histologically altered lesions with the propensity to develop into histologically detectable cancer may result. In the *migratory model*, continuous insult by external factors induce the formation of altered cells that may divide to some extent and form patches, but additionally develop the capability of migrating, thereby spreading the occurrence of altered cells and generating the field. In both models, these events can happen at multiple locations giving rise to polyclonal origins of altered fields, leading to heterogeneous fields described in Figure 9-2B.

The *migratory model* raises an additional question that may require a special view on cell motility. It is important to discern the type of cell migration that may be displayed by field cancerized cells forming the field from the invasive capabilities of cancer cells (Figure 9-4). Invasive cancer cells typically develop expressional changes that include the overproduction and secretion of extracellular proteases, such as matrix metalloproteinases (MMPs), urokinase plasminogen activator (uPA), cathepsins, and others [29,30,31,32], along with changes in expression of adhesion molecules, including integrins and cadherins [30,33]. These changes allow transformed cells to become anchorage independent, motile, and breach the basement membrane (basal lamina) and the underlying stromal compartment, giving rise to an altered structure typical for invasive carcinoma, as shown in Figure 9-4A.

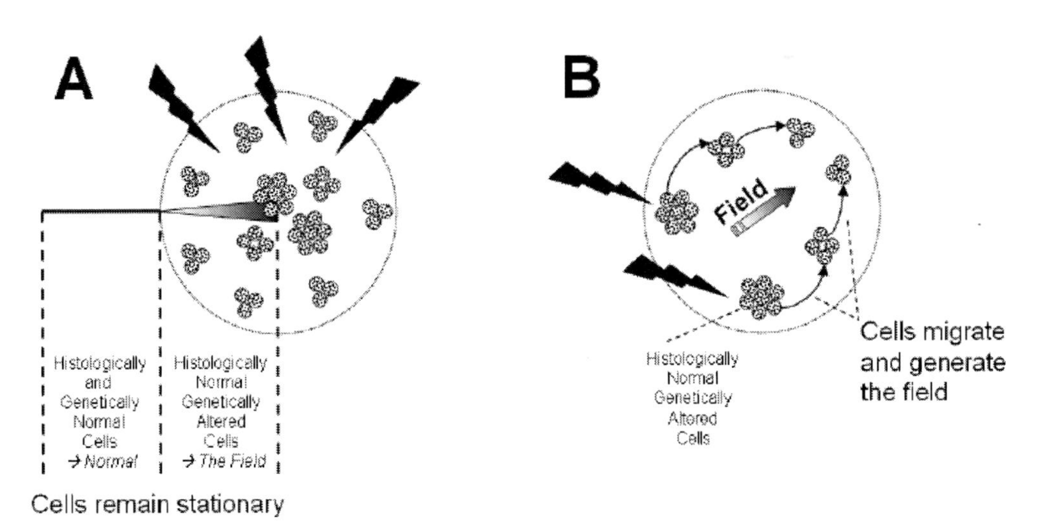

Figure 9.3. Concept models of field cancerization in mammary tissues. (A) *Stationary model*: Upon external insult (lightning bolts), cells undergo genetic/biochemical alterations, divide into patches, but remain stationary; regions with the highest level of alteration may develop histologically evident change. (B) *Migratory model:* External insult induces genetic/biochemical alterations leading to cell patches with migratory capabilities that form the field through spreading.

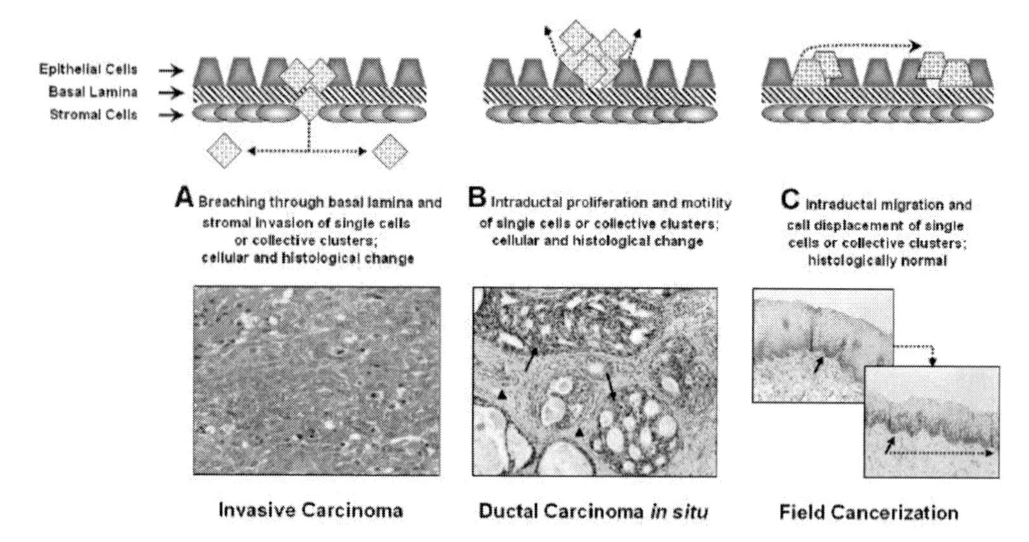

Figure 9.4. Types of cell migration occurring in or postulated for mammary tissues. (A) Histologically altered cells breach the basal lamina and invade stromal compartment (invasive carcinoma) leading to a chaotic histology. (B) Histologically altered cells proliferate, migrate, but remain within ducts leading to ductal carcinoma *in situ* (DCIS). Arrows denote areas of DCIS, arrowheads denote stroma. (C) Histologically normal yet genetically altered cells (patches) dislocate within epithelial sheets and expand the field according to the concept of "homologous positional information". Brown cell staining denotes immunohistochemical detection of p53 mutation. This concept is adapted from head and neck squamous cell carcinoma and is proposed by us as mechanism of field cancerization in mammary tissue (reproduced with permission from [4]).

Preceding or accompanying this frankly malignant phenotype may be conditions where cells are hyper-proliferative yet remain intraductal. This is the case for ductal carcinoma *in situ* (DCIS) as shown in Figure 9-4B or for atypical ductal hyperplasia (ADH), a proliferative alteration of mammary epithelial cells. It is important to note that for all of these conditions, the underlying cellular processes are microscopically visible as histological changes. In contrast, the migratory model applied to field cancerization in mammary tissues implies a type of intra-ductal cell motility that has to date not been established in mammary tissues, but stems from observations in head and neck squamous cell carcinoma [4], and has been hypothesized for other types of tumors with epithelial sheets [11] including breast cancer (Figure 9-4C). According to this model, phenotypically normal epithelial cells develop migrating capabilities and either individually or as collective clusters (often termed "patches") change location, thereby displacing other cells. It is postulated that this process, consisting of migration, survival (i.e. resistance to apoptosis/anoikis due to detachment), and proliferation is guided by intra-ductal tissue specific contacts and signals, possibly in partial combination with movement along paths of low mechanical resistance. Such cell dislocation would occur according to the concept of "homologous positional information" within tissues and along surfaces with "home-like" characteristics. Such information could be provided directly or indirectly by the local environment, including the basal lamina and various cells of the stroma, as shown for fibroblasts [34] and endothelial cells [35]. This concept is adapted here to explain possible mechanisms of field cancerization and stems from studies in embryology and fetal development, which may be retained in adult anatomic structures deriving from common precursor tissues representing homologous morphogenetic units (often termed "anlage" in developmental biology). Strong candidate molecules underlying these compartment-specific processes are by definition proteins engaged in cell-cell interaction and adhesion, such as integrins, as well as growth/survival and pro-migratory factors.

The exact mechanisms and molecules that permit such cell plasticity and migration without disrupting tissue structure remain largely elusive to date. However, these proposed processes are in excellent agreement with the second definition of field cancerization given in the introduction (section 9.1) of this chapter: "*The monoclonal or multiclonal displacement of normal epithelium by a genetically altered but microscopically undistinguishable homologue*". Furthermore, these processes also perfectly match the mammary anatomy reviewed in section 9.1.1, where cell displacement could happen over relatively large distances (centimeters) along the intertwined and highly branched ductal structures.

With these concepts in mind, we will now discuss the evidence for field cancerization in mammary tissues as reported in the literature by several groups working on this interesting and for breast disease, clinically important phenomenon. We have structured the content of the next sections according to the type of molecular alterations reported. While considering these data, it is hoped that the reader can refer back to the definitions and concepts provided in this introduction.

9.2. Genomic Aberrations in Histologically Normal Mammary Tissues

While section 9.1 defined and described the general concepts of field cancerization in mammary tissues, this section will focus on the genomic alterations that may accumulate in histologically normal breast tissues resulting from internal and external insults. It must be noted that mammary tissue comprises numerous cell types, including the mammary epithelium (including both myoepithelial and luminal cells), as well as the stromal cells (as outlined in Figure 9-1B). Cancer cells, as compared to normal cells, have been extensively studied and characterized for aberrations in genetic and molecular markers of their DNA. However, not until recently, have histologically normal mammary cells been extensively investigated. This section will focus on genomic alterations, including allelic imbalance, loss of heterozygosity, aneusomy, and telomere dysfunction in histologically normal breast tissues, including histologically normal tissues from both cancerous and disease-free mammary tissues. Numerous recent studies will be briefly discussed below.

9.2.1. Allelic Imbalance and Loss of Heterozygosity in Histologically Normal Mammary Tissues

Histological changes occur rather late in the malignant transformation process; however, molecular changes occur earlier and may reflect the earliest genetic changes underlying tumorigenesis. Genomic instability is the generation of chromosomal breakage and fusion throughout the genome and occurs in virtually all cancers. Genomic alterations, such as the loss or duplication of entire chromosomes or chromosomal regions, can be manifested as allelic imbalance. Allelic imbalance is a situation where one allele of a gene pair is lost or amplified resulting in a deviation from the normal 1:1 ratio of alleles. Allelic imbalance may be present as either the complete absence of one allele in a given locus (loss of heterozygosity, LOH), or the duplication or amplification of one or both alleles of a particular locus.

Several studies have focused on detecting allelic imbalance in histologically normal breast tissues. During the development of mammary tissue, genomic abnormalities may accumulate. Evidence for this was provided in previous studies that detected allelic imbalance in breast cancer precursors, such as proliferative breast lesions, for example atypical ductal hyperplasia [36,37]. Since it had been known that genetic alterations precede phenotypic changes, then it was postulated that these genetic abnormalities would be present in histologically normal tissue. Carol Rosenberg and her group sought to test the hypothesis that *"some genetic abnormalities may have occurred even earlier, i.e. before the development of histologically abnormal tissue and, therefore, might be detectable in normal-appearing breast ductal tissue"*. In a pilot study, this group analyzed normal-appearing breast ducts or terminal ductal lobular units (TDLUs) from twenty women that varied by risk of developing breast cancer [38]. The study included different risk groups, (i) women at no increased risk of breast cancer (reduction mammoplasty), (ii) women without a prior breast cancer but evidence of an atypical hyperplastic lesion at biopsy, and (iii) women already diagnosed with breast cancer (surgical specimens). DNA from microdissected tissues was examined with a panel of nine highly informative microsatellite markers. The authors found genetically abnormal clones in 22% of the normal-appearing samples from 50% of the women from all three risk groups. The authors concluded that *"genetic abnormalities potentially critical to breast tumorigenesis accumulate before pathological detection even of high-risk lesions and are detectable in tissue that is not only histologically benign but also completely normal."*

In a follow-up study, the same group sought to further characterize the presence of allelic imbalance in another set of women and try to correlate the presence of allelic imbalance in the histologically normal tissue to what was present in the adjacent cancer [39]. Again, allelic imbalance was determined in DNA from microdissected, histologically normal ducts or TDLUs and matched malignant epithelial-enriched samples from eighteen breast cancer cases. This study examined twenty-one microsatellite markers on ten different chromosome arms. The authors measured allelic imbalance in 13% of the normal ducts/TDLUs from 44% of the cases and these genetically abnormal ducts/TDLUs were found in cancerous breasts throughout the normal appearing epithelium. However, these clones were distinct from the co-existing cancer, meaning that these abnormalities could either be a consequence of normal development or could be a result of a pathological event. The authors speculated that "*the ducts/TDLUs with LOH form a reservoir from which cancers may develop if sufficient additional abnormalities accumulate*".

In a more recent investigation, Larson *et al.* followed up and asked the question whether the presence of allelic imbalance in normal-appearing breast epithelium is associated with cancer or cancer risk [40]. Using a panel of twenty microsatellite markers, the authors assessed allelic imbalance on a large set of histologically normal, microdissected breast TDLUs from three groups of women, (i) sporadic breast cancer patients, (ii) BRCA1 gene mutation carriers, and (iii) controls undergoing reduction mammoplasty. The study found that allelic imbalance was increased three-fold in the women with sporadic breast cancer or BRCA1 gene mutation, when compared to the women undergoing reduction mammoplasty. The authors concluded that "*the presence of AI* [allelic imbalance] *in normal-appearing breast epithelium from breast cancer patients and BRCA1 mutation-carriers may reflect ongoing, aberrant processes contributing to the development of malignancy, even while the tissue appears normal*".

In one of our own previous studies, we investigated the extent and spatial distribution of allelic imbalance in histologically normal tissues surrounding breast tumors [41]. We utilized a panel of sixteen unlinked microsatellite loci and analyzed twenty normal breast tissues obtained from reduction mammoplasties, as well as a group of twelve matched tumor adjacent, histologically normal (TAHN) breast tissues excised at sites 1cm and 5cm from the tumor margins and the corresponding tumor tissue. We observed low levels of allelic imbalance in the reduction mammoplasty tissue and in the TAHN tissue excised at 5cm. However, we observed a 5 times higher incidence in the TAHN tissue excised at 1cm, suggesting a field of cells surrounding the tumor (up to at least 1cm) that contain genetic abnormalities. As expected, the tumors contained high levels of allelic imbalance. Somewhat surprising though, was the observation that a substantial fraction of the unbalanced alleles in the TAHN tissues were conserved in the tumor, implying cellular clonal evolution. These data suggest that both tumors and TAHN (1cm) tissues are genetically distinct from TAHN (5cm) tissue, and that both are genetically unstable. We concluded that "*the finding that genomic instability occurs in fields of histologically normal tissues surrounding the tumor is of clinical importance, as it has implications for the definition of appropriate tumor margins and the assessment of recurrence risk factors in the context of breast-sparing surgery*". This study also included analysis of telomere length in these tissues and the results will be discussed later in this chapter (see section 9.2.3).

While the previous set of studies focused on allelic imbalance, the next group of investigations focuses on loss of heterozygousity (LOH). Whereas allelic imbalance can occur by either gaining or losing an allele, LOH is specifically the situation where there is a complete loss of one of the alleles at a particular locus. One of the initial studies came from Hemminki's group which assessed six monozygotic twin pairs [42]. LOH was measured in histologically normal, tumor adjacent breast tissues for markers located on chromosomes 1, 13 and 17. The authors concluded that these histologically normal, tumor-adjacent tissues contained genetic changes that resembled those found in tumors and that they may represent some of the earliest genetic changes in the initiation of a cancer.

The Ellsworth and Shriver group has been a major contributor of the data that supports the idea of field cancerization in the breast. In a series of studies, the group evaluated patterns of LOH and allelic imbalance in histologically normal breast tissues obtained from the quadrants of diseased breasts following surgical resection. Whereas, some of the previous studies utilized general microsatellite markers (*i.e.* non-disease associated), this group developed a high-throughput panel of microsatellite markers from 26 of the most commonly deleted regions in breast cancer [43]. Using this assay, the authors observed genomic instability in all the breast quadrants, but instability was increased in the outer quadrants as compared to the inner quadrants [44]. The authors speculated that "*greater genomic instability in outer quadrants can partially explain the propensity for breast cancers to develop there, rather than simple volume-related concepts*". In fact, in a follow-up review article [12], the authors speculated that "*carcinogenic agents could contribute to fields of genomic instability localised to specific areas of the breast*". This concept is outlined in Figure 9-5. Although not taken at defined distances from the tumors, this group also observed that genomic instability was increased in histologically normal tissue adjacent to the primary breast cancer, as compared to histologically normal tissue at a further distance within the same breast [45]. The authors concluded that "*genomic instability may be inherently greater in disease-free tissue close to developing tumors, which may have important implications for defining surgical margins and predicting recurrence*".

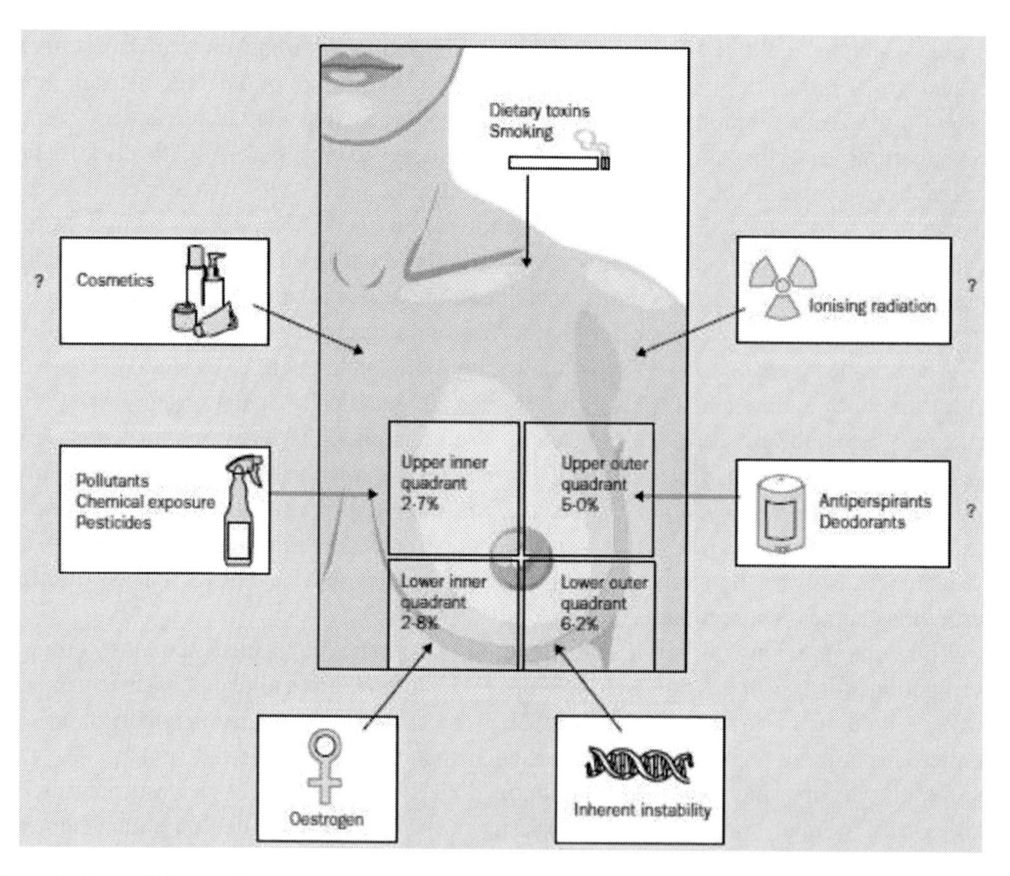

Figure 9.5. Possible contributing factors to genomic instability in histologically normal breast tissues. The average frequency of instability for each quadrant is shown (reproduced with permission from [12].

9.2.2. Aneusomy in Histologically Normal Mammary Tissues

Carcinogenesis is a multistep process driven by an accumulation of genetic alterations. We have previously focused on losses or gains of particular alleles; however, whole or large sections of chromosomes can also be amplified or lost in tumor cell populations. This process is referred to as aneusomy, a form of aneuploidy (incomplete chromosome sets), and is a major characteristic of most human tumors. Anna Maria Cianciulli and colleagues hypothesized that this process could be occurring in seemingly normal breast tissues. Therefore, they utilized a fluorescence *in situ* hybridization assay with centromere-specific probes for chromosomes 1 and 17 on tumor and matched histologically normal tissues [46]. The authors observed aneusomy in most primary tumors and in the majority of adjacent normal tissues. These data support the hypothesis of field cancerization in the breast.

9.2.3. Aberrations in Telomere Maintenance in Histologically Normal Mammary Tissues

One important factor in the progression of breast cancer is the generation and subsequent accumulation of genomic instability [47]. Telomere dysfunction is one mechanism that generates genomic instability [48,49]. In human somatic cells, telomeres are composed of 1,000 to 2,000 repeated copies of the DNA sequence, TTAGGG [50], and function to stabilize the ends of chromosomes and prevent them from being recognized by the cell as DNA double-strand breaks, thereby preventing degradation and recombination [51]. Short, dysfunctional telomeres can be generated by incomplete replication of the lagging strand during DNA synthesis [52], loss or alterations of telomere-binding proteins involved in telomere maintenance [53], or by DNA damage caused by oxidative stress [54]. Conversely, telomeres may be lengthened or maintained by the enzyme telomerase [55], or through a recombination pathway, know as alternative lengthening of telomeres (ALT) [56].

In a previous section (9.2.1) we described one of our own studies that assessed the extent and spatial distribution of allelic imbalance in histologically normal tissues surrounding breast tumors [41]. In the same investigation, we also measured telomere content, a surrogate for telomere length, using a slot-blot based chemiluminescence assay [57]. We determined telomere content in twenty normal breast tissues obtained from reduction mammoplasties, as well as from the group of twelve matched tumor adjacent, histologically normal (TAHN) breast tissues excised at sites 1cm and 5cm from the tumor margins and the corresponding tumor tissue. The telomere content in the reduction mammoplasty and TAHN (5cm) were nearly identical. Telomere shortening was observed in both the tumors and surrounding histologically normal tissues at distances at least 1cm from the visible tumor margins. Strikingly, the degree of telomere shortening in many TAHN 1cm tissues was comparable to that found in the matched tumor. We concluded that our results were "*in agreement with the concepts of "field cancerization" and "cancer field effect," concepts that were previously introduced to describe areas within tissues consisting of histologically normal, yet genetically aberrant, cells that represent fertile grounds for tumorigenesis*".

Another group that has been at the forefront of telomere research on human tissue is Angelo De Marzo's group. This group developed a highly sensitive telomere fluorescent *in situ* hybridization (TELI-FISH) assay that allows telomere length measurements with single cell resolution while conserving tissue architecture [58]. Using this *in situ* method, Alan Meeker and colleagues demonstrated that telomere shortening occurred in ~50% of the benign secretory (luminal) cells of histologically normal TDLUs; however, the myoepithelial cells in the same TDLUs did not exhibit telomere shortening (Figure 9-6) [59].

This finding was confirmed in a recent study by Kurabayashi and colleagues [60]. These authors observed telomere shortening in normal luminal and tumor cells, but did not observe telomere shortening in the myoepithelial or fibroblast cells. The finding that telomere length alterations occur in seemingly histologically normal breast tissues, both in normal TDLUs adjacent to a tumor and even in disease-free breast tissues obtained from reduction mammoplasties is extremely important and further investigation is warranted. In fact, the authors postulated "*that such shortening is the result of hormonally driven, physiological proliferation, and may delineate a population of epithelial cells at risk for subsequent malignant transformation*". In a related review article, Meeker and Argani argued that "*telomere shortening is therefore a strong candidate for the cause of structural chromosome defects that contribute to breast cancer development*" [61].

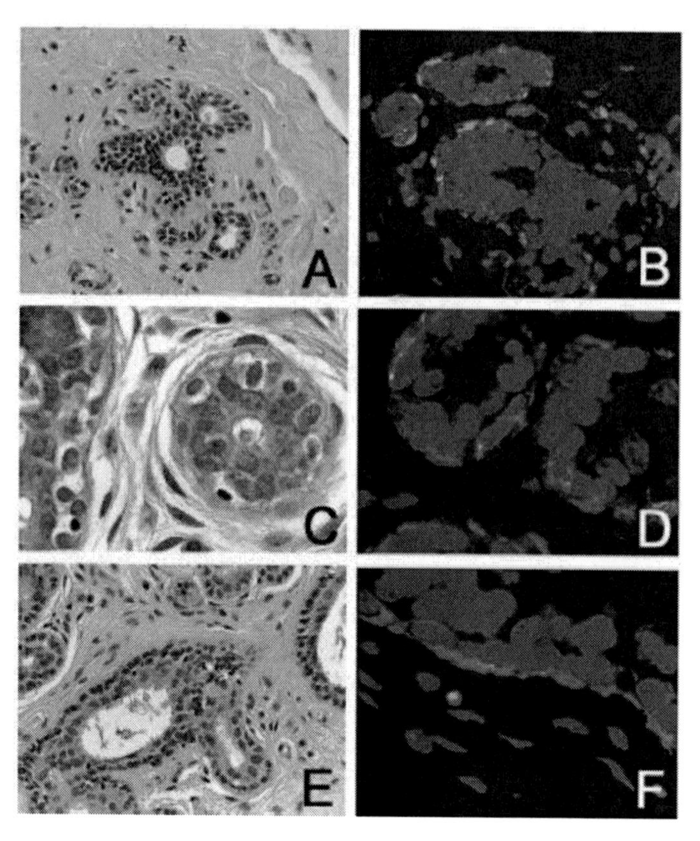

Figure 9.6. H&E staining and TELI-FISH analysis of telomere length in normal breast TDLU. The H&E stains (A, C, E) and the matched TELI-FISH (B, D, F) demonstrate normal breast TDLUs (reproduced with permission from [59]. In panels A and B, the luminal cells (negative for the green actin stain) show similar telomere signals (red) as the myoepithelial cells. In panels C and D, the luminal cells have diminished telomere signals as compared to the myoepithelial cells, and other TDLUs (panels E and F) even contain variation in telomere signals from cell to cell.

9.3. Epigenetic Field Cancerization in Mammary Tissues

As discussed in the introduction of this chapter, mammary epithelium can be affected by internal (metabolism, presence of tumor, etc.) and external (carcinogens, radiation, dietary components, etc.) factors which may be able to induce permanent biochemical changes in histologically normal tissue thereby generating the phenomenon of field cancerization. While section 9.2 focused on genomic alterations resulting from these types of exposure, *i.e.* the onset of allelic imbalance, loss of heterozygousity, and mutations, another prominent type of mechanisms that could be part of field cancerization are epigenetic aberrations, as defined for example by aberrant methylation and acetylation. While these mechanisms are abundantly described in breast cancer, and are in fact being proposed as important clinical biomarkers and therapeutic targets [62], they are under-researched in histologically normal and potentially field cancerized mammary tissue. However, reports on dietary factors and carcinogens capable of inducing epigenetic changes in normal mammary tissues are increasing in number and could explain the phenomenon of field cancerization. Some of these studies and their underlying concepts are briefly discussed here.

9.3.1. Dietary, Environmental, and Inflammatory Induction of Epigenetic Alterations

Countless studies on dietary and environmental mediators with carcinogenic and mutagenic effect in breast epithelial cells continue to be conducted and published, and their review exceeds the scope of this chapter [63]. In contrast, knowledge on the specific effect of such mediators on the *epigenetic status of mammary cells* is scarce. Yet, the induction of epigenetic aberrations in mammary and other tissues seems to be amenable to exposure of external and environmental factors. An example of a "dietary" ingredient capable of inducing epigenetic changes in breast tissues is alcohol. Anand and colleagues have indicated in a recent comprehensive review of cancer etiologies that approximately 3% of all breast cancer cases are associated with increased alcohol consumption [64]. At the mechanistic level, there is accumulating and convincing evidence that the first metabolite produced during alcohol degradation (by alcohol dehydrogenase), *i.e.* acetaldehyde, can have carcinogenic and mutagenic effects on DNA, including altered methylation. Among other mechanisms, acetaldehyde has been shown to inhibit the activity of O6-guanine-methyltransferase, an enzyme involved in epigenetic reactions pertaining to the DNA repair system [65]. Similarly, other dietary factors, including zinc, selenium, and vitamins, and their physiological imbalances have been implicated in nutrients-gene methylation interactions [66].

An example of a well-studied xenobiotic able to induce epigenetic changes is the synthetic nonsteroidal estrogen and clinically used drug, diethylstilbesterol (DES). Depending on the time and duration of exposure, DES has been shown to specifically affect promoter methylation of a number of genes, including the developmentally important homeobox genes Hoxa-10 and Hoxa-11, and the natural antimicrobial lactoferrin [67].

A prominent example of a widely occurring environmental pollutant able to induce epigenetic changes is benzopyrene, a five-ring polyclic aromatic hydrocarbon. Using genome-wide methylation profiling techniques, such as amplification of intermethylated sites (AIMS) analysis, dynamic and sequence-specific hypo- and hypermethylation events were shown in human mammary epithelial cells [68]. These alterations have been shown to induce carcinogenesis. Consequently, benzopyrene has been widely used to immortalize human mammary cells to generate *in vitro* cell culture models [69]. Important for field cancerization, benzopyrene and other dietary/environmental carcinogens including [2-amino-1-methyl-6-phenylimidazo[4,5b]pyridine (PhIP), 4-aminobiphenyl (ABP), and 2,3,7,8-tetrachl-orodibenzo-p-dioxin] were shown to affect the post-translational modification (including methylation) of histones in *normal human mammary epithelial cells* [70].

Finally, inflammatory processes have been recognized to be potential inducers of epigenetic alterations [71,72]. While the mechanisms remain largely unclear, recent *in vitro* studies have shown that inflammation-mediated halogenated cytosine damage products can mimic 5-methylcytosine and can direct enzymatic DNA methylation and affect the function of methyl-binding proteins, thereby interfering with normal epigenetic control of gene regulation [71]. This line of research is young for mammary tissues and associated diseases, and exact mechanisms are still elusive. Nevertheless, they are being increasingly addressed. For example, aberrant promoter methylation of the adenomatous polyposis coli (APC) gene, and others, has been previously studied in breast cancer and has even been used as a serum biomarker [73], but is now being specifically linked to inflammatory processes in the context of inflammatory breast disease [74].

9.3.2. Examples of Epigenetic Field Cancerization in Mammary Tissues

Promoter methylation and histone acetylation are epigenetic processes of physiological and developmental importance and are not exclusively linked to cancer development or progression. Why then should epigenetic and/or epigenomic analyses of normal human mammary tissues that are unaffected by disease be performed? One reason for a comprehensive epigenomic study of normal human mammary epithelium was recently presented by Bloushtain-Qimron and colleagues, and does not necessarily pertain to cancer at all. These authors aimed at characterizing cellular identity and differentiation in human mammary tissues in comparison with mammary stem cells [75]. Using a technology called methylation-specific digital karyotyping (MSDK), these authors have determined discrete methylation and concordant gene expression patterns specific for cell subpopulations, as specified by CD44 and CD24 positivity/negativity. Genes defining these patterns included HOXA10, TCF3, and FOXC1.

In revisiting the concepts of field cancerization depicted in Figure 9-2, an obvious reason to analyze normal mammary tissue for epigenetic alterations would be the presence of a histologically detectable lesion that induces such alterations in its surrounding field. Of note is the work by Tim Huang and his group, as published in two recent papers [76,77]. In their investigations, the status of genome-wide methylation (the "methylome"), and consequently of specific genes was analyzed in "geographic zones" of mammary tissues at defined distances (1-4 cm) from the grossly visible tumor margin of a number of breast tumors and in the four quadrants of disease-unaffected breasts. In the paper by Yan *et al.* [77], global methylation, as well as the methylation status of the RASSF1A promoter was analyzed in primary tumors, histologically normal adjacent tissues, and disease-free reduction mammoplasties. In support of field cancerization, the authors found elevated overall and RASSF1A methylation in tumor adjacent normal tissues compared with reduction mammoplasties, but not as elevated as in the tumors. Based on the distances from the visible tumor margin that were analyzed, the authors concluded that *"a more extensive field of epigenetically altered breast epithelia is present in breast cancer patients than previously thought"*. In Cheng *et al.* [76] the authors started out to study the imprinting effect of estrogen on genome-wide methylation using mammospheres of human mammary cells, and subsequently identified, among others, the tumor suppressor, RUNX3 as a prominent target. Similar to the previous study, in some of the tumors analyzed, RUNX3 hypermethylation was found to correlate with the distance from the tumor margin. Again, the authors concluded that *"RUNX3 methylation may precede morphologic transformation of normal breast epithelia"* and that such *"hypermethylation may create a large field of cancerization in the human breast"*.

Following the same concept of field cancerization, Umbricht and coworkers studied the hypermethylation of protein 14-3-3 σ (stratifin), a protein often lost during breast carcinogenesis, in a number of diseased and disease-free breast tissues [78]. As expected, 14-3-3 σ was hypermethylated in the majority of invasive and non-invasive carcinomas, but not in benign hyperplasias. The authors further stated that *"unexpectedly, patients with breast cancer showed 14-3-3 σ hypermethylation in adjacent histologically normal breast epithelium [from separate free-of-cancer tissues], while this was never observed in individuals without evidence of breast cancer"* and concluded that loss of expression of 14-3-3 σ is an early event in breast neoplastic transformation.

Other reports on epigenetic alterations in histologically normal mammary tissues link their findings to a potentially increased risk for developing cancerous lesions in the future, which conforms to the "field precedes tumor"-model depicted in Figure 9-2. Of note in this category is the work by Thea Tlsty and her group [6,7]. In this work, the widely studied tumor suppressor p16INK4a was investigated with respect to its promoter hypermethylation in normal mammary tissue. In particular, human mammary epithelial cells from healthy individuals were used to determine how early epigenetic and genetic events affect genomic integrity and induce carcinogenesis. The authors found that p16INK4a promoter hypermethylation in subpopulations of ductal and lobular epithelial cells occurs frequently, *i.e.* in about a third of randomly selected healthy, disease-free women. Importantly, since these alterations were found in healthy mammary tissues completely free of any conditions, the authors presented a model in which altered epigenetic events, including p16INK4a promoter hypermethylation were placed not only in the so-called *pre-clonal phase*, but also at the very beginning of it (Figure 9-7). Essentially, by all other known criteria, this "phase" corresponds to normal, differentiated and resting cells only affected by every day factors, including aging and diet consumption, and should perhaps not be called a "phase" at all. According to their model however, the authors expect this phase to give rise to more extensive dysfunctions, including the accumulation of genetic alterations in centromeres and telomeres (see section 9.2), ultimately leading to the "clonal phase", in which microscopically detectable changes (hyperplasia) become evident. Based on these observations, the authors place epigenetic alterations well before any pre-malignant induction in the sequence of events towards neoplasia. Collectively, these events as described by this group are in excellent agreement with the concept of field cancerization in human mammary tissues.

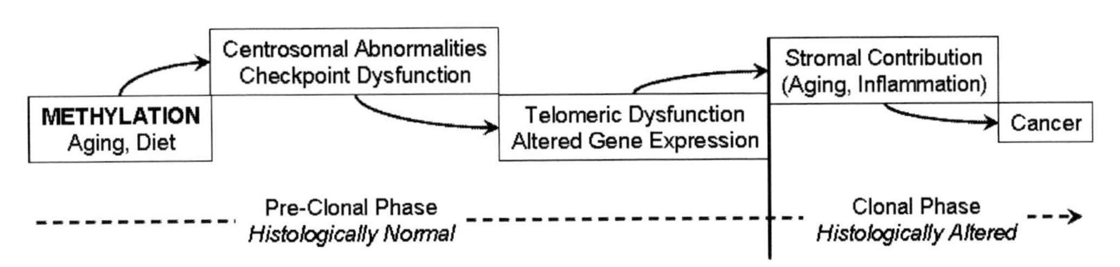

Figure 9.7. Timing of methylation events along the path to breast cancer. The model is based on reports from Thea Tlsty and her group [6,7] and may be specific for the tumor suppressor p16INK4a; the model does not exclude later methylation events. The pre-clonal phase consists of changes that do not induce proliferation or microscopically obvious tissue disruptions, which occurs in the clonal phase.

An important implication of this type of research is that such measurements may be used to assess the risk of developing breast cancer in the future, even in histologically normal and entirely disease-free individuals. This approach has recently been reported by Lewis and colleagues [79]. In this work, the promoter methylation status of the tumor suppressor genes RASSF1A, APC, H-cadherin, RARb2, and cyclin D2 which are frequently hypermethylated in breast cancer, was assessed in 55 disease-unaffected women with elevated risk of breast cancer calculated in mathematical models based on non-clinical, epidemiologic criteria. These criteria included factors such as age, age at menarche, age of first live birth, ethnicity, cancer family and reproductive history, and are frequently used in models (termed Gail, Claus, and BRCAPRO) to asses risk and make informed decisions of preventive measures. The authors not only found disease-free tissues to contain promoter methylation for RARb2, RASSF1A, and APC, but were also able to significantly associate these findings with the risks calculated by the mathematical models. The authors thus concluded that such markers could be used to assess risk of future breast disease in completely healthy women with elevated risk.

9.3.3. Concepts and Conclusions

The most comprehensive review of epigenetic field cancerization, although not specific for mammary tissues, was recently provided by T. Ushijima [80]. In this review, methylation in histologically normal tissues of liver, colon, lung, renal, Barrett's esophagus, gastric, and breast cancer (the study by Yan and coworkers outlined earlier) was reviewed. An interesting piece of information provided in this report is the nature of inducing factors for these alterations, which can include pathogen infection. For example, Ushijima reports *Helicobacter pylori*, an aerophilic gram-negative bacterium that resides in the stomach and duodenum and causes a low-level chronic infection, as a cause of aberrant methylation events that lead to gastric cancer, presumably through inflammatory mechanisms. Such events could then be used as diagnostic tool, either for an existing or past infection. A question emerging from this observation is whether infection could also induce epigenetic field cancerization in mammary tissues. While numerous studies link predominantly viral infections with the onset of breast cancer, (for a review see [81]), specific examples of epigenetic events are lacking. However, it is conceivable that viral components, either from external sources or expressed from endogenous retroelements found in the human genome, as implicated by Cho and colleagues [82], may affect the epigenetic molecular machinery, thereby generating an epigenetic field prone to further genetic alterations.

The possibility of migration of histologically normal yet genetically and perhaps epigenetically altered epithelial cells based on the concept of homologous positional information, as outlined in section 9.1.2 and Figure 9-4, should be considered. As briefly mentioned in section 9.1.2, cell adhesion molecules might be involved in this phenomenon. In support of this hypothesis, the expression of MUC1, a transmembrane mucin that is highly expressed in various cancers and correlates with malignant potential, has recently been shown to be controlled by methylation events [83]. More established is research on the methylation status of E-cadherin. For example, both invasive lobular carcinoma and lobular carcinoma *in situ* characteristically show loss of E-cadherin expression, and immunohistochemistry for E-cadherin is being increasingly used as a tool to differentiate between lobular and ductal lesions [84]. While it remains to be shown whether such epigenetic events could in part explain the presence of field cancerized cells in mammary tissues, these theories seem conceptually logical and investigations along these lines of thought are to be expected.

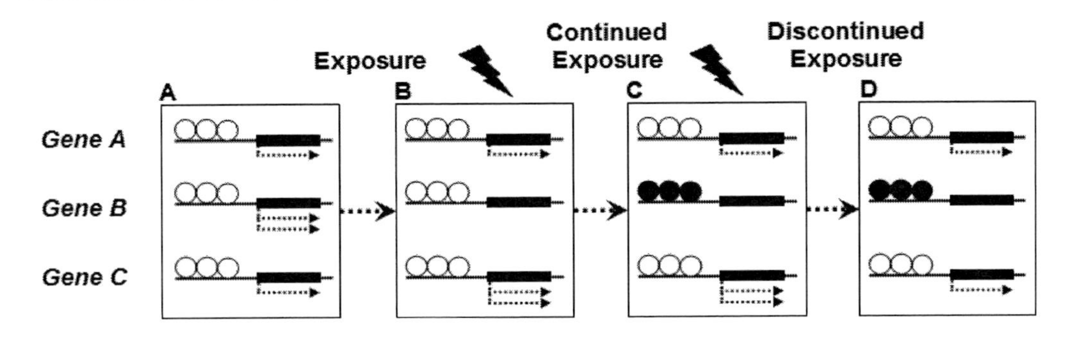

Figure 9.8. Preferential methylation of specific genes. (A) Expression (dotted arrows) and methylation (circles) status of three hypothetical genes. (B) Exposure (lightning bolt) to an inducer does not change Gene A, decreases Gene B, and increases Gene C in the absence of epigenetic changes (open circles). (C) Continued exposure leads to methylation of Gene B (closed circle). (D) When exposure discontinues, Gene C returns to normal (transient effect), while Gene B is permanently altered due to remaining epigenetic alterations. Model re-drawn from [80].

Lastly, we would like to revisit the model of epigenetic field cancerization presented by T. Ushijima [80], and link it to the heterogeneity of the subtypes of epithelial cells present in mammary tissues as presented in section 9.1.1. It is known that cellular heterogeneity is higher in tumor than in normal tissues due to the genetic and biochemical alterations cancer cells go through. A logical implication of this is that disease-free tissues across individuals are more similar to each other than cancerous tissues. In this context, Ushijima points out that methylation events in field cancerized tissues may occur preferentially at specific genes in specific organs, and that different genes are more or less prone or resistant to epigenetic changes induced by exposure to inducers (Figure 9-8). Accordingly, the expression of some genes are affected by exposure to inducing agents in a transient and reversible manner, while other genes undergo epigenetically irreversible alterations and are permanently changed in expression even if exposure discontinues. Whether such events occur in histologically normal mammary tissues and support field cancerization remains to be shown.

9.4. Expressional Aberrations in Histologically Normal Mammary Tissues

As outlined in more details in section 9.6, due to the size of human mammary tissue affected by disease, and its location in the human body, it is easily accessible and should render research focused on mammary field cancerization highly practical. It is thus rather surprising that in the era of the "-omics" sciences, genome-wide molecular signatures for field cancerized mammary tissues are scarce. This is in contrast to the relative wealth of knowledge on genomic instability (section 9.2), and most probably due to the fact that the focus still lies on cancerous tissues, and that the clinical importance of field cancerization in breast tissues has not yet been fully recognized and/or acknowledged (see section 9.5 for a more detailed discussion). The rationale for the expectations of expressional changes lies in the ample evidence for the occurrence of genetic and epigenetic changes in field cancerized mammary tissues, as described in detail in sections 9.2 and 9.3. While some of these genetic changes may be subtle in nature, it is doubtful that they are completely silent with respect to downstream effects, such as expression and even phenotypic behavior. The latter is also implied when considering the mechanistic and cellular concepts of field cancerization discussed in section 9.1.2. As with other analyses, the question of proper controls in research on field cancerization remains largely unresolved for breast tissues, too, as the object of attention in this case is what in many other studies is used as control [85] (see also section 9.6.1). What follows are examples of notable studies representing perhaps a new era of research into mammary field cancerization.

9.4.1. Expressional Changes in Field Cancerized Mammary Tissues

As predicted, a literature review attempting to find reports on proteomic and metabolomic analyses on human normal mammary tissues only identified studies in which structurally normal tissue adjacent to lesions was used as control. In contrast, we report here on at least two genomic approaches published to date and attempting to characterize normal breast tissue adjacent to breast carcinomas using laser capture microscopy (LCM) followed by whole transcriptome microarray analysis.

Finak and colleagues provided the first in depth analysis of gene expression in morphologically normal epithelium and stroma adjacent to breast cancers in comparison with tissues obtained from reduction mammoplasty specimens [86]. In discordance with the concepts of field cancerization, the authors noted that *"there are no significant differences between tumor derived* (morphologically normal, added by the author) *and reduction mammoplasty derived tissue"*. On the other hand, it is interesting that comparison of these signatures with other extensive breast cancer datasets revealed significant similarities with Her2/neu, estrogen receptor (ER), and progesterone receptor (PR)-negative subclusters of basal-like and normal-like cancer subtypes. This finding is somewhat contradictory as it indicates molecular similarities between normal breast epithelium and basal-like breast tumors with poor outcome.

Tripathi and colleagues [105] microdissected histologically normal terminal ductal-lobular units (TDLU) from tumor adjacent tissues and from age-matched reduction mammoplasties and subjected the isolated RNA to microarray analysis. This analysis revealed 105 transcripts differentially expressed between normal TDLU and reduction mammoplasty. Perhaps most importantly, ~60% of these transcripts, which included G-coupled chemokine receptors, signal transductors, and immediate early proteins, had been previously implicated in breast cancer according to the literature. In strong support of field cancerization, the authors of this study concluded that *"global gene expression abnormalities exist in normal epithelium of breast cancer patients"*, that *"cancer-related pathways may be perturbed in normal epithelium"*, and that *"these abnormalities could be markers of disease risk, occult disease, or the tissue's response to an existing tumor"*.

These seemingly contradictory studies emphasize the challenges accompanying research on mammary field cancerization. These include: (i) tissue heterogeneity and other patient population-dependent differences; (ii) different analysis platforms; (iii) different morphological material (*e.g.* terminal lobular ducts *vs.* indifferent); and (iv) different locations of tissue removal, such as distance from the tumor margin (2 mm in the study by Finak *et al vs.* 1-2 cm in the study by Tripathi *et al*). It is thus clear that studies of mammary field cancerization would greatly benefit from standardization methods allowing comparisons between different studies and patient populations.

9.4.2. Telomerase Positive Cells in Histologically Normal Mammary Tissues

Telomerase is a ribonucleoprotein that in combination with several other telomere-binding proteins regulates telomere length in eukaryotic cells by catalyzing the de novo synthesis of telomere repeats. Activation of the human telomerase reverse transcriptase (hTERT), the catalytic subunit of telomerase, plays a critical role in cellular immortalization and carcinogenesis, rendering it an important clinical biomarker and therapeutic target [87]. Human telomerase reverse transcriptase (hTERT), the catalytic domain of telomerase, is the rate-limiting factor for telomerase activity, is expressed in virtually all tumors, and has been identified as one of the minimal factors necessary to transform normal mammary epithelial into cancerous cells [88].

In our own studies [5] we have used quantitative (real-time) reverse transcriptase polymerase chain reaction (qRT-PCR) and *in situ* hybridization specific for hTERT to characterize its expression in both breast adenocarcinoma and matched structurally normal tumor adjacent mammary tissues. The *in situ* hybridization technique allows direct visualization and comparison of hTERT mRNA expression at the cellular level. Intense hTERT mRNA staining was confined to the epithelial cells within both breast tumors and several associated fields of histologically normal breast tissues. Although telomerase activity in normal breast tissue could be attributed to activated infiltrating lymphocytes or other contaminating cell types, our findings showed that hTERT was specifically expressed in some but not all normal breast epithelium indicating intra-tissue heterogeneity (Figure 9-9).

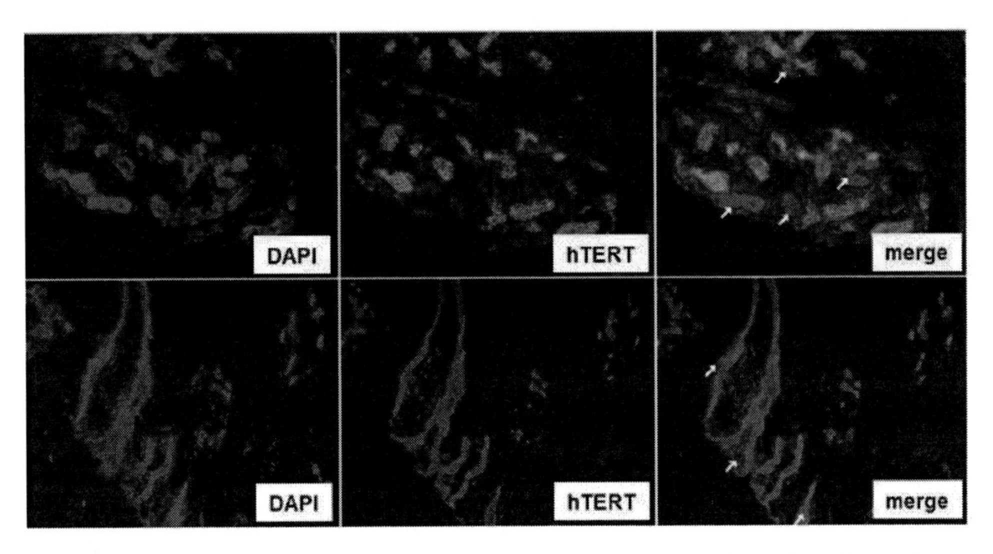

Figure 9.9. hTERT expression in normal human mammary tissue (tumor adjacent), as detected by *in situ* hybridization. hTERT probe-specific fluorescence appears green (Alexa Fluor 488), whereas nuclear counterstaining with DAPI appears blue. The results of representative normal terminal lobular unit (upper row) and ductal system (lower low) are shown. Epithelial cells lacking hTERT signal are indicated by arrows in the merged images. Magnification is 200x. Image is reproduced with permission from [5].

The main question arising from these studies is obvious: *What are the hTERT expressing epithelial cells in the histologically normal ducts adjacent to breast cancers?* While some telomerase activity has been shown to occasionally occur in normal mammary tissue [89,90], it is more so associated with cancer development and progression, and in fact a designated therapeutic target for breast cancer [91]. Therefore, its detection in normal mammary tissues could have important implications. Three possible and very different explanations for the presence of hTERT positive cells in normal breast tissue are the following:

i. *Field cancerized mammary epithelial cells:* According to some of the models of field cancerization depicted in section 9.1.2, altered cellular behavior may necessitate limited yet above average proliferative capacity, as conferred by expression of hTERT. This assumption is in agreement with the studies on the hypermethylation of the tumor suppressor p16INK4a in mammary tissues from healthy individuals (discussed in section 9.3). Together, these two expressional alterations could induce slightly elevated proliferation leading to a relative expansion of the field of modified cells. Possible inducing mechanisms of hTERT expression include inflammatory events or unknown carcinogens. These possible links are better described in prostate tumorigenesis [92], but similar mechanisms could be at play in mammary tissues. Alternatively, since telomere attrition has been observed in histologically normal breast tissues adjacent to cancers (see section 9.2), similar initiating events inducing telomere deregulation could lead to hTERT expression, either directly or indirectly through the induction of genomic instability and expressional changes. Parts of these possible pathways have been previously reported in mammary epithelial cells [93]. However, in almost all (of the few) reported examples of telomerase positive cells in normal breast tissues, it is obvious that the presence of the tumor may influence the surrounding tissues (see Figure 9-2) and induce hTERT expression through soluble factors, such as for example epidermal growth factor (EGF)[94]. These hypothesized possibilities of hTERT expression induction in normal mammary tissue are depicted in Figure 9-10.
ii. *Naturally occurring mammary epithelial cells expressing hTERT:* Our own data presented above is in strong agreement with the study by Liu and colleagues who by *in situ* hybridization found hTERT highly expressed in normal breast ductal-lobular units, even at higher levels than in ductal carcinoma *in situ* [95]. These authors acknowledged that their findings challenge the conventional view that hTERT expression is repressed in somatic cells but activated in neoplastic cells, and concluded that *"hTERT may play an important role in the homeostasis of normal breast epithelial cells"*. Earlier work seems to support these observations by reporting expression of hTERT in early premalignant lesions and a subset of cells in normal breast lobular epithelia [96]. Of note, menstrual information for the patients' tissues under investigation is usually not known, yet could influence the findings. While reports on menstrual cycle dependent hTERT expression are lacking, estrogen fluctuations could induce hTERT expression through activation of the estrogen receptor (ER), as previously reported [97].
iii. *Putative mammary epithelial stem cells:* Type I human mammary epithelial cells (HMEC) have been postulated to be candidate stem cells and shown to contain low levels of endogenous expression of telomerase [98]. However, their frequency of

occurrence is presumably orders of magnitudes lower than the cells from the reports outlined above, including our own [5].

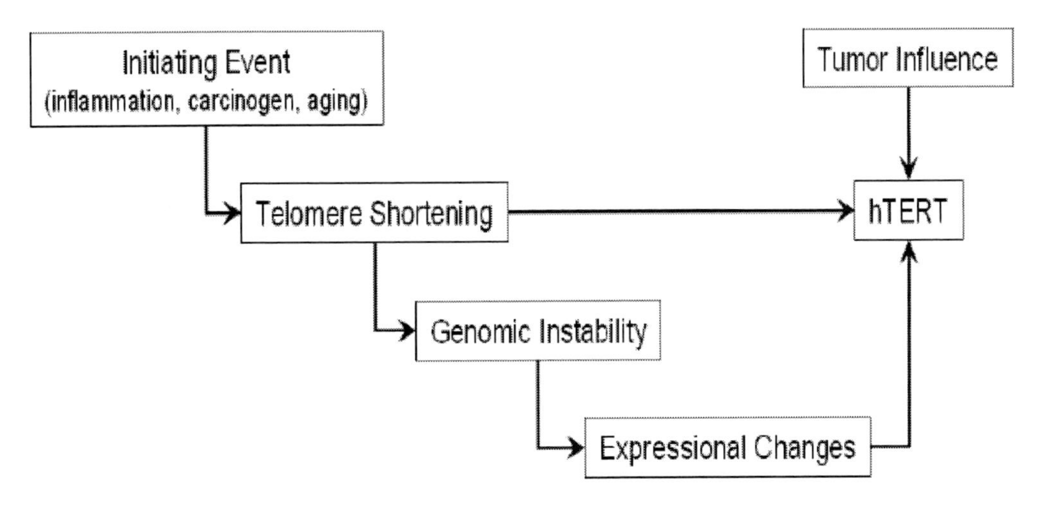

Figure 9.10. Hypothesized pathways of hTERT expression induction in normal mammary tissue. Initiating events could induce telomere deregulation leading to hTERT expression, either directly or indirectly through induction of genomic instability and expressional changes. Alternatively, hTERT may be induced by soluble factors secreted by the tumor.

9.5. Clinical Importance of Field Cancerization in Mammary Tissues

As mentioned several times in this chapter, it can be readily appreciated that field cancerization is of clinical importance in any cancer [10]. While the information given in the previous chapters is self-evident, we discuss here clinical scenarios specific to breast disease which are related to, or could greatly benefit from a better insight into the phenomenon of field cancerization. In particular, as outlined in the next paragraphs, such knowledge would provide objective criteria for better informed decision making in patient risk stratification and treatment.

9.5.1. Mammary Field Cancerization as a Source of Biomarkers

Diseased mammary tissue continues to be characterized at the molecular level with the intent of discovering highly informative biomarkers that can predict the course of disease or the response to a specific therapeutic intervention. In particular, the highly parallel "-omics" sciences including genomics, proteomics, and metabolomics are increasingly identifying molecular signatures with prognostic and predictive power, thereby identifying specific cancer subtypes and allowing better and refined patient stratification [99,100,101]. In fact, such novel efforts have been deemed highly necessary [102] in order to complement the current breast cancer stratification system, which is based entirely on clinical or pathological staging according to the Tumor-Node-Metastasis (TNM) system introduced in the 1950s and multiply revised thereafter [103]. Of course, such efforts are greatly supported by the proven clinical utility of prominent markers including the estrogen receptor (ER), the progesterone receptor (PR), and Her2/neu, for which quantitative immunohistochemical analyses are established in clinical laboratories [104]. However, these biomarkers are specific to tumors and are thus utilized primarily for patient stratification purposes to predict the efficiency of therapeutic intervention (Tamoxifen® and Herceptin®).

Similar protein biomarkers emerging from field cancerized mammary tissues are largely absent to date, yet it is readily conceivable that such markers may be present in such tissues. Furthermore, in contemplating the possible concept mechanisms of field cancerization outlined in section 9.1.2, it is clear that such biomarkers would be great assets towards a better diagnosis and perhaps even prognosis of breast disease. Studies such as the one by Tripathi and colleagues reviewed in section 9.4 [105] reflect some investigator's efforts to identify protein biomarkers in field cancerized mammalian tissues for the purpose of clinical use, although much controversy remains as to how consistent such biomarkers are in different patient populations, as shown by the study of Finak and colleagues also reviewed in section 9.4 [86]. As reviewed in section 9.2, DNA based and genomic alterations occurring in histologically intact mammary tissues adjacent to tumors are more established.

Regardless of the nature of the biomarker (protein *vs.* DNA), the following is a discussion of clinical utilities identified or projected for markers derived from field cancerized mammalian tissues.

9.5.2. Diagnosis of Aggressive Breast Cancers and Their Prognosis

Early diagnosis of breast disease relies entirely on self-examination (palpation) and imaging technologies, primarily mammography [106,107]. The latter can be routinely performed as part of medical check-ups and is continuously discussed as active screening tool, although its diagnostic specificity continues to be an issue [108], and its population-wide use has been deemed prohibitively costly [109,110]. Nevertheless, the widespread use of mammography has resulted in an increase in the detection of breast cancer at an early stage (i.e. *in situ* stage 0 and early stage 1). While these cancers are primarily of indolent nature, the absence of powerful prognostic markers leads to over-treatment, a clinical reality for many women initially diagnosed with early stage disease [111]. For example, "only" ~30% of women diagnosed with node-negative breast cancer will develop recurrent disease, yet because currently available prognostic markers are unable to reliably identify patients that will progress, most guidelines recommend adjuvant treatment for the majority of breast cancer patients [112,113]. Such treatments are often accompanied by severe physical and psychological side effects markedly reducing the quality of life without benefit in up to 70% of patients. This emphasizes the continuous need for biomarkers able to not only confirm the presence of a tumor (diagnosis), but especially to be informative about the course of disease (prognosis). Of note, the propensity to recur and metastasize has been recently revised at the molecular level by leaders in the field [114,115], providing novel concepts. These emerging concepts deviate from the dogmatic notion that molecular alterations enabling metastatic spread (leading to poor prognoses) occur late in tumor progression. Rather, recent findings seem to indicate that molecular signatures present at tumorigenesis are indicative of the tumor's course of progression. If field cancerized mammary tissue reflects in part its risk to develop into a malignancy (as outlined in section 9.1), this concept can be extended to pre-malignant statuses, as indicated by our findings on telomere dysfunction and genomic instability in field cancerized breast tissues outlined in section 9.2.

Along this line, we have previously shown in multiple studies and within several breast cancer patient populations that telomere shortening, measured as telomere DNA content (see section 9.2.3) is an independent predictor of clinical outcome and survival interval, and may discriminate by stage [2,116]. In particular, in a patient cohort of 530 patients, TC was independent of other commonly used risk factors such as tumor-node-metastasis stage, estrogen receptor, progesterone receptor, and p53 status [2]. As shown by the method of Kaplan and Meier in Figure 9-11, log-rank analysis showed a significant relationship between TC group and overall survival interval in all cases or invasive cases only ($p = 0.025$ and $p = 0.046$, respectively), with low TC predicting a shorter survival interval in both cohorts. In addition, multivariate Cox proportional hazards models that included TC, p53 status, tumor-node-metastasis stage, and estrogen receptor status low TC conferred an adjusted relative hazard of 2.88 (95% confidence interval, 1.16-7.15; $p = 0.022$) for breast cancer-related adverse events.

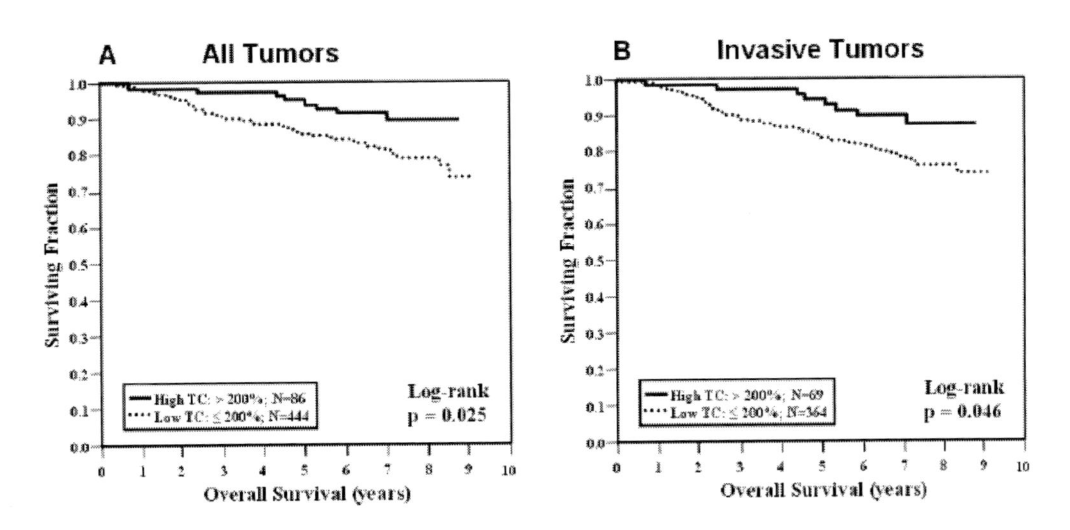

Figure 9.11. Prognostic power of telomere dysfunction. Telomere DNA content (TC), a proxy for telomere length was measured in 530 breast cancer cases and associated with time of patient survival by log-rank test. The set of all tumors (A) or invasive tumors only (B) was divided into two groups based on the low-TC and high-TC cutoff (200% of standard). Overall survival interval (in y) is shown on the x axis, and the surviving fraction is shown on the y axis. Subjects were censored at the time lost to follow-up. N, number of subjects in each group. Image is reproduced with permission from [2].

In conclusion, it is conceivable to propose the following: Telomere dysfunction and genomic instability are present in histologically normal breast tissue, as shown by us and others [41,59].As outlined above, telomere dysfunction holds prognostic power. By extrapolation, it seems possible that telomere dysfunction and other markers of genomic instability in field cancerized mammary tissues could act as prognosticators of disease.

9.5.3. Disease Recurrence after Breast Conservation Therapy

A more refined extension of the general discussion in the previous section is given by the evaluation of surgical margins in women who choose breast conservation therapy (BCT) as a treatment for early stage breast cancer, often followed by breast reconstruction. In fact, the majority of small breast cancers are treated today by BCT, which includes wide local excision and radiation treatment. However, prospective randomized clinical trials, including the National Surgical Adjuvant Breast and Bowel Project (NSABP), indicate that breast cancer patients younger than 35 years have higher rates of local recurrence and decreased rates of survival compared with women of 35 years and older [117,118,119], and that the overall incidence of local regional recurrence after BCT for stage 0-II breast cancer is 5-22% [120]. This leaves many patients who choose BCT with anxiety about local recurrence, repeated surgery, and treatment.

Hockel and Dornhofer have recently provided a detailed and mechanistic insight analysis into the concepts of local recurrence and second primary breast tumors [11]. Accordingly, two fundamentally different concepts explaining loco-regional tumor recurrences are (i) *in situ* recurrences that arise in the residual organ/organ system not involved in the surgery for the primary tumor, and (ii) scar recurrences that develop at the site of previous tumor resection. It is important to note that only the former relates to field cancerization, while the latter are regarded as the result of the interaction of minimal residual (microscopically occult) disease with the supporting surgical wound environment inside a developmentally defined tissue or organ compartment. In support for scar recurrence, but not in disagreement with *in situ* recurrences due to field cancerization, most breast cancer recurrences (63%) occur at the same site where surgery was performed. In addition, in strong support of field cancerization, 23% of all recurrences occur within the same quadrant, but not necessarily at the same site [120].

Surgical margins are typically examined histologically by specialized pathologists to determine the presence of infiltrative cancer cells in the surrounding tissues. However, according to the possible concepts of field cancerization, margins could contain cells that are genetically and biochemically altered. These concepts and their relation to surgical margins in breast cancer, and their importance for surgical practice is schematically shown in Figure 9-12. The concepts discussed in section 9.1.2, particularly as depicted in Figure 9-2, indicate the possibility of heterogeneous patches of histologically normal yet genetically altered cells. Within these patches, cancer may develop in areas where cells bear high levels of genomic instability. Surgical removal of tumors with close margins such as by lumpectomy may leave behind genetically unstable cells able to cause *in situ* recurrence at or close to the same site. Even if the presence of such fields is taken into account and surgical removal is extended to include more "normal" tissue, second primary tumors may develop due to extended fields in different quadrants.

In conclusion, it is evident that depending on the nature of the field, the extent of resection may determine the rate of residual "disease", and as a consequence, the rate of local recurrence. This line of research emphasizes the necessity of redefining the assessment of surgical margins, in particular by adding molecular markers to the already established and successful histological procedure. As mentioned in the introduction to this section, we make a case for field cancerized breast tissue to be a formidable source of such markers.

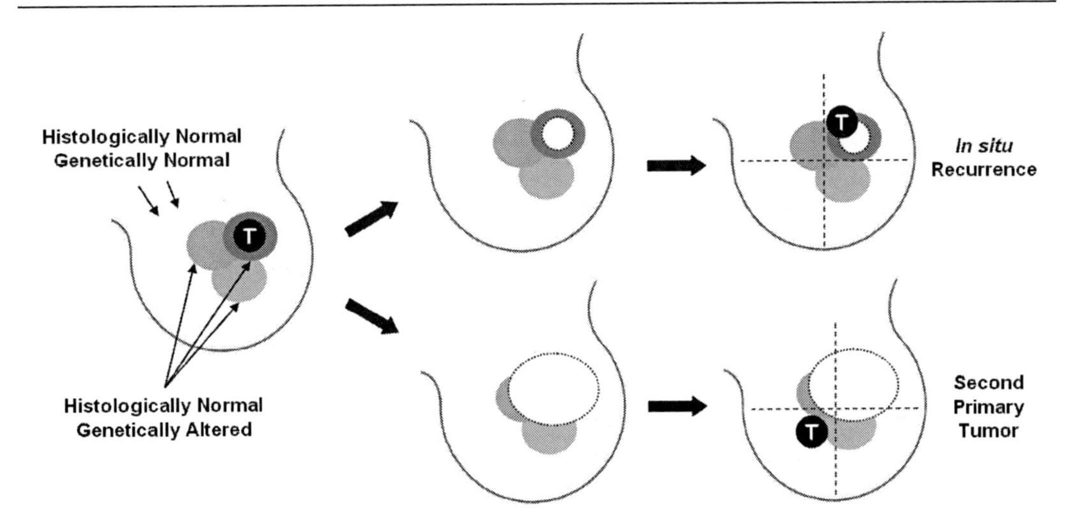

Figure 9.12. Relationship between field cancerization and surgical margins. Breast tissue may contain heterogeneous patches (see also Figure 9-2) of histologically normal yet genetically altered (field cancerized) cells. Tumors (T) may develop in areas with highest degree of genomic instability. Resection of tumor with close margins by lumpectomy may result in an *in situ* recurrence in the same quadrant (upper panel). Even in the case of a wider resection, a second primary tumor due to extended fields of genetically altered cells may develop, possibly in a different quadrant (lower panel). Quadrants are indicated by the dotted lines.

9.5.4. Development of Contralateral Breast Cancer

The previous discussion on second primary tumors and local recurrences was focused on the ipsilateral breast. The development of second tumors in the contralateral breast (also called bilateral breast cancer) occurs at 2-11% and has been associated with several risk factors, including family history, age at diagnosis of the primary tumor, and lobular-type histology of the primary tumor [121]. The development of second tumors in the unaffected breast strongly indicate truly independent events, and perhaps a hereditary condition, such as the high penetrance mutations in the BRCA1 gene [122]. Genome-wide molecular analyses, including the association between whole genome distributions of single nucleotide polymorphisms and risk of developing contralateral breast cancer, are underway [123].

Second primary tumors in the contralateral breast do not easily lend themselves to concepts of field cancerization, because of the breast morphology discussed in section 9.1 and the implied histological distances of centimeters rather that milli- or micrometers. On the other hand, mechanisms of field cancerization in the development of contralateral breast cancer cannot be entirely excluded, as the processes discussed in section 9.1.2, as well as our own studies on telomere dysfunction in tumor adjacent breast tissues [41], imply the possibility that these may happen over relatively large distances (centimeters) along the intertwined and highly branched ductal structures combined with additional intra-compartmental cell displacements.

Ultimately, the identification of unequivocal biomarkers of field cancerization achieved in other contexts may indicate in the future whether such markers are of any clinical value in the prediction of second primary tumors.

9.6. Conclusion and Future Directions

9.6.1. Methods to Study Breast Field Cancerization

The morphology of human mammalian tissue as reviewed in section 9.1.1 indicates a high complexity and heterogeneous consistency with multiple types of cells, including of the epithelial, stromal, adipocyte, endothelial, smooth muscle, and other types. Although breast adenocarcinoma ultimately originates from epithelial cells, field cancerization may affect all of these cells (see our discussion on reactive stroma in section 9.1.2). In addition, with respect to biomarkers of field cancerization and their clinical utility discussed in the previous section, these could originate in any of the above mentioned cell types.

Consequently, in order to identify informative biomarkers according to their exact origin, it may be necessary to study specific cell types or isolate them from human tissues using sophisticated technologies such as laser capture microscopy (LCM) and other, more physiological means (see below). On the other hand, omitting isolation of specific cell populations and deliberately analyzing bulk tissues consisting of naturally occurring mixtures of cells as present in human tissues may be of advantage for the identification of biomarkers. This is because of the well documented and previously discussed (section 9.1) stromal-epithelial and other cell-cell interactions leading most probably to unique molecular signatures, which are lost when cell types are separated. Much as systems biology attempts to integrate different sciences to unmask the "secrets" of breast cancer [124,125], it may take combinatorial and multiplatform "-omics" approaches to completely understand the nature of mammary field cancerization. Of course, these would include genomics, proteomics, metabolomics, and other highly parallel genome-wide analysis approaches including microRNAs and single nucleotide polymorphisms. However, considering the use in clinical laboratories, quantitative immunohistochemistry for protein biomarkers would be highly amenable to such a task. Studies such as the ones reported by Tripathi, and Finak and colleagues [86,105] (reviewed in section 9.4) reflect such efforts.

It is conceivable that markers of mammary field cancerization are primarily located in the affected tissues adjacent to the lesions, which implies their use in research (see below). However, it must be noted that new paradigms relating to cell dissemination are emerging. These paradigms are primarily discussed in the context of metastasis by leaders in the field [114,115] and state that genetically and biochemically altered cells may be capable of escaping their primary environments at early, even pre-malignant stages of tumor development. By extrapolation, the occurrence of early stage field cancerized mammary cells in other compartments such as serum would conceptually be in agreement with the possible mechanisms of cell displacement and movement reviewed in section 9.1.2 (especially Figure 9.4). Serum as a source of circulating malignant breast cancer cells has been previously identified, although the importance and utility of such cells remains to be shown [126]. In addition, it can be hypothesized that field cancerized mammary cells of all types; epithelial, stromal, etc. may change their "secretome", *i.e.* pattern of secreted or surface molecules (adhesion molecules, soluble factors, extracellular proteases, etc.). Theoretically, such secreted factors could be detected in serum by mass-spectrometric serum proteomics, again as shown for the attempted detection of bulk breast cancer [127]. A formidable challenge in all of these, so far speculative approaches would be to discern molecular signatures specific for field cancerization from those typical of fully developed cancer. While these methods and approaches may be possible in the future due to a better understanding of the molecular nature of mammary field cancerization, the current default for researching the mechanisms underlying breast field cancerization rely primarily on cells and tissues isolated from the field itself. This is discussed in more detail in the next chapters.

Finally, the study of field cancerization bears an inherent problem which is not easily resolved: The choice of proper controls. By default in numerous studies, typically one would choose the histologically normal tissues surrounding the cancer as control to study the biology of the latter. However, in studying field cancerization, this type of tissue is itself at the center of attention, and usually lacks a properly matched control. The latter is especially true for organs for which healthy donor tissue from volunteers are not meaningful, including breast tissue. This dilemma has led leaders in the field to make correct statements such as *"Using tissue adjacent to carcinoma as a normal control: an obvious but questionable practice"* [85]. While the procurement of healthy donor tissues from breast cancer-unrelated cases and autopsies is still possible through special programs (*e.g.* the Cooperative Human Tissue Network supported by the US National Cancer Institute), the study of breast field cancerization can benefit from the use of remnant tissue obtained from women undergoing reduction mammoplasty. However, two prominent problems remain: First, the normalcy of mammary tissue from reduction mammoplasty could be questioned. After all, the majority of patients undergoing reduction mammoplasty may be affected by hyperproliferative conditions in their mammary tissues. If not genetically altered, mammary tissues from reduction mammoplasties are perhaps affected by epigenetic and/or biochemical effects, rendering them different from truly normal tissues unaffected by any condition. Second, the necessity of using non-matched tissues as controls introduces substantial heterogeneity into the experimental system. While the careful choice of control parameters, such as matched age and exact tissue location can counteract some of these concerns, the effect of tissue heterogeneity must be taken into consideration as a blurring factor when attempting to characterize field cancerized mammary tissue.

9.6.2. Potential *In Vitro* Models of Mammary Field Cancerization

Regardless of the underlying mechanisms, field cancerization is understood as a phenomenon affecting histologically normal and structurally intact tissues. Therefore, naturally or artificially immortalized cell lines of mammary origin, even if non-tumorigenic and of pre-malignant nature, may not be suitable to study mechanisms of field cancerization, as their genetic and biochemical makeup have already reached transformative status. Fortunately, and as mentioned previously, given the size of human mammary tissue affected by disease, and its location in the human body, it is easily accessible and renders research focused on cancer biology and field cancerization highly practical. In fact, the isolation of human mammary tissues and primary cells from these tissues has long been established and previously reported in quite some detail [128]. It is thus possible to isolate primary cells and culture specific cell subpopulations from human breast tissues obtained from surgical material (as shown in Figure 9-13). This can be accomplished through combinatorial steps including mechanical (mincing) and enzymatic (proteases able to degrade extracellular matrix) disruption, followed by differential trypsinization and centrifugation, followed by culturing in special media conditioned to enrich specific cell populations utilizing directed growth factors supporting epithelial or other cell types. Of note, by definition primary cells from structurally intact non-cancerous but perhaps field cancerized breast tissues are expected to display a finite proliferative capacity according to the Hayflick limit and to the telomere based "molecular clock" [129]. In fact, proliferative capacity may disappear completely due to tissue structure disruption and the lack of growth and survival stimuli, leading to a special type of apoptosis, termed anoikis [130]. To circumvent such problems, primary mammary epithelial cells may be cultured as "mammospheres" in extracellular matrix support (consisting of basement membrane components, collagen, and laminin) as described in a recent review [8] and as shown in Figure 9-13. Under such conditions, primary cells undergo polarization and may display a more physiologically relevant phenotype leading to more meaningful molecular analyses. In fact, completely normal mammary epithelial cells are amenable to such systems and continue to provide insight into the processes of tumorigenesis [131].

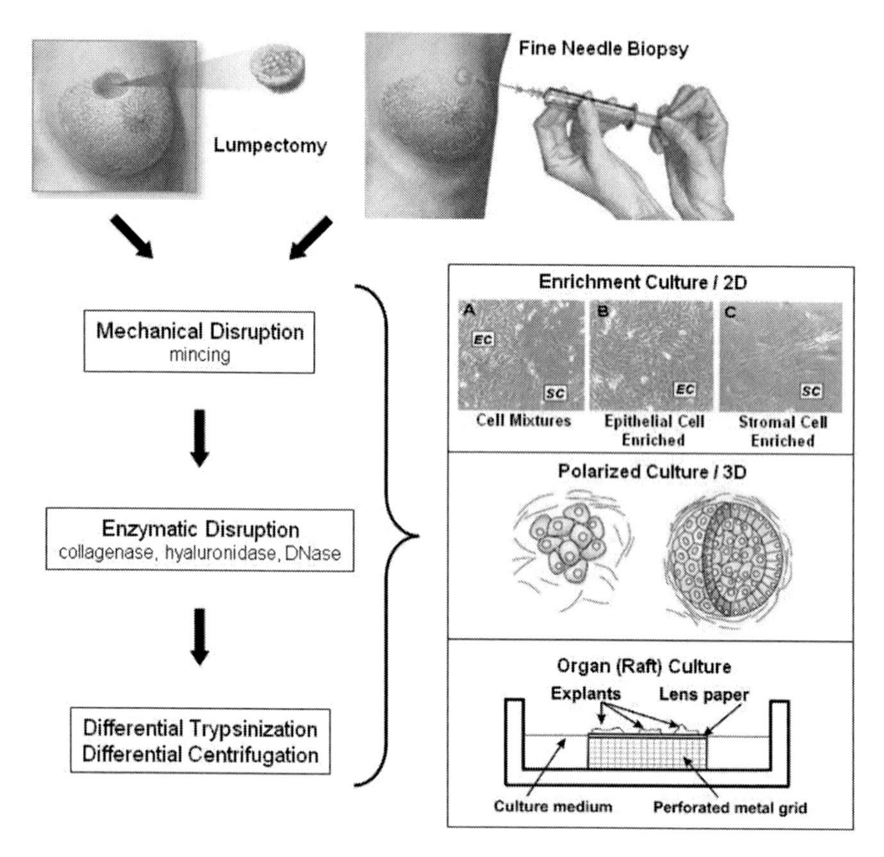

Figure 9.13. Possible *in vitro* models of mammary field cancerization. Human mammary cells of different types, including epithelial (EC) and stromal (SC) can be isolated from lumpectomies and fine needle aspirates through mechanical and enzymatic disruption followed by differential trypsinization and centrifugation. Single cells can be enriched in conventional 2D cultures in specific media, or cultured in 3D to induce cell polarization and mammospheres, or whole tissue explants can be cultured as rafts in humidified environments to preserve tissue structure. Some images are reproduced with permission from [8,9].

Finally, single cells do not necessarily need to be isolated and field cancerization could be studied in a *"semi-situ"* almost completely non-disruptive manner using the raft system for organ cultures reported by Eigeliene and colleagues [9], also shown in Figure 9-13. In this system, chunks or sections of freshly isolated human mammary breast tissues (explants) are placed on lens paper soaked in growth supporting medium placed in a humidified environment. Tissue structure and physiology are largely preserved under these conditions.

9.6.3. Potential *In Vivo* (Animal) Models of Mammary Field Cancerization

Some of the current and future *in vivo* mouse models that could be used for the study of mammary field cancerization are depicted graphically in Figure 9-14 and further discussed in the next sections.

The inherent nature of field cancerized mammary tissue, i.e. its non- or pre-malignant genotypic and phenotypic make-up puts substantial limitations to its use as xenotransplanted subcutaneous deposits in immunocompromised mice, a widely used *in vivo* model for many tumors. In fact, field cancerized mammary cells most probably are limited in proliferative capacity, and are by definition not transformed, rendering them by default non-tumorigenic. They thus lack the minimal molecular requirements for a transformed phenotype in mammary cells, including for example the expression of hTERT, explaining their limited proliferative capacity [6,88]. Consequently, they would not be able to induce angiogenesis, grow, or even survive as an independent cell mass in a subcutaneous environment. Nevertheless, it is not entirely inconceivable that deposits consisting of cell mixtures and extracellular matrices (such as reconstituted basement membrane, or Matrigel™), or even small intact tissue chunks, could survive subcutaneously for a certain amount of time during which cell interactions could be studied.

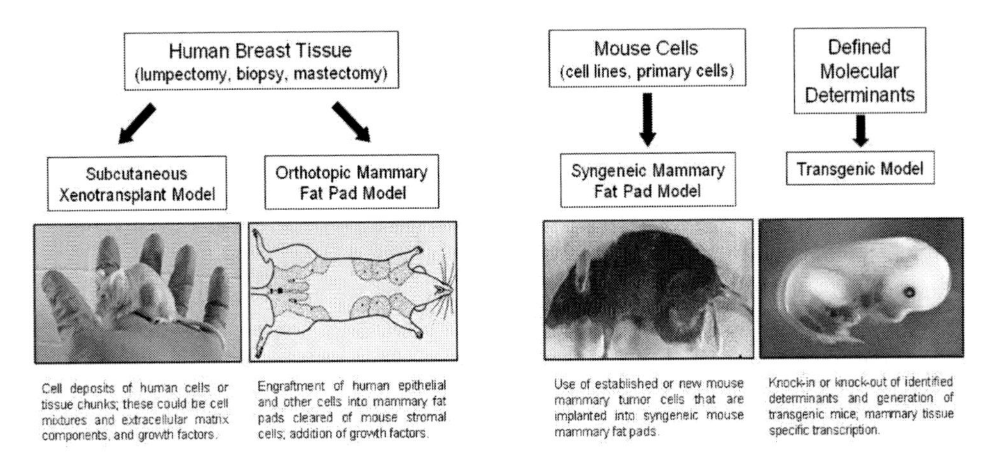

Figure 9.14. Possible *in vivo* models of mammary field cancerization. Human material (tissue, cells) from lumpectomies, biopsies, or mastectomies can be engrafted into subcutaneous deposits (xenotransplants) in immunocompromised mice, or as orthotopical implants into cleared mammary fat pads. Established or new cells can be implanted into the mammary fat pads of syngeneic mice. Finally, if molecular determinants and mediators of field cancerization are known, their action can be studied in transgenic mice under tissue-specific conditions.

Perhaps the most commonly used *in vivo* models for the study of mammary carcinogenesis are syngeneic mouse models, in which established or new mouse mammary cancer cell lines can be orthotopically engrafted into mouse mammary fad pads. The obvious major advantage of using syngeneic systems is the fact that the implanted cells are of the same species and genotype, thus negating the necessity of using artificially immunocompromised mice. As a consequence, observations made under such conditions tend to be more physiological. A prominent example of such systems is the 4T1 cell subline of a spontaneous mammary gland carcinoma from a Balb/cC3H mouse, although more are available [132]. However, the complete lack of human elements in this system may be regarded as major limitation. This is especially true currently for studies focused on mammary field cancerization, as most of the knowledge in this field has indeed been generated (perhaps correctly so) using human tissues, and no syngeneic mouse cells specific for mammary field cancerization exists to date. As a special type of syngeneic model, preneoplastic lesions can be induced in murine mammary tumorigenesis, especially alveolar hyperplasias represented by the classical hyperplastic alveolar nodule (HAN) and the ductal hyperplasias (DHs) represented by usual DH and ductal carcinoma *in situ* (DCIS) [133]. The former type of lesion is induced by viral, chemical and hormonal agents; the latter by chemical agents and specific genetic alterations. Such models can be used to study aspects of molecular alterations associated with tumorigenesis, immortalization and epithelial hyperplasia, and perhaps alterations specific for mammary field cancerization.

One notable *in vivo* model recently presented to the scientific community interested in mammary cell biology, and amenable to the study of field cancerization, is the orthotopic humanized mammary fad pad model reported by Kuperwasser and colleagues from Robert Weinberg's laboratory [134]. In this model, mammary fat pads in immunocompromised mice are cleared of mouse fibroblasts and reconstituted with irradiated telomerase-immortalized human mammary stromal fibroblasts. Adding radiation to the model led to the non-tumorigenic proliferation of these fibroblasts in the fad pads. Importantly, the human fibroblasts were observed to intersperse and integrate with murine adipose tissue, indicating successful tissue reconstitution. A remarkable observation in this model was that it generated a platform for engraftment of normal human mammary epithelial and non-irradiated human stromal cells as organoids to grow and undergo normal breast tissue morphology, primarily of the acinar shape, consisting of spherical structures with hollow lumina. A less commonly observed shape was of the linear ductal histology with side branching, also a normal phenotype. This orthotopic model also allows for manipulation using different growth factors, including hepatocyte growth factor (HGF) and transforming growth factor β (TGF-β). However, perhaps the most important finding from using this model was that some cases of reduction mammoplasties led to hyperplastic outgrowths with histology not dissimilar to *in situ* and even invasive carcinoma [134]. The latter result has important implications for the study of mammary field cancerization. If field cancerized mammary epithelial cells represent pre-malignant entities according to some of the concepts discussed in section 9.1.2, this orthotopic mammary fat pad model would be highly suitable for the study of field cancerized epithelial cells from human breast tissues.

Finally, the ultimate goal is to understand in full detail the mechanisms of field cancerization. Should these efforts reveal causative molecular mediators responsible for field cancerization, it should be possible to develop transgenic (knock-in, knock-out, conditional regulation) mouse models to study the mechanism of action of these mediators. This approach could be combined with mammary tissue specific expression of the mediators of interest, for example using whey acidic protein promoter controlled transcription.

9.7. Final Conclusions

The study of field cancerization in mammary tissues is clearly an emerging field of research driven by the increasing realization of its clinical importance and utility, once understood at the mechanistic level. The present chapter provides ample evidence for molecular alterations occurring in structurally intact tissues located at some distances adjacent to cancerous lesions. These alterations are of genetic (section 9.2), epigenetic (section 9.3), and expressional (section 9.4) nature. Thus, while the extension of the concept of field cancerization from the original observations in head and neck cancer to human mammary tissues has been accepted, there are unresolved and pressing issues that should be prioritized in the future. Some of these issues are listed below:

i. *Mechanisms:* As the major focus in breast tissue research lies on the characterization of cancers, research on field cancerization is rather recent and mostly of observational nature. While these observations are now substantial, especially in regard to markers of genomic instability, it is imperative to transition from observations to mechanisms, *i.e.* to elucidate the underlying pathways leading to or supporting this fascinating phenomenon. Only then will the full potential of clinical utility become evident. The latter may include means for diagnosis, prevention, and treatment stratification (see also section 9.5). The *in vitro* and *in vivo* models discussed in sections 9.6.2 and 9.6.3 could be part of this quest.
ii. *Standardization:* Some of the studies presented in this chapter clearly indicate the necessity for methods of standardization in order to allow meaningful comparisons between studies and patient populations. This pertains to multiple types of data, including biological measures, patient annotation information, literature referring, and others. This problem is of course not specific to research on mammary field cancerization, but inherent to all multi-Institutional and translational research utilizing material obtained from different patient populations. These efforts are clearly underway, as shown by the widely-used public databases and data repositories (*e.g.* the National Center for Biotechnology Information (NCBI)'s Gene Expression Omnibus (GEO) Database available at http://www.ncbi.nlm.nih.gov/geo/), and by numerous innovative data mining approaches reported in the literature. Of note, the integration of vast information stemming from research on mammary field cancerization should in theory benefit from the fact that field cancerized tissues are less heterogeneous than their cancerous counterparts, thus theoretically representing a "simplification" towards their analyses. This however, remains to be shown.
iii. *Extension:* Seemingly contradictory to the previous statement, it is also necessary to extend the current observations using additional technologies, perhaps in an integrative manner as strongly suggested by the concepts of systems biology. The latter is already being actively pursued in breast disease [124,125], and is believed to

hold the key to personalized medicine as a goal for the 21st century. Accordingly, and as mentioned previously, genetic observations of mammary field cancerization are plenty, while other biochemical and biological data is lacking. In addition, as indicated in section 9.1.2, the extent of the field of affected cells is to date poorly defined. As is true for the quest of mechanism identification, it is clear that in order to fully exploit the clinical utility of biomarkers of field cancerization as applied to breast disease, the field itself, *i.e.* its disease-dependent size variations and its possible pattern commonalities needs to be better defined.

In trying to integrate these ideas, we propose a "positive feed-forward approach" as shown in Figure 9-15, a cycle appropriately initiated by the use of human material as the most relevant source to date for the study of mammary field cancerization. This approach is designed to generate new knowledge of this phenomenon in the future, with the ultimate goal of developing clinical applications, such as the use of biomarkers and the discovery of targets.

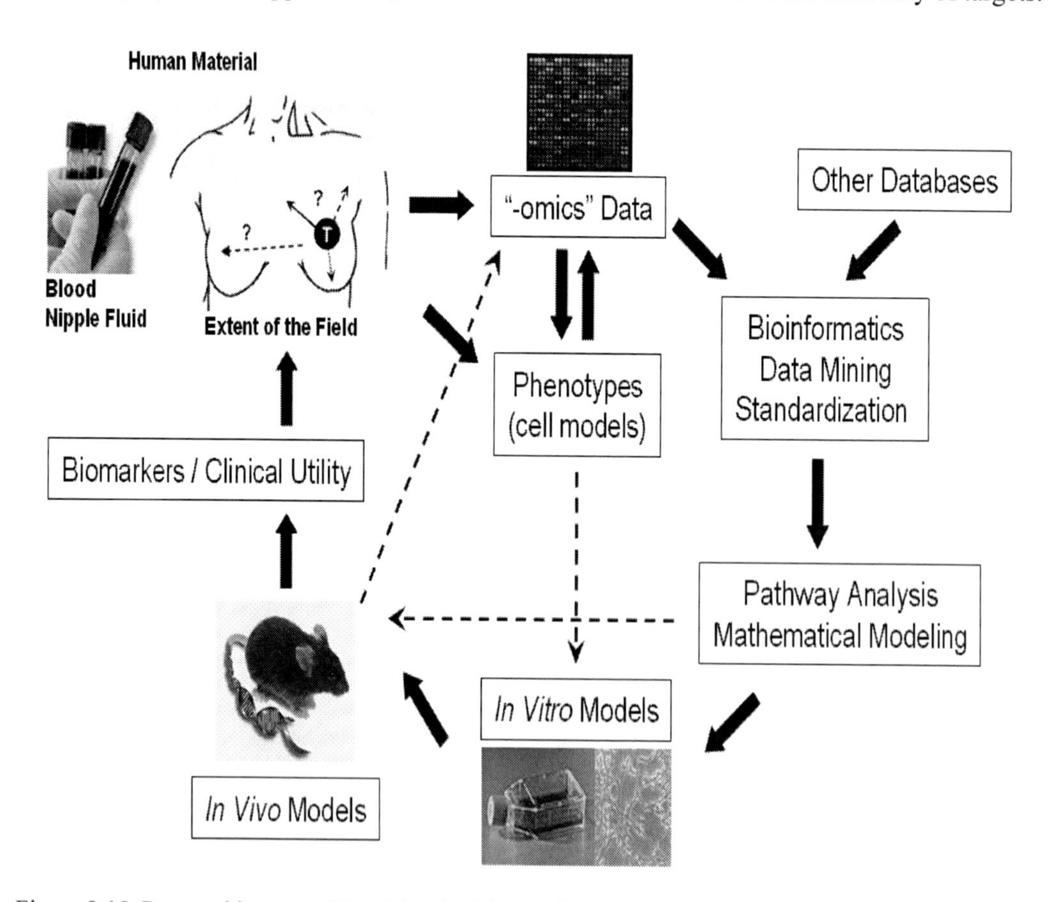

Figure 9.15. Proposed integrated "positive feed-forward approach" for research in mammary field cancerization. Human material (breast tissue, blood, nipple fluid) is highly appropriate and accessible as a source of complex "-omics" data. Bioinformatic data mining will lead to models and mechanisms that can be tested *in vitro* and *in vivo* systems, leading to the development of clinically useful devices (biomarkers, assays, targets) that in turn can be tested in human patients. Several possible shortcuts (dotted lines) are also shown.

References

[1] Sternlicht MD (2006) Key stages in mammary gland development: the cues that regulate ductal branching morphogenesis. *Breast Cancer Res.* 8: 201.

[2] Heaphy CM, Baumgartner KB, Bisoffi M, Baumgartner RN, Griffith JK (2007) Telomere DNA content predicts breast cancer-free survival interval. *Clin. Cancer Res.* 13: 7037-7043.

[3] Slaughter DP, Southwick HW, Smejkal W (1953) Field cancerization in oral stratified squamous epithelium; clinical implications of multicentric origin. *Cancer* 6: 963-968.

[4] Braakhuis BJ, Tabor MP, Kummer JA, Leemans CR, Brakenhoff RH (2003) A genetic explanation of Slaughter's concept of field cancerization: evidence and clinical implications. *Cancer Res.* 63: 1727-1730.

[5] Hines WC, Fajardo AM, Joste NE, Bisoffi M, Griffith JK (2005) Quantitative and spatial measurements of telomerase reverse transcriptase expression within normal and malignant human breast tissues. *Mol. Cancer Res.* 3: 503-509.

[6] Holst CR, Nuovo GJ, Esteller M, Chew K, Baylin SB, et al. (2003) Methylation of p16(INK4a) promoters occurs in vivo in histologically normal human mammary epithelia. *Cancer Res.* 63: 1596-1601.

[7] Tlsty TD, Crawford YG, Holst CR, Fordyce CA, Zhang J, et al. (2004) Genetic and epigenetic changes in mammary epithelial cells may mimic early events in carcinogenesis. *J. Mammary Gland Biol. Neoplasia* 9: 263-274.

[8] Debnath J, Brugge JS (2005) Modelling glandular epithelial cancers in three-dimensional cultures. *Nat Rev Cancer* 5: 675-688.

[9] Eigeliene N, Harkonen P, Erkkola R (2006) Effects of estradiol and medroxyprogesterone acetate on morphology, proliferation and apoptosis of human breast tissue in organ cultures. *BMC Cancer* 6: 246.

[10] Dakubo GD, Jakupciak JP, Birch-Machin MA, Parr RL (2007) Clinical implications and utility of field cancerization. *Cancer Cell Int.* 7: 2.

[11] Hockel M, Dornhofer N (2005) The hydra phenomenon of cancer: why tumors recur locally after microscopically complete resection. *Cancer Res.* 65: 2997-3002.

[12] Ellsworth DL, Ellsworth RE, Liebman MN, Hooke JA, Shriver CD (2004) Genomic instability in histologically normal breast tissues: implications for carcinogenesis. *Lancet Oncol.* 5: 753-758.

[13] Watson CJ, Khaled WT (2008) Mammary development in the embryo and adult: a journey of morphogenesis and commitment. *Development* 135: 995-1003.

[14] Mailleux AA, Overholtzer M, Brugge JS (2008) Lumen formation during mammary epithelial morphogenesis: insights from in vitro and in vivo models. *Cell Cycle* 7: 57-62.

[15] Lanigan F, O'Connor D, Martin F, Gallagher WM (2007) Molecular links between mammary gland development and breast cancer. *Cell Mol. Life Sci.* 64: 3159-3184.

[16] Kopans D (1998) Breast Imaging. Philadelphia, PA, USA: Lippincott Williams and Wilkins.

[17] Hayes D (2000) Atlas of Breast Cancer. St. Louis, MO, USA: Mosby (Elsevier).

[18] Soto AM, Vandenberg LN, Maffini MV, Sonnenschein C (2008) Does breast cancer start in the womb? *Basic Clin. Pharmacol. Toxicol.* 102: 125-133.

[19] De Wever O, Demetter P, Mareel M, Bracke M (2008) Stromal myofibroblasts are drivers of invasive cancer growth. *Int. J. Cancer* 123: 2229-2238.

[20] De Wever O, Mareel M (2003) Role of tissue stroma in cancer cell invasion. *J. Pathol.* 200: 429-447.

[21] Condon MS (2005) The role of the stromal microenvironment in prostate cancer. *Semin. Cancer Biol.* 15: 132-137.

[22] Rowley DR (1998) What might a stromal response mean to prostate cancer progression? *Cancer Metastasis Rev.* 17: 411-419.

[23] Tuxhorn JA, Ayala GE, Rowley DR (2001) Reactive stroma in prostate cancer progression. *J. Urol.* 166: 2472-2483.

[24] Radisky ES, Radisky DC (2007) Stromal induction of breast cancer: inflammation and invasion. *Rev. Endocr. Metab. Disord.* 8: 279-287.

[25] Fukino K, Shen L, Matsumoto S, Morrison CD, Mutter GL, et al. (2004) Combined total genome loss of heterozygosity scan of breast cancer stroma and epithelium reveals multiplicity of stromal targets. *Cancer Res.* 64: 7231-7236.

[26] Fukino K, Shen L, Patocs A, Mutter GL, Eng C (2007) Genomic instability within tumor stroma and clinicopathological characteristics of sporadic primary invasive breast carcinoma. *Jama* 297: 2103-2111.

[27] Kurose K, Hoshaw-Woodard S, Adeyinka A, Lemeshow S, Watson PH, et al. (2001) Genetic model of multi-step breast carcinogenesis involving the epithelium and stroma: clues to tumour-microenvironment interactions. *Hum. Mol. Genet.* 10: 1907-1913.

[28] Moinfar F, Man YG, Arnould L, Bratthauer GL, Ratschek M, et al. (2000) Concurrent and independent genetic alterations in the stromal and epithelial cells of mammary carcinoma: implications for tumorigenesis. *Cancer Res.* 60: 2562-2566.

[29] Brooks SA, Lomax-Browne HJ, Carter TM, Kinch CE, Hall DM (2009) Molecular interactions in cancer cell metastasis. *Acta Histochem.*

[30] McSherry EA, Donatello S, Hopkins AM, McDonnell S (2007) Molecular basis of invasion in breast cancer. *Cell Mol. Life Sci.* 64: 3201-3218.

[31] Stallings-Mann M, Radisky D (2007) Matrix metalloproteinase-induced malignancy in mammary epithelial cells. *Cells Tissues Organs* 185: 104-110.

[32] Han B, Nakamura M, Mori I, Nakamura Y, Kakudo K (2005) Urokinase-type plasminogen activator system and breast cancer (Review). *Oncol. Rep.* 14: 105-112.

[33] White DE, Muller WJ (2007) Multifaceted roles of integrins in breast cancer metastasis. *J. Mammary Gland Biol. Neoplasia* 12: 135-142.

[34] Chang HY, Chi JT, Dudoit S, Bondre C, van de Rijn M, et al. (2002) Diversity, topographic differentiation, and positional memory in human fibroblasts. *Proc. Natl. Acad. Sci. USA* 99: 12877-12882.

[35] Cleaver O, Melton DA (2003) Endothelial signaling during development. *Nat. Med.* 9: 661-668.

[36] Larson PS, de las Morenas A, Cerda SR, Bennett SR, Cupples LA, et al. (2006) Quantitative analysis of allele imbalance supports atypical ductal hyperplasia lesions as direct breast cancer precursors. *J. Pathol.* 209: 307-316.

[37] O'Connell P, Pekkel V, Fuqua SA, Osborne CK, Clark GM, et al. (1998) Analysis of loss of heterozygosity in 399 premalignant breast lesions at 15 genetic loci. *J. Natl. Cancer Inst.* 90: 697-703.

[38] Larson PS, de las Morenas A, Cupples LA, Huang K, Rosenberg CL (1998) Genetically abnormal clones in histologically normal breast tissue. *Am. J Pathol.* 152: 1591-1598.

[39] Larson PS, de las Morenas A, Bennett SR, Cupples LA, Rosenberg CL (2002) Loss of heterozygosity or allele imbalance in histologically normal breast epithelium is distinct from loss of heterozygosity or allele imbalance in co-existing carcinomas. *Am. J. Pathol.* 161: 283-290.

[40] Larson PS, Schlechter BL, de las Morenas A, Garber JE, Cupples LA, et al. (2005) Allele imbalance, or loss of heterozygosity, in normal breast epithelium of sporadic breast cancer cases and BRCA1 gene mutation carriers is increased compared with reduction mammoplasty tissues. *J. Clin. Oncol.* 23: 8613-8619.

[41] Heaphy CM, Bisoffi M, Fordyce CA, Haaland CM, Hines WC, et al. (2006) Telomere DNA content and allelic imbalance demonstrate field cancerization in histologically normal tissue adjacent to breast tumors. *Int. J. Cancer* 119: 108-116.

[42] Forsti A, Louhelainen J, Soderberg M, Wijkstrom H, Hemminki K (2001) Loss of heterozygosity in tumour-adjacent normal tissue of breast and bladder cancer. *Eur. J. Cancer* 37: 1372-1380.

[43] Ellsworth RE, Ellsworth DL, Lubert SM, Hooke J, Somiari RI, et al. (2003) High-throughput loss of heterozygosity mapping in 26 commonly deleted regions in breast cancer. *Cancer Epidemiol. Biomarkers Prev.* 12: 915-919.

[44] Ellsworth DL, Ellsworth RE, Love B, Deyarmin B, Lubert SM, et al. (2004) Outer breast quadrants demonstrate increased levels of genomic instability. *Ann. Surg. Oncol.* 11: 861-868.

[45] Ellsworth DL, Ellsworth RE, Love B, Deyarmin B, Lubert SM, et al. (2004) Genomic patterns of allelic imbalance in disease free tissue adjacent to primary breast carcinomas. *Breast Cancer Res. Treat.* 88: 131-139.

[46] Botti C, Pescatore B, Mottolese M, Sciarretta F, Greco C, et al. (2000) Incidence of chromosomes 1 and 17 aneusomy in breast cancer and adjacent tissue: an interphase cytogenetic study. *J. Am. Coll Surg.* 190: 530-539.

[47] Lengauer C, Kinzler KW, Vogelstein B (1998) Genetic instabilities in human cancers. *Nature* 396: 643-649.

[48] Desmaze C, Soria JC, Freulet-Marriere MA, Mathieu N, Sabatier L (2003) Telomere-driven genomic instability in cancer cells. *Cancer Lett.* 194: 173-182.

[49] Hackett JA, Feldser DM, Greider CW (2001) Telomere dysfunction increases mutation rate and genomic instability. *Cell* 106: 275-286.

[50] Moyzis RK, Buckingham JM, Cram LS, Dani M, Deaven LL, et al. (1988) A highly conserved repetitive DNA sequence, (TTAGGG)n, present at the telomeres of human chromosomes. *Proc. Natl. Acad. Sci. USA* 85: 6622-6626.

[51] Maser RS, DePinho RA (2004) Telomeres and the DNA damage response: why the fox is guarding the henhouse. *DNA Repair* (Amst) 3: 979-988.

[52] Olovnikov AM (1971) [Principle of marginotomy in template synthesis of polynucleotides]. *Dokl. Akad. Nauk SSSR* 201: 1496-1499.

[53] Smogorzewska A, van Steensel B, Bianchi A, Oelmann S, Schaefer MR, et al. (2000) Control of human telomere length by TRF1 and TRF2. *Mol. Cell Biol.* 20: 1659-1668.

[54] Bohr VA, Anson RM (1995) DNA damage, mutation and fine structure DNA repair in aging. *Mutat. Res.* 338: 25-34.

[55] Kim NW, Piatyszek MA, Prowse KR, Harley CB, West MD, et al. (1994) Specific association of human telomerase activity with immortal cells and cancer. *Science* 266: 2011-2015.

[56] Neumann AA, Reddel RR (2002) Telomere maintenance and cancer -- look, no telomerase. *Nat. Rev. Cancer* 2: 879-884.

[57] Fordyce CA, Heaphy CM, Griffith JK (2002) Chemiluminescent measurement of telomere DNA content in biopsies. *Biotechniques* 33: 144-146, 148.

[58] Meeker AK, Gage WR, Hicks JL, Simon I, Coffman JR, et al. (2002) Telomere length assessment in human archival tissues: combined telomere fluorescence in situ hybridization and immunostaining. *Am. J. Pathol.* 160: 1259-1268.

[59] Meeker AK, Hicks JL, Gabrielson E, Strauss WM, De Marzo AM, et al. (2004) Telomere shortening occurs in subsets of normal breast epithelium as well as in situ and invasive carcinoma. *Am. J. Pathol.* 164: 925-935.

[60] Kurabayashi R, Takubo K, Aida J, Honma N, Poon SS, et al. (2008) Luminal and cancer cells in the breast show more rapid telomere shortening than myoepithelial cells and fibroblasts. *Hum. Pathol.*

[61] Meeker AK, Argani P (2004) Telomere shortening occurs early during breast tumorigenesis: a cause of chromosome destabilization underlying malignant transformation? *J. Mammary Gland Biol. Neoplasia* 9: 285-296.

[62] Lo PK, Sukumar S (2008) Epigenomics and breast cancer. *Pharmacogenomics* 9: 1879-1902.

[63] Coyle YM (2004) The effect of environment on breast cancer risk. *Breast Cancer Res.* Treat 84: 273-288.

[64] Anand P, Kunnumakkara AB, Sundaram C, Harikumar KB, Tharakan ST, et al. (2008) Cancer is a preventable disease that requires major lifestyle changes. *Pharm. Res.* 25: 2097-2116.

[65] Seitz HK, Stickel F (2007) Molecular mechanisms of alcohol-mediated carcinogenesis. *Nat. Rev. Cancer* 7: 599-612.

[66] Friso S, Choi SW (2002) Gene-nutrient interactions and DNA methylation. *J. Nutr.* 132: 2382S-2387S.

[67] Li S, Hursting SD, Davis BJ, McLachlan JA, Barrett JC (2003) Environmental exposure, DNA methylation, and gene regulation: lessons from diethylstilbesterol-induced cancers. *Ann. N. Y. Acad. Sci.* 983: 161-169.

[68] Sadikovic B, Rodenhiser DI (2006) Benzopyrene exposure disrupts DNA methylation and growth dynamics in breast cancer cells. *Toxicol. Appl. Pharmacol.* 216: 458-468.

[69] Gudjonsson T, Villadsen R, Ronnov-Jessen L, Petersen OW (2004) Immortalization protocols used in cell culture models of human breast morphogenesis. *Cell Mol. Life Sci.* 61: 2523-2534.

[70] Bradley C, van der Meer R, Roodi N, Yan H, Chandrasekharan MB, et al. (2007) Carcinogen-induced histone alteration in normal human mammary epithelial cells. *Carcinogenesis* 28: 2184-2192.

[71] Valinluck V, Sowers LC (2007) Inflammation-mediated cytosine damage: a mechanistic link between inflammation and the epigenetic alterations in human cancers. *Cancer Res.* 67: 5583-5586.

[72] Kanai Y (2008) Alterations of DNA methylation and clinicopathological diversity of human cancers. *Pathol. Int.* 58: 544-558.

[73] Dulaimi E, Hillinck J, Ibanez de Caceres I, Al-Saleem T, Cairns P (2004) Tumor suppressor gene promoter hypermethylation in serum of breast cancer patients. *Clin. Cancer Res.* 10: 6189-6193.
[74] Van der Auwera I, Van Laere SJ, Van den Bosch SM, Van den Eynden GG, Trinh BX, et al. (2008) Aberrant methylation of the Adenomatous Polyposis Coli (APC) gene promoter is associated with the inflammatory breast cancer phenotype. *Br. J. Cancer* 99: 1735-1742.
[75] Bloushtain-Qimron N, Yao J, Snyder EL, Shipitsin M, Campbell LL, et al. (2008) Cell type-specific DNA methylation patterns in the human breast. *Proc. Natl. Acad. Sci. USA* 105: 14076-14081.
[76] Cheng AS, Culhane AC, Chan MW, Venkataramu CR, Ehrich M, et al. (2008) Epithelial progeny of estrogen-exposed breast progenitor cells display a cancer-like methylome. *Cancer Res.* 68: 1786-1796.
[77] Yan PS, Venkataramu C, Ibrahim A, Liu JC, Shen RZ, et al. (2006) Mapping geographic zones of cancer risk with epigenetic biomarkers in normal breast tissue. *Clin. Cancer Res.* 12: 6626-6636.
[78] Umbricht CB, Evron E, Gabrielson E, Ferguson A, Marks J, et al. (2001) Hypermethylation of 14-3-3 sigma (stratifin) is an early event in breast cancer. *Oncogene* 20: 3348-3353.
[79] Lewis CM, Cler LR, Bu DW, Zochbauer-Muller S, Milchgrub S, et al. (2005) Promoter hypermethylation in benign breast epithelium in relation to predicted breast cancer risk. *Clin. Cancer Res.* 11: 166-172.
[80] Ushijima T (2007) Epigenetic field for cancerization. *J. Biochem. Mol. Biol.* 40: 142-150.
[81] Lawson JS, Gunzburg WH, Whitaker NJ (2006) Viruses and human breast cancer. *Future Microbiol.* 1: 33-51.
[82] Cho K, Lee YK, Greenhalgh DG (2008) Endogenous retroviruses in systemic response to stress signals. *Shock* 30: 105-116.
[83] Yamada N, Nishida Y, Tsutsumida H, Hamada T, Goto M, et al. (2008) MUC1 expression is regulated by DNA methylation and histone H3 lysine 9 modification in cancer cells. *Cancer Res.* 68: 2708-2716.
[84] Da Silva L, Parry S, Reid L, Keith P, Waddell N, et al. (2008) Aberrant expression of E-cadherin in lobular carcinomas of the breast. *Am. J. Surg. Pathol.* 32: 773-783.
[85] Braakhuis BJ, Leemans CR, Brakenhoff RH (2004) Using tissue adjacent to carcinoma as a normal control: an obvious but questionable practice. *J. Pathol.* 203: 620-621.
[86] Finak G, Sadekova S, Pepin F, Hallett M, Meterissian S, et al. (2006) Gene expression signatures of morphologically normal breast tissue identify basal-like tumors. *Breast Cancer Res.* 8: R58.
[87] Baird DM (2008) Mechanisms of telomeric instability. *Cytogenet. Genome Res.* 122: 308-314.
[88] Elenbaas B, Spirio L, Koerner F, Fleming MD, Zimonjic DB, et al. (2001) Human breast cancer cells generated by oncogenic transformation of primary mammary epithelial cells. *Genes. Dev.* 15: 50-65.
[89] Baykal A, Rosen D, Zhou C, Liu J, Sahin AA (2004) Telomerase in breast cancer: a critical evaluation. *Adv. Anat. Pathol.* 11: 262-268.

[90] Hiyama E, Gollahon L, Kataoka T, Kuroi K, Yokoyama T, et al. (1996) Telomerase activity in human breast tumors. *J. Natl. Cancer Inst.* 88: 116-122.
[91] Herbert BS, Wright WE, Shay JW (2001) Telomerase and breast cancer. *Breast Cancer Res*. 3: 146-149.
[92] De Marzo AM, Meeker AK, Zha S, Luo J, Nakayama M, et al. (2003) Human prostate cancer precursors and pathobiology. *Urology 62*: 55-62.
[93] Soler D, Genesca A, Arnedo G, Egozcue J, Tusell L (2005) Telomere dysfunction drives chromosomal instability in human mammary epithelial cells. *Genes Chromosomes Cancer* 44: 339-350.
[94] Maida Y, Kyo S, Kanaya T, Wang Z, Yatabe N, et al. (2002) Direct activation of telomerase by EGF through Ets-mediated transactivation of TERT via MAP kinase signaling pathway. *Oncogene* 21: 4071-4079.
[95] Liu J, Baykal A, Fung KM, Thompson-Lanza JA, Hoque A, et al. (2004) Human telomerase reverse transcriptase mRNA is highly expressed in normal breast tissues and down-regulated in ductal carcinoma in situ. *Int. J. Oncol.* 24: 879-884.
[96] Kolquist KA, Ellisen LW, Counter CM, Meyerson M, Tan LK, et al. (1998) Expression of TERT in early premalignant lesions and a subset of cells in normal tissues. *Nat. Genet.* 19: 182-186.
[97] Kyo S, Takakura M, Fujiwara T, Inoue M (2008) Understanding and exploiting hTERT promoter regulation for diagnosis and treatment of human cancers. *Cancer Sci.* 99: 1528-1538.
[98] Chang CC, Sun W, Cruz A, Saitoh M, Tai MH, et al. (2001) A human breast epithelial cell type with stem cell characteristics as target cells for carcinogenesis. *Radiat. Res.* 155: 201-207.
[99] Hondermarck H, Tastet C, El Yazidi-Belkoura I, Toillon RA, Le Bourhis X (2008) Proteomics of breast cancer: the quest for markers and therapeutic targets. *J. Proteome Res.* 7: 1403-1411.
[100] Culhane AC, Howlin J (2007) Molecular profiling of breast cancer: transcriptomic studies and beyond. *Cell Mol. Life Sci.* 64: 3185-3200.
[101] Claudino WM, Quattrone A, Biganzoli L, Pestrin M, Bertini I, et al. (2007) Metabolomics: available results, current research projects in breast cancer, and future applications. *J. Clin. Oncol.* 25: 2840-2846.
[102] Sawyers CL (2008) The cancer biomarker problem. *Nature* 452: 548-552.
[103] Burke HB (2004) Outcome prediction and the future of the TNM staging system. *J. Natl. Cancer Inst.* 96: 1408-1409.
[104] Dowsett M, Dunbier AK (2008) Emerging biomarkers and new understanding of traditional markers in personalized therapy for breast cancer. *Clin. Cancer Res*. 14: 8019-8026.
[105] Tripathi A, King C, de la Morenas A, Perry VK, Burke B, et al. (2008) Gene expression abnormalities in histologically normal breast epithelium of breast cancer patients. *Int. J. Cancer* 122: 1557-1566.
[106] Wallis M, Tardivon A, Helbich T, Schreer I (2007) Guidelines from the European Society of Breast Imaging for diagnostic interventional breast procedures. *Eur. Radiol.* 17: 581-588.
[107] Smith JA, Andreopoulou E (2004) An overview of the status of imaging screening technology for breast cancer. *Ann. Oncol.* 15 Suppl 1: I18-I26.

[108] Esserman LJ, Shieh Y, Park JW, Ozanne EM (2007) A role for biomarkers in the screening and diagnosis of breast cancer in younger women. *Expert Rev. Mol. Diagn* 7: 533-544.
[109] Baines CJ (2005) Are there downsides to mammography screening? *Breast J.* 11 Suppl 1: S7-10.
[110] Feig SA (2005) Screening mammography controversies: resolved, partly resolved, and unresolved. *Breast J.* 11 Suppl 1: S3-6.
[111] Paci E, Warwick J, Falini P, Duffy SW (2004) Overdiagnosis in screening: is the increase in breast cancer incidence rates a cause for concern? *J. Med. Screen* 11: 23-27.
[112] Goldhirsch A, Glick JH, Gelber RD, Coates AS, Thurlimann B, et al. (2005) Meeting highlights: international expert consensus on the primary therapy of early breast cancer 2005. *Ann. Oncol.* 16: 1569-1583.
[113] Goldhirsch A, Wood WC, Gelber RD, Coates AS, Thurlimann B, et al. (2007) Progress and promise: highlights of the international expert consensus on the primary therapy of early breast cancer 2007. *Ann. Oncol.* 18: 1133-1144.
[114] Bernards R, Weinberg RA (2002) A progression puzzle. *Nature* 418: 823.
[115] Klein CA (2008) Cancer. The metastasis cascade. *Science* 321: 1785-1787.
[116] Fordyce CA, Heaphy CM, Bisoffi M, Wyaco JL, Joste NE, et al. (2006) Telomere content correlates with stage and prognosis in breast cancer. *Breast Cancer Res. Treat* 99: 193-202.
[117] Fisher ER, Anderson S, Tan-Chiu E, Fisher B, Eaton L, et al. (2001) Fifteen-year prognostic discriminants for invasive breast carcinoma: National Surgical Adjuvant Breast and Bowel Project Protocol-06. *Cancer* 91: 1679-1687.
[118] Fisher B, Anderson S, Bryant J, Margolese RG, Deutsch M, et al. (2002) Twenty-year follow-up of a randomized trial comparing total mastectomy, lumpectomy, and lumpectomy plus irradiation for the treatment of invasive breast cancer. *N. Engl. J. Med.* 347: 1233-1241.
[119] Veronesi U, Cascinelli N, Mariani L, Greco M, Saccozzi R, et al. (2002) Twenty-year follow-up of a randomized study comparing breast-conserving surgery with radical mastectomy for early breast cancer. *N. Engl. J. Med.* 347: 1227-1232.
[120] Huston TL, Simmons RM (2005) Locally recurrent breast cancer after conservation therapy. *Am. J. Surg.* 189: 229-235.
[121] Chen Y, Thompson W, Semenciw R, Mao Y (1999) Epidemiology of contralateral breast cancer. *Cancer Epidemiol. Biomarkers Prev.* 8: 855-861.
[122] Robson ME (2007) Treatment of hereditary breast cancer. *Semin. Oncol.* 34: 384-391.
[123] Roukos DH (2008) Genetics and genome-wide association studies: surgery-guided algorithm and promise for future breast cancer personalized surgery. *Expert. Rev. Mol. Diagn.* 8: 587-597.
[124] Celis JE, Moreira JM, Gromova I, Cabezon T, Ralfkiaer U, et al. (2005) Towards discovery-driven translational research in breast cancer. *Febs J.* 272: 2-15.
[125] Li J, Gromov P, Gromova I, Moreira JM, Timmermans-Wielenga V, et al. (2008) Omics-based profiling of carcinoma of the breast and matched regional lymph node metastasis. *Proteomics* 8: 5038-5052.
[126] Ignatiadis M, Georgoulias V, Mavroudis D (2008) Circulating tumor cells in breast cancer. *Curr. Opin. Obstet. Gynecol.* 20: 55-60.

[127] Garrisi VM, Abbate I, Quaranta M, Mangia A, Tommasi S, et al. (2008) SELDI-TOF serum proteomics and breast cancer: which perspective? *Expert Rev. Proteomics* 5: 779-785.

[128] Burdall SE, Hanby AM, Lansdown MR, Speirs V (2003) Breast cancer cell lines: friend or foe? *Breast Cancer Res.* 5: 89-95.

[129] Holliday R (1996) Endless quest. *Bioessays* 18: 3-5.

[130] Marastoni S, Ligresti G, Lorenzon E, Colombatti A, Mongiat M (2008) Extracellular matrix: a matter of life and death. *Connect Tissue Res.* 49: 203-206.

[131] Bissell MJ (2007) Modelling molecular mechanisms of breast cancer and invasion: lessons from the normal gland. *Biochem. Soc. Trans.* 35: 18-22.

[132] Ottewell PD, Coleman RE, Holen I (2006) From genetic abnormality to metastases: murine models of breast cancer and their use in the development of anticancer therapies. *Breast Cancer Res. Treat.* 96: 101-113.

[133] Medina D (2002) Biological and molecular characteristics of the premalignant mouse mammary gland. *Biochim. Biophys. Acta* 1603: 1-9.

[134] Kuperwasser C, Chavarria T, Wu M, Magrane G, Gray JW, et al. (2004) Reconstruction of functionally normal and malignant human breast tissues in mice. *Proc. Natl. Acad. Sci. USA* 101: 4966-4971.

In: Field Cancerization: Basic Science and Clinical Applications ISBN 978-1-61761-006-6
Editor: Gabriel D. Dakubo

Chapter 10

Field Cancerization in Gastric Cancer

Toshikazu Ushijima and Takeichi Yoshida

Abstract

Frequent occurrence of multiple gastric cancers became clear as their endoscopic resection became popular. As an important mechanism, accumulation of aberrant DNA methylation of various genes, both driver and passenger genes, in "normal-appearing" gastric mucosae has been revealed.

Aberrant DNA methylation is induced by inflammation caused by *Helicobacter pylori* infection, a major causative agent of gastric cancers, and consists of permanent and temporary components that will remain and disappear, respectively, after discontinuance of *Helicobacter pylori* infection. Permanent methylation is almost absent in gastric mucosae of healthy individuals, and is present at low levels in gastric mucosae of patients with a single gastric cancer and at high levels in those of patients with multiple gastric cancers.

The presence of microsatellite instability in gastric cancers, mostly due to *MLH1* methylation, is also known to be associated with multiple gastric cancers. Accumulation of aberrant DNA methylation in gastric mucosae constitutes the major mechanism of field defect for gastric cancers.

10.1. Introduction

Gastric cancer is a major cause of cancer deaths world-wide [1]. Its incidence has markedly declined in the last century in the US and Europe [2], as shown by its crude mortality rate in Caucasian males at 33/100,000 in the early 20th century and at 5 in the late 20th century. However, gastric cancer incidence is still high in many Asian countries and Russia [1]. Histologically, gastric cancers are classified into intestinal and diffuse types, established by Lauren, in Western countries, and these two types largely correspond to differentiated and undifferentiated types in Japanese classification [3].

Early gastric cancers used to be treated by gastrectomy (total and partial gastrectomy), but now early intestinal-type gastric cancers are treated by endoscopic resection (ER), including endoscopic mucosal resection and endoscopic submucosal dissection [4,5]. ER conserves a much larger part of gastric mucosae than partial gastrectomy, and brought a dramatic improvement of quality of life after treatment. At the same time, it became clear that metachronous gastric cancers occur in 8.5-14.0 % of patients after ER [6,7], which was much higher than the incidence after partial gastrectomy (1.8 – 2.4 %) [8,9]. Also, patients with multiple gastric cancers are known to have a higher risk of developing another gastric cancer than patients with a single gastric cancer [10,11]. The very high incidence of metachronous gastric cancers and high risk of gastric cancer patients with multiple gastric cancers strongly indicate that "field cancerization" or "field defect" is involved in gastric carcinogenesis. As its molecular basis, accumulation of aberrant DNA methylation in "normal-appearing" gastric mucosae is now recognized to be deeply involved [12,13]. The aberrant DNA methylation is induced by *H. pylori* infection, a major etiologic factor for gastric cancers [14], mainly through inflammation [12,15]. In this chapter, we will describe both epigenetic and genetic field defects, placing emphasis on the epigenetic field defect.

10.2. Conventional Changes Indicative of the Presence of Field Defect

The presence of individuals with high risk of gastric cancers has been known for a long time, and suggested that a field defect for gastric cancers is present. Conventionally, the presence of gastric atrophy and/or intestinal metaplasia in the stomach of gastric cancer patients has been well known [16]. Recently, much effort has been made to develop serum and other molecular markers to detect individuals with high risk of gastric cancers.

10.2.1. Histological Changes Associated with Increased Risk

Gastric atrophy is characterized by loss of gastric glandular cells, and appearance of fibrous tissue. Intestinal metaplasia is characterized by the appearance of intestinal-type epithelia in the stomach, and is considered as an abnormal differentiation. Gastric atrophy and intestinal metaplasia are produced as a result of chronic inflammation due to *H. pylori* infection. A prospective study involving 5,373 subjects for more than 10 years revealed that subjects with moderate atrophy at the baseline had a hazard ratio of 2.22 to develop gastric cancers [17].

10.2.2. Serum and Molecular Markers for Increased Risk

Most serum markers to detect individuals at high risk for gastric cancers are related to atrophy of gastric mucosae [18]. Among these, the pepsinogen concentrations are most widely used. Pepsinogen I is produced in chief and mucous neck cells, and Pepsinogen II is produced in not only chief and mucous neck cells but also in cardiac, pyloric, and duodenal Brunner gland cells. Since gastric atrophy advances from the pyloric glands towards the cardiac glands, the level of pepsinogen I and the ratio of pepsinogen I/II decrease with the advancement [19]. If individuals are classified according to *H. pylori* infection status and the presence of atrophy, gastric cancer risk increases in the order of Group A (*H. pylori*-negative, atrophy-negative), Group B (*H. pylori*-positive, atrophy-negative), Group C (*H. pylori*-positive, atrophy-positive), and then Group D (*H. pylori*-negative, atrophy-positive) [20]. Groups B, C, and D have hazard ratios of 3.0, 3.7, and 32 compared with Group A [20,21].

Molecular risk markers that can be assessed in gastric biopsy specimens are still analyzed for research purpose, and their clinical usefulness has not been established. For example, expression of brain-type glycogen phosphorylase in non-cancerous gastric mucosae has been reported to be useful to predict occurrence of another gastric cancer [22]. *CDX2* is known as a master regulator of the intestinal phenotype, and is expressed in intestinal metaplasia. However, its expression has been shown to progressively decrease from intestinal metaplasia, dysplasia, and then cancers [23].

10.3. Epigenetic Field for Cancerization

Epigenetic mechanisms are deeply involved in gastric cancers because tumor-suppressor genes that can be inactivated by genetic or epigenetic mechanisms are more frequently inactivated by epigenetic mechanisms in gastric cancers [24]. Now, the deep involvement is underlain by a mechanism, induction of aberrant DNA methylation by *H. pylori* infection in gastric mucosae and formation of "epigenetic field defect".

10.3.1. Epigenetic Alterations

Epigenetic modifications are characterized by their inheritance upon somatic cell division, and represented by DNA methylation and histone modifications. They control development, cellular differentiation, and reprogramming by establishing gene usage patterns. DNA methylation of a promoter CpG island (CGI) is known to cause silencing of its downstream gene (figure 10-1) [25].

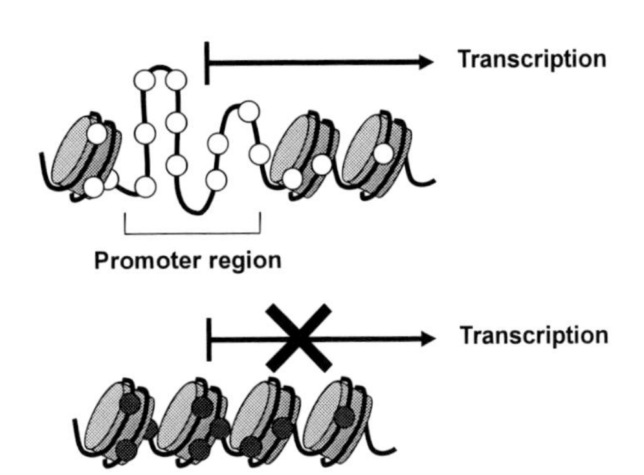

Figure 10.1. Silencing effect of DNA methylation of a CGI in promoter region. Most CGIs in gene promoter regions lack DNA methylation, and no nucleosome is formed. Therefore, transcription factors and RNA polymerase can have access to DNA, and the gene is transcribed. In contrast, if the CGI is methylated, a nucleosome is formed. Therefore, transcription machinery does not have access to DNA, and the gene is silenced.

When a promoter CGIs of a tumor-suppressor gene is aberrantly methylated, it leads to inactivation of the gene and can be causally involved in cancer development [26,27,28]. Therefore, aberrant methylation of promoter CGIs is considered to be equivalent to point mutations and chromosomal deletions.

Recent genome-wide studies on aberrant DNA methylation in cancers revealed that a large number of genes are methylated in their promoter CGIs in a single cancer cell [29,30,31]. Methylation of some genes, such as *CDKN2A*, *CDH1*, *MLH1*, *RUNX3*, *LOX*, and *MiR-124a*, is considered to be causally involved in cancer development [24,32,33], and these genes are designated as drivers. Methylation of other genes, such as *HAND1*, *FLNc*, and *THBD*, are unlikely to be involved in cancer development considering their low expression in normal gastric mucosae and known functions [12], and these genes are designated as passengers. The distinction between the drivers and passengers is just as in mutations.

10.3.2. Epigenetic Field for Cancerization, or Epigenetic Field Defect

Aberrant methylation of some genes, especially that of passenger genes, is accumulated in a large fraction of epithelial cells of the stomach, reaching up to several tens % [12,13,15]. The accumulation levels of methylation of specific passenger genes correlate with those of methylation of driver genes, and can be quantified more precisely because their methylation levels are high (figure 10-2).

Healthy people without *H. pylori* infection have very low methylation levels in their gastric mucosae, but gastric cancer patients without *H. pylori* infection have 5- to 300-fold higher methylation levels in their non-cancerous gastric mucosae (not in cancer tissues) (figure 10-2) [12].

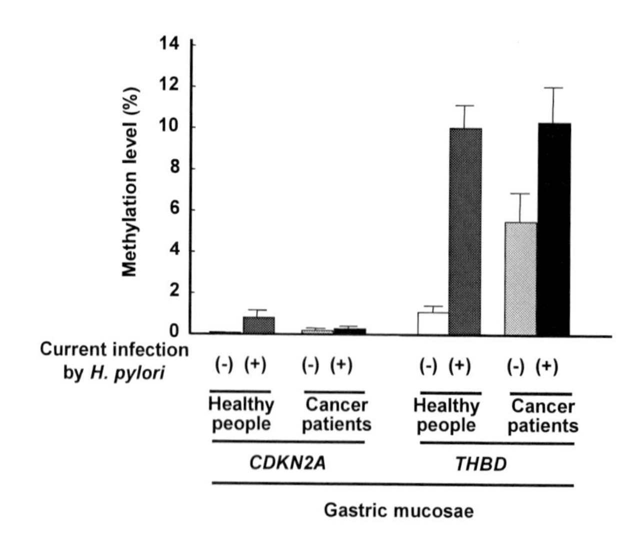

Figure 10.2. DNA methylation levels of *CDKN2A* and *THBD* in gastric mucosae of healthy people and cancer patients with and without *H. pylori* infection. Modified from Maekita et al [12]. Among healthy people, methylation levels were high in individuals with *H. pylori* infection, suggesting that *H. pylori* infection induce aberrant DNA methylation. Among individuals without *H. pylori* infection, gastric cancer patients showed higher methylation levels than healthy people, indicating that accumulation of aberrant DNA methylation is involved in formation of field defect.

Further, among individuals without *H. pylori* infection, patients with multiple gastric cancers have higher methylation levels in their non-cancerous gastric mucosae than those with a single gastric cancer, showing methylation levels in gastric mucosae are correlated with gastric cancer risk [13]. This shows that accumulation of aberrant DNA methylation of various genes in non-cancerous gastric mucosae forms an epigenetic field for cancerization, or epigenetic field defect.

10.3.3. Temporal Profile of Formation of Epigenetic Field Defect

Individuals with *H. pylori* infection have a very high methylation level irrespective of their cancer status and cancer risk. Since the vast majority of gastric cancer patients without current *H. pylori* infection are known to have had this infection in their past [14], the very high methylation level in individuals with *H. pylori* infection is expected to decrease when *H. pylori* infection discontinues. Temporal analysis of methylation levels in individuals who underwent eradication therapy for *H. pylori* confirmed that methylation levels decrease after eradication [34,35]. In other words, a methylation level in gastric mucosae is composed of two components – a temporary component that disappears when *H. pylori* infection discontinues and a permanent component that persists even after *H. pylori* infection discontinues.

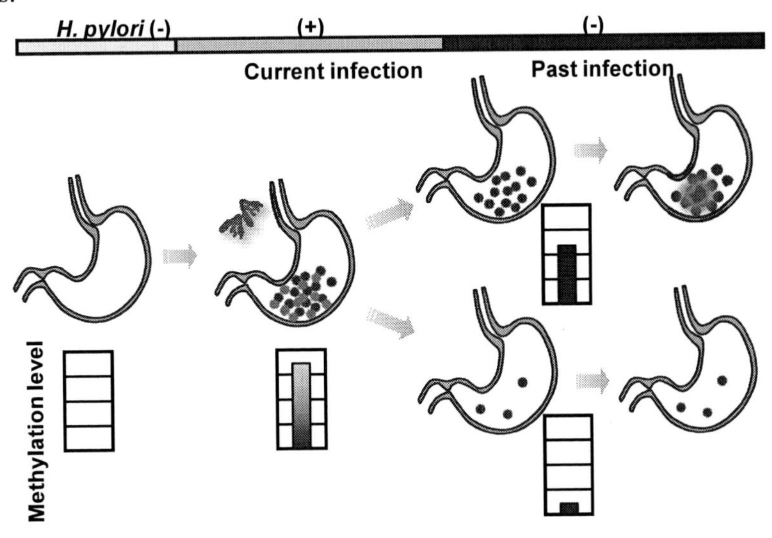

Figure 10.3. Induction of temporary and permanent components of methylation by *H. pylori* infection, and correlation between the permanent component and gastric cancer risk. Almost no methylation is present in gastric mucosae of individuals without any *H. pylori* infection. In gastric mucosae of individuals with *H. pylori* infection, very high levels of aberrant DNA methylation is induced, consisting of temporary and permanent components. When *H. pylori* infection discontinues by eradication or progression of atrophy, the temporary component, which is likely to be methylation in progenitor or differentiated cells, will disappear. In contrast, the permanent component, which is likely to be methylation in stem cells, will remain, and its level correlates with gastric cancer risk.

Based on these findings, a methylation level in gastric mucosae in one's life can be inferred to be very low before *H. pylori* infection takes place, to be very high while *H. pylori* infection is present, and to decrease when *H. pylori* infection discontinues (figure 10-3). If one's methylation level decreases to a low level, this indicates that his gastric mucosa has limited epigenetic damage in stem cells and has a low risk for gastric cancers. If one's methylation level shows little decrease, this indicates that his gastric mucosa has already accumulated a lot of epigenetic damage in stem cells and has a high risk for gastric cancers.

10.3.4. Mechanisms of Methylation Induction by *H. Pylori* Infection

The observations in humans described above strongly indicate that *H. pylori* infection induces aberrant methylation in gastric mucosae, but lack demonstration of a causal relationship.

Now, the causal role of *H. pylori* infection in methylation induction has been demonstrated by use of Mongolian gerbils. Infection of gerbils with *H. pylori* induced aberrant methylation in gastric mucosae while little methylation was induced in non-infected age-matched gerbils [15].

Mechanisms how *H. pylori* infection induces aberrant DNA methylation were also unclear in humans. *H. pylori* has endogenous methyltransferases and the type IV secretion system that allows its endogenous proteins to infect epithelial cells [36,37], and there was a possibility that bacterial methyltransferase was directly involved in methylation induction.

However, such a direct role was excluded since suppression of inflammation without decreasing number of *H. pylori* in the stomach markedly suppressed methylation induction [15]. It is still unknown what component of inflammation induced by *H. pylori* is responsible for methylation induction.

10.3.5. Gene Specificity in Methylation Induction

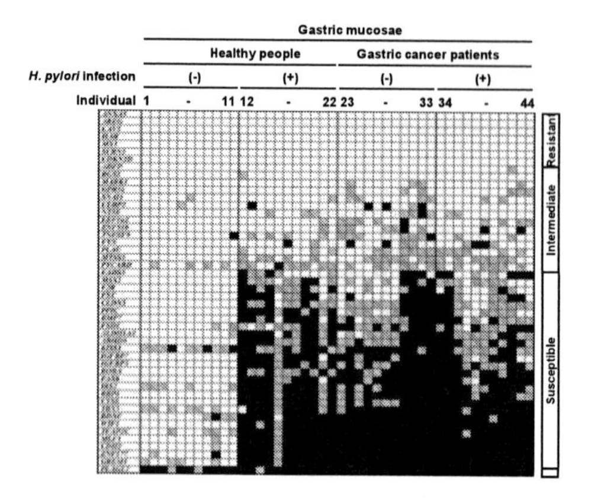

Figure 10.4. The presence of target gene specificity in methylation induction. Modified from Nakajima et al [38]. The presence of aberrant DNA methylation was analyzed by a high-sensitivity method, methylation-specific PCR, in gastric mucosae of healthy people and gastric cancer patients with and without *H. pylori* infection. Filled box, high levels of methylation detected; hatched box, low levels of methylation detected; and open box, no methylation detected. Some genes were easily methylated by *H. pylori* infection, and their methylation persisted in gastric cancer patients. The other genes were resistant to methylation induction.

Both driver and passenger genes are methylated in gastric mucosae, but there is a gene specificity in methylation induction [38]. A panel of genes was analyzed for methylation induction in gastric mucosae of individuals with and without *H. pylori* infection, and it was found that only a fraction of the genes were methylated in individuals with *H. pylori* infection (figure 10-4).

Similar target gene specificity has been found in esophageal mucosae of tobacco smokers [39]. Target genes for methylation induction are known to be determined by low transcription, the presence of a specific histone modification (trimethylation of lysine 27 of histone H3), and the lack of stalled RNA polymerase II [40,41].

10.4. Genetic Changes in Gastric and Other Tissues Associated with Gastric Cancers

Germline mutations and genetic polymorphisms are known to be associated with increased inborn risk of gastric cancers, and thus can be considered to be involved in the formation of "genetic field defect" of gastric cancers. Germline mutations have high penetrance and odds ratios, but are very rare. In contrast, genetic polymorphisms are commonly observed in general populations, but their effects on gastric cancer susceptibility are very weak.

10.4.1. Germline Mutations Associated with Gastric Cancers

Germline mutations of *CDH1* (E-cadherin) were first found in a large family from New Zealand in which diffuse-type gastric cancers took place at an early age [42,43]. *CDH1* germline mutations are very rare, but have been found in other areas in the world [44]. An individual with a *CDH1* germline mutation starts to accumulate a number of small foci of signet ring cells, most of which have methylation of the wild-type allele, and a small fraction of the foci develop into diffuse type cancers [45].

Since the penetrance of *CDH1* germline mutations is very high, prophylactic gastrectomy is a treatment option [42].

In families with hereditary nonpolyposis colorectal cancer (HNPCC), caused by germline mutations of mismatch repair genes, such as *MLH1*, *MSH2*, and *MSH6*, there used to be cases of gastric cancers. The gastric manifestation used to be common in older generations of HNPCC families [46], and is common in Asian populations who have high incidence of gastric cancers[47]. Patients with familial adenomatous polyposis, which is caused by *APC* germline mutations, often present gastric polyps, and also have increased risk for gastric cancers [48].

10.4.2. Genetic Polymorphisms Associated with Gastric Cancer

Genes whose genetic polymorphisms are most widely analyzed are pro-inflammatory cytokine, IL1b, and its receptor antagonist, *IL1RN*. It was initially reported that a single nucleotide polymorphism (SNP) in the *IL1b* promoter was associated with approximately 10-

fold higher risk of gastric atrophy and 2- to 3-fold higher risk of gastric cancers [49]. A SNP in *IL1RN* was also associated with increased gastric cancer risk. Many studies followed this initial study, and a meta-analysis reports that overall gastric cancer risk associated with *IL1b* and *IL1RN* are 1.26 and 1.20 folds, respectively [50].

It is noteworthy that *IL1b* is one of the candidate cytokines involved in methylation induction [15], and that frequent methylation in gastric cancers (CGI methylator phenotype; CIMP) was associated with a SNP in *IL1b* [51]. Taken together, the SNPs in cytokines can be involved in the susceptibility in methylation induction, and thus in gastric cancer susceptibility.

A SNP in the first exon of *PSCA* was identified by a large-scale genome-wide association study, and was associated with 1.62-fold increased risk of diffuse-type gastric cancers [52]. A meta-analysis showed that a SNP in *EGFR* is associated with 1.54-fold increased risk of gastric cancers [53].

Another meta-analysis supported that there is 1.42-fold increased risk for a SNP in folate metabolizing enzyme, *MTHFR* [54]. SNPs in *IL8*, *IL10*, and *TP53* might be risk factors for gastric cancer, but definitive conclusions cannot be made [55,56,57].

10.4.3. Somatic Genetic Changes Associated with Field Defect

Microsatellite instability (MSI) is caused by inactivation of mismatch repair genes, such as *MLH1* and *MSH2*. Especially, *MLH1* is known to be inactivated by its promoter methylation, and one of the important drivers involved in epigenetic field defect. By analysis of cancer tissues, cancers of patients with multiple gastric cancers have been reported to exhibit a higher incidence of MSI than cancers of patients with a single gastric cancer [58]. Since the major mechanism of *MLH1* inactivation is its promoter methylation [24], the presence of MSI in cancer tissues indicates that the patient has high levels of methylation and thus epigenetic field defect. It is difficult to analyze the presence of MSI in non-cancerous gastric mucosae since the fraction of cells with MSI is expected to be very small, and individual gastric glands with MSI are expected to have different types of microsatellite mutation. However, *MLH1* methylation can be detected using a sensitive method, methylation-specific PCR (MSP), and was shown to be present in non-cancerous gastric mucosae of gastric cancer patients with MSI [59].

Activation-induced cytidine deaminase (AID) is a member of the cytidine-deaminase family that acts as a DNA- and RNA-editing enzyme. Infection of gastric epithelial cells with *H. pylori* is known to induce aberrant expression of AID via the IkB kinase-dependent nuclear factor-kB activation pathway. Upregulation of AID is reported to lead to increased *TP53* mutations in gastric epithelial cells *in vitro*, and it seems to contribute to formation of field defect for gastric cancers [60].

Conclusion

Gastric cancer is closely associated with *H. pylori* infection. It induces aberrant methylation of various but specific genes in gastric mucosae mainly through inflammation, and produces an epigenetic field defect (figure 10-5).

Methylation levels of some genes are correlated with gastric cancer risk, and are promising cancer risk markers. *H. pylori* infection can also induce AID expression, which leads to induction of mutations in gastric epithelial cells. Germline mutations of *CDH1*, *MLH1*, and *APC* are involved in gastric cancer susceptibility, but all these are very rare. In contrast, SNPs of some cytokines, such as *IL1b* and *IL1RN*, are common but only weakly associated with gastric cancer risk. These could be involved in the differential responses to *H. pylori* infection and thus in how "efficiently" epigenetic field defect is formed.

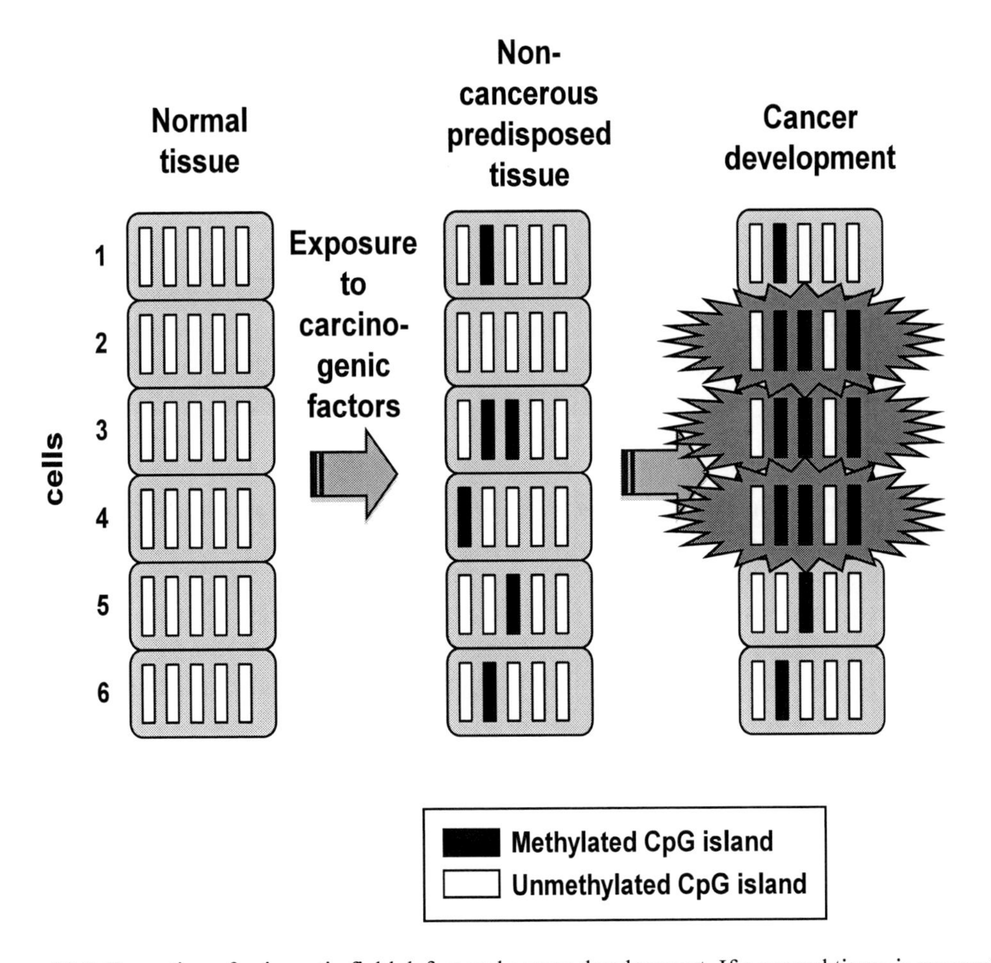

Figure 10.5. Formation of epigenetic field defect and cancer development. If a normal tissue is exposed to an inducer of aberrant DNA methylation, such as *H. pylori* infection, methylation of various but specific genes is induced (non-cancerous predisposed tissue). Both driver and passenger genes (genes A, B, and C) are methylated, but driver genes usually have very low methylation levels. If a predisposed cell harbors an additional hit (e. g. methylation of gene E), a cancer is considered to develop.

References

[1] Marugame T, Dongmei Q (2007) Comparison of time trends in stomach cancer incidence (1973-1997) in East Asia, Europe and USA, from Cancer Incidence in Five Continents Vol. IV-VIII. *Jpn J. Clin. Oncol.* 37: 242-243.

[2] Jemal A, Siegel R, Ward E, Hao Y, Xu J, et al. (2009) *Cancer statistics*, 2009. CA *Cancer J. Clin.* 59: 225-249.

[3] Tatematsu M, Tsukamoto T, Inada K (2003) Stem cells and gastric cancer: role of gastric and intestinal mixed intestinal metaplasia. *Cancer Sci.* 94: 135-141.

[4] Ono H, Kondo H, Gotoda T, Shirao K, Yamaguchi H, et al. (2001) Endoscopic mucosal resection for treatment of early gastric cancer. *Gut* 48: 225-229.

[5] Oda I, Gotoda T, Hamanaka H (2005) Endoscopic submucosal dissection for early gastric cancer: technical feasibility, operation time and complications from a large consecutive cases. *Dig. Endosc.* 17: 54-58.

[6] Nasu J, Doi T, Endo H, Nishina T, Hirasaki S, et al. (2005) Characteristics of metachronous multiple early gastric cancers after endoscopic mucosal resection. *Endoscopy* 37: 990-993.

[7] Nakajima T, Oda I, Gotoda T, Hamanaka H, Eguchi T, et al. (2006) Metachronous gastric cancers after endoscopic resection: how effective is annual endoscopic surveillance? *Gastric Cancer* 9: 93-98.

[8] Takeda J, Toyonaga A, Koufuji K, Kodama I, Aoyagi K, et al. (1998) Early gastric cancer in the remnant stomach. *Hepatogastroenterology* 45: 1907-1911.

[9] Hosokawa O, Kaizaki Y, Watanabe K, Hattori M, Douden K, et al. (2002) Endoscopic surveillance for gastric remnant cancer after early cancer surgery. *Endoscopy* 34: 469-473.

[10] Aoi T, Marusawa H, Sato T, Chiba T, Maruyama M (2006) Risk of subsequent development of gastric cancer in patients with previous gastric epithelial neoplasia. *Gut* 55: 588-589.

[11] Arima N, Adachi K, Katsube T, Amano K, Ishihara S, et al. (1999) Predictive factors for metachronous recurrence of early gastric cancer after endoscopic treatment. *J. Clin. Gastroenterol.* 29: 44-47.

[12] Maekita T, Nakazawa K, Mihara M, Nakajima T, Yanaoka K, et al. (2006) High levels of aberrant DNA methylation in Helicobacter pylori-infected gastric mucosae and its possible association with gastric cancer risk. *Clin. Cancer Res.* 12: 989-995.

[13] Nakajima T, Maekita T, Oda I, Gotoda T, Yamamoto S, et al. (2006) Higher methylation levels in gastric mucosae significantly correlate with higher risk of gastric cancers. *Cancer Epidemiol. Biomarkers Prev.* 15: 2317-2321.

[14] Uemura N, Okamoto S, Yamamoto S, Matsumura N, Yamaguchi S, et al. (2001) Helicobacter pylori infection and the development of gastric cancer. *N. Engl. J. Med.* 345: 784-789.

[15] Niwa T, Tsukamoto T, Toyoda T, Mori A, Tanaka H, et al. (2010) Inflammatory processes triggered by *Helicobacter pylori* infection cause aberrant DNA methylation in gastric epithelial cells. *Cancer Res.* 70: 1430-1440.

[16] Correa P (1992) Human gastric carcinogenesis: a multistep and multifactorial process--First American Cancer Society Award Lecture on Cancer Epidemiology and Prevention. *Cancer Res.* 52: 6735-6740.

[17] Inoue M, Tajima K, Matsuura A, Suzuki T, Nakamura T, et al. (2000) Severity of chronic atrophic gastritis and subsequent gastric cancer occurrence: a 10-year prospective cohort study in Japan. *Cancer Lett.* 161: 105-112.

[18] di Mario F, Cavallaro LG (2008) Non-invasive tests in gastric diseases. *Dig. Liver Dis.* 40: 523-530.

[19] Mukoubayashi C, Yanaoka K, Ohata H, Arii K, Tamai H, et al. (2007) Serum pepsinogen and gastric cancer screening. *Intern. Med.* 46: 261-266.

[20] Ohata H, Kitauchi S, Yoshimura N, Mugitani K, Iwane M, et al. (2004) Progression of chronic atrophic gastritis associated with Helicobacter pylori infection increases risk of gastric cancer. *Int. J. Cancer* 109: 138-143.

[21] Yanaoka K, Oka M, Mukoubayashi C, Yoshimura N, Enomoto S, et al. (2008) Cancer high-risk subjects identified by serum pepsinogen tests: outcomes after 10-year follow-up in asymptomatic middle-aged males. *Cancer Epidemiol. Biomarkers Prev.* 17: 838-845.

[22] Shimada S, Shiomori K, Honmyo U, Maeno M, Yagi Y, et al. (2002) BGP expression in gastric biopsies may predict the development of new lesions after local treatment for early gastric cancer. *Gastric Cancer* 5: 130-136.

[23] Liu Q, Teh M, Ito K, Shah N, Ito Y, et al. (2007) CDX2 expression is progressively decreased in human gastric intestinal metaplasia, dysplasia and cancer. *Mod. Pathol.* 20: 1286-1297.

[24] Ushijima T, Sasako M (2004) Focus on gastric cancer. *Cancer Cell* 5: 121-125.

[25] Bird A (2002) DNA methylation patterns and epigenetic memory. *Genes. Dev.* 16: 6-21.

[26] Laird PW, Jaenisch R (1996) The role of DNA methylation in cancer genetic and epigenetics. *Annu. Rev. Genet.* 30: 441-464.

[27] Robertson KD (2005) DNA methylation and human disease. *Nat. Rev. Genet.* 6: 597-610.

[28] Jones PA, Baylin SB (2007) The epigenomics of cancer. *Cell* 128: 683-692.

[29] Costello JF, Fruhwald MC, Smiraglia DJ, Rush LJ, Robertson GP, et al. (2000) Aberrant CpG-island methylation has non-random and tumour-type-specific patterns. *Nat. Genet.* 24: 132-138.

[30] Rauch TA, Zhong X, Wu X, Wang M, Kernstine KH, et al. (2008) High-resolution mapping of DNA hypermethylation and hypomethylation in lung cancer. *Proc. Natl. Acad. Sci. USA* 105: 252-257.

[31] Yamashita S, Hosoya K, Gyobu K, Takeshima H, Ushijima T (2009) Development of a novel output value for quantitative assessment in methylated DNA immunoprecipitation-CpG island microarray analysis. *DNA Res.* 16: 275-286.

[32] Kaneda A, Wakazono K, Tsukamoto T, Watanabe N, Yagi Y, et al. (2004) *Lysyl oxidase* is a tumor suppressor gene inactivated by methylation and loss of heterozygosity in human gastric cancers. *Cancer Res.* 64: 6410-6415.

[33] Ando T, Yoshida T, Enomoto S, Asada K, Tatematsu M, et al. (2009) DNA methylation of microRNA genes in gastric mucosae of gastric cancer patients: its

possible involvement in the formation of epigenetic field defect. *Int. J. Cancer* 124: 2367-2374.

[34] Miyazaki T, Murayama Y, Shinomura Y, Yamamoto T, Watabe K, et al. (2007) E-cadherin gene promoter hypermethylation in H. pylori-induced enlarged fold gastritis. *Helicobacter* 12: 523-531.

[35] Nakajima T, Enomoto S, Yamashita S, Ando T, Nakanishi Y, et al. (2010) Persistence of a component of DNA methylation in gastric mucosae after Helicobacter pylori eradication. *J. Gastroenterol.* 45: 37-44.

[36] Hatakeyama M (2004) Oncogenic mechanisms of the Helicobacter pylori CagA protein. *Nat. Rev. Cancer* 4: 688-694.

[37] Vitkute J, Stankevicius K, Tamulaitiene G, Maneliene Z, Timinskas A, et al. (2001) Specificities of eleven different DNA methyltransferases of Helicobacter pylori strain 26695. *J. Bacteriol.* 183: 443-450.

[38] Nakajima T, Yamashita S, Maekita T, Niwa T, Nakazawa K, et al. (2009) The presence of a methylation fingerprint of *Helicobacter pylori* infection in human gastric mucosae. *Int. J. Cancer* 124: 905-910.

[39] Oka D, Yamashita S, Tomioka T, Nakanishi Y, Kato H, et al. (2009) The presence of aberrant DNA methylation in noncancerous esophageal mucosae in association with smoking history: a target for risk diagnosis and prevention of esophageal cancers. *Cancer* 115: 3412-3426.

[40] Takeshima H, Ushijima T (2010) Methylation destiny: Moira takes account of histones and RNA polymerase II. Epigenetics 5.

[41] Takeshima H, Yamashita S, Shimazu T, Niwa T, Ushijima T (2009) The presence of RNA polymerase II, active or stalled, predicts epigenetic fate of promoter CpG islands. *Genome Res.* 19: 1974-1982.

[42] Guilford P, Blair V, More H, Humar B (2007) A short guide to hereditary diffuse gastric cancer. *Hered Cancer Clin Pract* 5: 183-194.

[43] Guilford P, Hopkins J, Harraway J, McLeod M, McLeod N, et al. (1998) E-cadherin germline mutations in familial gastric cancer. *Nature* 392: 402-405.

[44] Kaurah P, MacMillan A, Boyd N, Senz J, De Luca A, et al. (2007) Founder and recurrent CDH1 mutations in families with hereditary diffuse gastric cancer. *JAMA* 297: 2360-2372.

[45] Humar B, Blair V, Charlton A, More H, Martin I, et al. (2009) E-cadherin deficiency initiates gastric signet-ring cell carcinoma in mice and man. *Cancer Res.* 69: 2050-2056.

[46] Lynch HT, Smyrk T (1996) Hereditary nonpolyposis colorectal cancer (Lynch syndrome). An updated review. *Cancer* 78: 1149-1167.

[47] Park YJ, Shin KH, Park JG (2000) Risk of gastric cancer in hereditary nonpolyposis colorectal cancer in Korea. *Clin. Cancer Res.* 6: 2994-2998.

[48] Oberhuber G, Stolte M (2000) Gastric polyps: an update of their pathology and biological significance. *Virchows Arch.* 437: 581-590.

[49] El-Omar EM, Carrington M, Chow WH, McColl KE, Bream JH, et al. (2000) Interleukin-1 polymorphisms associated with increased risk of gastric cancer. *Nature* 404: 398-402.

[50] Wang P, Xia HH, Zhang JY, Dai LP, Xu XQ, et al. (2007) Association of interleukin-1 gene polymorphisms with gastric cancer: a meta-analysis. *Int. J. Cancer* 120: 552-562.

[51] Chan AO, Chu KM, Huang C, Lam KF, Leung SY, et al. (2007) Association between Helicobacter pylori infection and interleukin 1beta polymorphism predispose to CpG island methylation in gastric cancer. *Gut* 56: 595-597.

[52] Sakamoto H, Yoshimura K, Saeki N, Katai H, Shimoda T, et al. (2008) Genetic variation in PSCA is associated with susceptibility to diffuse-type gastric cancer. *Nat. Genet.* 40: 730-740.

[53] Zhang YM, Cao C, Liang K (2010) Genetic polymorphism of epidermal growth factor 61A>G and cancer risk: A meta-analysis. *Cancer Epidemiol.*

[54] Sun L, Sun YH, Wang B, Cao HY, Yu C (2008) Methylenetetrahydrofolate reductase polymorphisms and susceptibility to gastric cancer in Chinese populations: a meta-analysis. *Eur. J. Cancer Prev.* 17: 446-452.

[55] Wang J, Pan HF, Hu YT, Zhu Y, He Q (2009) Polymorphism of IL-8 in 251 Allele and Gastric Cancer Susceptibility: A Meta-Analysis. *Dig. Dis. Sci.*

[56] Zhuang W, Wu XT, Zhou Y, Liu L, Liu GJ, et al. (2009) Interleukin10 -592 Promoter Polymorphism Associated with Gastric Cancer Among Asians: A Meta-Analysis of Epidemiologic Studies. *Dig. Dis. Sci.*

[57] Zhou Y, Li N, Zhuang W, Liu GJ, Wu TX, et al. (2007) P53 codon 72 polymorphism and gastric cancer: a meta-analysis of the literature. *Int. J. Cancer* 121: 1481-1486.

[58] Miyoshi E, Haruma K, Hiyama T, Tanaka S, Yoshihara M, et al. (2001) Microsatellite instability is a genetic marker for the development of multiple gastric cancers. *Int. J. Cancer* 95: 350-353.

[59] Sakata K, Tamura G, Endoh Y, Ohmura K, Ogata S, et al. (2002) Hypermethylation of the hMLH1 gene promoter in solitary and multiple gastric cancers with microsatellite instability. *Br. J. Cancer* 86: 564-567.

[60] Matsumoto Y, Marusawa H, Kinoshita K, Endo Y, Kou T, et al. (2007) Helicobacter pylori infection triggers aberrant expression of activation-induced cytidine deaminase in gastric epithelium. *Nat. Med.* 13: 470-476.

In: Field Cancerization: Basic Science and Clinical Applications ISBN 978-1-61761-006-6
Editor: Gabriel D. Dakubo

Chapter 11

Field Cancerization in Colorectal Cancer

Jun Kato

Abstract

It has been shown that there are two ways by which colorectal cancer (CRC) develops: sporadic CRC and colitis-associated CRC. The former is cancer that is seen in ordinary people, while the latter occurs in patients with inflammatory bowel disease, in particular, ulcerative colitis.

Although similar multistep carcinogenesis occurs in both types of cancer development, there are clinical and biological differences between the two: so-called adenoma-carcinoma sequence and dysplasia-carcinoma sequence, respectively. In terms of field cancerization, therefore, there are unique biologic alterations in normal colonic mucosa in each type of cancer occurrence.

In the past, field cancerization in sporadic carcinogenesis was demonstrated using histological and immunohistochemical methods. Later, genetic and epigenetic alterations in normal mucosa around tumors have been detected. In particular, epigenetic alterations such as methylation have been featured, because methylation profiles have been elucidated in sporadic colorectal carcinogenesis.

On the other hand, in carcinogenesis based on inflammatory bowel disease, a broad inflamed area of colorectal mucosa is regarded as the "field" predisposed to neoplasitic transformation, and multiple dysplasia and/or cancer arise from such mucosa. The inflamed mucosa harbors several biological changes such as aneuploidy, chromosomal and microsatellite instability, as well as epigenetic changes.

Enthusiastic efforts have been made to elucidate the biologic mechanisms of field cancerization in colorectal carcinogenesis. The knowledge accrued from such studies not only facilitate elucidating mechanisms of initiation and development of CRC, but is applicable to early detection and treatment of CRC, particularly, colitis-associated CRC.

The development of an expanding prenoeplastic field appears to be a critical step in colorectal carcinogenesis with important clinical implications. For example, diagnosis and treatment of CRCs should not only be focused on the tumor, but also on the normal mucosa from which it developed.

11.1. Introduction

The presence of mucosa that is predisposed to cancer development was initially described for oral cancers by Slaughter et al. using the term "field cancerization" [1]. Later, this phenomenon has also been designated as "field effect" or "field defect". Although the predisposed mucosa can display some histological changes, they are essentially made of epithelial cells of polyclonal origins and have few monoclonal lesions. Field cancerization was proposed to explain the development of multiple primary tumors and locally recurrent tumors. In the field of colorectal cancer (CRC), it had been demonstrated as histological or immunohistochemical changes in the normal mucosa around tumors.

As our knowledge and technology of molecular biology progress, the molecular mechanisms of colorectal carcinogenesis are being elucidated. It is now generally accepted that CRC develops by accumulation of multiple genetic alterations. In addition, recently, it has been shown that epigenetic alterations such as DNA methylation play an important role in colorectal carcinogenesis. In terms of field cancerization, therefore, genetic and epigenetic alterations in normal colonic mucosa have recently been highlighted.

11.1.1. Genetic Alterations

It is now well established that an accumulation of genetic alterations transforms a normal cell from normalcy to cancerous progression, referred to as the process of multistep carcinogenesis [2]. Until now, the number of genetic alterations has been known to increase with the level of malignancy as judged by histopathologic examination. The process of field cancerization can also be defined in molecular terms, and its position in the process of multistep carcinogenesis can be delineated. Several lines of evidence indicate that the presence of a field lesion with genetically altered cells is a distinct biologic stage in epithelial carcinogenesis with important clinical implications. Loss of heterozygosity, microsatellite alterations, chromosomal instability (CIN), and genomic mutations are genetic alterations, which frequently occur in colorectal field cancerization.

11.1.2. Epigenetic Alterations

In contrast to genetic changes that involve DNA alterations, epigenetic changes are defined as changes in genetic information or expression "above – or epi" DNA mutations. Prototypical examples are DNA methylation at CpG islands, histone modifications and polypcomb complex formation [3]. DNA methylation, for example replicates at a high fidelity in mammalian cells [4-6], and serves as a long-term memory of cells [7]. DNA methylation in promoter CpG islands consistently induces the repression of transcription of their downstream genes [3,8], mainly by inducing changes in histone modifications, such as deacetylation of histones and methylation of lysine 9 of histone H3 [9]. Methylation in gene bodies does not block transcription, and is sometimes associated with active transcription [3,10]. Even when methylation of a gene body is associated with decreased transcription, such association has many exceptions, and does not have a causal role in gene silencing [8].

In cancer cells, "genome-overall hypomethylation" and "regional hypermethylation" are present. The genome-overall hypomethylation is almost always observed in cancers, and is mainly due to hypomethylation of repetitive sequences, which comprise more than 40% of the human genome, and are normally heavily methylated [11]. The hypomethylation can lead to genomic instability and is considered to be involved in tumor progression [12]. "Genome-overall hypomethylation" can also involve normally methylated CpG islands, which can induce aberrant transcription of their downstream genes, such as melanoma antigen genes (MAGEs) [13].

Regional hypermethylation has been extensively analyzed in various cancers because methylation of promoter CpG islands of various tumor-suppressor genes can cause their inactivation [3,8]. Similarly, methylations of CpG islands outside gene promoter regions are present in cancers, and it is still unclear whether or not such methylation has any biological consequences. In colorectal cancers, *CDKN2A, hMLH1, HIC1, SFRP1*, and many other genes are inactivated by methylation [3]. Notably, methylation of some tumor-suppressor genes, such as *SFRP1*, whose inactivation enhances WNT signaling, was observed in aberrant crypt foci of very early lesions of colon carcinogenesis [14].

Field cancerization caused by certain epigenetic alterations is denoted as "epigenetic field". We recently showed that methylation levels of age-related methylation loci in normal colon mucosa were correlated with the tumors arising from the mucosa [15]. In addition, we also reported that genomewide hypomethylation in normal mucosa is correlated with the occurrence and development of colorectal neoplasia [16]. These findings unequivocally demonstrate the presence of "an epigenetic field for cancerization" in colorectal carcinogenesis.

11.1.3. Sporadic and Colitis-Associated Colorectal Cancer

It has been shown that CRC develops by two processes. One is sporadic cancer that occurs in ordinary people, and most of CRCs are assigned to this type. The other is colitis-associated CRC that arises from the inflammatory mucosa due to inflammatory bowel disease (IBD) including ulcerative colitis (UC) and Crohn's disease. Biological and clinical features of carcinogenesis of colitis-associated CRC are quite different from those of sporadic CRC. In terms of field cancerization therefore, there are quite different characteristics between sporadic and colitis-associated CRCs. In this chapter, we describe field cancerization of each type of cancer, separately. In each type, after a description of the clinical features and molecular mechanisms of colorectal carcinogenesis, genetic and epigenetic alterations in normal (non-neoplastic) colonic mucosa are particularly highlighted. In addition, inducers of field cancerization and perspective for its clinical application in the future are discussed.

11.2. Field Cancerization in Sporadic Colorectal Cancer

At least some sporadic CRC cases have colorectal mucosa that do not have any tumors but are already predisposed to developing CRCs. Although the predisposed mucosa does not display any significant histological changes, multiple adenomas and CRCs can develop from it. This phenomenon largely implies the presence of field cancerization in sporadic colorectal carcinogenesis. The field cancerization in sporadic CRC has formerly been demonstrated histologically or immunohistochemically, and later explained by the presence of cells with genetic alterations [17]. Recently, however, the involvement of epigenetic alterations in field cancerization in CRC has also been shown [18].

11.2.1. Clinical Features

There are several clinical features suggestive of the presence of field cancerization in the colorectum.

- There are significant predisposing risk factors for occurrence and development of CRC.
- Patients with multiple precursor lesions (i.e., adenomas) and those who have a history of CRC are likely to develop CRC.
- There are clinical differences with regards to the tumor location (i.e., differences between left-side and right-side colon cancers).

Risk factors: Older age (usually > 50 years), male gender, smoking and/or drinking habits, obesity, diabetes, high meat intakes etc. have been shown to be risk factors for development of CRC [19]. The presence of definite risk factors implies that the colonic mucosa of subjects with such risk factors is more susceptible to neoplasia transformation than mucosa of those without such factors. Thus, these risk factors may directly or indirectly create field cancerization in normal colorectal mucosa.

Multiple precursors and history of colorectal cancer: In general, CRC develops from benign adenoma (adenoma-carcinoma sequence). Accumulating evidences have shown that patients with multiple adenomas are likely to develop CRC [20]. In addition, those who have a history of CRC have an elevated risk for developing another CRC [21]. These suggest that there are patients who are likely to develop neoplasia in the colorectum. With regards to field cancerization, the colorectal mucosa of these patients harbors predisposing factors for neoplastic changes.

Distinct characteristics according to tumor location: Recently, it has been shown that there are clinical and biological differences between cancers occurring in the left side of the colorectum (rectum, sigmoid colon, and descending colon) and those arising from the right side of the colon (transverse colon, ascending colon, and cecum). For example, right-side colon cancer is frequently observed in female and older patients, while left-side colon cancer is dominant in male and relatively younger patients [22]. Moreover, right-side colon cancer is more likely to be microsatellite unstable with wildtype *p53*, while left-side cancer is characterized by the presence of chromosomal instability (CIN) with mutated *p53* [23]. In addition, epigenetic characteristics of CRCs differ between right and left parts of the colon. Colorectal cancer with highly methylated phenotype (CpG island methylator phenotype (CIMP)-high or CIMP+) is frequently observed in the right-side colon [24]. We also reported that a laterally spreading type of colorectal adenoma exhibited high frequency of CIMP-high and *K-ras* mutations especially on the right-side colon [25].

In addition to these observations, we previously reported that synchronous and metachronous cancers are likely to occur in the same side of the colon [20]. We also indicated that the characteristics and timing of alterations in Ras signaling pathway during the development of colorectal neoplasia are different with regards to the location of the neoplastic changes [26]. All of these findings suggest that clinical and biological characteristics of colorectal tumors are different with regards to tumor location, and that there are distinct field cancerizations in each of the two regions of the colon.

11.2.2. Molecular Mechanisms of Sporadic Colorectal Cancer

Before describing the biology of filed cancerization of the colorectum, we have to know the molecular mechanisms of how CRCs develop. There are two major pathways in sporadic colorectal carcinogenesis. One is the chromosomal instability (CIN, also known as microsatellite stable (MSS)) pathway (adenoma-carcinoma sequence), which is characterized by allelic losses, and the other is a pathway involving microsatellite instability (MSI).

Fearon and Vogelstein (2) proposed a multistep model of colorectal carcinogenesis, in which mutations in the *APC* gene occur early during the development of polyps. *K-ras* mutations arise during the adenomatous stage, and mutations of *p53* and deletions of chromosome 18q occur concurrently with the transition to malignancy. This pathway is characterized by allelic losses on chromosome 5q (*APC*), 7p (*p53*), and 18q (*DCC/SMAD4*), and is therefore called the CIN pathway. One of the cornerstones of the CIN pathway is the model presented by familial adenomatous polyposis (FAP), in which multiple small adenomas form and initiate tumorigenesis. In this model, two hits in the *APC* gene, followed by mutations of *K-ras*, and subsequently mutations of *p53* and deletion on chromosome 18q lead to cancer formation. It has been surmised that this same mechanism is also applicable to sporadic colorectal carcinogenesis. Approximately 85% of sporadic CRCs develop through the CIN pathway.

Microsatellite instability is characterized by expansions or contractions in the number of tandem repeats of simple DNA sequences (microsatellites). Microsatellite instability has been identified in CRC associated with hereditary nonpolyposis colorectal cancer (HNPCC) syndrome [27], and DNA mismatch repair (MMR) enzymes, including *hMSH2, hMLH1, hPMS2,* and *hMSH6* have since been shown to be responsible for the MSI [28]. Moreover, mutations in microsatellites of genes such as the type II receptor of transforming growth factor-β (*TGF-β*), and *Bax* have also been identified in MSI positive tumors [29]. Loss of function of the target genes becomes a trigger for cancer development. Approximately 15% of sporadic CRC have characteristics of MSI, and most sporadic-MSI cancers are correlated with loss of expression of *hMLH1* caused by hypermethylation of its promoter region [30].

In addition to the increasing knowledge of genetic pathways, recent studies have suggested that epigenetic alterations are also involved in the development of CRC. In the early 1990's, methylation of promoter CpG islands of tumor suppressor genes was discovered [3,31]. CpG-rich regions located at the 5' ends of coding sequences can undergo hypermethylation, leading to gene silencing. Silencing of the gene induced by promoter CpG methylation has been shown to play important role in the biology of human cancers. In CRCs, several tumor suppressor genes are inactivated frequently by promoter methylation as well as by mutations. Moreover, recent genome-wide screening techniques have revealed that promoter CpG island of many genes are methylated in cancers, and that only a fraction of them are tumor suppressor genes [8].

In addition to the functional relevance of DNA methylation, Toyota et al. proposed the concept of CpG island methylator phenotype (CIMP) [32]. Cancers demonstrating methylation and silencing of multiple genes are described as CIMP-high or CIMP-positive. CIMP-positive CRCs exhibit unique clinical and pathological features that include their frequent location in the proximal colon, higher frequency in female subjects and poorly differentiated, mucinous histology [32]. As described above, the *hMLH1* gene is a frequent target of hypermethylation, which leads to the MSI phenotype, and therefore, most of MSI sporadic cancers exhibit CIMP-positive phenotype. Whether the unique properties arise because of aberrant DNA hypermethylation or as a consequence of MSI phenotype has been highly contentious.

Field cancerization of the colorectum has recently been described in correlation with genetic and epigenetic alterations. Because several mechanisms mediate different types of cancer development, there should be several types of field cancerization, field effects associated with CIN pathway, MSI pathway, and/or CIMP.

11.2.3. Biological Features of Field Cancerization of Sporadic Colorectal Cancer

In the 70s, when genetic or epigenetic alterations were not yet enthusiastically investigated, field cancerization of CRC had been described using morphological and histochemical terms [33-35]. Subsequently, additional methods including flow cytometry [36] and uptake of tritium labeled thymidine [37] were used to study CRC field defects. Using these methodologies, field effects have been shown by sialomucin production [33], cellular protein synthesis [37], stage-specific embryonic antigen [38], carcinoemboryonic antigen expression [39], oncogene activation [40], ornithine decarboxylase activity [41], DNA ploidy [36], and mucosal cell proliferation [42-44]. Even in recent days, immunohistochemical approach is still being used, and TGF-α expression in the normal-appearing colorectal mucosa was statistically significantly associated with accepted risk factors for colorectal neoplasias [45].

Among these studies, cell proliferation and apoptosis have particularly been highlighted. Anti et al. reported that patients with resected large adenomas and thus were at an increased risk of CRC, had imbalance of proliferation and apoptosis in the left colon compared to patients who never had a tumor [46]. In this context, expression of *Bcl-*x_L, an anti-apoptotic protein that inhibits apoptosis by preventing release of cytochrome c from the mitochondria, increased at 1 cm and 10 cm distances away from colorectal adenocarcinomas in non-neoplastic colorectal mucosa. This finding suggests the presence of an apoptosis resistant field [47]. A similar finding was also reported for the anti-apoptotic protein *Bcl-2* [48].

Recently, along with progress in molecular biology, analysis of normal colon mucosa for field defects has been examined genetically and/or epigenetically. Proteomic approach for study of field defects has also been reported [49]. Epigenetic alterations, in particular, have recently been examined enthusiastically. Because genetic changes, such as mutations and allelic losses are often correlated with morphological change, such alterations in non-neoplastic mucosa are relatively rarely observed. In contrast, epigenetic change can occur in morphologically normal mucosa, because it is not necessarily accompanied by genome sequence alteration.

Genetic alterations: Although there have been few reports regarding genetic alterations in normal colonic mucosa, mutations of *K-ras* and *p53*, key molecular targets of colon carcinogenesis, have been reported (figure 11-1). *K-ras* mutation frequently occurs in colorectal adenoma and cancer, and 15% - 68% of adenomas and 40% - 65% of carcinomas have *K-ras* mutations [26,50]. *K-ras* mutations usually occur in codon 12 or 13. In contrast to the neoplastic tissue, the reports regarding mutations in the non-neoplastic colorectal mucosa have been scarce. Minamoto et al. reported that *K-ras* mutations were detected in 18% - 25% of non-neoplastic colorectal mucosa from CRC patients [51]. Shen et al. reported that 12% of normal mucosa adjacent to CRC, which harbored O^6-methylguanine-DNA methyltransferase (*MGMT*) methylation as "epigenetic field" showed *K-ras* mutation [18]. Yamada et al. showed that approximately 30% of CRC patients exhibited *K-ras* mutations in normal mucosa, but none of control subjects exhibited it [52].

All of these three reports used very sensitive PCR-based methods, although *K-ras* mutations in neoplastic tissues are usually examined by direct sequencing. In addition and interestingly, the sequences of mutant allele in the normal mucosa were not necessarily identical to those in the CRC arising from the mucosa, therefore, it remains to be elucidated whether the mutated *K-ras* genes indentified in non-neoplastic mucosa truly represent *de novo* mutations, which lead to neoplasia, or these mutations might be initiated by different etiologic factors. Thus, *K-ras* mutation in normal colorectal mucosa as a player of field cancerization needs further examinations.

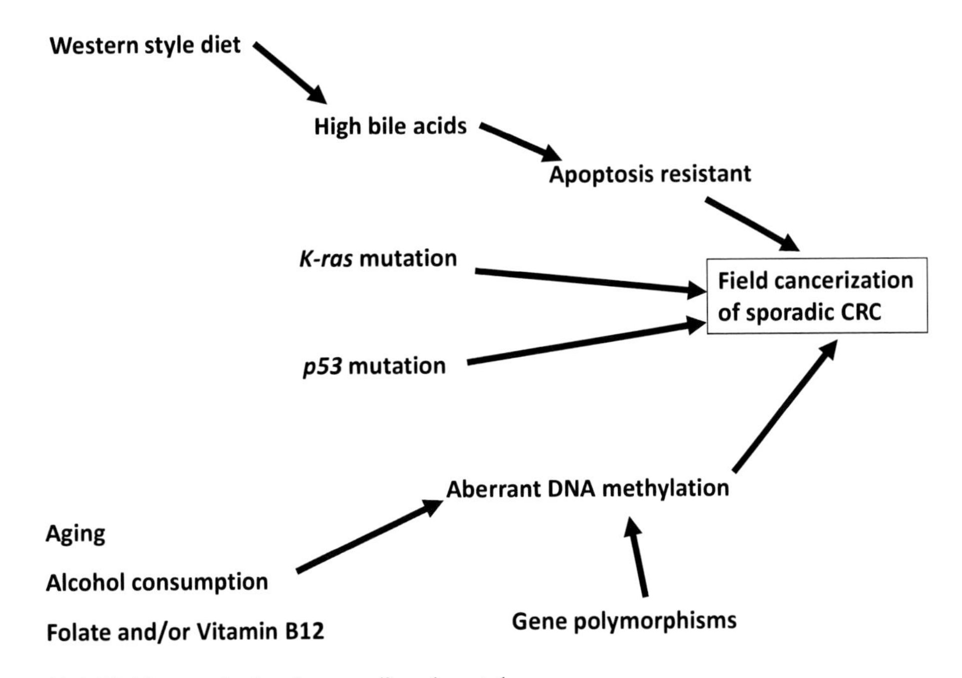

Figure 11.1. Field cancerization in sporadic colorectal cancer.

p53 mutation is also rarely observed in non-neoplastic colorectal mucosa. Visca et al. showed weakly positive *p53* immunostaining in 17/100 adjacent-to-tumor non-neoplastic mucosa [53]. However, *p53* immunostaining does not always indicate *p53* gene mutation. In general, *p53* mutation has been shown to be a late event in colorectal multistep tumorigenesis, and therefore, *p53* mutation in normal colorectal mucosa would be scarce. The Visca's study reported that immunostaining of other proteins in normal mucosa such as *Bcl-2* and *c-myc* also correlated with field effect of sporadic CRC carcinogenesis.

There have been fewer reports regarding other genetic alterations as field cancerization. Bian et al. reported that *TGFB1*6A*, a hypomorphic variant of the type I TGF-β receptor, is somatically acquired by stromal and epithelial cells adjacent to colorectal tumors [54].

Epigenetic alterations: The methylation of some CpG islands in the normal colonic mucosa has been shown to increase with age (figure 11-1) [55-57]. This has led to a proposal by Toyota et al. [32] that methylation of some genes in this tissue is age-related (Type A genes), whereas for other genes the methylation is cancer-specific (Type C genes). Type A genes are sometimes methylated in normal cells, while methylation of type C genes is relatively rare. In terms of field cancerization, therefore, methylation of type A genes has particularly been highlighted.

Kawakami et al. reported that multiple genes including both type A and type C genes were highly methylated in normal mucosa with CIMP or MSI positive cancer [58]. We have previously reported that age-related methylation status of normal colon mucosa differs between proximal and distal colon, and that lower methylation status of *ESR1* is correlated with advanced features of colorectal neoplasia in distal colon [15]. In addition, in the distal colon, methylation of the age-related loci in normal colon mucosa decreased as the stage of neoplasia arising from the mucosa increased, while in the proximal colon, such correlation was not observed [16].

These results suggest that age-related methylation in the normal mucosa does not always correlate with neoplasia susceptibility, but that hypomethylation may correlate with neoplasia, at least in the distal colon. In general, MSI/CIMP-high cancer is frequently observed in the proximal colon, whereas MSS/CIMP-low cancer is prevalent in the distal colon. Taken together, proximal and distal colon may have distinct epigenetic field, respectively. In the distal colon, low methylation status of age-related loci may generate epigenetic field for neoplasia with low methylation characteristics (MSS/CIMP-low), while in the proximal colon, higher methylation status may generate epigenetic field for neoplasia with high methylation characteristics (MSI/CIMP-high).

Epigenetic field has usually been shown by methylation status of the genes; however, in most cases the biologic meanings of the methylation are not defined. In contrast, Shen et al. quantified *MGMT* methylation levels in colonic mucosa of CRC cases and healthy individuals, and unequivocally showed the presence of epigenetic field defect [18]. *MGMT* functions to remove alkyl group from the O^6-position of guanine damaged by alkylating agents. The loss of its function, therefore, causes increased genomic mutation rate and risk of cancer [59]. Silencing of *MGMT* has been shown to be associated with and to precede the appearance of G-to-A point mutations in *K-ras* during colorectal tumorigenesis [60]. Although the Shen's report did not show definite influence of methylation of *MGMT* in normal mucosa, the methylation may be an initial step of *K-ras* G-to-A mutation in cancer tissue.

In terms of genome-overall hypomethylation, Pufulete et al. reported that hypomethylation of colonic mucosa correlated with neoplastic transformation [61], while we reported that in the distal colon genome-wide methylation in normal mucosa becomes higher as the stage of neoplasia arising from the mucosa increased [16]. Thus, the correlation between genome-wide methylation in normal mucosa and neoplasia susceptibility is still unsettled. As a comprehensive approach of CpG island methylation, Belshaw et al. examined methylation status of 18 genes in normal mucosa of patients with and without neoplasia, and performed statistical analysis for predicting the presence of neoplasia, and also identified changes likely to be early in colorectal carcinogenes [62].

The observations regarding epigenetic field suggest that methylation levels in the normal colonic mucosa could serve as markers of risk for the development of CRC, and moreover, the methylation may be an initial step of CRC development.

11.2.4. Inducers of Field Cancerization in Sporadic Colorectal Cancer

Some CRC risk factors may be responsible for presence of field cancerization in the normal colonic mucosa (figure 11-1). One of the candidates of such risk factors is a Western style diet. A high fat, low fiber Western style diet, as well as elevated fecal bile acid concentration is an important risk factor for CRC [63]. Bile acids induce oxidative/nitrosative stress, DNA damage and apoptosis in the colonic epithelium. Epithelial cells of the non-neoplastic colonic mucosa of individuals with CRC often have reduced capacity to undergo induction of apoptosis by bile acid compared to epithelial cells of individuals without neoplasia [64,65]. These findings suggest that repeated exposure to high levels of bile acids as a consequence of a Western style diet may select for cells resistant to induction of apoptosis giving rise to a field of apoptosis-resistant epithelium that may further evolve to become malignant. Western style diet was shown to be responsible for high recurrence rate of CRC after surgical resection [66]. This finding also suggests the correlation between diet and field cancerization.

Although there are epigenetic field changes in colonic epithelium of CRC patients, the factors that regulate both global DNA methylation and site-specific hypermethylation in normal and neoplastic tissues are largely unknown. Age clearly has some influence, with dietary folate and/or vitamin B12 status, alcohol consumption and gender also likely to be important factors [67-70]. Age-related methylation has been considered to be a functional link to the neoplasia susceptibility due to aging. However, we recently showed that low (not high) methylation status of age-related loci in normal colon mucosa was correlated with neoplasia susceptibility [15]. Therefore, the concept that age-related methylation in normal mucosa is linked to neoplasia susceptibility should be reevaluated. Folate, vitamin B12, and alcohol consumption are collectively responsible for intracellular folate status, which works as a methyl group donor during DNA methylation reaction.

Genetic factors could also play a role in determining the level of normal tissue DNA methylation, and hence the risk of cancer. In particular, functional polymorphisms have been described for several genes involved in methyl group metabolism. Most attention has so far been focused on variants in methylenetetrahydrofolate reductase (*MTHFR*), thymidylate synthase (*TS*), methionine synthese (*MS*), DNA methyltransferase (*DNMT3B*) and methylenetetrahydrofolate dehydrogenase (*MTHFD1*) genes [71-75]. In particular, polymorphism of *MTHFR* 677C allele has been implicated in the level of global DNA methylation in normal tissues [71,72].

11.2.5. Perspective for Clinical Application

One of the important clinical implications of colonic field cancerization is that fields often remain after surgery of the primary tumor, and may lead to new cancers, designated presently by clinicians as "second primary tumors" or "local recurrences", depending on the exact site and time interval between the two tumors. It is a well-known clinical experience that after surgical removal of a tumor, there is still a high risk for another tumor in the same anatomical area. For some cases, the new tumor is explained by the growth of incompletely resected carcinoma. However, for the cases where the tumor had been removed by radical surgical procedures, it seems logical to assume that a genetically/epigenetically-altered field is the cause of a new cancer. The presence of a field with genetically/epigenetically-altered cells appears to be a continuous risk factor for cancer.

Moreover, genetic/epigenetic alterations in field cancerization may be useful as a marker for determining surgically clean or safe margins. When genetic/epigenetic alterations of normal surrounding mucosa of surgically resected tumor specimens are examined, the remainder of the field defect can be determined, and whether sufficient surgical safety margin is present or not can be estimated. This may help estimate risk of local recurrence. In addition, some of the field effects may have spread over surgical margins into the remnant colon, and patients with such field effects may be at risk of a second primary cancer. Moreover, the clinical definition of "local recurrence" needs to be reconsidered in molecular terms. This type of lesion can be the result of remaining tumor cells, but also the local remnants of a field may develop into cancer.

Not only occurrence of a second primary cancer or local recurrence, but occurrence of the first primary cancer may be predicted by examining colorectal field cancerization. Namely, there may be some effective markers (particularly epigenetic alterations) predicting occurrence of colorectal neoplasia in the field. If so, biopsy from normal appearing mucosa during screening colonoscopy can predict occurrence of colorectal neoplasia in the future. In addition, if inducers of field cancerization that predict occurrence of neoplasia are discovered, prophylaxis of neoplasia may be possible by restricting the intake of such inducers.

Additional research is needed to identify the fields that carry the highest risk for cancer. Besides host factors, like the amount of cigarettes smoked, alcohol consumption etc., the biological characteristics of the field itself might be of importance for CRC development.

11.3. Field Cancerization in Colitis-Associated Colorectal Cancer

Chronic inflammation is closely correlated with cancer development. For example, chronic inflammation in the liver and stomach is almost necessary for development of hepatocellular carcinoma and gastric cancer, respectively. In these cancers, microorganisms such as hepatitis virus and *Helicobacter pylori* (*H. pylori*) are considered to play an important role in inflammation-related carcinogenesis. Ulcerative colitis (UC), a chronic inflammation in colonic mucosa, is also causative of CRC, although related microorganisms have not yet been identified. In colitis-associated CRC, the biological and clinical features are quite different from those of sporadic CRC that arise from non-inflammatory mucosa. Ulcerative colitis patients are at risk of developing colitis-associated CRC, and the mucosa that is involved in the inflammatory change can be considered a wide-spreading field cancerization.

11.3.1. Clinical Features

Individuals with long-standing UC have an increased risk of development of CRC. This increased risk begins after 7 - 10 years of disease duration, and is even much increased with earlier age of disease onset, longer disease duration, the degree of inflammation, and the presence of concomitant inflammatory conditions such as primary sclerosing cholangitis [76]. Thus, it is likely that the acquired cancer risk in UC is a consequence of the inflammatory process, rather than a common genetic link between inflammation and neoplasia in the colon.

Compared with sporadic CRC, colitis-associated CRC has several distinguishing clinical features. Colitis-associated CRC arises in a younger population, often from flat rather than polyploid dysplasia. There is a greater frequency of mucinous or signet cell histology and a higher incidence of multiple synchronous lesions [77]. During the development of CRC, sporadic tumors tend to follow the adenoma-carcinoma sequence [78], whereas colitis-associated CRC usually develops from low-grade and high-grade dysplasia.

Thus, colitis-associated CRC has unique characteristics, and the inflamed colonic mucosal due to UC is even predisposed to different type of cancer including sporadic CRC. Therefore, field cancerization of colitis-associated CRC definitely exists, but that seems quite different from field cancerization of sporadic CRC.

11.3.2. Molecular Mechanisms of Developing Colitis-Associated Colorectal Cancer

Although the carcinogenesis pathway in UC is less well defined than the carcinogenesis of sporadic CRC, the neoplastic transformation in inflammatory bowl disease (IBD) is thought to be similar to the adenoma-carcinoma sequence in sporadic CRC. However, unlike sporadic CRC, where dysplastic lesions arise in one or two focal areas of the colon, in inflammatory mucosa, it is not unusual for dysplasia or cancer to be multifocal, reflecting a broader "field effect". Many of the molecular alterations responsible for sporadic CRC development also play a role in colitis-associated colon carcinogenesis. The emerging evidence suggests that the two major pathways of CIN and MSI also apply to colitis-associated cancers and with roughly the same frequencies (85% CIN and 15% MSI). Distinguishing features of colitis-associated CRC, however, are differences in timing and frequency of these alterations. For example, *APC* loss of function that is considered a very common early event in sporadic CRC is much less frequent and usually occurs late in the colitis-associated dysplasia-carcinoma sequence. Conversely, *p53* mutations in sporadic neoplasia usually occur late in the adenoma-carcinoma sequence, whereas in patients with colitis, *p53* mutations occur early, and are often detected in mucosa that is non-dysplastic or indefinite for dysplasia.

Epigenetic change is assuming increasing importance as a mechanism contributing to the genetic alterations in colitis-associated cancer. Methylation of CpG islands in several genes seems to precede dysplasia, and is more widespread throughout the mucosa of UC patients. However, details of genetic/epigenetic alterations that are definitely involved in colitis-associated carcinogenesis still remain to be elucidated.

11.3.3. Biological Features of Field Cancerization in Colitis-Associated Colorectal Cancer

11.3.3.1. Genetic Alterations

The genetic alterations in colitis-associated colorectal cancer are illustrated in figure 11-2, and discussed below.

CIN: Normal cells possess mechanisms that preserve gene integrity and prevent mutations both at the nucleotide sequence and chromosomal levels. The fidelity of these mechanisms means that the spontaneous point mutation rate of normal cells is approximately 1.4×10^{-10} per base pair per cell generation [79]. Tissue from patients with IBD, however, has a far higher mutation load, both in dysplastic and inflamed tissue, and these mutations occur across a scale from individual nucleotide substitutions to gross chromosomal changes that can result in loss of heterozygosity of important tumor suppressor genes.

Numerous studies suggest that gross chromosomal mutations leading to changes in chromosome number or aneuploidy are the most frequent form of genomic instability in IBD [80-82]. Chromosomal abnormalities increase with histologic progression from dysplasia to cancer. In addition, CIN was also seen in 36% of non-dysplastic tissue [81]. Chromosomal instability seems to occur early in UC and can be detected in histologically non-dysplastic tissue from high-risk patients (extensive disease distribution and duration) by comparative genomic hybridization [82], image and flow cytometry [83,84], and is thought to precede the development of dysplasia in these patients. Therefore, identification of DNA aneuploidy from colonic biopsies identified a subgroup of patients without dysplasia who were at greater risk of subsequent development of dysplasia [85]. Moreover, Clausen et al. [86] showed similar patterns of chromosome gains and losses by flow cytometry and comparative genomic hybridization in synchronous colitis-associated tumors, widely separated in the bowel, and suggested that this may be the consequence of a colon-wide field effect.

It has been proposed that CIN results from the effect of inflammation and reactive oxygen species promoting telomere shortening and thus allowing chromosomal end fusion. This results in cycles of chromatin bridge breakage and fusion promoting the accumulation of chromosomal aberrations [87]. Different researchers working on colorectal cancer cell lines have proposed that key regulatory proteins in the mitotic spindle checkpoint are defective, preventing chromosomal segregation during mitosis [88]. The mechanisms responsible for the high level of aneuploidy seen in IBD are not clear, but the presence of CIN in non-dysplastic tissue suggests this process may be an early step in tumorigenesis in these conditions.

p53: Identification of mutations in tumor-suppressor genes that are involved early in the pathogenesis of a dysplastic lesion can be used as true clonal markers, because these lesions are likely to be the original founding mutations that occur at the initiation of a progenitor clone [89]. As well as early CIN, painstaking research has shown that dysplastic lesions may be surrounded by larger regions of cells with *p53* mutations [90,91], suggesting that *p53* inactivation may also be an early event in colitis-associated dysplasia. Yoshida et al. [92] identified *p53* mutations from single crypts obtained from multiple lesions in 3 different colitis colectomy specimens. They showed *p53* point mutation in dysplastic and non-dysplastic regenerating crypts, although many of the latter mutations were noncoding silent mutations. Identification of a variety of coding and noncoding *p53* mutations in a dysplasia-associated lesion or mass led them to suggest that low-grade, colitis-associated dysplasia has a polyclonal origin with subsequent monocloncal outgrowth in high-grade dysplasia and cancer.

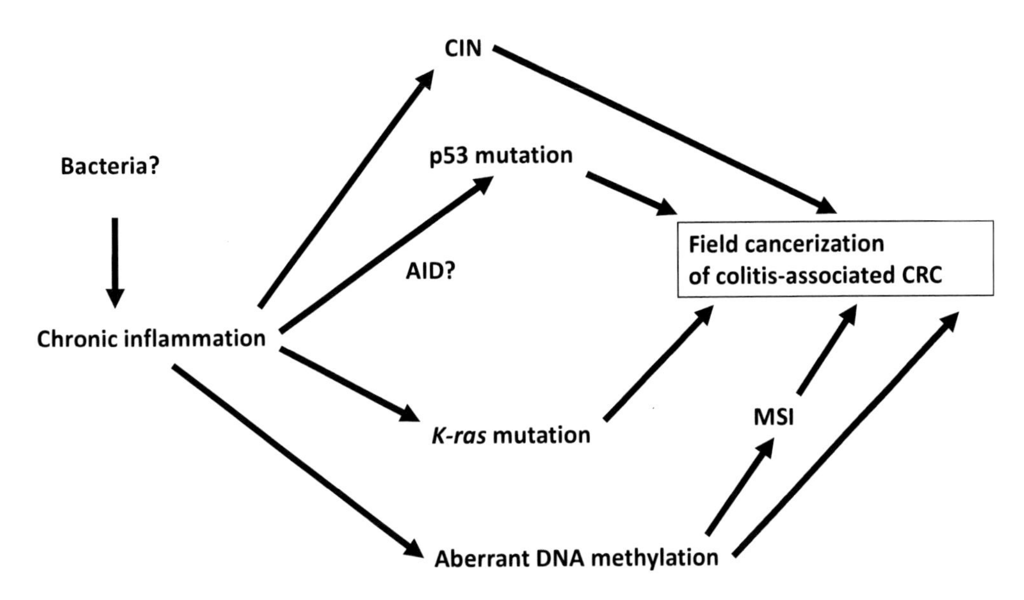

Figure 11.2. Field cancerization in colitis-associated colorectal cancer.

Leedham et al. recently examined *p53* mutations in dysplastic and/or cancerous tissues as well as surrounding non-dysplastic mucosa of 10 UC patients. They showed that 8 patients carried *p53* mutations in dysplastic lesions, and moreover, 2 of these 8 patients carried *p53* mutations even in non-dysplastic mucosa [93]. Therefore, they indicated that in colitis-associated tumours, *p53* was the most common single founding mutation. It is easy to understand why *p53* may act as an initiating mutation in colitis. If the main tumorigenic driving force in colitis is the underlying CIN throughout the colon, then early *p53* inactivation would be selected, on the basis that disruption of a mitotic checkpoint would permit the survival and selection of clones with gross chromosomal changes.

Recently, Endo et al. reported that activation-induced cytidine deaminase (AID), which was originally identified as an inducer of somatic hypermutations in the immunoglobulin gene, was aberrantly expressed in the inflamed colonic mucosa of UC patients, and that its expression may be involved in mutation of the *p53* genes in colonic cells [94]. Their result also suggests that *p53* mutation is an early event of carcinogenesis in colitis-associated cancer.

K-ras: Leedham et al. also reported that *K-ras* mutation is another gatekeeping mutation in colitis-associated carcinogenesis [93]. In the analyses of colectomied samples, *K-ras* mutation was detected in non-dysplastic inflammatory mucosa, as well as in dysplastic or cancerous mucosa. [95-97].

Mutational activation of the *K-ras* gene plays a definite role in the genesis of sporadic colorectal carcinomas, mainly during the step from small adenoma to large adenoma. *K-ras* mutation may be involved in an earlier step of UC-mediated colorectal carcinogenesis. Regarding frequency of the mutation, some groups have found mutations in carcinomas and dysplasia in UC to be lower than in sporadic adenocarcinoma and adenomas [95,98], while others showed *K-ras* mutation frequency in carcinoma in UC to be about the same as in sporadic CRC [96,99]. Holzmann et al. reported that *K-ras* mutation was detected in inflammatory mucosa of UC patients without any dysplasia [100], suggesting that *K-ras* mutation in UC mucosa is not correlated with neoplasia occurrence. Thus, the relevance of *K-ras* mutation in non-dysplastic mucosa of long-standing UC patients is still unclear.

MSI: MSI can also be detected in a small subset of colitis-associated CRC. The prevalence of MSI in IBD varies, with frequencies of 8% to 21% in colitis-associated CRC, 13% to 19% in dysplasia, and 8.9% to 50% in inflamed, non-dysplastic mucosa [101]. The wide variation in reported rates is a consequence of the use of different techniques to detect MSI and different definitions of low and high level MSI, based upon the number of affected markers. Microsatellite instability tends to occur in a subset of about 10% to 15% of IBD tumors that retain their diploid chromosome number (i.e., have a low level of CIN), and it was suggested that this subtype may exhibit a genetic predisposition towards MSI, perhaps as a consequence of mismatch repair mutation (an HNPCC variant) [102] or saturation as a consequence of increased oxidative stress [103]. Gene mutation is unlikely, because low level MSI was not associated with any loss of expression of *hMLH2* or *hMLH1* protein in UC [104]. Therefore, in UC-associated carcinogenesis, aberrant methylation in the promoter of *hMLH1* should also be considered as described below.

11.3.3.2. Epigenetic Alterations

Two types of gene methylation are recognized as described in the prior section. Type A is seen normally in aging epithelial cells, whereas type C is cancer cell restricted methylation. Increased levels of C type methylation in the promoters of tumor suppressor genes, such as *p16* [105] and $p14^{ARF}$ [106,107], cell adhesion molecules such as *E-cadherin* [108], and mismatch repair genes, such as *hMLH1* [109], have all been described in UC. However, the frequencies of methylation in these genes vary widely among studies, maybe because of differences in experimental methods employed for the detection of methylation. For example, Issa et al. were unable to detect any methylation within the *p16* gene promoter (C type) but did detect significant methylation within exon 1 of the *p16* gene. In addition, they observed methylation of the estrogen receptor gene and *MyoD* regions that characteristically undergo A type methylation [110].

Higher levels of gene methylation were present both in dysplastic tissue and neighboring normal appearing epithelium from patients with UC dysplasia or cancer, compared with normal controls and UC patients without dysplasia [110]. In addition, Fujii et al. showed that the estrogen receptor gene was extensively methylated in non-neoplastic epithelia throughout the colorectum compared with those in UC without neoplasia [111]. These results led the researchers to suggest that chronic inflammation is responsible for premature A type methylation in the colon, and that the associated cancer risk is related to the premature aging of the tissue.

11.3.3.3. Other Field Markers

In colitis-associated CRC, reports using immunohistochemistry to detect field cancerization are relatively scarce, compared to sporadic CRC. However, the expressions of Sialyl-Tn antigen [112], and laminin-5 gamma 2 chain [113] have been reported to be a marker for increased risk for cancer development.

11.3.4. Inducers of Field Cancerization in Colitis-Associated Carcinogenesis

Although inflammation in both the liver and stomach has specific carcinogenic factors (i.e., hepatitis virus and *H. pylor,i* respectively), such specific carcinogenic factors have not been determined in UC. Bacteria in the gut flora have been proposed as a candidate, but specific microorganisms have not yet been identified. Therefore, whether a specific carcinogenic factor (i.e., virus, bacteria etc.) or chronic inflammation status is responsible for generation of field cancerization is still unsettled.

Activation-induced cytidine deaminase (AID), which is aberrantly expressed in colorectal mucosa of UC, and was shown to be involved in *p53* mutations, is also expressed in chronic gastritis caused by *H. pylori* infection [114]. AID is induced in response to microorganisms or inflammation itself, and is capable of contributing to the generation of somatic mutations in tumor-related genes including *p53* in both gastric and colorectal epithelial cells. Thus, inflammation-mediated AID expression might underlie the development of colitis-associated CRC as well as *H. pylori*-related gastric cancer.

In addition, with regards to epigenetic field, both chronic hepatitis from hepatitis virus infection [115] and chronic gastritis due to *H. pylori* [116] have been shown to be causative of aberrant methylation. Although there certainly seems epigenetic field also exists in UC, the inducers of aberrant methylation are largely unknown, and may be the inflammatory reaction itself. Further studies regarding this issue would elucidate not only specific causal factors of field cancerization in UC but factors causative of chronic inflammation in UC.

11.3.5. Perspective for Clinical Application

For patients with long-standing UC, colonoscopic surveillance for colitis-associated dysplasia/CRC is currently recommended. Identification of patients with UC carrying an increased cancer risk is based on histological demonstration of dysplasia during colonoscopic surveillance. Dysplasia has been defined as an unequivocally neoplastic transformation of the colonic epithelium [117]. Although the criteria for the classification of dysplasia have been described in detail, the diagnosis is problematic and is often poorly reproducible. Classification of dysplasia is influenced by the degree of inflammation and is subject to inter- and intra-observer variation [118]. Because of these difficulties in morphological decision of dysplasia, there is still a demand for other methods for the detection of patients prone to carcinoma development.

In addition, because coexisting chronic inflammatory changes modifies the colonoscopic findings, it is not always easy to identify dysplastic lesion by colonoscopic observation. Therefore, in surveillance colonoscopy, taking a minimum of 4 biopsies from every 10 cm of the colon is recommended [119]. Although it has been shown that target biopsies with chromoendoscopy are superior to the random biopsy in detecting dysplasia [120], effective detection of dysplasia is still challenging for enodoscopists. Therefore, detecting genetic and/or epigenetic alterations indicating the existence of field cancerization using biopsy specimens taken during colonoscopy would be of much clinical importance.

Finally, the standard operation method for UC patients with CRC is total colectomy. In terms of elimination of field susceptible to giving rise to cancer, the method seems reasonable. However, establishment of a definite marker of field cancerization may change the strategy. If partial resection of only the region with field cancerization becomes allowable, quality of life of UC patients after undergoing colonic resection may be improved.

Conclusion

In conclusion, the development of an expanding pre-neoplastic field appears to be a critical step in colorectal carcinogenesis with important clinical consequences. Diagnosis and treatment of CRCs should not only be focused on the tumor, but also on the normal mucosa form which it developed. Detection and monitoring of field may have profound implications for cancer prevention.

References

[1] Slaughter DP, Shouthwick HW, Smejkal W. Field cancerization in oral starified squamous epithelium; clinical implications of multicentric origin. *Cancer* 1953; 6:963-968.

[2] Fearon ER, Vogelstein B. A genetic model for colorectal tumorigenesis. *Cell* 1990;61:759-767.

[3] Baylin SB, Ohm JE. Epigenetic gene silencing in cancer - a mechanism for early oncogenic pathway addiction? *Nat. Rev. Cancer* 2006;6:107-116.

[4] Ushijima T, Watanabe N, Okochi E, Kaneda A, Sugimura T, Miyamoto K. Fidelity of the methylation pattern and its variation in the genome. *Genome Res.* 2003;13:868-874.

[5] Riggs AD, Xiong Z. Methylation and epigenetic fidelity. *Proc. Natl. Acad. Sci. USA* 2004;101:4-5.

[6] Laird CD, Pleasant ND, Clark AD, Sneeden JL, Hassan KM, Manley NC, Vary JC Jr., Morgan T, Hansen RS, Stoger R. Hairpin-bisulfite PCR: assessing epigenetic methylation patterns on complementary strands of individual DNA molecules. Proc. Natl. Acad. Sci. *USA* 2004;101:204-209.

[7] Li E. Chromatin modification and epigenetic reprogramming in mammalian development. *Nat. Rev. Genet* 2002;3:662-673.

[8] Usihijima T, Detection and interpretation of altered methylation patterns in cancer cells. *Nat. Rev. Cancer* 2005;5:223-231.

[9] Richards EJ, Elgin SC. Epigenetic codes for heterochromatin formation and silencing: rounding up the usual suspects. *Cell* 2002;108:489-500.

[10] Miyamoto K, Asada K, Fukutomi T, Okochi E, Yagi Y, Hasegawa T, Asahara T, Sugimura T, Ushijima T. Methylation-associated silencing of heparin sulfate D-glucosaminyl 3-O-sulfotransferase-2 (3-OST-2) in human breast, colon, lung and pancreatic cancers. *Oncogene* 2003;22:274-280.

[11] Kaneda A, Tsukamoto T, Takamura-Enya T, Watanabe N, Kaminishi M, Sugimura T, Tatematsu M, Ushijima T. Frequent hypomethylation in multiple promoter CpG islands is associated with global hypomethylation, but not with frequent promoter hypermethylation *Cancer Sci.* 2004;95:58-64.

[12] Eden A, Gaudet F, Waghmare A, Jaenisch R. Chromosomal instability and tumors promoted by DNA hypomethylation. *Science* 2003;300:455.

[13] de Smet C, Lurquin C, Lethe B, Martelange V, Boon T. DNA methylation is the primary silencing mechanism for a set of germ line- and tumor-specific genes with a CpG-rich promoter. *Mol. Cell Biol.* 1999;19:7327-7335.

[14] Suzuki H, Watkinss DN, Jair KW, Schuebel KE, Markowitz SD, Chen WD, Pretlow TP, Yang B, Akiyama Y, Van Engeland M, Toyota M, Tokino T, Hinoda Y, Imai K, Herman JG, Baylin SB. Epigenetic inactivation of SFRP genes allows constitutive WNT signaling in colorectal cancer. *Nat. Genet.* 2004;36:417-422.

[15] Horii J, Hiraoka S, Kato J, Harada K, Kuwaki K, Fujita H, Toyooka S, Yamamoto K. Age-related methylation in normal colon mucosa differs between the proximal and distal colon in patients who underwent colonoscopy. *Clin. Biochem.* 2008;41:1440-1448.

[16] Hiraoka S, Kato J, Horii J, Saito S, Harada K, Fujita H, Motoaki K, Takemoto K, Uraoka T, Yamamoto K. Methylation status of normal background mucosa is correlated with occurrence and development of neoplasia in the distal colon. *Hum. Pathol.* 2010;41:38-47.

[17] Braakhuis BJ, Tabor MP, Kummer JA, Leemans CR, Brakenhoff RH. A genetic explanation of Slaughter's concept of field cancerization: evidence and clinical implications. *Cancer Re.s* 2003;63:1727-1730.

[18] Shen L, Kondo Y, Roser GL, Xiao L, Hernandez NS, Vilaythong J, Houlihan PS, Krouse RS, Prasad AR, Einspahr JG, Buckmeier J, Alberts DS, Hamilton SR, Issa JP. MGMT promoter methylation and field defect in sporadic colorectal cancer. *J. Natl. Cancer Inst.* 2005;97:1330-1338.

[19] Huxley RR, Ansary-Moghaddam A, Clifton P, Czernichow S, Parr CL, Woodward M. The impact of dietary and lifestyle risk factors on risk of colorectal cancer: a quantitative overview of the epidemiological evidence. *Int. J. Cancer* 2009;125:171-180.

[20] Fukatsu H, Kato J, Nasu J-I, Kawamoto H, Okada H, Yamamoto H, Sakaguchi K, Shiratori Y. Clinical characteristics of synchronous colorectal cancer are different according to tumour location. *Dig. Liver Dis.* 2007;39:40-46.

[21] Ringland CL, Arkenau HT, O'Connell DL, Ward RL. Second primary colorectal cancers (SPCRCs): experiences from a large Australian Cancer Registry. *Ann. Oncol.* 2010;21:92-97.

[22] Nawa T, Kato J, Kawamoto H, Okada H, Yamamoto H, Kohno H, Endo H, Shiratori Y. Differences between right- and left-sided colon cancer in patient characteristics, cancer morphology and histology. *J. Gastoenterol. Hepatol.* 2008;23:418-423.

[23] Iacopetta B. Are there two sides to colorectal cancer? *Int. J. Cancer* 2002;101:403-408.

[24] Shen L, Toyota M, Kondo Y, Li E, Zhang L, Guo Y, Hernandez NS, Chen X, Ahmed S, Konishi K, Hamilton SR, Issa JP. Integrated genetic and epigenetic analysis identifies three different subclasses of colon cancer. *Proc. Natl. Acad. Sci. USA* 2007;104:18654-18659.

[25] Hiraoka S, Kato J, Tatsukawa M, Harada K, Fujita H, Morikawa T, Shiraha H, Shiratori Y. Laterally spreading type of colorectal adenoma exhibits a unique methylation phenotype an K-ras mutations. *Gastroenterology* 2006;131:379-389.

[26] Harada K, Hiraoka S, Kato J, Horii J, Fujita H, Sakaguchi K, Shiratori Y. Genetic and epigenetic alterations of Ras signaling pathway in colorectal neoplasia: analysis based on tumour clinicopathological features. *Br. J. Cancer* 2007;97:1425-1431.

[27] Thibodeau SN, Bren G, Schaid D. Microsatellite instability in cancer of the proximal colon. *Science* 1993;260:816-819.

[28] Nicolaides NC, Carter KC, Shell BK, Papadopoulos N, Vogelstein B, Kinzler KW. Genomic organization of the human PMS2 gene family. *Genomics* 1995;30:195-206.

[29] Rampino N, Yamamoto H, Ionov Y, Li Y, Sawai H, Reed JC, Perucho M. Somatic frameshift mutations in the BAX gene in colon cancers of the microsatellite mutator phenotype. *Science* 1997;275:967-969.

[30] Cunningham JM, Christensen ER, Tester DJ, Kim CY, Roche PC, Burgart LJ, Thibodeau SN. Hypermethylation of the hMLH1 promoter in colon cancer with microsatellite instability. *Cancer Res.* 1998;58:3455-3460.

[31] Ohtani-Fujita N, Fujita T, Aoike A, Osifchin NE, Robbins PD, Sakai T. CpG methylation inactivates the promoter activity of the human retinoblastoma tumor-suppressor gene. *Oncogene* 1993;8:1063-1067.

[32] Toyota M, Ahuja N, Ohe-Toyota M, Herman JG, Baylin SB, Issa JP. CpG island methylator phenotype in colorectal cancer. *Proc. Natl. Acad. Sci. USA* 1999;96:8681-8686.

[33] Filipe MI, Branfoot AC, Abnormal patterns of mucus secretion in apparently normal mucosa of large intestine with carcinoma. *Cancer* 1974;34:282-290.

[34] Dawson PA, Filipe MI. An ultrastructural and histochemical study of the mucous membrane adjacent to and remote from carcinoma of the colon. *Cancer* 1976;37:2388-2398.

[35] Saffos RO, Rhatigan RM. Benign (non-polypoid) mucosal changes adjacent to carcinomas of the colon: A light microscopic study of 20 cases. *Hum. Pathol.* 1977;8:441-449.

[36] Ngoi SS, Staiano-Coico L, Godwin TA, Wong RJ, DeCosse JJ. Abnormal DNA ploidy and proliferative patterns in superficial colonic epithelium adjacent to colorectal cancer. *Cancer* 1990;66:953-959.

[37] Dawson PA, Filipe MI. Uptake of ^{3}H threonine in human colonic mucosa associated with carcinoma: An autoradiographic analysis at the ultrastructural level. *Histochem. J.* 1982;14:385-401.

[38] Gong EC, Hirohashi S, Shimosato Y, Watanabe M, Ino Y, Teshima S, Kodaira S. Expression of carbohydrate antigen 19-9 and stage-specific embryonic antigen 1 in nontumorous and tumorous epithelia of the human colon and rectum. *J. Natl. Cancer Inst.* 1985;75:447-454.

[39] Jothy S, Slesak B, Harlozinska A, Lapinska J, Adamiak J, Rabczynski J. Field cancerization of human colon carcinoma on normal mucosa: relevance of carcionembryonic antigen expression. *Tumor Biol.* 1996;17:58-64.

[40] Mariani-Costantini R, Theillet C, Hutzell P, Merlo G, Schlom J, Callahan R. In situ detection of c-myc mRNA in adenocarcinomas, adenomas, and mucosa of human colon. *J. Histochem. Cytochem.* 1989;37:293-298.

[41] Koo HB, Sigurdson ER, Daly JM, Beckenseon M, Groshen S, DeCosse JJ. Ornithine decarboxylase levels in the rectal mucosa of patients with colonic neoplasia. *J. Surg. Oncol.* 1988;38:240-243.

[42] Maskens AP, Deschner EE. Tritiated thymidine incorporation into epithelial cells of normal-appearing colorectal mucosa of cancer patients. *J. Natl. Cancer Inst.* 1977;58:1221-1224.

[43] Romagnoli P, Filipponi F, Bandettini L, Brugnola D. Increase of mitotic activity in the colorectal mucosa of patients with colorectal cancer. *Dis. Colon Rectum* 1984;27:305-308.

[44] Ponz de Leon M, Roncucci L, Di Donato P, Tassi L, Smerieri O, Amorico MG, Malagoli G, De Maria D, Antonioli A, Chahin NJ, Perini M, Rigo G, Barberini G, Manenti A, Biasco G, Barbara L. Pattern of epithelial cell proliferation in colorectal mucosa of normal subjects and of patients with adenomatous polyps or cancer of the large bowel. *Cancer Res.* 1988;48:4121-4126.

[45] Daniel CR, Bostick RM, Flanders WD, Long Q, Fedirko V, Sidelnikov E, Seabrook ME. TGF-a expression as a potential biomarker of risk within the normal-appearing colorectal mucosa of patients with and without incident sporadic adenoma. *Cancer Epidemiol. Biomarkers Prev.* 2009;18:65-73.

[46] Anti M, Armuzzi A, Morini S, Iascone E, Pignataro G, Coco C, Lorenzetti R, Paolucci M, Covino M, Gasbarrini A, Vecchio FM, Gasbarrini G. Severe imbalance of cell proliferation and apoptosis in the left colon and in the rectosigmoid tract in subjects with a history of large adenomas. *Gut* 2001;48:238-246.

[47] Bradvie S, Hanna-Morris A, Andreyev HJN, Cohen P, Saini S, Allen-Mersh TG, A "field change" of inhibited apoptosis occurs in colorectal mucosa adjacent to colorectal adenocarcinoma. *J. Clin. Pathol.* 2006;59:942-946.

[48] Bronner MP, Culin C, Reed JC, Furth EE. The bcl-2 proto-oncogene and the gastrointestinal epithelial tumor progression model. *Am. J. Pathol.* 1995;146:20-26.

[49] Polley AC, Mulholland F, Pin C, Williams EA, Bradburn DM, Mills SJ, Mathers JC, Johnson IT. Proteomic analysis reveals field-wide changes in protein expression in the morphologically normal mucosa of patients with colorectal neoplasia. *Cancer Res.* 2006;66:6553-6562.

[50] Takayama T, Ohi M, Hayashi T, Miyanishi K, Nobuoka A, Nakajima T, Satoh T, Takimoto R, Kato J, Sakamaki S, Niitsu Y. Analysis of K-ras, APC, b-catenin in aberrant crypt foci in sporadic adenoma, cancer, and familial adenomatous polyposis. *Gastroenterology* 2001;121:599-611.

[51] Minamoto T, Yamashita N, Ochiai A, Mai M, Sugimura T, Ronai Z, Esumi H. Mutant K-ras in apparently normal mucosa of colorectal cancer patients. *Cancer* 1995;75:1520-1526.

[52] Yamada S, Yashiro M, Maeda K, Nishiguchi Y, Hirakawa K. A novel high-specificity approach for colorectal neoplasia: Detection of K-ras2 oncogene mutation in normal mucosa. *Int. J. Cancer* 2005;113:1015-1021.

[53] Visca P, Alo PL, Nonno FD, Botti C, Trombetta G, Marandino F, Filippi S, Tondo UD, Donnorso RP. Immunohistochemical expression of fatty acid synthase, apoptotic-regulating genes, proliferating factors, and ras protein product in colorectal adenomas, carcinomas, and adjacent nonneoplastic mucosa. *Clin. Cancer Res.* 1999;5:4111-4118.

[54] Bian Y, Knobloch TJ, Sadim M, Kaklamani V, Raji A, Yang G-Y, Weghorst CM, Pasche B. Somatic acquisition of TGFBR1*6A by epithelial and stromal cells during head and neck and colon cancer development. *Hum. Mol. Genet.* 2007;16:3128-3135.

[55] Issa JP, Ottaviano YL, Celano P, Hamilton SR, Davidson NE, Baylin SB. Methylation of the oestrogen receptor CpG island links ageing and neoplasia in human colon. *Nat. Genet.* 1994;7:536-540.

[56] Ahuja N, Li Q, Mohan AL, Baylin SB, Issa JP. Aging and DNA methylation in colorectal mucosa and cancer. *Cancer Res.* 1998;58:5489-5494.

[57] Nakagawa H, Nuovo GJ, Zervos EE, Martin EW Jr., Salovaara R, Aaltonen LA, de la Chappelle A. Age-related hypermethylation of the 5' region of MLH1 in normal colonic mucosa is associated with microsatellite-unstable colorectal cancer development. *Cancer Res.* 2001;61:6991-6995.

[58] Kawakami K, Ruszkiewicz A, Bennett G, Moore J, Grieu F, Watanabe G, Iacopetta B. DNA hypermethylation in the normal colonic mucosa of patients with colorectal cancer. *Br. J. Cancer* 2006;94:593-598.

[59] Povey AC, Badawi AF, Cooper DP, Hall CN, Harrison KL, Jackson PE, Lees NP, O'Connor PJ. Margison GP. DNA alkylation and repair in the large bowel: animal and human studies. *J. Nutr.* 2002;132:3518S-3521S.

[60] Esteller M, Toyota M, Sanchez-Cespedes M, Capella G, Peinado MA, Watkins DN, Issa JP, Sidransky D, Baylin SB, Herman JG. Inactivation of the DNA repair gene O^6-methylguanine-DNA methyltransferase by promoter hypermethylation in associated with G to A mutations in K-ras in colorectal tumorigenesis. *Cancer Res.* 2000;60:2368-2371.

[61] Pufulete M, Al-Ghnaniem R, Leather AJ, Appleby P, Gout S, Terry C, Emery PW, Sanders TA. Folate status, genomic DNA hypomethylation, and risk of colorectal adenoma and cancer: a case control study. *Gastroenterology* 2003;114:1240-1248.

[62] Belshaw NJ, Elliott GO, Foxall RJ, Dainty JR, Pal N, Coupe A, Garg D, Bradburn DM, Mathers JC, Johnson IT. Profiling CpG island field methylation in both morphologically normal and neoplastic human colonic mucosa. *Br. J. Cancer* 2008;99:136-142.

[63] Bernstein H, Bernstein C, Payne CM, Dvorakova K, Garewal H. Bile acids as carcinogens in human gastrointestinal cancers. *Mutat. Res.* 2005;589;47-65.

[64] Garewal H, Bernstein H, Bernstein C, Sampliner R, Payne C. Reduced bile acid-induced apoptosis in "normal" colorectal mucosa: a potential biological marker for cancer risk. *Cancer Res.* 1996;56:1480-1483.

[65] Bernstein H, Holubec H, Warneke JA, Garewal H, Earnest DL, Payne CM, Roe DJ, Cui H, Jacobson EL, Bernstein C. Patch field defects of apoptosis resistance and dedifferentiation in flat mucosa of colon resections from colon cancer patients. *Ann. Surg. Oncol.* 2002;9:505-517.

[66] Meyerhardt JA, Niedzwiecki D, Hollis D, Saltz LB, Hu FB, Mayer RJ, Nelson H, Whittom R, Hantel A, Thomas J, Fuchs CS. Association of dietary patterns with cancer recurrence and survival in patients with stage III colon cancer. *JAMA* 2007;298:754-764.

[67] Choi SW, Mason JB. Folate status: effects on pathways of colorectal carcinogenesis. *J. Nutr.* 2002;132:2413S-2418S.

[68] Kim YI. Folate and DMA methylation: a mechanistic link between folate deficiency and colorectal cancer? *Cancer Epidemiol. Biomarkers Prev.* 2004;13:511-519.

[69] Al-Ghenaniem R, Peters J, Foresti R, Heaton N, Pufulete M. Methylation of estrogen receptor a and mutL homolog 1 in normal colonic mucosa: association with folate and vitamin B-12 status in subjects with and without colorectal neoplasia. *Am. J. Clin. Nutr.* 2007.

[70] Pufulete M, Al-Ghenaniem R, Rennie JA, Appleby P, Harris N, Gout S, Enery PW, Sanders TA. Influence of folate status on genomic DNA methylation in colonic mucosa of subjects without colorectal adenoma or cancer. *Br. J. Cancer* 2005;92:838-842.

[71] Friso S, Choi SW, Girelli D, Mason JB, Dolnikowski GG, Bagley PJ, Olivieri O, Jacques PF, Rosenberg IH, Corrocher R, Selhub J. A common mutation in the 5,10-methylenetetrahydrofolate reductase gene affects genomic DNA methylation through an interaction with folate status. *Proc. Natl. Acad. Sci. USA* 2002;99:5606-5611.

[72] Paz MF, Avila S, Fraga MF, Pollan M, Capella G, Peinado MA, Sanchez-Cespedes M, Herman JG, Esteller M. Germ-line variants in methyl-group metabolism genes and susceptibility to DNA methylation in normal tissues and human primary tumours. *Cancer Res.* 2002;62:4519-4524.

[73] Kawakami K, Watanabe G. Identification and functional analysis of single nucleotide polymorphism in the tandem repeat sequence of thymidylate synthase gene. *Cancer Res.* 2003;63:6004-6007.

[74] Chen J, Kyte C, Valcin M, Chan W, Wetmur JG, Selhub , Hunter DJ, Ma J. Polymorphism in the one-carbon metabolic pathway, plasma folate levels and colorectal cancer in a prospective study. *Int. J. Cancer* 2004;110:617-620.

[75] Sharp L, Little J. Polymorphisms in genes involved in folate metabolism and colorectal neoplasia: a HuGE review. *Am. J. Epidemiol.* 2004;159:423-443.

[76] Eaden JA, Abrams KR, Mayberry JF. The risk of colorectal cancer in ulcerative colitis: a meta-analysis. *Gut* 2001;48:526-535.

[77] Itzkowitz SH, Yio X, Inflammation and cancer IV. Colorectal cancer in inflammatory bowel disease: the role of inflammation. *Am. J. Physiol. Gastrointest. Liver Physiol.* 2004;287:G7-G17.

[78] Vogelstein B, Fearon ER, Hamilton SR, Kern SE, Preisinger AC, Leppert M, Nakamura Y, White R, Smits AM, Bos JL. Genetic alterations during colorectal-tumor development. *N. Engl. J. Med.* 1988;319:525-532.

[79] Loeb K, Loeb L. Genetic instability and the mutator phenotype. Studies in ulcerative colitis. *Am. J. Pathol.* 1999;154:1621-1626.

[80] Aust DE, Willenbucher RF, Terdiman JP, Ferrell LD, Chang CG, Moore DH 2nd, Molinaro-Clark A, Baretton GB, Loehrs U, Waldman FM. Chromosomal alterations in ulcerative colitis-related and sporadic colorectal cancers by comparative genomic hybridization. *Hum. Pathol.* 2000;31:109-114.

[81] Willenbucher RF, Aust DE, Chang CG, Zelman SJ, Ferrell LD, Moore DH 2nd, Waldman FM. Genomic instability is an early event during the progression pathway of ulcerative-colitis-related neoplasia. *Am. J. Pathol.* 1999;154:1825-1830.

[82] Willenbucher RF, Zelman SJ, Ferrell LD, Moore DH 2nd, Waldman FM. Chromosomal alterations in ulcerative colitis-related neoplastic progression. *Gastroenterology* 1997;113:791-801.

[83] Keller R, Foerster EC, Kohler A, Floer B, Winde G, Terpe HJ, Domschke W. Diagnostic value of DNA image cytometry in ulcerative colits. *Dig. Dis. Sci.* 2001;46:870-878.

[84] Befrits R, Hammarberg C, Rubio C, Jaramillo E, Tribukait B. DNA aneuploidy and histologic dysplasia in long-standing ulcerative colitis. A 10-year follow-up study. *Dis. Colon Rectum* 1994;37:313-320.

[85] Rubin C, Haggitt R, Burmer G, Brentnall TA, Stevens AC, Levine DS, Dean PJ, Kimmey M, Perera DR, Rabinovitch PS. DNA aneuploidy in colonic biopsies predicts future development of dysplasia in ulcerative colitis. *Gastroenterology* 1992;103:1611-1620.

[86] Clausen OP, Andersen SN, Stroomkjaer H, Nielsen V, Rognum TO, Bolund L, Koolvraa S. A strategy combining flow sorting and comparative genomic hybridization for studying genetic aberrations at different stages of colorectal tumorigenesis in ulcerative colitis. *Cytometory* 2001;43:46-54.

[87] O'Sullivan JN, Bronner MP, Brentnall TA, Finley JC, Shen WT, Emerson S, Emond MJ, Gollahon KA, Moskovitz AH, Crispin DA, Potter JD, Rabinovitch PS. Chromosomal instability in ulcerative colitis is related to telomere shortening. *Nat. Genet.* 2002;32:280-284.

[88] Cahill D, Lengauer C, Yu J, Riggins GJ, Willson JK, Markowitz SD, Kinzler KW, Vogelstein B. Mutations of mitotic checkpoint genes in human cancers. *Nature* 1998;392:30-303.

[89] Leedham SJ, Wright NA. Human tumour clonality assessment – flawed but necessary. *J. Pathol.* 2008;215:351-354.

[90] Brentnall TA, Crispin DA, Rabinovitch PS, Haggitt RC, Rubin CE, Stevens AC, Burmer GC. Mutations in the p53 gene: an early marker of neoplastic progression in ulcerative colitis. *Gastroenterology* 1994;107:369-378.

[91] Lashner BA, Shapiro BD, Husain A, Goldblum JR. Evaluation of the usefulness of testing for p53 mutations in colorectal cancer surveillance for ulcerative colitis. *Am. J. Gastroenterol.* 1999;94:456-462.

[92] Yoshida T, Mikami T, Mitomi H, Okayasu I. Diverse p53 alterations in ulcerative colitis-associated low-grade dysplasia: full-length gene sequencing in microdissected single crypts. *J. Pathol.* 2003;199:166-175.

[93] Leedham SJ, Graham TA, Oukrif D, McDonald SAC, Rodriguez-Justo M, Harrison RF, Shepherd NA, Novelli MR, Jankowski JAZ, Wright NA. Clonality, founder mutations, and field cancerization in human ulcerative colitis-associated neoplasia. *Gastroenterology* 2009;136:542-550.

[94] Endo Y, Marusawa H, Kou T, Nakase H, Fujii S, Fujimori T, Kinoshita K, Honjo T, Chita T. Activation-induced cytidine deaminase links between inflammation and the development of colitis-associated colorectal cancers. *Gastroenterology* 2008;135:889-898.

[95] Chaubert P, Benhattar J, Saraga E, Costa J. K-ras mutations and p53 alterations in neoplastic and nonneoplastic lesions associated with longstanding ulcerative colitis. *Am. J. Pathol.* 1994;144:767-775.
[96] Redston MS, Papadopoulos N, Caldas C, Kinzler KW, Kern SE. Common occurrence of APC and K-ras gene mutations in the spectrum of colitis-associated neoplasias. *Gastroenterology* 1995;108:383-392.
[97] Andersen SN, Loving T, Clausen OPF, Bakka A, Fausa O, Rognum TO. Villous, hypermucinous mucosa in long standing ulcerative colitis shows high frequency of K-ras mutations. *Gut* 1999;45:686-692.
[98] Bell SM, Kelly SA, Hoyle JA, Lewis FA, Taylor GR, Thompson H, Dixon MF, Quirke P. c-Ki-ras gene mutations in dysplasia and carcinomas complicating ulcerative colitis. *Br. J. Cancer* 1991;64:174-178.
[99] Chen J, Compton C, Cheng E, Fromowitz F, Viola MV. c-Ki-ras mutations in dysplastic fields and cancers in ulcerative colitis. *Gastroenterology* 1992;102:1983-1987.
[100] Holzmann K, Weis-Klemm M, Klump B, Hsieh C-J, Borchard F, Gregor M, Porschen R. Comparison of flow cytometry and histology with mutational screening for p53 and Ki-ras mutations in surveillance of patients with long-standing ulcerative colitis. *Scand. J. Gastroenterol.* 2001;36:1320-1326.
[101] Seril DN, Liao J, Yang GY, Yang CS. Oxidative stress and ulcerative colitis-associated carcinogenesis: studies in humans and animal models. *Carcinogenesis* 2003;24:353-362.
[102] Brentnall TA, Rubin CE, Crispin DA, Stevens A, Batchelor RH, Haggitt RC, Bronner MP, Evans JP, McCahill LE, Billir N, Boland CR, Rabinovitch PS. A germline substitution in the human MSH2 gene is associated with high-grade dysplasia and cancer in ulcerative colitis. *Gastroenterology* 1995;109:151-155.
[103] Brentnall TA, Crispin DA, Bronner MP, Cherian SP, Hueffed M, Rabinovitch PS, Rubin CE, Haggitt RC, Boland CR. Microsatellite instability in nonneoplastic mucosa from patients with chronic ulcerative colitis. *Cancer Res.* 1996;56;1237-1240.
[104] Cawkwell L, Sutherland F, Murgatroyd H, Jarvis P, Gray S, Cross D, Shepherd N, Day D, Quirke P. Defective hMSH2/hMLH1 protein expression is seen infrequently in ulcerative colitis associated colorectal cancers. *Gut* 2000;46:367-369.
[105] Hsieh CJ, Klump B, Hozmann K, Borchard F, Gregor M, Porschen R. Hypermethylation of the p16^{INK4a} promoter in colectomy specimens of patients with longstanding and extensive ulcerative colitis. *Cancer Res.* 1998;58:3942-3945.
[106] Sato F, Harpaz N, Shibata D, Xu Y, Yin J, Mori Y, Zou TT, Wang S, Desai K, Leytin A, Selaru FM, Abraham JM, Meltzer SJ. Hypermethylation of the p14(ARF) gene in ulcerative colitis-associated colorectal carcinogenesis. *Cancer Res.* 2002;62:1148-1151.
[107] Moriyama T, Matsumoto T, Nakamura S, Jo Y, Mibu R, Yao T, Iida M. Hypermethylation of p14(ARF) may be predictive of colitic cancer in patients with ulcerative colitis. *Dis. Colon Recum* 2007;50:1384-1392.
[108] Wheeler J, Kim H, Efstathiou J, Ilyas M, Mortensen NJ, Bodmer WF. Hypermethylation of the promoter region of the E-cadherin gene (CDH1) in sporadic and ulcerative colitis associated colorectal cancer. *Gut* 2001;48:367-371.
[109] Fleisher A, Esteller M, Harpaz N, Leytin A, Rashid A, Xu Y, Liang J, Stine OC, Yin J, Zou TT, Abraham JM, Kong D, Wilson KT, James SP, Herman JG, Meltzer SJ.

Microsatellite instability in inflammatory bowel disease-associated neoplastic lesions is associated with hypermethylation and diminished expression of the DNA mismatch repair gene, hMLH1. *Cancer Res.* 2000;60:4864-4868.

[110] Issa JP, Ahuja N, Toyota M, Bronner M, Brentnall TA. Accelerated age-related CpG island methylation in ulcerative colitis. *Cancer Res.* 2001;61:3573-3577.

[111] Fujii S, Tominaga K, Kitajima K, Takeda J, Kusaka T, Fujita M, Ichikawa K, Tomita S, Ohkusa Y, Ono Y, Imura J, Chiba T, Fujimori T. Methylation of the oestrogen receptor gene in non-neoplastic epithelium as a marker of colorectal neoplasia risk in longstanding and extensive ulcerative colitis. *Gut* 2005;54:1287-1292.

[112] Karlen P, Young E, Brostrom O, Lofberg R, Tribukait B, Ost K, Bodian C, Itzkowitz S. Sialyl-Tn antigen as a marker of colon cancer risk in ulcerative colitis: relation to dysplasia and DNA aneuploidy. *Gastroenterology* 1998;115:1395-1404.

[113] Habermann J, Lenander C, Roblick UJ, Kruger S, Ludwig D, Alaiya A, Freitag S, Dumbgen L, Bruch HP, Stange E, Salo S, Tryggvason K, Auer G, Shimmelpenning H. Ulcerative colitis and colorectal carcinoma: DNA-profile, laminin-5 gamma 2 chain and cyclin A expression asearly markers for risk assessment. *Scand. J. Gastroenterol.* 2001;36:751-758.

[114] Matsumoto Y, Marusawa H, Kinoshita K, Endo Y, Kou T, Morisawa T, Azuma T, Okazaki IM, Honjo T, Chiba T. Helicobacter pylori infection triggers aberrant expression of activation-induced cytidine deaminase in gastric epithelium. *Nat. Med.* 2007;13:470-476.

[115] Kondo Y, Kanai Y, Sakamoto M, Mizokami M, Ueda R, Hirohashi S. Genetic instability and aberrant DNA methylation in chronic hepatitis and cirrhosis - A comprehensive study of loss of heterozygosity and microsatellite instability at 39 loci and DNA hypermethylation on 8 CpG islands in microdissected specimens from patients with hepatocellular carcinoma. *Hepatology* 2000;32:970-979.

[116] Ushijima T. Epigenetic field for cancerization. *J. Biochem. Mol. Biol.* 2007;40:142-150.

[117] Riddell RH, Goldman H, Ransohoff DF, Appelman HD, Fenoglio CM, Haggitt RC, Ahren C, Correa P, Hamilton SR, Morson BC, Sommers SC, Yardley JH. Dysplasia in inflammatory bowel disease: standardized classification with provisional clinical applications. *Hum. Pathol.* 1983;14:931-968.

[118] Melville DM, Jass JR, Shepherd NA, Northover JM, Capellaro D, Richman PI, Lennard-Jones JE, Ritchie JK, Andersen SN. Dysplasia and deoxyribonucleic acid aneuploidy in the assessment of precancerous changes in chronic ulcerative colitis. Observer variation and correlations. *Gastroenterology* 1988;95:668-675.

[119] Winawer S, Fletcher R, Rex D, Bond J, Burt R, Ferrucci J, Ganiats T, Levin T, Woolf S, Johnson D, Kirk L, Litin S, Simmang C; Gastrointestinal Consortium Panel. Colorectal cancer screening and surveillance: clinical guidelines and rationale-Update based on new evidence. *Gastroenterology* 2003;124:544-560.

[120] Marion JF, Waye JD, Present DH, Israel Y, Bodian C, Harpaz N, Chapman M, Itzkowtz S, Steinlauf AF, Abreu MT, Ullman TA, Aisenberg J, Mayer L. Chromoendoscopy-targeted biopsies are superior to standard colonoscopic surveillance for detecting dysplasia in inflammatory bowel disease patients: A prospective endoscopic trial. *Am. J. Gastroenterol.* 2008;103:2342-2349.

In: Field Cancerization: Basic Science and Clinical Applications ISBN 978-1-61761-006-6
Editor: Gabriel D. Dakubo

Chapter 12

Epigenetic Changes in Hepatic Tissues: Evidence of Field Cancerization

Yutaka Kondo

Abstract

Epigenetic abnormities, such as DNA methylation and histone modifications, alter the pattern of gene expression and play a key role in tumorigenesis. Around 70-80% of hepatocellular carcinomas (HCCs) develop in liver tissues with chronic hepatitis or cirrhosis due to continuous viral infections. While the connection between inflammation and tumorigenesis was suspected a long time ago, key factors linking these two processes were not completely understood. Ample evidence shows that during hepatocarcinogenesis, genetic and epigenetic abnormalities accumulate, which may be fundamental mechanisms underlying tumor formation. With the recent advanced technologies for assessing DNA methylation on a genome-wide scale, it now possible to examine the global patterns of DNA methylation in cancers as well as precancerous conditions. These studies suggest that aberrant epigenetic regulation of subsets of genes occur sequentially from precancerous conditions to HCC. In this chapter, aberrant DNA methylation as a field cancerization in chronic hepatitis or cirrhosis are mainly focused on and discussed.

12.1. Introduction

Hepatocellular carcinoma (HCC) is one of the most common human malignancies worldwide. Epidemiological studies indicate that the majority of HCCs are associated with chronic viral infection and aflatoxin B1 exposure, which have been recognized as carcinogens for HCCs, and may influence the genetic and/or epigenetic alterations [1]. The prevalence of HCCs differs in various countries, with incidences of about 3 to 4/100,000 in Western countries, and up to 120/100,000 in Asian and African countries where hepatitis B virus (HBV) and hepatitis C virus (HCV) infections and aflatoxin B1 exposure are more common [2]. Although the molecular mechanisms that connect chronic inflammation and cancer are not completely understood, multi-step nature of HCC is suggested by the long period of preneoplastic stage caused by chronic viral infection. "Field cancerization" may be present in liver cancer progression, in which cells accumulate genetic and epigenetic alterations and are therefore predisposed to tumor development [3]. A common finding in chronic inflammatory liver diseases is the activation of growth factor expression and signaling [4]. Chronic stimulation of such growth factors might contribute to neoplastic transformation of hepatic cells through a series of molecular and functional changes. However, considering the long period of precancerous conditions indicated by chronic hepatitis and liver cirrhosis, a simple and direct association between the dysregulation of these signaling pathways and HCC tumorigenesis seems unlikely (figure 12-1).

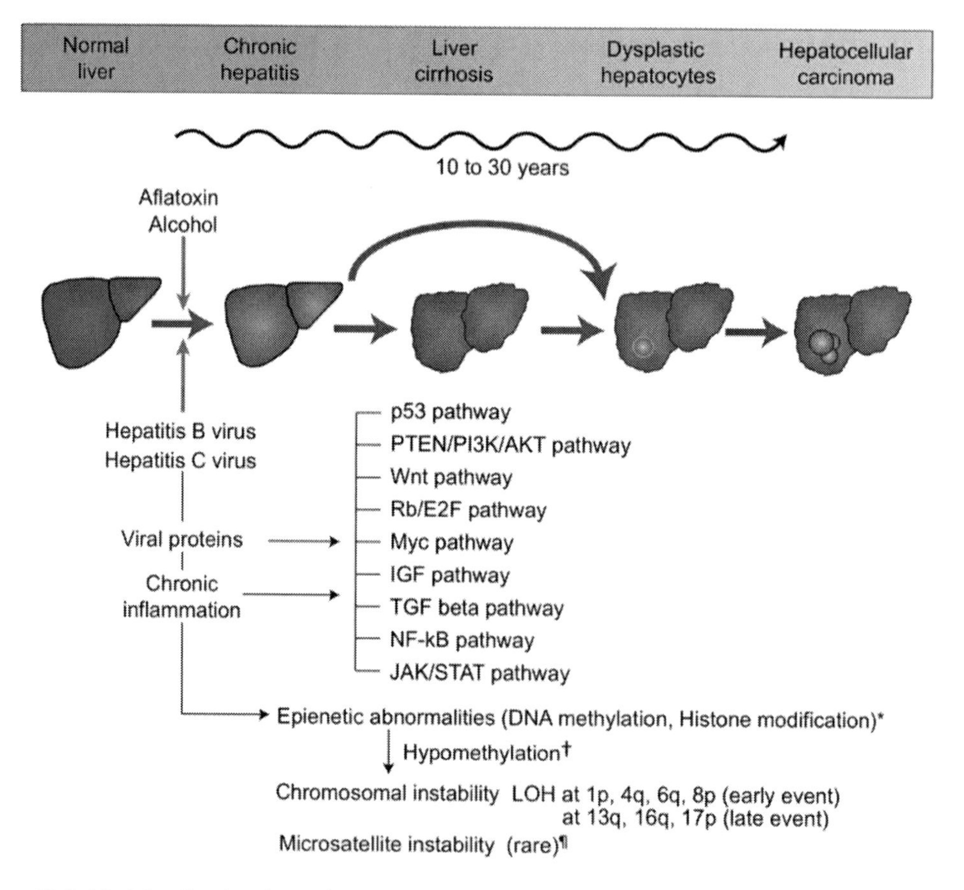

Figure 12.1. Models of molecular pathogenesis of human HCC. Accumulation of genetic and epigenetic changes in multiple molecular pathways underlies the evolution of HCC. *Candidate targets of hypermethylation are shown in Table 12-2. †Association between hypomethylation and chromosomal instability in HCC is not conclusive. Conclusive results of inactivation of mismatch repair system have not been demonstrated.

A long-term follow-up study revealed that liver cell dysplasia or adenomatous hyperplasia, both of which are precancerous lesions of the liver with histological findings of chronic hepatitis and/or liver cirrhosis, transformed into cancer [5]. These findings suggest that a developmental sequence of genomic changes, and possibly multiple molecular pathways may be involved in the process of hepatocarcinogenesis [1]. Indeed, genetic alterations in HCCs are numerous and varied [6]. Mutations in the critical tumor suppressor genes, *TP53* or *Rb*, were observed in late stage HCC [7], while loss of heterozygosity (LOH) was detected even in chronic hepatitis or liver cirrhosis [8,9]. Thus, HCC displays multiple genetic abnormalities, as gross genomic alterations including chromosomal instability, DNA rearrangements associated with hepatitis B virus DNA integration, and to a lesser degree of microsatellite instability [10].

In addition to these genetic abnormalities, HCC may be induced by epigenetic alterations that compromise more than one regulatory pathway. Aberrant DNA methylation and/or histone modifications on the promoter regions of genes have been described in many human cancers. These epigenetic alterations are associated with gene silencing, sometimes together with point mutations and deletions, serving as mechanisms leading to the inactivation of tumor suppressor genes and critical cancer-related genes in human cancers. Dysregulation of these target genes has been connected with essential tumor properties such as tumor cell proliferation, anti-apoptosis, neo-angiogenesis, invasive behavior and chemotherapy resistance [11,12]. The relationship between promoter DNA hypermethylation and inflammation has been documented in many types of cancers, including HCC [9,13,14,15,16]. Studies in several candidate genes demonstrated that aberrant methylation was detected even in adjacent non-cancerous liver tissues, indicating that DNA methylation is an early event during hepatocarcinogenesis [9,17,18]. Recent advanced microarray-based technology for assessing DNA methylation in a genome-wide scale revealed that a large number of CpG islands (CGIs) could be methylated *de novo* at an early stage of tumorigenesis [19,20].

In this chapter, epigenetic abnormalities in precancerous tissues as well as HCCs are focused on, and the significance of these epigenetic mechanisms in HCCs is discussed.

12.2. Significance of DNA Methylation in Mammalian Cells

Promoter DNA methylation is widely recognized as an epigenetic modification [21]. DNA methylation occurs in the cytosine-guanine sequence (CpG) in the DNA strand in mammals. Whole genome analysis revealed that CpG sites are unevenly distributed in the mammalian genome. While approximately 70% of CpG dinucleotides are methylated and scattered throughout the genome, short unmethylated CpG rich regions (up to 2kb) are found and called "CpG islands (CGI)" [22,23]. A recent study proposed a criterion for CGI that is more likely to be associated with the 5' regions of genes, and this definition excluded most *Alu*-repetitive elements (table 12-1) [24]. About 60% of genes have CGI in their promoter regions where DNA methylation takes place to maintain the repressive chromatin state and stably silence promoter activity. Inhibition of gene expression in CpG rich promoters is dependent on the density of methylation, and this is typically irreversible. CpG poor promoters are often methylated, but this do not seem to be associated with gene silencing [19,25]. Intermediate CpG promoters may also be regulated in part by DNA methylation, possibly with other regulatory mechanisms (histone modifications) or through inhibition of transcription factor binding. This light methylation is reversible, and is part of the normal mechanisms of regulation of gene expression for some tissue specific genes [26].

Table 12.1. Criteria for CpG island

	Gardiner-Garden [27]	Takai et al. [24]
Sequence length examined (bp)	200	500
GC content (%)	50	55
Observed CpG /expected CpG	0.6	0.65

CpG islands are also found in non-promoter regions. Large-scale analysis revealed that around 50% of CGIs are not coincident with annotated promoters. A fraction of these CGIs are exceptionally methylated in normal somatic tissues and may play significant roles in gene regulation. Although interest of the non-promoter CGI methylation is increasing, precise biological functions of such CGI methylation are not well understood [26].

12.3. DNA Methylation in Hepatocellular Carcinomas

Cancer cells generally demonstrate global hypomethylation and regional hypermethylation simultaneously, especially at selected gene-associated CGIs that are normally unmethylated. Cancer hypomethylation has been reported to involve repetitive elements localized in satellite sequences or pericentromeric regions, which comprise more than 40% of the human genome and are normally heavily methylated [28]. It has been shown that hypomethylation results in karyotypic instability, as in the immunodeficiency, centromere instability and facial anomalies (ICF) syndrome caused by DNA methyltransferase 3b (Dnmt 3b) mutation through global hypomethylation [29]. Genomic instability induced by hypomethylation is also considered to be involved in tumor progression [30,31].

In HCC, it has been shown that DNA hypomethylation on pericentromeric satellite regions is an early event associated with heterochromatin instability during human hepatocarcinogenesis [32]. In contrast, another study has also demonstrated that Dnmt1-deficient cells do not show an increased rate of chromosomal changes [33]. Although, global hypomethylation might be expected to lead to genomic instability in some cases, clear association between hypomethylation and genomic instability in cancer cells remains to be clarified.

Hypomethylation in CpG promoter regions is associated with the derepression in some cancer-associated genes. Hypomethylation in normally methylated CGIs has been reported to induce aberrant gene expression, such as *melanoma antigen genes* (*MAGEs*), in cancer cells [34].

Loss of imprinting (LOI), leading to pathological biallelic expression of *IGF2,* is another well-known cause for tumorigenesis [35]. Abnormal gene imprinting and/or activating cancer-associated genes may be linked to the early aberrant clonal expansion of cells and development of tumors.

Accumulating evidence indicates that aberrant DNA methylation on promoter CGIs has been found in most human cancers including HCC. As was described above, this epigenetic alteration is associated with silencing of many classic tumor suppressor genes.

Therefore, many cancers appear to have genes silenced by DNA methylation associated with loss of function, indicating a more epigenetic genetic causes of cancer [12,36]. Since multiple molecular pathways may be involved during the process of hepatocarcinogenesis, simultaneous silencing of many genes by epigenetic mechanism may be a strong driving force for transformation.

Continuous inflammation from viral infection seems to induce hypermethylation in HCCs, and an association between the presence of viral protein and aberrant DNA methylation has been suggested [37,38,39,40,41,42]. Summary of hypermethylated genes that have been reported in the previous studies are shown in table 12-2.

Inactivation of the cyclin-dependent kinase inhibitor *p16/CDKN2A* or *p15/CDKN2B* by methylation leads to disruption of cell-cycle regulation and potentially provides a growth advantage to affected cells [43,44].

p14/ARF activates P53 through interactions with mouse double minute 2 (MDM2), and loss of P14/ARF negatively affects P53 function. Cadherin 1 (CDH1), which has a potent invasive suppressor role, is involved in mechanisms regulating cell-cell adhesions, mobility and proliferation of epithelial cells [45].

Inactivation by methylation has also been found in DNA repair gene, *O-6-methylguanine-DNA methyltransferase* (*MGMT*) [46]. Epigenetic silencing of *secreted frizzled-related protein* (*SFRP*), which act as soluble modulators of Wnt signaling, leads to deregulated activation of the Wnt-pathway that is associated with cancer [47]. By contrast, another type of DNA repair gene, human *MutL protein homolog 1* (*hMLH1*), appears to be rarely methylated in HCC [9,18,20,48], which is consistent with the low frequency of microsatellite instability in HCCs [10,49]. *Thrombospondin 1* (*THBS1*) that has been shown to play roles in platelet aggregation, angiogenesis, and tumorigenesis, seems not to be a silencing target of DNA methylation in HCC [9,48]. These results suggest that DNA methylation is not a random event, and that the targets of DNA methylation may be determined by a pre-programmed targeting mechanism.

Intriguingly, the frequency of DNA methylation in non-cancerous tissues varies between genes (table 12-2).

Some genes (e.g. *achaete-scute complex-like* (*ASCL*), *cyclin A1* (*CCNA1*), *cyclooxygenase-2* (*COX2*), *p16* etc.) show no or low frequency of methylation in non-cancerous tissues, while other genes (e.g. *MGMT*, *developing brain homeobox 1* (*DBX1*), *hypermethylated in cancer 1* (*HIC1*), etc.) demonstrate similar methylation frequency between non-cancerous and cancerous tissues. The findings of DNA methylation in some developmental genes argue for a dynamic and age dependent epigenetic changes in the genome of precancerous tissues, in which increasing DNA methylation may drive tumor formation.

In adjacent precancerous lesions, DNA methylation did not involve all genes uniformly, suggesting that methylation of each gene may contribute differently to the pathogenesis of HCC.

Table 12.2. Genes affected by promoter methylation in non-cancerous liver and HCCs

Genes	Methylation in Non-cancerous tissues (%)	Methylation in cancerous tissues (%)	References
ASCL	0	24	[50]
CCNA1	0	36	[20]
COX2	0	18-38	[18,48,51,52]
hMLH1	0	0	[9,18,20]
NS3TP2	0	30	[20]
P15	0	47	[53]
P16	0-33	16-80	[9,17,18,20,40,48,51,52,53,54,55]
P73	0	6	[53]
SOCS3	0	33	[56]
THBS1	0	0	[9]
TIMP3	0	13	[18]
CACNA1G	1	21	[48,52]
BMP6	3	27	[20]
DAPK	10	10	[18]
APC	13-30	53-91	[18,51,52,53]
RARb2	13	7-12	[53,54]
SFRP2	13	11-30	[52]
GSTP1	13-35	41-86	[18,40,51,52,53]
RIZ1	16	5-33	[52]
SFRP1	16	45	[20]
RUNX3	18	39-82	[52]
PRDM14	19	70	[20]
RASSF1A	0-76	67-93	[18,20,51,52,54]
SOCS1	0-69	60-67	[52,53,57]
MMP14	24	53	[20]
CDH1	7-64	13-64	[18,40,51,52,53,54,58,59]
CASP8	34	50	[52]
MGMT	41	22	[40]
DBX1	43	52	[20]
TP53I11	50	65	[20]
TNFRSF10C	52	70	[20]
PENK	57	62	[20]
GNA14	60	94	[20]
HIC1	64	86	[52]
SLC16A5	79	93	[20]
ER	81	62	[48,55]
CIDEA	96	86	[20]
TBX4	97	93	[20]
P14	0-74	6-35	[40,53]

12.4. Causes of DNA Methylation

How might the aberrant DNA methylation be induced in hepatocytes? Hepatitis B virus (HBV) is a DNA virus that can integrate into the host genome, altering the expression of endogenous genes and also leading to genomic instability [60,61]. Because the integrated viral DNA is known to alter the DNA methylation status in several adjacent cellular genes and DNA segments, this might partially explain the induction of DNA methylation in HBV infected cells [62,63,64]. Hepatitis B virus X (HBx) protein activates several signal transduction pathways that lead to the transcriptional regulation of a number of cancer-related genes [65,66,67]. The involvement of the HBx protein in epigenetic modifications during hepatocarcinogenesis has also been suggested [37,38,39,40,41,42,68]. Recent study showed that HBx expression increases DNMT activity by up-regulation of DNMT1, DNMT3A1 and DNMT3A2, and selectively promoted regional hypermethylation of specific tumor suppressor genes [39]. Hepatitis C virus (HCV) is a single-stranded RNA virus that may not directly integrate into the host genome. At least four of the HCV gene products (core, NS3, NS4B, and NS5A) interact with proteins in the host cells and exhibit oncogenic activity [69]. By contrast to HBV, the direct association between DNMTs and HCV gene products has been suggested by just a few studies [70].

It appears reasonable that HBV, in particular HBx protein could modulate the transcriptional activation of DNMTs to epigenetically silence the expression of some genes. Considering this interrelationship, HBV infection could be a powerful trigger for DNA methylation. However, comparison between HBV-related HCC and HCV-related HCC has shown that the frequency of aberrant DNA methylation was almost similar between the two [9,20,52,53]. It remains an open question as to whether HBx-mediated increases in DNMT activity leads to aberrant DNA methylation in tumor suppressor genes on a genome-wide scale, rather than in specific tumor suppressor genes.

DNA methylation analysis in autoimmune hepatitis and primary biliary cirrhosis showed no aberrant DNA methylation, while aberrant DNA methylation occurred in non-neoplastic liver cells from patients with hereditary hemochromatosis [17,71]. There is compelling evidence that patients with hemochromatosis have a 20- to 200-fold increased risk of developing HCCs, while patients with autoimmune hepatitis or primary biliary cirrhosis rarely develop HCC [72,73]. Long-standing severe iron overload is frequently associated with epigenetic defects (probably caused by oxidative stress reactions) characteristic of HCC. Several studies demonstrate that reactive oxygen species (ROS) promote DNA methylation [74,75,76,77]. This might be key to understanding the contributions of chronic inflammation to aberrant DNA methylation in the process of carcinogenesis, because both HBV and HCV may cause oxidative stress in infected cells [78,79]. The compensatory proliferation of surviving hepatocytes under inflammatory and oxidative stress conditions increases epigenetic alterations and the risk of malignant transformation. Nevertheless, these multiple mechanisms lead to the accumulation of aberrant DNA methylation that are possible early events preceding morphological alterations of malignant transformation.

12.5. Multistep Accumulation of DNA Methylation during Hepatocarcinogenesis

Studies in multiple types of cancers and corresponding normal tissues demonstrate the involvement of epigenetic alterations as a fundamental event of field cancerization in gastric cancers [13,14], colon cancers [80], esophageal cancers [15], and lung cancers [81]. With respect to HCCs, we reported the presence of field cancerization using 8 DNA methylation markers [9]. Another comprehensive study that examined 19 loci in paired cancerous and noncancerous tissues from HCC patients with HCV infection suggests that infection may accelerate the methylation process in a set of genes in the liver [52].

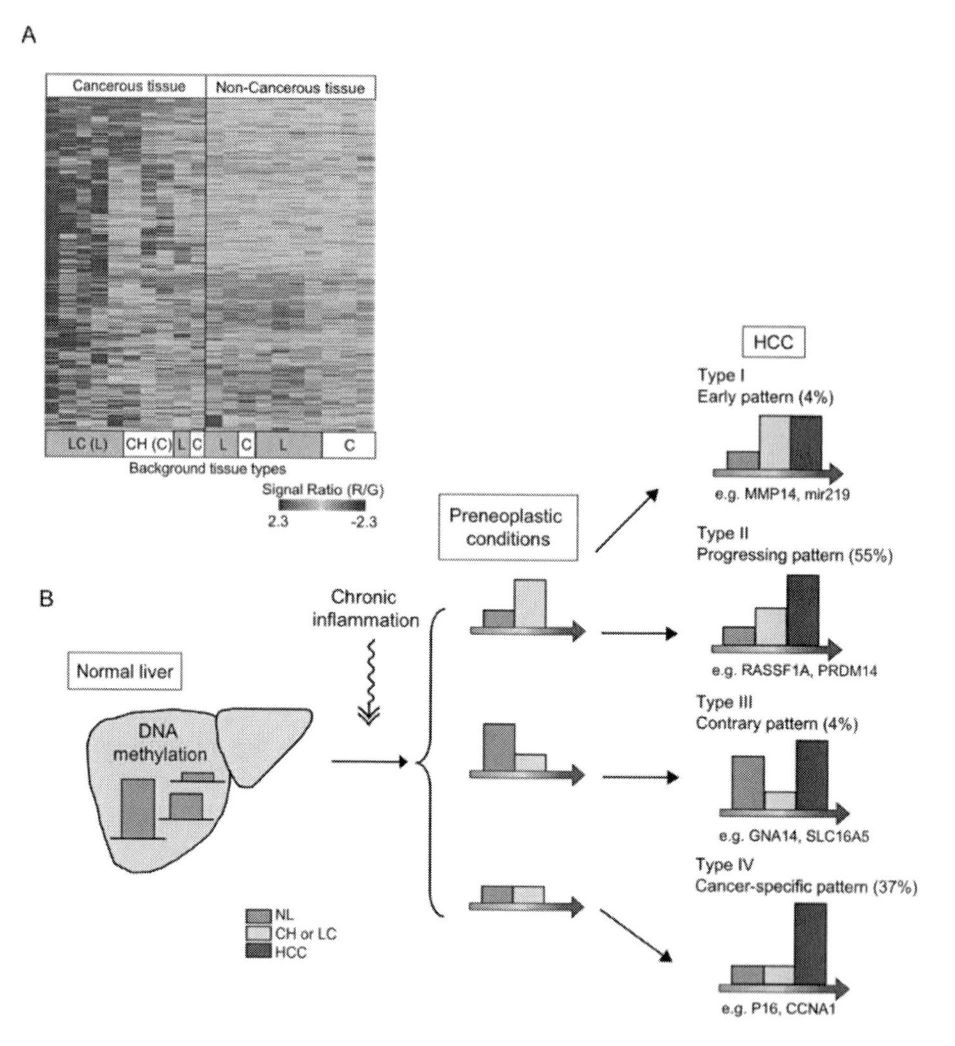

Figure 12.2. Global DNA methylation analysis in paired cancerous and adjacent precancerous tissues from HCC samples. A, Heat-map overview of hierarchical cluster analysis (unsupervised learning) of DNA methylation data in cancerous and adjacent tissues from HCCs. Each cell in the matrix represents the DNA methylation status of a gene in an individual sample. Red and blue in cells reflect high and low methylation level, respectively, as indicated in the scale bar below the matrix (left matrix; log2-transformed scale). Gray box and in white box indicate sample from liver cirrhosis (LC) patient and that from chronic hepatitis (CH) patient, respectively. B, Schema of DNA methylation changes observed in the process of HCC tumorigenesis. Most CGIss in normal liver tissue from young individuals are unmethylated except a subset of genes, which was methylated according to the age or tissue specifically. DNA methylation in some genes starts in the earliest phases of tumor progression and is established even in non-cancerous liver tissue (Type I), while that in the other genes might begin gradually (Type II) or emerge only in cancer (Type IV). Intriguingly, in some genes, the methylation level was decreased in CH or LC and was increased again in cancer (Type III). These distinct patterns of methylation likely represent different pathophysiologic processes. Pink colored box, yellow colored box and green colored box indicate methylation level in normal liver (NL), in chronic hepatitis (CH) or liver cirrhosis (LC) and cancer (HCC), respectively.

Deciphering the global epigenetic alterations in preneoplastic condition may be a key to determining the timing of events in malignant transformation of the liver, and to investigate the role of known risk factors for HCC. We therefore conducted global DNA methylation analysis using promoter microarray and classified the types of DNA methylation [20]. In examination of 6,458 CpG islands in cancerous and adjacent precancerous tissues, we found that DNA methylation did not occur uniformly in each gene, we were able to classify them into 4 characteristic types (figure 12-2).

The variations in the DNA methylation patterns may depend on the intrinsic susceptibility of each gene to *de novo* methylation [82] as a consequence of the specific mechanism mediating epigenetic changes in specific genes, and could reflect events that are selected during tumor progression [83].

Among them, DNA methylation in the gene groups (59%, type I and II) was observed in precancerous lesions, while some genes (37%, type IV) were specifically affected in progressed cancerous lesions (figure 12-2). These data suggest that a subset of cells that acquired DNA methylation in these promoters (type I and II genes) could be prone to cancer formation.

In contrast, type IV genes includes genes, which have been known for their key role in tumorigenesis, such as *CDKN2A* and *CCNA1*, suggesting that methylation of these genes is relevant to cancer and appears to be required for the establishment and progression of cancers. Methylation of these different types of genes was observed in a different stage of the disease, suggesting that susceptibility to DNA methylation of each gene is different or multiple mechanisms regulate the acquisition of epigenetic changes during hepatocarcinogenesis.

Conclusion

Several recent studies clearly indicate that liver cancer cells have global epigenetic changes, and that entire pathways relevant to cell renewal are subject to epigenetic dysregulation. Although treatments of chronic viral hepatitis have improved, there are still patients who do not respond favorably to these treatments. In addition, some patients may have "genetic/epigenetic scars" in their hepatocytes after successful treatments. Therefore, it is imperative to reevaluate the approaches to liver cancer prevention, detection, and therapy. Aberrant DNA methylation appears to be very early events in the process of tumorigenesis. This gives an important window to be exploited for therapeutic intervention through prevention strategies. As a risk marker of developing HCCs, assessment of DNA methylation in hepatitis or cirrhotic liver tissues is potential valuable clinical practice. Regarding the prevention of aberrant DNA methylation, antioxidants might be potent agents to use in chronic hepatitis. Research on the etiology and mechanisms of epigenetic changes, as well as discover and development of new agents to counteract these changes not only in HCC but also in many types of cancers is very important. Discoveries in such studies may provide new strategies for cancer treatments, and perhaps in future make it possible to reset epigenetic abnormalities and to control cancers.

References

[1] Thorgeirsson SS, Grisham JW (2002) Molecular pathogenesis of human hepatocellular carcinoma. *Nat. Genet.* 31: 339-346.

[2] Stickel F, Schuppan D, Hahn EG, Seitz HK (2002) Cocarcinogenic effects of alcohol in hepatocarcinogenesis. *Gut* 51: 132-139.

[3] Slaughter DP, Southwick HW, Smejkal W (1953) Field cancerization in oral stratified squamous epithelium; clinical implications of multicentric origin. *Cancer* 6: 963-968.

[4] Berasain C, Castillo J, Perugorria MJ, Latasa MU, Prieto J, et al. (2009) Inflammation and liver cancer: new molecular links. *Ann. N. Y. Acad. Sci.* 1155: 206-221.

[5] Lencioni R, Caramella D, Bartolozzi C, Di Coscio G (1994) Long-term follow-up study of adenomatous hyperplasia in liver cirrhosis. *Ital. J. Gastroenterol.* 26: 163-168.

[6] Feitelson MA, Sun B, Satiroglu Tufan NL, Liu J, Pan J, et al. (2002) Genetic mechanisms of hepatocarcinogenesis. *Oncogene* 21: 2593-2604.

[7] Murakami Y, Hayashi K, Hirohashi S, Sekiya T (1991) Aberrations of the tumor suppressor p53 and retinoblastoma genes in human hepatocellular carcinomas. *Cancer Res.* 51: 5520-5525.

[8] Kanai Y, Ushijima S, Tsuda H, Sakamoto M, Hirohashi S (2000) Aberrant DNA methylation precedes loss of heterozygosity on chromosome 16 in chronic hepatitis and liver cirrhosis. *Cancer Lett.* 148: 73-80.

[9] Kondo Y, Kanai Y, Sakamoto M, Mizokami M, Ueda R, et al. (2000) Genetic instability and aberrant DNA methylation in chronic hepatitis and cirrhosis--A comprehensive study of loss of heterozygosity and microsatellite instability at 39 loci and DNA hypermethylation on 8 CpG islands in microdissected specimens from patients with hepatocellular carcinoma. *Hepatology* 32: 970-979.

[10] Herath NI, Leggett BA, MacDonald GA (2006) Review of genetic and epigenetic alterations in hepatocarcinogenesis. *J. Gastroenterol. Hepatol.* 21: 15-21.

[11] Baylin SB, Herman JG, Graff JR, Vertino PM, Issa JP (1998) Alterations in DNA methylation: a fundamental aspect of neoplasia. *Adv. Cancer Res.* 72: 141-196.

[12] Jones PA, Baylin SB (2002) The fundamental role of epigenetic events in cancer. *Nat. Rev. Genet.* 3: 415-428.

[13] Maekita T, Nakazawa K, Mihara M, Nakajima T, Yanaoka K, et al. (2006) High levels of aberrant DNA methylation in Helicobacter pylori-infected gastric mucosae and its possible association with gastric cancer risk. *Clin. Cancer Res.* 12: 989-995.

[14] Nakajima T, Maekita T, Oda I, Gotoda T, Yamamoto S, et al. (2006) Higher methylation levels in gastric mucosae significantly correlate with higher risk of gastric cancers. *Cancer Epidemiol. Biomarkers Prev.* 15: 2317-2321.

[15] Eads CA, Lord RV, Kurumboor SK, Wickramasinghe K, Skinner ML, et al. (2000) Fields of aberrant CpG island hypermethylation in Barrett's esophagus and associated adenocarcinoma. *Cancer Res.* 60: 5021-5026.

[16] Kanai Y, Ushijima S, Tsuda H, Sakamoto M, Sugimura T, et al. (1996) Aberrant DNA methylation on chromosome 16 is an early event in hepatocarcinogenesis. *Jpn J. Cancer* Res 87: 1210-1217.

[17] Kaneto H, Sasaki S, Yamamoto H, Itoh F, Toyota M, et al. (2001) Detection of hypermethylation of the p16(INK4A) gene promoter in chronic hepatitis and cirrhosis associated with hepatitis B or C virus. *Gut* 48: 372-377.
[18] Lee S, Lee HJ, Kim JH, Lee HS, Jang JJ, et al. (2003) Aberrant CpG island hypermethylation along multistep hepatocarcinogenesis. *Am. J. Pathol.* 163: 1371-1378.
[19] Weber M, Davies JJ, Wittig D, Oakeley EJ, Haase M, et al. (2005) Chromosome-wide and promoter-specific analyses identify sites of differential DNA methylation in normal and transformed human cells. *Nat. Genet.* 37: 853-862.
[20] Gao W, Kondo Y, Shen L, Shimizu Y, Sano T, et al. (2008) Variable DNA methylation patterns associated with progression of disease in hepatocellular carcinomas. *Carcinogenesis* 29: 1901-1910.
[21] Jones PA, Baylin SB (2007) The epigenomics of cancer. *Cell* 128: 683-692.
[22] Bestor TH, Gundersen G, Kolsto AB, Prydz H (1992) CpG islands in mammalian gene promoters are inherently resistant to de novo methylation. *Genet. Anal. Tech. Appl.* 9: 48-53.
[23] Cross SH, Bird AP (1995) CpG islands and genes. *Curr. Opin. Genet. Dev.* 5: 309-314.
[24] Takai D, Jones PA (2002) Comprehensive analysis of CpG islands in human chromosomes 21 and 22. *Proc. Natl. Acad. Sci. USA* 99: 3740-3745.
[25] Weber M, Hellmann I, Stadler MB, Ramos L, Paabo S, et al. (2007) Distribution, silencing potential and evolutionary impact of promoter DNA methylation in the human genome. *Nat. Genet.* 39: 457-466.
[26] Illingworth R, Kerr A, Desousa D, Jorgensen H, Ellis P, et al. (2008) A novel CpG island set identifies tissue-specific methylation at developmental gene loci. *PLoS Biol.* 6: e22.
[27] Gardiner-Garden M, Frommer M (1987) CpG islands in vertebrate genomes. *J. Mol. Biol.* 196: 261-282.
[28] Kaneda A, Tsukamoto T, Takamura-Enya T, Watanabe N, Kaminishi M, et al. (2004) Frequent hypomethylation in multiple promoter CpG islands is associated with global hypomethylation, but not with frequent promoter hypermethylation. *Cancer Sci.* 95: 58-64.
[29] Okano M, Bell DW, Haber DA, Li E (1999) DNA methyltransferases Dnmt3a and Dnmt3b are essential for de novo methylation and mammalian development. *Cell* 99: 247-257.
[30] Eden A, Gaudet F, Waghmare A, Jaenisch R (2003) Chromosomal instability and tumors promoted by DNA hypomethylation. *Science* 300: 455.
[31] Cadieux B, Ching TT, VandenBerg SR, Costello JF (2006) Genome-wide hypomethylation in human glioblastomas associated with specific copy number alteration, methylenetetrahydrofolate reductase allele status, and increased proliferation. *Cancer Res.* 66: 8469-8476.
[32] Saito Y, Kanai Y, Sakamoto M, Saito H, Ishii H, et al. (2002) Overexpression of a splice variant of DNA methyltransferase 3b, DNMT3b4, associated with DNA hypomethylation on pericentromeric satellite regions during human hepatocarcinogenesis. *Proc. Natl. Acad. Sci. USA* 99: 10060-10065.

[33] Chan MF, van Amerongen R, Nijjar T, Cuppen E, Jones PA, et al. (2001) Reduced rates of gene loss, gene silencing, and gene mutation in Dnmt1-deficient embryonic stem cells. *Mol. Cell Biol.* 21: 7587-7600.

[34] De Smet C, Lurquin C, Lethe B, Martelange V, Boon T (1999) DNA methylation is the primary silencing mechanism for a set of germ line- and tumor-specific genes with a CpG-rich promoter. *Mol. Cell Biol.* 19: 7327-7335.

[35] Sakatani T, Kaneda A, Iacobuzio-Donahue CA, Carter MG, de Boom Witzel S, et al. (2005) Loss of imprinting of Igf2 alters intestinal maturation and tumorigenesis in mice. *Science* 307: 1976-1978.

[36] Ting AH, McGarvey KM, Baylin SB (2006) The cancer epigenome--components and functional correlates. *Genes. Dev.* 20: 3215-3231.

[37] Zhong S, Yeo W, Tang MW, Wong N, Lai PB, et al. (2003) Intensive hypermethylation of the CpG island of Ras association domain family 1A in hepatitis B virus-associated hepatocellular carcinomas. *Clin. Cancer Res.* 9: 3376-3382.

[38] Lee JO, Kwun HJ, Jung JK, Choi KH, Min DS, et al. (2005) Hepatitis B virus X protein represses E-cadherin expression via activation of DNA methyltransferase 1. *Oncogene* 24: 6617-6625.

[39] Park IY, Sohn BH, Yu E, Suh DJ, Chung YH, et al. (2007) Aberrant epigenetic modifications in hepatocarcinogenesis induced by hepatitis B virus X protein. *Gastroenterology* 132: 1476-1494.

[40] Su PF, Lee TC, Lin PJ, Lee PH, Jeng YM, et al. (2007) Differential DNA methylation associated with hepatitis B virus infection in hepatocellular carcinoma. *Int. J. Cancer* 121: 1257-1264.

[41] Zhu R, Li BZ, Li H, Ling YQ, Hu XQ, et al. (2007) Association of p16INK4A hypermethylation with hepatitis B virus X protein expression in the early stage of HBV-associated hepatocarcinogenesis. *Pathol. Int.* 57: 328-336.

[42] Jung JK, Arora P, Pagano JS, Jang KL (2007) Expression of DNA methyltransferase 1 is activated by hepatitis B virus X protein via a regulatory circuit involving the p16INK4a-cyclin D1-CDK 4/6-pRb-E2F1 pathway. *Cancer Res.* 67: 5771-5778.

[43] Herman JG, Merlo A, Mao L, Lapidus RG, Issa JP, et al. (1995) Inactivation of the CDKN2/p16/MTS1 gene is frequently associated with aberrant DNA methylation in all common human cancers. *Cancer Res.* 55: 4525-4530.

[44] Herman JG, Jen J, Merlo A, Baylin SB (1996) Hypermethylation-associated inactivation indicates a tumor suppressor role for p15INK4B. *Cancer Res* 56: 722-727.

[45] Oda T, Kanai Y, Oyama T, Yoshiura K, Shimoyama Y, et al. (1994) E-cadherin gene mutations in human gastric carcinoma cell lines. *Proc. Natl. Acad. Sci. USA* 91: 1858-1862.

[46] Costello JF, Futscher BW, Tano K, Graunke DM, Pieper RO (1994) Graded methylation in the promoter and body of the O6-methylguanine DNA methyltransferase (MGMT) gene correlates with MGMT expression in human glioma cells. *J. Biol. Chem.* 269: 17228-17237.

[47] Suzuki H, Watkins DN, Jair KW, Schuebel KE, Markowitz SD, et al. (2004) Epigenetic inactivation of SFRP genes allows constitutive WNT signaling in colorectal cancer. *Nat. Genet.* 36: 417-422.

[48] Shen L, Ahuja N, Shen Y, Habib NA, Toyota M, et al. (2002) DNA methylation and environmental exposures in human hepatocellular carcinoma. *J. Natl. Cancer Inst.* 94: 755-761.

[49] Kondo Y, Kanai Y, Sakamoto M, Mizokami M, Ueda R, et al. (1999) Microsatellite instability associated with hepatocarcinogenesis. *J. Hepatol.* 31: 529-536.

[50] Kubo T, Yamamoto J, Shikauchi Y, Niwa Y, Matsubara K, et al. (2004) Apoptotic speck protein-like, a highly homologous protein to apoptotic speck protein in the pyrin domain, is silenced by DNA methylation and induces apoptosis in human hepatocellular carcinoma. *Cancer Res.* 64: 5172-5177.

[51] Katoh H, Shibata T, Kokubu A, Ojima H, Fukayama M, et al. (2006) Epigenetic instability and chromosomal instability in hepatocellular carcinoma. *Am. J. Pathol.* 168: 1375-1384.

[52] Nishida N, Nagasaka T, Nishimura T, Ikai I, Boland CR, et al. (2008) Aberrant methylation of multiple tumor suppressor genes in aging liver, chronic hepatitis, and hepatocellular carcinoma. *Hepatology* 47: 908-918.

[53] Yang B, Guo M, Herman JG, Clark DP (2003) Aberrant promoter methylation profiles of tumor suppressor genes in hepatocellular carcinoma. *Am. J. Pathol.* 163: 1101-1107.

[54] Schagdarsurengin U, Wilkens L, Steinemann D, Flemming P, Kreipe HH, et al. (2003) Frequent epigenetic inactivation of the RASSF1A gene in hepatocellular carcinoma. *Oncogene* 22: 1866-1871.

[55] Kondo Y, Shen L, Suzuki S, Kurokawa T, Masuko K, et al. (2007) Alterations of DNA methylation and histone modifications contribute to gene silencing in hepatocellular carcinomas. *Hepatol. Res.* 37: 974-983.

[56] Niwa Y, Kanda H, Shikauchi Y, Saiura A, Matsubara K, et al. (2005) Methylation silencing of SOCS-3 promotes cell growth and migration by enhancing JAK/STAT and FAK signalings in human hepatocellular carcinoma. *Oncogene* 24: 6406-6417.

[57] Okochi O, Hibi K, Sakai M, Inoue S, Takeda S, et al. (2003) Methylation-mediated silencing of SOCS-1 gene in hepatocellular carcinoma derived from cirrhosis. *Clin Cancer Res.* 9: 5295-5298.

[58] Kanai Y, Ushijima S, Hui AM, Ochiai A, Tsuda H, et al. (1997) The E-cadherin gene is silenced by CpG methylation in human hepatocellular carcinomas. *Int. J. Cancer* 71: 355-359.

[59] Matsumura T, Makino R, Mitamura K (2001) Frequent down-regulation of E-cadherin by genetic and epigenetic changes in the malignant progression of hepatocellular carcinomas. *Clin. Cancer Res.* 7: 594-599.

[60] Edman JC, Gray P, Valenzuela P, Rall LB, Rutter WJ (1980) Integration of hepatitis B virus sequences and their expression in a human hepatoma cell. *Nature* 286: 535-538.

[61] Laurent-Puig P, Zucman-Rossi J (2006) Genetics of hepatocellular tumors. *Oncogene* 25: 3778-3786.

[62] Doerfler W (1995) The insertion of foreign DNA into mammalian genomes and its consequences: a concept in oncogenesis. *Adv. Cancer Res.* 66: 313-344.

[63] Heller H, Kammer C, Wilgenbus P, Doerfler W (1995) Chromosomal insertion of foreign (adenovirus type 12, plasmid, or bacteriophage lambda) DNA is associated with enhanced methylation of cellular DNA segments. *Proc. Natl. Acad. Sci. USA* 92: 5515-5519.

[64] Remus R, Kammer C, Heller H, Schmitz B, Schell G, et al. (1999) Insertion of foreign DNA into an established mammalian genome can alter the methylation of cellular DNA sequences. *J. Virol.* 73: 1010-1022.

[65] Kim CM, Koike K, Saito I, Miyamura T, Jay G (1991) HBx gene of hepatitis B virus induces liver cancer in transgenic mice. *Nature* 351: 317-320.

[66] Feitelson MA, Duan LX (1997) Hepatitis B virus X antigen in the pathogenesis of chronic infections and the development of hepatocellular carcinoma. *Am. J. Pathol.* 150: 1141-1157.

[67] Wang XW, Forrester K, Yeh H, Feitelson MA, Gu JR, et al. (1994) Hepatitis B virus X protein inhibits p53 sequence-specific DNA binding, transcriptional activity, and association with transcription factor ERCC3. *Proc. Natl. Acad. Sci. USA* 91: 2230-2234.

[68] Zheng DL, Zhang L, Cheng N, Xu X, Deng Q, et al. (2009) Epigenetic modification induced by hepatitis B virus X protein via interaction with de novo DNA methyltransferase DNMT3A. *J. Hepatol.* 50: 377-387.

[69] Levrero M (2006) Viral hepatitis and liver cancer: the case of hepatitis C. *Oncogene* 25: 3834-3847.

[70] Arora P, Kim EO, Jung JK, Jang KL (2008) Hepatitis C virus core protein downregulates E-cadherin expression via activation of DNA methyltransferase 1 and 3b. *Cancer Lett.* 261: 244-252.

[71] Lehmann U, Wingen LU, Brakensiek K, Wedemeyer H, Becker T, et al. (2007) Epigenetic defects of hepatocellular carcinoma are already found in non-neoplastic liver cells from patients with hereditary haemochromatosis. *Hum. Mol. Genet.* 16: 1335-1342.

[72] Niederau C, Fischer R, Sonnenberg A, Stremmel W, Trampisch HJ, et al. (1985) Survival and causes of death in cirrhotic and in noncirrhotic patients with primary hemochromatosis. *N. Engl. J. Med.* 313: 1256-1262.

[73] Elmberg M, Hultcrantz R, Ekbom A, Brandt L, Olsson S, et al. (2003) Cancer risk in patients with hereditary hemochromatosis and in their first-degree relatives. *Gastroenterology* 125: 1733-1741.

[74] Weitzman SA, Turk PW, Milkowski DH, Kozlowski K (1994) Free radical adducts induce alterations in DNA cytosine methylation. *Proc. Natl. Acad. Sci. USA* 91: 1261-1264.

[75] Romanenko A, Morell-Quadreny L, Lopez-Guerrero JA, Pellin A, Nepomnyaschy V, et al. (2002) P16INK4A and p15INK4B gene alteration associated with oxidative stress in renal cell carcinomas after the chernobyl accident (pilot study). *Diagn Mol. Pathol.* 11: 163-169.

[76] Belinsky SA, Snow SS, Nikula KJ, Finch GL, Tellez CS, et al. (2002) Aberrant CpG island methylation of the p16(INK4a) and estrogen receptor genes in rat lung tumors induced by particulate carcinogens. *Carcinogenesis* 23: 335-339.

[77] Lim SO, Gu JM, Kim MS, Kim HS, Park YN, et al. (2008) Epigenetic changes induced by reactive oxygen species in hepatocellular carcinoma: methylation of the E-cadherin promoter. *Gastroenterology* 135: 2128-2140, 2140 e2121-2128.

[78] Schwarz KB (1996) Oxidative stress during viral infection: a review. *Free Radic. Biol. Med.* 21: 641-649.

[79] Larrea E, Beloqui O, Munoz-Navas MA, Civeira MP, Prieto J (1998) Superoxide dismutase in patients with chronic hepatitis C virus infection. *Free Radic. Biol. Med.* 24: 1235-1241.

[80] Shen L, Kondo Y, Rosner GL, Xiao L, Hernandez NS, et al. (2005) MGMT promoter methylation and field defect in sporadic colorectal cancer. *J. Natl. Cancer Inst.* 97: 1330-1338.

[81] Guo M, House MG, Hooker C, Han Y, Heath E, et al. (2004) Promoter hypermethylation of resected bronchial margins: a field defect of changes? *Clin. Cancer Res.* 10: 5131-5136.

[82] Feltus FA, Lee EK, Costello JF, Plass C, Vertino PM (2003) Predicting aberrant CpG island methylation. *Proc. Natl. Acad. Sci. USA* 100: 12253-12258.

[83] Myöhänen SK, Baylin SB, Herman JG (1998) Hypermethylation can selectively silence individual p16ink4A alleles in neoplasia. *Cancer Res.* 58: 591-593.

In: Field Cancerization: Basic Science and Clinical Applications ISBN 978-1-61761-006-6
Editor: Gabriel D. Dakubo

Chapter 13

Molecular Genetic Alterations in Preneoplastic and Neoplastic Lesions of the Gallbladder

Juan C. Roa and Jonathan Castillo

13.1. Epidemiology of Gallbladder Cancer

Gallbladder cancer (GBC) represents 3% of malignant tumors worldwide and is the fifth most frequent malignant neoplasia of the digestive tract, after stomach, colon, rectal and esophageal cancers [1]. This neoplasia is not frequent in developed countries and is not included in the World Health Organization [2] and International Agency for Research on Cancer [3] databases. Gallbladder carcinoma affects women two to six times more than men, and it's incidence increases progressively with age in both sexes. It is most frequent in the seventh decade of life [4,5,6,7,8]. Susceptibility in native North and South American women, who also present an increased risk of cholelithiasis, may be explained by common ancestral origins, suggesting a genetic component may be responsible for the greater risk in Chilean [9]. High incidence rates of GBC have been detected in indigenous Chilean Mapuches (35/100,000), in women in Delhi, India (21.5/100,000), women in La Paz, Bolivia (15.5/100,000), women in South Karachi, Pakistan (13.8/100,000) and Quito, Ecuador (12.9/100,000)[5,6,7]. It is also relatively frequent in north of India, Korea, Japan and some Eastern European countries such as Slovakia, Poland, the Czech Republic and the former Yugoslavia. Gallbladder cancer is not frequent in North America, except for Indians of New Mexico (11.3/100,000) and female immigrants from Latin America, confirming a role for both genetic and environmental [8]. The incidence of gallbladder carcinoma also varies within a country. In India, for example, the incidence is very high in the north compared to the south; similar geographical variations can be found in Japan, where the highest incidence is observed in the north. Within countries, there are also variations in the incidence according to race and ethnic group. In the United States, there is a greater incidence in white people of both sexes than in the black population. The geographical zone and ethnic and cultural variations in the incidence of gallbladder carcinoma suggest that there is a considerable genetic and environmental influence on the development of the disease, which includes diet and lifestyle [5,10]. In Chile, it is the main cause of cancer death in women over age 40, with a mortality rate of 7 deaths per 100,000 in men and 15.6 deaths per 100,000 in women, and this pattern has remained constant over the last 18 years.

13.2. Etiology of Gallbladder Cancer

13.2.1. Cholelithiasis (Gallstones)

The most significant risk factor for GBC is cholelithiasis [5,11]. The link between cholelithiasis and GBC has been known since 1861 [12]. The theoretical foundation for this phenomenon is that inflammation, chronic trauma and infection that is inherent in approximately one-third of patients with gallstones promotes epithelial dysplasia and the progression to adenocarcinoma [13].

Lithiasis is the only element present in over 95% of chronic cholecystitis, and in 65-90% of patients with gallbladder carcinoma [11]. The study of stones in the gallbladder with cancer has shown that patients with a total stone volume higher than 10 ml have a relative risk of more than 11 times of developing cancer compared to patients whose stones have a volume lower than this number. Diehl also disclosed that in subjects with gallstones larger than three centimeters, the risk of GBC is ten times greater than in subjects with gallstones smaller than one centimeter [14]. The stones present in gallbladders with cancer attain larger sizes and volumes than those in gallbladders without cancer. This finding strongly suggests that stones precede the appearance of cancer, and that the volume attained in the vesicular lumen is greater in subjects with cancer [15]. Therefore, it has been suggested that larger stones have a greater impact on the risk of developing GBC, possibly reflected in the longer duration and intensity of the epithelial [11]. Cholesterol gallstones represent approximately 80 to 90 percent of all gallstones in the Western world. There is little information available as to whether pigment or cholesterol gallstones act as promoters in the development of GBC. It is however, known that some components of bile can be endogenous carcinogens [16,17,18].

One potential connection between genetic predisposition to stones and incidence of GBC has been suggested by studies on populations where there is a predominance of gallstones. In a study that included three ethnic groups (Mapuches, Chilean Hispanics and Maoris on Easter Island), it was concluded that lithogenic genes are very frequent among Chilean indigenous peoples and the Hispanic populations with the highest rates of GBC mortality [19]. These studies strongly support the thesis that genetic factors play an important role in some specific populations, contributing to lithogenic bile production [15]. Specific polymorphisms of apoproteins and plasma cholesterol ester transfer proteins seem to correlate with cholesterol cholelithiasis [20].

Although it is certain that a high percentage of cholelithiasis cases are associated with gallbladder carcinomas, close to 10-25% of patients with this disease have no cholelithiasis, and only a small proportion (1-3%) of patients with gallstones develop cancer. It is estimated that in Chile cholelithiasis is present in 47% of female adults [21]. Various studies have shown that of all the gallbladders operated on for cholelithiasis, between 3 and 4% present with GBC at different stages in [22,23]. For this reason, it has been suggested that cholecystectomy is the fundamental intervention for reducing GBC in high-risk areas [23,24].

13.2.2. Calcified Gallbladder or Porcelain Gallbladder

The term "porcelain gallbladder" refers to a fragile gallbladder with a bluish coloration as a result of excessive calcification of the organ wall. Porcelain gallbladder has been associated with carcinoma in 12.5 to 62% of patients. The extensive calcification can be detected by ultrasound examination [25].

13.2.3. Gallbladder Polyps

The presence of polyps is another predisposing factor for GBC. Recent evidence suggests that polyps larger than 10 millimeters in diameter have the potential to become malignant. If it is diagnosed in asymptomatic patients, even in the absence of gallstones, removal of the gallbladder is recommended. Small polyps (less than 10 millimeters in diameter) must be removed if they are producing symptoms or are associated with gallstones [10,26].

13.2.4. Anomalous Pancreaticobiliary Ductal Junction

An anomalous pancreaticobiliary ductal junction (APBDJ) is associated with the development of gallbladder carcinoma. This anomalous ductal junction is seen in close to 17% of patients with carcinoma, compared to less than 3% of patients with other hepatobiliary disorders. The APBDJ between the common bile duct and the pancreatic duct are not under sphincteric control when situated outside the duodenal wall. Therefore, the pancreatic juice can flow freely into the gallbladder, which causes bile stasis leading to precancerous changes in the gallbladder mucosa. Patients who have APBDJ with no dilatation of the bile duct develop gallbladder stasis. These patients have a higher incidence of gallbladder carcinoma than patients with dilatation of the bile duct. Patients who develop gallbladder carcinoma in association with APBDJ are generally young, have a low incidence of gallstones, and are more frequently Asians rather than Westerners [10,27].

13.2.5. Carcinogens

Carcinogens are probably involved in the development of GBC. Studies have shown that methylcholanthrene, o-aminoazotoluene and nitrosamines can produce gallbladder carcinoma in animal experiments [28]. Occupational exposure to chemical carcinogens in individuals who work in the rubber industry suggests these compounds may play a role in gallbladder carcinogenesis. In northern India, the use of mustard oil loaded with carcinogenic impurities has been proposed as an etiological factor for GBC. In addition, a high concentration of the products of free radical oxidation and secondary bile acids has been reported in patients with gallbladder carcinoma compared to a control group of patients with cholelithiasis [29,30]. In other analyses conducted on workers who handle cellulose acetate or who work in industries exposed to radon, a higher risk of suffering from GBC was also found [31,32].

13.2.6. Chronic Gallbladder Infection

During the last two decades, epidemiological evidence has linked chronic infections to several cancers; examples include hepatitis B and hepatitis C with liver cancer; *H. pylori* with gastric cancer; and Apolobothrium sp. with cholangiocarcinoma of the liver [33,34]. Although the participation of chronic bacterial infections like *Salmonella* [35,36,37] and *Helicobacter* [38,39] are implicated in gallbladder carcinogenesis, there are contradictory evidences. This association has been assumed particularly in countries like India, where typhoid fever is endemic [36]. With regards to *Helicobacter*, findings are not consistent and do not support a significant role with respect to the presence of this bacterium in gallbladder carcinogenesis [40,41].

13.2.7. Other Factors

Epidemiological studies have proven that there is a strong association between gallbladder carcinoma, obesity and [42]. Gallbladder adenomyomatosis segmentaria, chronic inflammation of the intestine and polyposis coli have also been linked to gallbladder carcinoma. Among others risk factors, a number of genetic, dietary, endo-and exobiotic factors have also been associated with familial adenomatous polyposis or Gardner's syndrome and with Peutz-Jeghers syndrome [43,44].

13.3. Pathogenesis of Gallbladder Cancer

13.3.1. Carcinogenic Pathways

In most epithelial tumors, particularly glandular tumors or adenocarcinomas, two models of malignant progression are proposed: The *metaplasia-dysplasia-carcinoma* and the *adenoma-carcinoma* sequences [45,46,47,48,49,50]. The first is based on alterations to the normal gallbladder epithelium, whereby metaplasia first appears as an adaptive process secondary to chronic irritation or inflammation. Dysplasia develops in the metaplastic epithelium, progresses to a carcinoma in situ and subsequently to invasive cancer [51,52,53]. The second pathway presents the malignant transformation process from an initially benign glandular tumor called adenoma [45,50]. Experimental and clinical evidences support both models; however, in specific organs both pathways are of distinct importance and connotation. The evolution and transformation of each one of these lesions to more aggressive forms requires different conditions and duration. Finally, the evidence at the genetic-molecular level also demonstrates that the two pathways correspond to two different biological events [54,55].

13.3.2. Metaplasia-Dysplasia-Carcinoma Sequence

In gallbladder carcinogenesis model, the initial lesions on the epithelium of the mucosa are attributable to inflammation. The formation of stones may be the primary initiating process. According to our observations, epithelial hyperplasia does not seem to be an important process in gallbladder carcinogenesis. Most of the mucosa adjacent to early tumors shows metaplasia and atrophies, not hyperplasia. Two types of metaplasia can be observed in the gallbladder mucosa, and these are comparable to those found in the stomach: the pyloric and intestinal type metaplasias [56]. Gallbladder cancers are most frequently associated with the pyloric type of metaplasia. In fact, at least 50% of GBCs present a "gastric" phenotype with pepsinogen I and II expression by tumor cells [57].

Epithelial dysplasia has been found adjacent to gallbladder carcinomas in situ [46,51,56]. In other organs, these frequently multiple lesions have been considered as precursors to GBC. Over 80% of infiltrative GBCs show foci of carcinoma in situ and epithelial dysplasia [58,59,60]. Initial morphological evidence and its molecular characterization support this transformation [61,62]. Practically all dysplasias are lesions that go undetected upon macroscopic examination. A study involving long series of early carcinomas did not reveal the presence of adenomatous lesions [63,64], providing strong evidence in support of the notion that gallbladder carcinogenesis occurs through the transformation of the normal epithelium and not through the transformation of a pre-existing benign tumor (adenoma). On the other hand, patients with dysplasia and carcinoma in situ are 15 and 5 years younger than those with invasive cancer, suggesting a progression from intraepithelial lesions to carcinoma. According to our observations, the period required to progress from dysplasia to advanced gallbladder carcinoma is ~15 years, because we observed a continuum in the progression of the lesions over such period (see figure 13-1, top) [46].

13.3.3. Adenoma-Carcinoma Sequence

Some investigators have demonstrated in the presence of adenomatous foci in carcinomas, as well as the presence of malignant foci in gallbladder adenomas. The malignant transformation of gallbladder adenomas, just as in the large intestine, would keep in proportion with the size of the adenoma. The adenoma-carcinoma carcinogenic sequence was suggested by Kozuka [45], who reviewed the histology of 1605 GBCs and found 11 benign adenomas, 7 adenomas with signs of malignancy and 79 adenomas with invasive carcinomas. His theory was also supported by the following observations:

- The Presence of histological transition from adenoma to carcinoma,
- The Association of adenomatous components with the carcinoma in situ, and in 19% with invasive cancer,
- The Close relation between the size of the lesion and the malignant change; all the benign adenomas were less than 12mm in diameter and all the adenomas with signs of malignancy were larger than 12mm; the invasive carcinomas were more than 30mm in diameter;

- The Progression of age in relation to the diagnosis: 50 years for benign adenomas, 58 years for the adenomas with malignant changes and 64 for the invasive carcinoma.

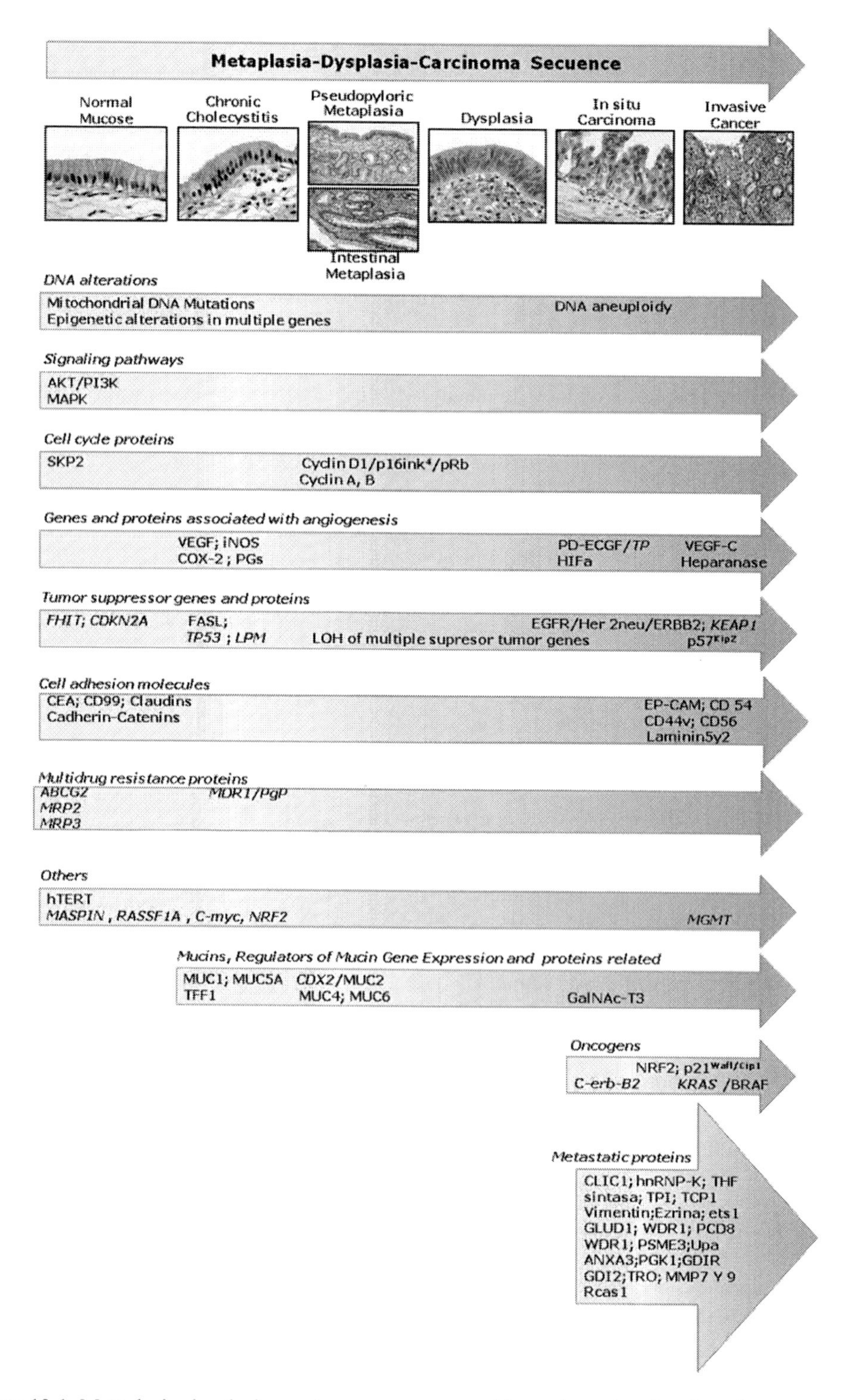

Figure 13.1. Metaplasia-dysplasia-carcinoma sequence and its main molecular alterations.

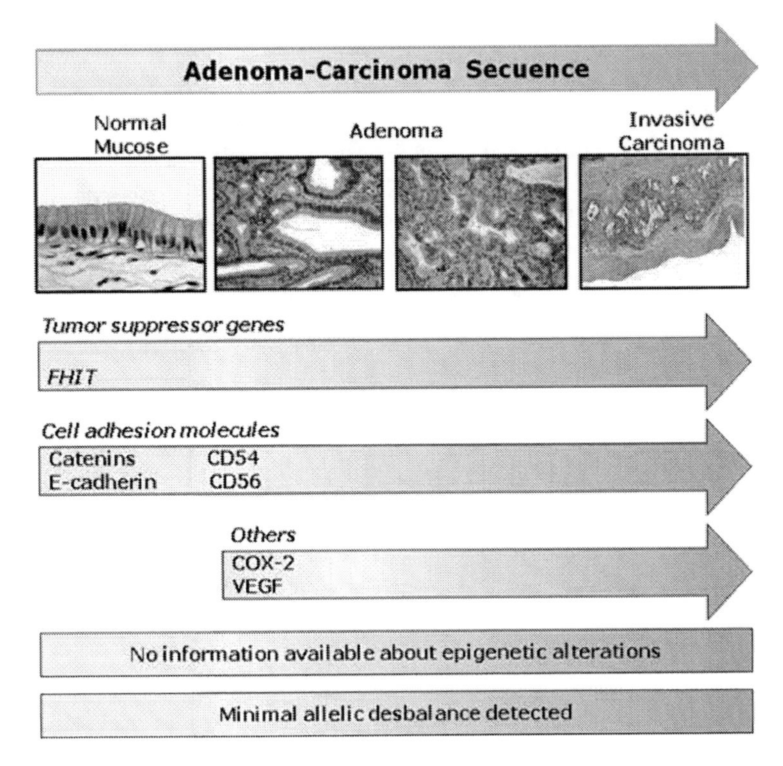

Figure 13.2. Adenoma-Carcinoma sequence and its main molecular alterations.

This phenomenon can also be seen in other malignant gastrointestinal tumors, such as colorectal cancer, where adenomatous residue is observed in up to 32% of cases, and in ampullary cancer, where an adenomatous component can be seen in up to 90% of cases (see figure 13-2).

13.4. Infiltration of Immune Cells in Gallbladder Cancer

In GBC, lymph node metastasis and deep invasion of the primary tumor significantly affect patients who undergo surgery [65]. A strong correlation between these pathological factors and the number of infiltrating cells suggests that the anti-tumor immune response can influence the prognosis of patients with GBC. It was determined that large infiltrations of TCD4+, CD8+ and DC cells are in themselves favorable [66]. Tumor-associated antigens (TAA) can be recognized by T CD8+ cells in the context of tumors expressing MHC class I [67]. The total immune responses, however, were very weak and transients to eradicate carcinogenic cells in the majority of the patients receiving immunization; therefore, analysis of growth has focused on the value of T CD4+[68,69] and [70] in anti-tumor immunity. There is a correlation between DC infiltration and lymph node metastasis in GBC. In addition, an important correlation was observed between CD4+ and CD8+ T cells and CD4+ T cells and DCs [66]. Compared to benign diseases, high levels of infiltration of CD4+, CD8+ T cells and DCs were observed in cancer specimens. These results provide evidence that these immune cells possess specific activities in GBC. NKCs were frequently identified in cancer specimens and not in benign diseases; NKCs may have the ability to recognize cancerous cells. NKC infiltration, however, does not correlate with tumor progression or prognosis in this study. NKCs constitute only a small portion of lymphocytes [71] and are a component of the innate immune system, able to kill white cells without previous [70]. Thus, the incapacity of NKCs to influence the outcome of the disease may depend on the low proportion of the total cells and their weak anti-cancer specificity. Nakakubo et al. [66] concludes that the prognoses associated with the infiltration of T cells are not always good; infiltration of T cells CD4+, CD8+ and the infiltration of DC more than NKCs are correlated with tumor progression, serving as a good prognostic predictor in patients with gallbladder adenocarcinomas.

13.5. Genetic Alterations in Gallbladder Cancer

DNA Ploidy

Yamamoto et al. [72] observed that the incidence of aneuploidy in the DNA of GBC cells was 46.3%, and the diploidy patterns were 53.7%. No correlation was observed between DNA ploidy patterns and histological type of cancer. Sato et al. [73] demonstrated that 36% of GBC samples were diploid and 64% were aneuploid. Histological subtypes were not associated with nuclear DNA content except for specimens of poorly differentiated adenocarcinomas, which were all aneuploid. Mitotic indices of aneuploid tumors were higher than those of diploid cancers even in those cancers with the same histological subtype or the same level of invasiveness. There was, therefore, a significant correlation between nuclear DNA content and mitotic index. The patients who had diploidy patterns survived significantly longer than those with aneuploidy or high mitotic indices. Roa et al found that aneuploidy is a condition present in around 26% to 30% of subserosal gallbladder carcinomas and 80% of GBC [74,75]. This finding shows that there are differences in the neoplastic cells of tumors confined to the gallbladder and those at metastatic sites. The lack of association of ploidy with clinical and morphological variables (such as degree of differentiation, compromised blood vessels and nerves, as well as patient survival) raises the possibility that the alteration in DNA content in subserosal gallbladder carcinoma corresponds to an epiphenomenon rather than to a primary alteration. On the other hand, it was determined that aneuploidy is not related to any clinical or morphological variables in the series of patients analyzed (figures 13-1 and 13-2).

Mitochondrial DNA Mutations

Wistuba and coworkers [76] demonstrated that at the regulatory region or displacement loop specifically in the nucleotide 310 (D310) mutations were relatively frequent abnormality (47 of 123; 38%) in GBC. A very high frequency of mutations was detected in gallbladder dysplasia (8 of 14; 57%) and an apparently normal gallbladder epithelium (10 of 22; 46%) accompanying GBC, showing a clonal relationship compared to the corresponding tumor. Mutations (D-loop D310) were also detected in dysplasia (8 of 39; 21%) and normal epithelium (17 of 68; 25%) obtained from cholecystitis. A unique case of 15 normal gallbladders showed abnormality of D310. Altogether, deletions (67 of 91; 74%) in D310 were more frequent than insertions. The authors concluded that D310 mutations in the mtDNA displacement loop are relatively frequent and early events in the sequential pathogenesis of GBC, being detected in apparently normal epithelia from chronic cholecystitis (see figures 13-1 and 13-2).

Inducible Nitric Oxide Synthase

Zhang et al. [77] determined that the degree of iNOS expression in benign and malignant gallbladder diseases was 87.5% in cholecystitis, 100% in cholecystitis with adenomyoma and a 70.8% in adenocarcinoma. This study indicated that iNOS expression was not related to benign and malignant phases of gallbladder. It is suggested from this study that NO has a biphasic effect on the development of gallbladder tumor. The excessive NO induced by iNOS was a significant tumor-inducing factor in chronic cholecystitis and cholecystitis with adenomyoma. Furthermore, NO has an antitumor effect: low iNOS expression in gallbladder adenocarcinomas has been associated with early metastasis and poor prognosis (figures 13-1 and 13-2).

Loss of Heterozygosity and Microsatellite Instability

In a larger series of cases (59 samples) conducted in our laboratory [78], an MSI incidence of 10.1% was found in GBC, which is slightly less frequent than the incidence in colon and gastric cancers. Instability was found in 33% of intestinal metaplasias and 83% of dysplastic areas were associated with MSI-H tumors. In over 90% of cases, the pattern found in these preneoplastic lesions matched the one found in the normal tissue adjacent to the tumor, suggesting that MSI may be significant in the initial stages of gallbladder carcinogenesis. In general terms, it is accepted that although MSI is present from the initial stages of the gallbladder carcinogenic process, this is limited to a restricted sub-group of patients. Nevertheless, results obtained in our laboratory have shown that microsatellite alterations do not occur in inflammatory lesions (see figures 13-1 and 13-2) [78,79,80].

Human Telomerase Reverse Transcriptase (hTERT)

Luzar et al. [81] established the immunohistochemical expression of hTERT in GBC. The results indicated that nuclear signals increased progressively with the degree of abnormality in the gallbladder epithelium. The immunoreactivity was 3% in a normal epithelium, 4% in regenerative epithelium, 25% in low-grade dysplasia, 82% in high-grade dysplasia, and 93% in adenocarcinomas. Hansel et al. [82] identified telomere shortening in metaplastic (63%) and dysplastic (90%) gallbladder epithelium, and intrahepatic and extrahepatic bile duct adenocarcinoma infiltrations (98%). They showed therefore the reduction in the size of the telomeres in preneoplastic and neoplastic lesions in the gallbladder, specifically in gallbladder metaplasia and dysplasia as well as in invasive carcinoma of the biliary tract. This telomere shortening seems to be specific to cells involved in neoplastic transition and progression more than in cells involved in regenerative or reactive processes. Therefore, the authors concluded that the shortening of telomeres is an early and consistent finding in the development of biliary tract carcinoma (see figures 13-1 and 13-2).

DNA Repair System

In a series of gallbladder carcinoma samples analyzed, Kohya et al. [80] observed negative MGMT immunostaining in 59.0% and 60.0% of specimens with gallbladder and extrahepatic biliary duct carcinomas. In gallbladder carcinoma, negative staining for hMLH1 and hMSH2 were observed in 51.3% and 59.0% respectively, whereas in the extrahepatic bile duct carcinoma, the respective values were 57.1% and 65.7%. Negative MGMT staining was correlated with hepatic invasion in gallbladder carcinoma and with poor prognosis in both gallbladder and extrahepatic biliary duct carcinomas. Moreover, a combined status of MGMT and MMR were shown to be more significant biomarkers of prognosis in both types of tumors, which is why the authors concluded that MGMT and MMR are prognostic markers that probably reflect the accumulation of genetic mutations (see figures 13-1 and 13-2).

Epidermal Growth Factor Receptor and erbb2

Overexpression of epidermal growth factor receptor (EGFR, HER-1) occurs in 12.4%-100% of GBCs [83,84,85,86]. These results are complemented by several studies done in Asia, Europe, Australia and the United States, where EGFR expression has been examined in GBC and all of these obtained similar results, where the increased frequency of expression is linked to increased incidence of malignancy and, furthermore, the increase in expression is related to a decrease in life expectancy [87]. Ooi et al. [88] revealed that genomic instability due to amplification of Myc could cause the specific amplification of EGFR and/or ERBB2 in GBC. In another study, 63.6% of gallbladder adenocarcinomas showed overexpression of ErbB-2 proteins [89]. Yukawa et al. [90] reported expression of ErbB-2 protein in 69% of GBC, yet expression of ErbB-2 protein was undetectable in more advanced tumors. These data suggest that amplification of *ErbB-2* and/or overexpression may be involved in the development of GBC (see figures 13-1 and 13-2).

Ras

Gallbladder carcinomas associated with anomalous pancreaticobiliary muljunction are most frequently associated with K-ras mutation, suggesting the reflux of pancreatic juice constitutes a risk factor for developing GBC [91,92]. Results obtained by our laboratory indicate that approximately half of pancreatic-biliary tumors have mutation at codon 12 of the K-ras gene (46.4%). The mutation frequency was dependent upon the type of tumor ($p < 0.05$), being present in 29% of gallbladder adenocarcinomas, 56% and 50% of pancreatic and biliary tract carcinomas respectively, and in 80% of the ampulla of [93] (see figures 13-1 and 13-2).

B-raf

Saeta et al. showed that mutations in exon 15 of *B-raf* were observed in 33% of gallbladder carcinomas examined, [94]. It is possible to hypothesize that the activation at several levels of the RAS/RAF/MEK/ERK pathway may constitute an event secondary to Ras activation or that it may be due to the activation of points still not studied in gallbladder carcinogenesis. Future studies are necessary to determine conclusively whether the MAP kinase RAS/RAF/MEK/ERK signaling pathway could have an important role in the pathogenesis of GBC, although Saeta et al. have indicated that the disruption of this pathway occurs in around 65% of gallbladder carcinomas, and could therefore be considered one of the most common defects in the pathogenesis of this disease [95] (See figures 13-1 and 13-2).

ERK 1/2 and PI3K Signaling Pathway

Li et al. [96] examined the immunohistochemical expression of p-ERK1/2 and PI3-K in 108 samples of GBC. A strong positive stain was established for p-ERK1/2 and PI3-K at 58.3% and 50.9%, respectively, indicating that both p-ERK1/2 and PI3-K/AKT could be potential markers in GBC. Compared with benign lesions and peritumoral tissues, positive staining for p-ERK1/2 and PI3-K in gallbladder adenocarcinoma was significantly higher. The expression of p-ERK1/2 and PI3-K was correlated with a low degree of differentiation in adenocarcinoma. Additionally, p-ERK1/2 and PI3-K staining was more frequently detected in gallbladder adenocarcinomas with a larger tumor size, lymph node metastasis and invasion of the surrounding tissue compared with cases with a small tumor size and no metastasis or tissue invasion. These findings suggest that the activation of the p-ERK1/2 and PI3-K/AKT signaling pathways could be involved in malignant process and the progression of gallbladder adenocarcinoma (see figures 13-1 and 13-2).

RASSF1

Kee et al. [97] examined the methylation and protein expression of RASSF1A, and the correlation between these with the clinicopathological characteristics of GBC in 30 Korea patients. The results showed that there was a relatively moderate frequency of aberrant hypermethylation of *RASSF1A* in gallbladder carcinoma and adenoma, whereas methylation was rarely detected in histologically normal gallbladder tissues. They also revealed that the CpG islands of the promoter region in exon 1 of *RASSF1A* are hypermethylated in GBC and repress *RASSF1A* expression. In addition, three GBC cell lines expressing *RASSF1A* contained non-methylated promoter regions and exon 1. Although Kee et al studied a small number of tumor samples, the results they obtained suggest that deregulation of *RASSF1A* expression by DNA hypermethylation could be involved in gallbladder carcinogenesis and that hypermethylation of *RASSF1A* could provide a reliable marker for GBC (see figures 13-1 and 13-3).

Mucopolysaccharides 1,2,4,5A and 6

Among the determinations of mucopolysaccharide expression in the gallbladder, the expression of MUC1, MUC2, MUC4, MUC5A and MUC6 has been observed. It was verified that MUC1 expression was significantly higher in cancerous tissue than in normal tissue or with cholecystitis. It has been demonstrated that MUC1 expression is related to GBC progression and lymphatic invasion [98]. MUC2 was rarely expressed in gallbladder carcinoma and its immunoreactivity was detected in goblet cell cancer [99] study showed that MUC2 was expressed focally in non-dysplastic as well as dysplastic tissue, and was only more frequent in well-differentiated gallbladder adenocarcinoma. Positive MUC2 cells resembled goblet cells in non-dysplastic epithelium, dysplasia or carcinoma, and MUC2 expression is also related to low proliferative activity and reflects differentiation towards goblet [100]. Determinations have been made of MUC4 expression in GBC. It was established that the levels of MUC4 expression and messenger RNA were increased in GBC specimens. Immunoprecipitation experiments showed an interaction between MUC4 and ERBB2. This interaction was associated with ERBB2, MAPK and AKT hyperphosphorylation. MUC4 was detected in the apical surface of cancerous epithelium and it partially co-localized with ERBB2. Transfection studies also showed that MUC4 amplifies cell proliferation in the presence of heregulin by harnessing the phosphorylation of ERBB2 and its downstream signaling pathway [101]. Finally, it was shown that in preneoplastic lesions of the gallbladder, inflammation was dependent upon signaling pathways induced by EGFR overproducing MUC5AC, a gel-forming mucin that accumulates in cholecystitis produced by cholesterol stones [102]. Moreover, Sasaki et al. [103] determined that MUC6 expression was very frequent in pseudopyloric metaplasia just as in dysplasia and carcinoma (see figures 13-1 and 13-3).

CDX2

It has been reported that CDX2 is bound directly to *MUC2* promoter, and therefore regulates *MUC2* expression [100]. Wu et al. [104] observed *CDX2* and *MUC2* expression in intestinal metaplasia in the gallbladder, suggesting this preneoplastic lesion may be a premalignant condition not only in gastric carcinoma but also in gallbladder carcinoma. They speculated that the transcriptional control of *CDX2* may be changed by abnormal stimulation by inflammation and/or regeneration and consequently *CDX2* is induced following intestinal differentiation of gallbladder cells. Clinically this is important for future analyses of intestinal metaplasia as a premalignant condition in gallbladder carcinogenesis where *CDX2* may be a key factor in carcinogenesis with intestinal differentiation (see figures 13-1 and 13-3).

UDP-N-Acetyl-a-D-Galactosamine

Nomoto et al. [105] performed a retrospective analysis, where they determined the immunohistochemical expression of GalNAc-T3 in gallbladder carcinomas at different depths of invasion (pT1-pT4). In 34 cases of pT2 carcinoma, there was a correlation between the immunohistochemical location of GalNAc-T3 and the depth of invasion in the subserosal layer of the pT2 carcinoma. The results obtained by this group suggest that an increase in the expression levels of GalNAc-T3 in the subserosal layer of pT2 GBC cases is correlated with the aggressiveness of the disease. This phenotype may serve as a biological characteristic associated with malignant behavior, and may help early identification of those patients who need more aggressive treatments. It might be possible to determine that GalNAc-T3 expression is an independent prognostic factor in pT2 carcinomas (see figures 13-1 and 13-3).

Trefoil Factor Family Protein 1

Kornprat et al. [106] showed that the TFF1 protein is not present in healthy gallbladder mucosa, but present and upregulated in the inflamed gallbladder epithelium and expressed in large amounts in both primary and metastatic GBC. Trefoil factor family protein 1 expression in primary tumors decreased as the tumor stage and grade increased. Furthermore, patients with TFF1-positive tumors showed a more favorable outcome compared to TFF1-negative tumors in univariate analyses. It is also suggested that TFF1 may play a role in the relation between gallstones, chronic cholecystitis and GBC (see figures 13-1 and 13-3).

Skp2

Sanada et al. concluded that the overexpression of Skp2 is a poor independent prognostic factor in a small series of cancers of the biliary tract, where samples of gallbladder carcinoma were included. Skp2 levels increased in association with the number of the Skp2 genes on chromosome 5p11-13. This amplification was observed in 53% of the cases studied [107].

Li et al. [108] also determined that the overexpression of Skp2 was significantly correlated with vascular invasion, advanced T-stage, high histological grade and range of proliferation, indicating its importance in the progression of the disease and the inherent biological aggressiveness of gallbladder carcinoma. They determined that in gallbladder carcinoma it is not uncommon for there to be protein aberration within the proteolytic pathway associated with Skp2/p27Kip1. The overexpression of Skp2 is an independent indication of poor prognosis, and is associated with intrinsic biological aggressiveness in gallbladder carcinoma.

Cyclin E

Li et al. [108] also found that overexpression of cyclin E was detected more in women, and in gallbladder carcinomas with vascular invasion, tumor necrosis, high histological grade and range of proliferation. In addition, the overexpression of cyclin E was also predictive of patient survival as determined by univariate analyses (see figures 13-1 and 13-3).

Cyclin D1/p16/Rb Pathway

Using immunohistochemical methods, Ma et al. [109] analyzed the expression of cyclin D1, p16 and Rb pathway in gallbladder carcinomas, adenomas and cholecystitis. Disruption of the cyclin D1/p16[INK4]-pRb pathway plays an important role in the progression of gallbladder carcinoma. Loss or reduction in p16 and pRb expression has an obvious correlation with the malignant grade and gallbladder metastasis. Overexpression of cyclin D1 is an early event in gallbladder carcinogenesis. Mutations of p16 and Rb genes could be correlated with the progression of gallbladder carcinoma. Analyses of p16 and Rb can estimate the prognosis of gallbladder carcinoma and the expression of both may be correlated with the Nevin stage and the pathological grade in gallbladder carcinoma (see figures 13-1 and 13-3)

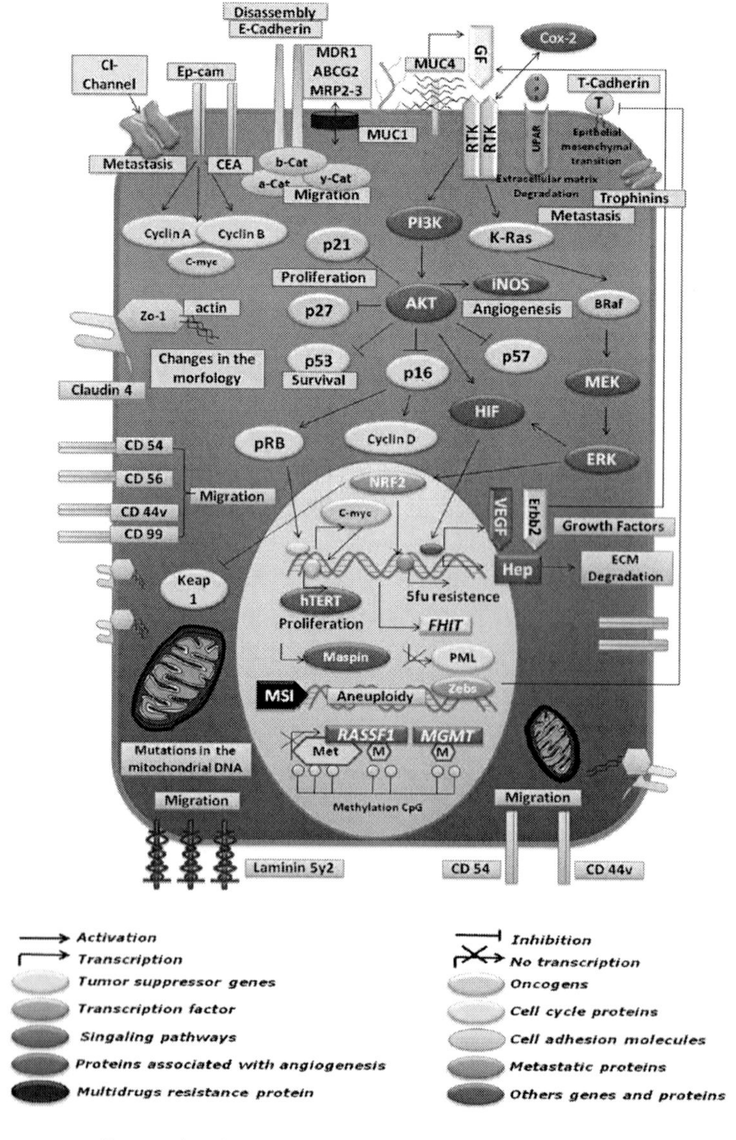

Figure 13.2. Summary of key molecular aspects involved in gallbladder cancer.

Prostaglandin and Cyclooxygenase

Legan et al. [110] reported that COX-2 plays an important role in gallbladder carcinogenesis and that its overexpression seems to be an early event, occurring at preneoplastic stages of epithelial changes (for example high-grade dysplasia) and, perhaps, its overexpression could be related to the dysfunction of p53. The observation of Legan et al. supports the fact that high overexpression of COX-2 in high-grade dysplasia is related to the hypothesis of the role of COX-2 in early carcinogenesis. Zhi et al. [111] found that some pathological variables such as Nevin stage and metastasis had a significant correlation with the high expression of COX-2 in GBC. In addition, their studies showed that the intensity of COX-2 expression correlated with lymph node metastasis. Moreover, prostaglandin (PGE2) produced by carcinoma cells expressing COX-2 and stromal cells could also be playing an important role in tumor growth and progression. This is because PGE2 can stimulate cancer cell proliferation through induction and phosphorylation of the Akt PI3-kinase pathways [112,113] or through the expression of insulin-like growth factor-I reception via PI3/Akt[114]. Another report suggests PGE2 could be related to the MAP kinase cell proliferation pathway [115] (see figures 13-1 and 13-2).

Vascular Endothelial Growth Factor

Quan et al. [116] determined that VEGF expression is directly related to the Nevin stage in gallbladder tumors, which means that as the degree of tumor invasion increases, the greater the vascularity produced by the tumor.

Tian et al. [117] examined the expression of p53 and VEGF as well as the amount of microvascular cells (MVC) in gallbladder carcinoma. Their findings suggest that tumor angiogenesis induced by VEGF plays an important role not only in tumor progression but also metastasis. In order to investigate the relation between the expression of vascular endothelial growth factor (VEGF) and C-myc with the development and metastasis of gallbladder carcinoma, Liu et al. [118] showed that the positive ranges of VEGF and C-myc in tissues with gallbladder carcinoma were 80% and 63.3% respectively, and 45% and 25% respectively in normal gallbladder tissue. The positive ranges of VEGF and C-myc were significantly higher in gallbladder carcinoma than in normal tissue. They determined that VEGF and C-myc expression in gallbladder carcinoma is related to metastasis (see figures 14-1 and 14-2).

Platelet-Derived Endothelial Cell Growth Factor and Thymidine Phosphorylase

Yamamoto et al. [119] showed that PD-ECGF/TP is expressed in carcinoma and infiltrating cells and its levels of were associated with advanced disease. They also showed that VEGF and *TP* were isolated as growth factors, but their actions were different; they noticed that VEGF acted in endothelial cells to increase microvascular permeability.

As was reported by other authors [120,121], *TP* does not induce angiogenesis by directly stimulating endothelial cell proliferation; it stimulates chemotaxis of endothelial cells in vitro and causes angiogenic activity in vivo. These different actions of VEGF and *TP* can be explained because there was no correlation between the expression of the *TP* gene and VEGF in this study. In conclusion the gene expression of *TP* in gallbladder carcinoma is associated with angiogenesis and this expression may be an independent prognostic factor (see figures 13-1 and 13-2).

Hypoxia-Inducible Factors

Hypoxic conditions within tumors should lead to a stabilization of HIFa in cancer cells, leading to increased VEGF expression. Hypoxia may be, therefore, the biggest cause of VEGF regulation and increased tumor angiogenicity. Giatromanolaki et al. [122] determined that HIF-1a and HIF-2a were independently related to VEGF overexpression and high microvascular density in GBC. It is of interest that HIF-2a was also related to high TP expression. Whether HIF-2 is also up-regulated under such conditions is unknown (see figures 13-1 and 13-2).

Heparanase

In a study reported by Wu et al. [123], it was established that the presence of heparanase was associated with tumor size, frequency of tumor invasion and poor survival in patients with GBC. They showed that large tumor sizes and lymph node metastasis were often more positive for heparanase than small cases with no metastasis. Wu et al. provide the first evidence in humans that heparanase expression is associated with larger tumor sizes and lymph node metastasis (see figures 13-1 and 13-2).

Fas and Fas Ligand Mechanisms of Action in Immune Escape

Xu et al. [124] determined the levels of FasL expression in gallbladder carcinoma chronic cholecystitis. Expectedly, the levels were significantly higher in gallbladder cancer than in chronic cholecystitis.

The apoptosis index of infiltrating lymphocytes in well-differentiated carcinoma was significantly lower than in poorly differentiated carcinoma. These results indicate that FasL protein expression in malignant gallbladder tissue is significantly higher than in normal tissue, and the amounts of apoptotic lymphocytes in malignant tissue are significantly higher than in normal tissue.

Over-regulation of FasL expression allows the tumor cell to escape the body's immune monitoring by inducing infiltrating lymphocyte apoptosis in gallbladder carcinoma tissues. In our study, the effect of Fas on immune escape was not confirmed. Up-regulation of FasL expression plays an important role in the invasiveness, histological classification and metastasis of gallbladder carcinoma (see figures 13-1 and 13-2).

Flip and Trail

Zhong et al. [125] showed that c-FLIP is over-expressed in 26 of the 35 gallbladder carcinomas studied and was not expressed in normal or adenomatous tissues. Small interfering RNA (siRNA) application substantially deregulated the levels of c-FLIP mRNA expression and produced significant apoptosis in gallbladder carcinoma cells (GBC-SD and SGC-996) in a TRAIL-dependent fashion. Also observed was the increase in picnosis, caspase-3/7 activity and chromatin condensation. Thus the mediated deregulation of c-FLIP by siRNA mediated the sensitivity for TRAIL-induced apoptosis. In conclusion, the expression of c-FLIP is up-regulated in gallbladder carcinoma and the deregulation of c-FLIP sensitizes TRAIL-induced apoptosis. The present study provides a powerful strategy for the treatment of gallbladder carcinoma by blocking c-FLIP (see figure 13-1)

CDKN2A (p16)

In thirty eight of our cases, we observed p16 inactivation in 41%, whether by LOH (11%) or methylation (24%) [126]. Other studies show the protein loss from p16/^{INK4} in 75% of GBCs associated with an overexpression of the retinoblastoma gene [127]. A greater immunostaining was found in normal epithelial tissue of GBC (50-90% of cells), decreasing in dysplasia-adenoma (over 50%) and carcinoma (10-50%) [128]. Inactivation of the p16 gene is associated with a poor prognosis in GBCs as well as its frequent association with mutation of the K-ras gene [116,127] (see figures 13-1 and 13-2).

P53

The loss of heterozygosity (LOH) from the alleles of TP53 has been proven in GBC in 92% of cases, and in the same study, LOH preceded the immunohistochemical expression of the protein produced by this gene [129]. Quan et al. [116] showed that there is positive immunoreactivity for p53 in 62% of GBCs, 25% in gallbladder adenomas and 16.7% of cholecystitis. Tian et al. [117] showed that in 61.2% of gallbladder carcinoma cases, there is positive immunoreactivity for p53. When classifying them according to the system proposed by Nevin, major immunohistochemical expression is observed as the degree of malignancy increase, with 47.4% being found between S1-S3, 70% between S4-S5 and 74% in metastasis with lymphatic compromise (see figures 13-1 and 13-2).

Fragile Histidine Triad

Studies have been conducted to determine the frequency of the abnormalities of FHIT during the gradual GBC carcinogenesis by determining FHIT loss of heterozygosity (LOH) and its comparison with the immunohistochemical expression of this gene. The reduction in the IHC expression of FHIT together with the loss of the alleles is almost universal in GBC, which is why these alterations are detected early in the sequential development of this neoplasia. This suggests that the FHIT gene is a possible tumor suppressor gene involved in the pathogenesis of this neoplasia [130] (see figures 13-1, 13-2 and 13-3).

KEAP1 and Nrf2

Shibata et al. [131] explained the alteration of the Keap1-Nrf2 pathway in tumors of the biliary tract for the first time. They revealed that the *Keap1* mutation occurs more frequently in GBC than in cancer of the bile duct. These mutations result in the accumulation and activation of Nrf2, an important transcriptional factor for many genes. Nrf2 provides cytoprotection against oxidative agents and increases cell growth, and can partially provide resistance to 5-FU in cancer cells (see figures 13-1 and 13-2).

Vascular Endothelial Growth Factor C

Vascular endothelial growth factor C (VEGF-C) is a lymphangiogenic polypeptide that has been involved in several solid human cancers. Nakashima et al., use immunohistochemistry to determine the expression of VEGF-C in samples of GBC, and correlated the expression with microvascular density (MVD), and clinical characteristics. Thirty-three (63%) of the 52 GBCs studied were highly positive for the VEGF-C protein by immunohistochemistry. The VEGF-C expression significantly correlated with the involvement of lymphatic vessels, lymph node metastasis and poor prognosis after surgery. Therefore, they suggest VEGF-C may play an important role in tumor progression through lymphangiogensis and lymph node metastasis in human gallbladder carcinoma [132] (see figure 13-1).

CLIC1

Wang et al. [133] found that CLIC1 expression is significantly up-regulated in highly metastatic GBC-SD18H cell line compared to the poorly metastatic GBC-SD18L cell line. In this study, the overexpression of CLIC1 significantly increased cell motility and invasiveness of the poorly metastatic GBC-SD18L cell lines, and knockdown of CLIC1 was shown to markedly deregulate cell migration and invasion of the highly metastatic GBC-SD18H cells. These results strongly demonstrate that CLIC1 plays an important role in tumor metastasis. But further investigation is necessary to explain the mechanism of how CLIC1 promotes tumorigenesis (see figures 13-1 and 13-2).

Urokinase-Type Plasminogen Activator Receptor

Yue et al. [134] determined the levels of uPAR and VEGF expression in GBC tissues, and established that the expression of both was significantly related to metastasis, but not with the state of differentiation and size of the tumor. Therefore, uPAR and VEGF may be considered an invasive phenotype of GBC and may be used for prognostication and as an evaluation marker for treatment effectiveness (see figures 13-1 and 13-2).

Claudins

Nemeth et al. [135] found that the claudin expression differs in groups of normal samples and those with gallbladder carcinoma: the normal gallbladder strongly expresses claudin-2, -3, -4 and -10, but only a weak reaction was seen in normal intrahepatic bile ducts. Although each type of cancer expresses various claudins with various intensities, only claudin-4 presented a strong immunoreaction in cancer of the intrahepatic bile duct and GBC, whereas claudin-1 and -10 appeared in cancer of the intrahepatic bile duct. Comparing the normal groups and the group with carcinoma, the most significant decrease was detected in the expression of claudin-10. Hence they conclude that the patterns of claudin expression are different in the different normal and carcinoma groups studied, and a decrease in immunoexpression is found in carcinomas compared to the normal samples (see figures 13-1 and 13-2).

EP-CAM

Prince et al. [136] examined the expression of EpCam in gallbladder carcinoma and its correlation with the disease stage and patient survival in order to explain the utility of Ep-cam as a prognosticator and its use for future treatments with antibodies. Similar studies were obtained conducted by Varga et al. [137], who concluded that Ep-Cam is an independent prognostic marker that constitutes an attractive target in the search for new therapies. The results of Prince et al. [136], on the other hand, determined that the expression of EpCAM did not correlate with the degree of the tumor or stage of the disease. The expression of EpCAM in gallbladder tumors also served as a prognostic factor for poor survival (see figures 13-1 and 13-2).

E-Cadherin-Catenin Complex

Puhalla et al. [138] examined the expression of E-cadherin and beta-catenina in mucosa, chronic inflammation and GBC tissues. The beta-catenin expression in the membrane differed between cholecystitis and malignant tissue, as well as between normal epithelium and carcinoma. The expression of E-cadherin was reduced in normal gallbladder epithelium and increased with the degree of malignancy, progressing from cholecystitis to carcinoma. Therefore, significant differences were detected between inflamed normal tissue and tissue with cancer. Similar results were obtained by Nemeth et al. [139]. This group found that E-cadherin and the protein zonula ocludens (ZO-1) were deregulated in carcinomas of several compartments of the biliary tract (intra- and extrahepatic bile duct and gallbladder) compared with the normal tissues of origin. The changes to the cadherin-catenin complex have been related to the loss of cell-cell adhesion, which leads to the formation of cell populations with a high probability of invading tissues distant from the primary neoplastic source. It has been suggested that the reduction in the expression of A, B and Y catenins is an early event in tumor progression, while the decrease in E-cadherin expression seems to be a late event [140]. Results obtained in our laboratory showed that the immunoexpression in subserosal GBC was 76% for alpha catenins, 71% for beta catenins and 72% for E-cadherin indicating that in tumor lesions, these adhesion molecules present a significant disappearance in up to 30% in the subserosa of the gallbladder [141] (see figures 13-1 and 13-2).

CD54, CD56, CD44, CD99 and CEA

Studies of the immunohistochemical expression of CD54, CD56, CD44, CD99 and CEA in the gallbladder were conducted by Choi et al. [140]. When IHC expression of CD54 was determined, there was only positive immunoreactivity in 14.3% of adenomas and in 39.1% of carcinomas. This shows that the aberrant expression of CD54 could be related to advanced stages of malignancy in the gallbladder [140] (see figures 14-1, 14-2 and 14-3). They showed the expression of CD56 in only gallbladder carcinoma (10.9%) and adenoma (50%). The frequency of CD56 expression was particularly high in the latter diseas stage (see figures 14-1, 14-2 and 14-3). The expression of CD44 and CD44v6 was examined in preneoplastic and neoplastic gallbladder lesions and it was verified that the immunoexpression of CD44 was found in 20% of normal tissues studied, in 33% of metaplasias, in 36.7% of low-grade dysplasias, 42.9% of adenomas and 23.9% of carcinomas. Furthermore, its CD44v6 variant was found only in late stages of 14.3% of adenomas and 39.1% of carcinoma (see figures 14-1 and 14-3). The IHC expression of CEA was demonstrated by Choi et al., where 3% positivity was demonstrated in normal tissues, 11.1% in metaplasia, 33.3% in low-grade dysplasia and 70.5% in carcinoma (see figure 14-1 and 14-3). The immunohistochemical expression of CD99 was 95% in a normal gallbladder, 87.5% in metaplasia, 85.7% in adenoma and 67.4% in carcinoma. These results mirror the change of adhesion molecule expression, and are normal events in the evolution of gallbladder carcinomas (see figures 13-1 and 13-2).

T-Cadherin and Zeb1

Takahashi et al., using genomic DNA from frozen tissue, reported aberrant methylation of the T-cadherin promoter in 44% of the GBC specimens, many of which were in an invasive state (45 of 50 cases) [142]. Some findings suggest that Zeb1 can repress T-cadherin expression in several cancers, including GBC. Recent studies have shown that Zeb1 is one of the key molecules responsible for EMT and the invasive activity of cancers [143]. Adachi et al[144] reported that the transcriptional regulator Zeb1 repressed the transcription activity of T-cadherin in order to increase the invasive activity in GBC cells. Zeb1 physically binds to the T-cadherin promoter, repressing the promoter activity in E-box through a form depending on the sequence, and thus suppresses T-cadherin expression. In GBC tissues, Zeb1 was expressed during cancer invasion, whereas T-cadherin was exclusively expressed in non-invasive foci. Thus, these findings suggest that Zeb1 represses T-cadherin expression, thereby increasing the activity of invasive GBC (see figures 13-1 and 13-2).

Laminin 5

Okada et al. [145] identified laminin-5y2 expression patterns in gallbladder carcinoma, and determined through univariate analyses that the stromal staining of laminin-5y2 is a strong predictor of lymphatic and venous invasion, subserosal neural infiltration and lymph node status; multivariate analyses revealed that laminin-5y2 is a strong predictor of stromal invasion. In conclusion, a high degree of proliferation and stromal staining of laminin-5y2 were significantly correlated with a pattern of invasion in the wall and the aggression of gallbladder carcinoma with destructive growth (see figures 13-1 and 13-2).

Trophinins

Chang et al. [146] showed that there was overexpression of trophinins in GBC cells compared to the parental counterpart. The up-regulation of trophinins increased cell invasion in vitro. The increase was associated with an increase in proteins found in metastasis, such as alpha3 integrin, MMP-7, MMP-, and Ets-1 (see figures 13-1 and 13-2).

RCAS1

In 110 resected gallbladder carcinomas, a high immunohistochemical expression of RCAS1 was observed in 32 of 46 cancers (70%). Positive expression in non-tumor tissue was not observed. The positivity of RCAS1 was associated with the depth of tumor invasion, metastasis in lymph nodes, lymphatic infiltration, infiltration of blood vessels and perineural infiltration. Even though RCAS1 expression can be considered a late event in gallbladder carcinogenesis, its expression is an independent predictive factor of survival [147] (see figures 13-1).

Maspin

Using DNA microarray, Kim et al. [148] analyzed more than 16,000 human genes to visualize whether those genes had an altered expression in tissues with GBC compared to normal tissue. They determined that SERPINB5 (maspin) was the most interesting gene. In this study, the gene that encodes maspin was up-regulated in GBC tissue when compared with normal tissue and was also up-regulated in early GBC tissue compared with advanced GBC. Thus, Kim et al [148] assume that maspin expression is associated with early stages of gallbladder carcinogenesis with a decrease in expression levels in advanced GBC (see figures 13-1 and 13-2).

Promyelocytic Leukemia

Chang et al. [149] showed PML together with p53 as potential markers of independent prognosis. Patients with PML expression and p53 showed favorable outcome, compared with abnormal expression of either of the two proteins. Therefore, it is considered that PML and p53 are potential candidates for development as molecular markers applicable to clinical practice that may be effective for this disease in the future (see figure 13-1).

13.6. Epigenetic Alterations in Gallbladder Cancer

Epigenetics is understood as all those heritable changes in gene expression that are not the result of alterations in the nucleotide sequence [150]. The main components of the epigenetic code that act as transcription repressors are: DNA methylation, histone modification (phosphorylation, acetylation and methylation), and altered regulation mechanisms using miRNA. The latter comprise a small family of non-codifying RNAs that negatively regulate gene expression at post-transcriptional level, and whose regulation is unknown.

Gene promoter region hypermethylation is a frequent epigenetic mechanism in the carcinogenic process. The inactivation of tumor suppressor genes by methylation seems to be an early, progressive and cumulative event in gallbladder carcinogenesis, increasing from chronic cholecystitis without metaplasia to chronic cholecystitis with metaplasia, which might provide supportive evidence that this morphological adaptation is likely, a premalignant lesion of the gallbladder mucosa. The presence of methylation has been used as a tumor marker for prognosis and in therapy selection [150]. Takashi et al. [142] found that in GBC, the frequencies of gene methylation varied from 0 to 80%. Ten genes showed a relatively high frequency of aberrant methylation: *SHP1* (80%), *3-OST-2* (72%), *CDH13* (44%), *P15INK4B* (44%), *CDH1* (38%), *RUNX3* (32%), *APC* (30%), *RIZ1* (26%), *P16INK4A* (24%) and *HPP1* (20%). Eight genes (*P73*, *RARbeta2*, *SOCS-1*, *DAPK*, *DcR2*, *DcR1*, *HIN1*, and *CHFR*) showed a low methylation frequency (2-14%), and methylation was not found in the remaining six genes studied (*TIMP-3*, *P57*, *RASSF1A*, *CRBP1*, *SYK* and *NORE1*). In chronic cholecystitis, methylation was detected for seven genes: *SHP1* (88%), *P15INK4B* (28%), *3-OST-2* (12%), *CDH1* (12%), *CDH13* (8%), *DcR2* (4%) and *P16INK4A* (4%). Significantly high methylation frequencies in GBC compared to chronic cholecystitis were detected for eight genes (*3-OST-2*, *CDH13*, *CDH1*, *RUNX3*, *APC*, *RIZ1*, *P16INK4A* and *HPP1*). The average methylation index of the cases studied was relatively high for GBC (0.196 +/- 0.013), compared to chronic cholecystitis (0.065 +/- 0.008; $P < 0.001$).

In a series of 109 advanced cancers examined in our laboratory, a significant association with survival was found in the methylation of *p73* ($p<0.006$), *MGMT* ($p< 0,006$) and *DCL1* ($p<0,044$), and a non-significant tendency for *CDH13* ($p< 0.06$) and *FHIT* ($p<0.1$). Subserosal tumors with methylation indices equal to or greater than 0.4 were associated with worse survival outcomes ($p<0.001$). A multivariate analysis found methylation of *MGMT* to be a prognostic factor independent of survival ($p<0.01$) [151]. Other studies have shown a high methylation frequency in *SEMA3B* (92%) and *FHIT* (66%), an intermediate incidence in *BLU* (26%) and *DUTT1* (22%) and a very low frequency in *RASSF1A* (8%) and *hMLH1* (4%) on chromosome 3p, a tumor suppressor gene candidate locus [152]. Studies published by our laboratory have demonstrated that *DAPK1*, *DLC1*, *TIMP3*, and *RARb2* show a progressive increase in their methylation state from chronic cholecystitis without metaplasia to advanced carcinoma that invades the serosal layer [151]. In addition, an increase in methylation of *p15*, *APC*, *DLC1*, and *CDH13* is related to poor survival. This finding illustrates the important role that epigenetic process may play in gallbladder carcinogenesis, and the use of epigenetic changes as prognostic factors as well as in the potential selection of alternative treatments for GBC (figures 13-1 and 13-2) [151,153].

13.7. Chemotherapy Resistance by Multiple Drug Resistance Proteins

Since the completion of the human genome, 49 different ABC transporters have been identified in humans. These have been divided in their phylogenetic characteristics within seven subfamilies, ABCA, ABCB, ABCC, ABCD, ABCE, ABCF and ABCG. At least 21 human ABC transporters have been described and have been associated with the transport of drugs in vitro, so it seems likely that the expression patterns of ABC transporters play an important role in individual differences in drug sensitivity tumor [175].

Several members of the family B are known to produce multidrug resistance in cancer, so this subfamily has been called "MDR subfamily of ABC transporters". MDR1 is the drug resistance protein mainly expressed in neoplastic lesions of the ABCB family. Chemotherapeutic agents that are substrates of MDR1 are: doxorubicin, daunorubicin, vincristine, vinblastine, actinomycin D, paclitaxel, docetaxol, etoposide, teniposide, bisantreno and homoharringtonine [176].

The multiple drug resistance proteins MRP/CFTR are part of the C family of the superfamily of ABC proteins (ABCC). This family includes a total of nine human MRP genes (MRP1 to MRP9), the defective gene in cystic fibrosis (CFTR) and both sulfonylurea receptor genes (SUR1, SUR2) [154,155,156].

The G subfamily comprises at least five genes, of which the most studied has been the ABCG2, protein involved in resistance to drugs such as doxorubicin, anthracyclines, daunorubicin, mitoxantrone and topotecan [176].

The main treatment for GBC is surgery, radiotherapy and chemotherapy. Adjuvant chemotherapies are one of the main cancer treatments that has been disappointing, without significant much positive results even in patients receiving postoperative treatment [157]. The failure of chemotherapy is mainly due to multiple drug resistance (MDR) proteins. In the past years, the expression of MDR1 in several tumors has been considered to play an important role in resistance to adjuvant chemotherapies [158,159]. The expression of the MDR1 gene has been related to resistance to chemotherapy for colon [160], ovarian [161], breast [162], [163] and bladder [164] cancer. Several studies have shown that the expression of MDR1 is a significant prognostic factor for some tumors [160,165].

The *MDR1* gene is widely expressed in normal gallbladder tissues [169]. The expression of MDR1 in the gallbladder is related to such physiological effects as antagonizing the excretion of extrinsic toxin products, and transforming steroid hormones [170]. Many of the tumors originating from normal tissues with a high MDR1 expression show a high expression of the *MDR1* gene, which is called an intrinsic resistance to drugs [171].

In order to better understand the relation between tumor chemotherapy, patient prognosis and MDR1 expression in GBC, Cao et al. [172] detected the expression of MDR1 in tumors and tissues with cholecystitis. The results obtained were that the percentage of cases positive for MDR1 between both groups was significantly different ($P<0.05$). The levels of MDR1 expression in gallbladder carcinomas in Nevin stage I-III were higher than in cholecystitis ($P<0.05$). This indicates that the expression levels are related to the Nevin stage or cancerous changes in the gallbladder or early development of carcinoma [172]. Another mechanism of resistance to multiple drugs in tumor cells is the product of the expression of the P-glycoprotein (P-gp), which is codified by the MDR1 gene. In many human neoplasias, the expression of MDR1 is a common phenomenon and represents a greater therapeutic problem in chemotherapy. In 53 cases of GBC with no previous treatment, positive expression of P-gp and mRNA-MDR1 was observed in 60.3% and 71.7%, respectively [173]. In well and moderately differentiated tumors the expression was 79.5% and 69.2% compared to 50% and 35.7% in poorly differentiated tumors ($p<0.05$). The high expression of P-glycoprotein and MDR could explain in part the poor response to treatment in GBC [172,174] (see figures 13-1 and 13-2).

MRP1 and MRP2 transport compounds, which are conjugated to anionic ligands like glutathione, glucuronate or sulfate or unmodified together with glutathione. MRP1 and MRP2 also are called GS-X pumps. MRP3 is closely related to MRP1, and is also a GS-X pump as has been shown experimentally by the transport of *S*-(2, 4-dinitrophenyl)-glutathione [166]. In cell lines transfected with MRP3, the range of drugs for which resistance has been observed is more limited compared to MRP1 [167]. In continuous exposure experiments, resistance to etoposide and teniposide was found but not to other drugs. In a panel of lung cancer cell lines, however, the association between *MRP3* expression and resistance was observed, not only for etoposide, but also for doxorubicin, vincristine and cisplatin [168]. Additionally, using short exposure times, the cells overproduced MRP3 and thus were highly resistant to methotrexate (MTX) [166]. Rost and colleagues [177] determined the expression of MRP2 and MRP3 which were analyzed by (RT-PCR) and immunofluorescence. This group identified the transporters MRP2 and MRP3 in gallbladder samples studied. Immunofluorescence showed that expression of MRP2 was found in the apical membrane and MRP3 in the basolateral membrane of gallbladder epithelium. They do not detect the expression of MRP1. So they concluded that MRP2 and MRP3 may be playing an important role in the export of conjugated xenobiotics and endogenous anionic one hand MRP3 to blood components and on the other hand MRP2 into the bile ducts.

Finally Aust et al. [178] determined the expression of ABCG2 in gallbladder tissues of both normal and malignant specimens. They demonstrated that ABCG2 is present in the luminal membrane of gallbladder epithelial cells. It concluded that ABCG2 has a role as an efflux pump ATP dependent and can prevent the accumulation of anticancer drugs (see figures 13-1 and 13-2).

Conclusion

There are numerous epidemiological, morphological and molecular studies that have characterized this neoplasia, providing significant prognostic associations that have made it possible, on the one hand, to select higher-risk groups and, on the other, to identify groups that must receive differentiated therapies. The molecular genetic characterization of this disease has begun to classify sub-groups of patients who cannot be routinely distinguished using the analysis of morphological patterns and who will benefit from the use of targeted therapies in the near future.

References

[1] Andia M, Gederlini A, Ferrecio C (2006) Cáncer de vesícula biliar: Tendencia y distribución del riesgo en Chile. *Rev. méd. Chile* 134: 565-574. .

[2] GLOBOCAN (2000) Cancer Incidence, Morality and Prevalence Worldwide. *IARC Cancer Base N°5.*

[3] WHO WCR, World Health Organization - International Agency for Research on Cancer, IARC Press (2003).

[4] Dixon E, Vollmer CM, Jr., Sahajpal A, Cattral M, Grant D, et al. (2005) An aggressive surgical approach leads to improved survival in patients with gallbladder cancer: a 12-year study at a North American Center. *Ann. Surg.* 241: 385-394.

[5] Lazcano-Ponce EC, Miquel JF, Munoz N, Herrero R, Ferrecio C, et al. (2001) Epidemiology and molecular pathology of gallbladder cancer. *CA Cancer J. Clin.* 51: 349-364.

[6] Randi G, Franceschi S, La Vecchia C (2006) Gallbladder cancer worldwide: geographical distribution and risk factors. *Int. J. Cancer* 118: 1591-1602.

[7] Kiran RP, Pokala N, Dudrick SJ (2007) Incidence pattern and survival for gallbladder cancer over three decades--an analysis of 10301 patients. *Ann. Surg. Oncol.* 14: 827-832.

[8] Barakat J, Dunkelberg JC, Ma TY (2006) Changing patterns of gallbladder carcinoma in New Mexico. *Cancer* 106: 434-440.

[9] Carey MC, Paigen B (2002) Epidemiology of the American Indians' burden and its likely genetic origins. *Hepatology* 36: 781-791.

[10] Misra S, Chaturvedi A, Misra NC, Sharma ID (2003) Carcinoma of the gallbladder. *Lancet Oncol.* 4: 167-176.

[11] Roa I, de Aretxabala X, Roa J, Araya JC, Villaseca M, et al. (2002) [Is gallbladder cancer a disease with bad prognosis?]. *Rev. Med. Chil.* 130: 1295-1302.

[12] Hart J, Modan B, Shani M (1971) Cholelithiasis in the aetiology of gallbladder neoplasms. *Lancet* 1: 1151-1153.

[13] Paz B, Kunakow N, Montiel F, Nervi F, (1986) Incidence of Salmonella typhi infection in symptomatic cholelithiasis in an endemic area. A prospective study. *Gastroenterol. Hepatol.* 9: 121-124.

[14] Attili AF, Capocaccia R, Carulli N, Festi D, Roda E, et al. (1997) Factors associated with gallstone disease in the MICOL experience. Multicenter Italian Study on Epidemiology of Cholelithiasis. *Hepatology* 26: 809-818.

[15] Apstein MD, Carey MC (1996) Pathogenesis of cholesterol gallstones: a parsimonious hypothesis. *Eur. J. Clin. Invest.* 26: 343-352.

[16] Everhart JE (1993) Contributions of obesity and weight loss to gallstone disease. *Ann. Intern. Med.* 119: 1029-1035.

[17] Petitti DB, Friedman GD, Klatsky AL (1981) Association of a history of gallbladder disease with a reduced concentration of high-density-lipoprotein cholesterol. *N. Engl. J. Med.* 304: 1396-1398.

[18] Lowenfels AB (1978) Does bile promote extra-colonic cancer? *Lancet* 2: 239-241.

[19] Ferreccio C, Chianale J, González C, Nervi F (1995) Epidemiología descriptiva del cáncer digestivo en Chile (1982-1991): una aproximación desde la mortalidad. . Alfabeta Impresores, Santiago, Chile 1995

[20] Juvonen T, Savolainen MJ, Kairaluoma MI, Lajunen LH, Humphries SE, et al. (1995) Polymorphisms at the apoB, apoA-I, and cholesteryl ester transfer protein gene loci in patients with gallbladder disease. *J. Lipid. Res.* 36: 804-812.

[21] Fernandez M, Csendes A, Yarmuch J, Diaz H, Silva J (2003) Management of common bile duct stones: the state of the art in 2000. *Int. Surg.* 88: 159-163.

[22] Roa I, de Aretxabala X, Araya JC, Villaseca M, Roa J, et al. (2001) [Incipient gallbladder carcinoma. Clinical and pathological study and prognosis in 196 cases]. *Rev. Med. Chil.* 129: 1113-1120.

[23] Levi F, Lucchini F, Negri E, La Vecchia C (2003) The recent decline in gallbladder cancer mortality in Europe. *Eur. J. Cancer Prev.* 12: 265-267.

[24] Serra I (2001) [Has gallbladder cancer mortality decrease in Chile?]. *Rev. Med. Chil.* 129: 1079-1084.

[25] Towfigh S, McFadden DW, Cortina GR, Thompson JE, Jr., Tompkins RK, et al. (2001) Porcelain gallbladder is not associated with gallbladder carcinoma. *Am. Surg.* 67: 7-10.

[26] Aldridge MC, Bismuth H (1990) Gallbladder cancer: the polyp-cancer sequence. *Br. J. Surg.* 77: 363-364.

[27] Chijiiwa K, Kimura H, Tanaka M (1995) Malignant potential of the gallbladder in patients with anomalous pancreaticobiliary ductal junction. The difference in risk between patients with and without choledochal cyst. *Int. Surg.* 80: 61-64.

[28] Kowalewski K, Todd EF (1971) Carcinoma of the gallbladder induced in hamsters by insertion of cholesterol pellets and feeding dimethylnitrosamine. *Proc. Soc. Exp. Biol. Med.* 136: 482-486.

[29] Shukla VK, Tiwari SC, Roy SK (1993) Biliary bile acids in cholelithiasis and carcinoma of the gall bladder. *Eur. J. Cancer Prev.* 2: 155-160.

[30] Pandey M, Shukla VK, Singh S, Roy SK, Rao BR (2000) Biliary lipid peroxidation products in gallbladder cancer: increased peroxidation or biliary stasis? *Eur. J. Cancer Prev* 9: 417-422.

[31] Goldberg MS, Theriault G (1994) Retrospective cohort study of workers of a synthetic textiles plant in Quebec: I. General mortality. *Am. J. Ind. Med.* 25: 889-907.

[32] Tomasek L, Darby SC, Swerdlow AJ, Placek V, Kunz E (1993) Radon exposure and cancers other than lung cancer among uranium miners in West Bohemia. *Lancet* 341: 919-923.

[33] Kato K, Akai S, Tominaga S, Kato I (1989) A case-control study of biliary tract cancer in Niigata Prefecture, Japan. *Jpn J. Cancer Res.* 80: 932-938.

[34] Coursaget P, Munoz N (1999) Vaccination against infectious agents associated with human cancer. *Cancer Surv.* 33: 355-381.

[35] Welton JC, Marr JS, Friedman SM (1979) Association between hepatobiliary cancer and typhoid carrier state. *Lancet* 1: 791-794.

[36] Dutta U, Garg PK, Kumar R, Tandon RK (2000) Typhoid carriers among patients with gallstones are at increased risk for carcinoma of the gallbladder. *Am. J. Gastroenterol.* 95: 784-787.

[37] Roa I, Ibacache G, Carvallo J, Melo A, Araya J, et al. (1999) [Microbiological study of gallbladder bile in a high risk zone for gallbladder cancer]. *Rev. Med. Chil.* 127: 1049-1055.

[38] Fox JG, Dewhirst FE, Shen Z, Feng Y, Taylor NS, et al. (1998) Hepatic Helicobacter species identified in bile and gallbladder tissue from Chileans with chronic cholecystitis. *Gastroenterology* 114: 755-763.

[39] Leong RW, Sung JJ (2002) Review article: Helicobacter species and hepatobiliary diseases. *Aliment Pharmacol. Ther.* 16: 1037-1045.

[40] Metz DC (1998) Helicobacter colonization of the biliary tree: commensal, pathogen, or spurious finding? *Am. J. Gastroenterol.* 93: 1996-1998.

[41] Mendez-Sanchez N, Pichardo R, Gonzalez J, Sanchez H, Moreno M, et al. (2001) Lack of association between Helicobacter sp colonization and gallstone disease. *J. Clin. Gastroenterol.* 32: 138-141.

[42] Strom BL, Soloway RD, Rios-Dalenz JL, Rodriguez-Martinez HA, West SL, et al. (1995) Risk factors for gallbladder cancer. An international collaborative case-control study. *Cancer* 76: 1747-1756.

[43] Walsh N, Qizilbash A, Banerjee R, Waugh GA (1987) Biliary neoplasia in Gardner's syndrome. *Arch. Pathol. Lab. Med.* 111: 76-77.

[44] Wada K, Tanaka M, Yamaguchi K (1987) Carcinoma and polyps of the gallbladder associated with Peutz-Jeghers syndrome. *Dig. Dis. Sci.* 32: 943-946.

[45] Kozuka S, Tsubone N, Yasui A, Hachisuka K (1982) Relation of adenoma to carcinoma in the gallbladder. *Cancer* 50: 2226-2234.

[46] Roa I, Araya JC, Villaseca M, De Aretxabala X, Riedemann P, et al. (1996) Preneoplastic lesions and gallbladder cancer: an estimate of the period required for progression. *Gastroenterology* 111: 232-236.

[47] Roa I, Araya JC, Villaseca M, Roa J, de Aretxabala X, et al. (1999) Gallbladder cancer in a high risk area: morphological features and spread patterns. *Hepatogastroenterology* 46: 1540-1546.

[48] Laitio M (1983) Histogenesis of epithelial neoplasms of human gallbladder I. Dysplasia. *Pathol Res Pract* 178: 51-56.

[49] Laitio M (1983) Histogenesis of epithelial neoplasms of human gallbladder II. Classification of carcinoma on the basis of morphological features. *Pathol. Res. Pract.* 178: 57-66.

[50] Harbison J, Reynolds JV, Sheahan K, Gibney RG, Hyland JM (1997) Evidence for the polyp-cancer sequence in gallbladder cancer. *Ir. Med. J.* 90: 98.

[51] Roa I, Araya JC, Wistuba I, Villaseca M, de Aretxabala X, et al. (1993) [Epithelial lesions associated with gallbladder carcinoma. A methodical study of 32 cases]. *Rev. Med. Chil.* 121: 21-29.

[52] Smok G, Cervilla K, Bosch H, Csendes A (1986) [Precancerous lesions of invasive carcinoma of the gallbladder]. *Rev. Med. Chil.* 114: 954-958.

[53] Albores-Saavedra J, Alcantra-Vazquez A, Cruz-Ortiz H, Herrera-Goepfert R (1980) The precursor lesions of invasive gallbladder carcinoma. Hyperplasia, atypical hyperplasia and carcinoma in situ. *Cancer* 45: 919-927.

[54] Yokoyama N, Watanabe H, Ajioka Y, Nishikura K, Date K, et al. (1998) [Genetic alterations in gallbladder carcinoma: a review]. *Nippon Geka Gakkai Zasshi* 99: 687-695.

[55] Wistuba, II, Miquel JF, Gazdar AF, Albores-Saavedra J (1999) Gallbladder adenomas have molecular abnormalities different from those present in gallbladder carcinomas. *Hum. Pathol.* 30: 21-25.

[56] Duarte I, Llanos O, Domke H, Harz C, Valdivieso V (1993) Metaplasia and precursor lesions of gallbladder carcinoma. Frequency, distribution, and probability of detection in routine histologic samples. *Cancer* 72: 1878-1884.

[57] Roa I, Araya JC, Shiraishi T, Yatani R, Wistuba I, et al. (1992) [Immunohistochemical demonstration of pepsinogens I and II in the gallbladder]. *Rev. Med. Chil.* 120: 1351-1358.

[58] Yamamoto M, Nakajo S, Tahara E (1989) Dysplasia of the gallbladder. Its histogenesis and correlation to gallbladder adenocarcinoma. *Pathol. Res. Pract.* 185: 454-460.

[59] Yamamoto M, Nakajo S, Tahara E (1989) Carcinoma of the gallbladder: the correlation between histogenesis and prognosis. *Virchows Arch. A Pathol. Anat. Histopathol.* 414: 83-90.

[60] Yamagiwa H, Tomiyama H (1986) [Significance of dysplasia of the gallbladder]. *Rinsho Byori* 34: 328-332.

[61] Sasatomi E, Tokunaga O, Miyazaki K (2000) Precancerous conditions of gallbladder carcinoma: overview of histopathologic characteristics and molecular genetic findings. *J. Hepatobiliary Pancreat Surg.* 7: 556-567.

[62] Wistuba, II, Albores-Saavedra J (1999) Genetic abnormalities involved in the pathogenesis of gallbladder carcinoma. *J. Hepatobiliary Pancreat Surg.* 6: 237-244.

[63] Medina E, Kaempffer AM (2001) [Cancer mortality in Chile: epidemiological considerations]. *Rev. Med. Chil.* 129: 1195-1202.

[64] Roa I, de Aretxabala X, Araya JC, Villaseca M, Roa J, et al. (2002) [Morphological prognostic elements in gallbladder cancer]. *Rev. Med. Chil.* 130: 387-395.

[65] Tsukada K, Kurosaki I, Uchida K, Shirai Y, Oohashi Y, et al. (1997) Lymph node spread from carcinoma of the gallbladder. *Cancer* 80: 661-667.

[66] Nakakubo Y, Miyamoto M, Cho Y, Hida Y, Oshikiri T, et al. (2003) Clinical significance of immune cell infiltration within gallbladder cancer. *Br. J. Cancer* 89: 1736-1742.

[67] Schumacher K, Haensch W, Roefzaad C, Schlag PM (2001) Prognostic significance of activated CD8(+) T cell infiltrations within esophageal carcinomas. *Cancer Res.* 61: 3932-3936.

[68] Marzo AL, Kinnear BF, Lake RA, Frelinger JJ, Collins EJ, et al. (2000) Tumor-specific CD4+ T cells have a major "post-licensing" role in CTL mediated anti-tumor immunity. *J. Immunol.* 165: 6047-6055.

[69] Beatty G, Paterson Y (2001) IFN-gamma-dependent inhibition of tumor angiogenesis by tumor-infiltrating CD4+ T cells requires tumor responsiveness to IFN-gamma. *J. Immunol.* 166: 2276-2282.

[70] Cooper MA, Fehniger TA, Caligiuri MA (2001) The biology of human natural killer-cell subsets. *Trends Immunol.* 22: 633-640.

[71] Ishigami S, Natsugoe S, Tokuda K, Nakajo A, Xiangming C, et al. (2000) Clinical impact of intratumoral natural killer cell and dendritic cell infiltration in gastric cancer. *Cancer Lett.* 159: 103-108.

[72] Yamamoto M, Oda N, Tahara E (1990) DNA ploidy patterns in gallbladder adenocarcinoma. *Jpn J. Clin. Oncol.* 20: 83-86.

[73] Sato Y, Tanaka J, Yoshioka H, Koyama K (1991) [Evaluation of the malignancy in gallbladder cancer assessed by nuclear DNA contents and mitotic indices--with special reference to the prognosis of the patients with cancer involvement to the subserosal layer]. *Nippon Geka Gakkai Zasshi* 92: 46-51.

[74] Roa I, de Aretxabala X, Fuentealba P, Cabrera ME, Araya JC, et al. (2004) [DNA content and survival in subserous gallbladder carcinoma]. *Rev. Med. Chil.* 132: 794-800.

[75] Roa I, Araya JC, Shiraishi T, Yatani R, Wistuba I, et al. (1993) DNA content in gallbladder carcinoma: a flow cytometric study of 96 cases. *Histopathology* 23: 459-464.

[76] Tang M, Baez S, Pruyas M, Diaz A, Calvo A, et al. (2004) Mitochondrial DNA mutation at the D310 (displacement loop) mononucleotide sequence in the pathogenesis of gallbladder carcinoma. *Clin. Cancer Res.* 10: 1041-1046.

[77] Zhang M, Pan JW, Ren TR, Zhu YF, Han YJ, et al. (2003) Correlated expression of inducible nitric oxide synthase and P53, Bax in benign and malignant diseased gallbladder. *Ann. Anat.* 185: 549-554.

[78] Roa JC, Roa I, Correa P, Vo Q, Araya JC, et al. (2005) Microsatellite instability in preneoplastic and neoplastic lesions of the gallbladder. *J. Gastroenterol.* 40: 79-86.

[79] Saetta AA (2006) K-ras, p53 mutations, and microsatellite instability (MSI) in gallbladder cancer. *J. Surg. Oncol.* 93: 644-649.

[80] Kohya N, Miyazaki K, Matsukura S, Yakushiji H, Kitajima Y, et al. (2002) Deficient expression of O(6)-methylguanine-DNA methyltransferase combined with mismatch-repair proteins hMLH1 and hMSH2 is related to poor prognosis in human biliary tract carcinoma. *Ann. Surg. Oncol.* 9: 371-379.

[81] Luzar B, Poljak M, Cor A, Klopcic U, Ferlan-Marolt V (2005) Expression of human telomerase catalytic protein in gallbladder carcinogenesis. *J. Clin. Pathol.* 58: 820-825.

[82] Hansel DE, Meeker AK, Hicks J, De Marzo AM, Lillemoe KD, et al. (2006) Telomere length variation in biliary tract metaplasia, dysplasia, and carcinoma. *Mod. Pathol.* 19: 772-779.

[83] Nakazawa K, Dobashi Y, Suzuki S, Fujii H, Takeda Y, et al. (2005) Amplification and overexpression of c-erbB-2, epidermal growth factor receptor, and c-met in biliary tract cancers. *J. Pathol.* 206: 356-365.

[84] Altimari A, Fiorentino M, Gabusi E, Gruppioni E, Corti B, et al. (2003) Investigation of ErbB1 and ErbB2 expression for therapeutic targeting in primary liver tumours. *Dig. Liver Dis.* 35: 332-338.

[85] Ito Y, Takeda T, Sasaki Y, Sakon M, Yamada T, et al. (2001) Expression and clinical significance of the erbB family in intrahepatic cholangiocellular carcinoma. *Pathol. Res. Pract.* 197: 95-100.

[86] Lee CS, Pirdas A (1995) Epidermal growth factor receptor immunoreactivity in gallbladder and extrahepatic biliary tract tumours. *Pathol. Res. Pract.* 191: 1087-1091.

[87] Kaufman M, Mehrotra B, Limaye S, White S, Fuchs A, et al. (2008) EGFR expression in gallbladder carcinoma in North America. *Int. J. Med. Sci.* 5: 285-291.

[88] Ooi A, Suzuki S, Nakazawa K, Itakura J, Imoto I, et al. (2009) Gene amplification of Myc and its coamplification with ERBB2 and EGFR in gallbladder adenocarcinoma. *AntiCancer Res.* 29: 19-26.

[89] Chow NH, Huang SM, Chan SH, Mo LR, Hwang MH, et al. (1995) Significance of c-erbB-2 expression in normal and neoplastic epithelium of biliary tract. *AntiCancer Res.* 15: 1055-1059.

[90] Yukawa M, Fujimori T, Hirayama D, Idei Y, Ajiki T, et al. (1993) Expression of oncogene products and growth factors in early gallbladder cancer, advanced gallbladder cancer, and chronic cholecystitis. *Hum. Pathol.* 24: 37-40.

[91] Hanada K, Itoh M, Fujii K, Tsuchida A, Ooishi H, et al. (1996) K-ras and p53 mutations in stage I gallbladder carcinoma with an anomalous junction of the pancreaticobiliary duct. *Cancer* 77: 452-458.

[92] Matsubara T, Funabiki T, Jinno O, Sakurai Y, Hasegawa S, et al. (1999) p53 gene mutations and overexpression of p53 product in cancerous and noncancerous biliary epithelium in patients with pancreaticobiliary maljunction. *J. Hepatobiliary Pancreat. Surg.* 6: 286-293.

[93] Roa JC, Anabalon L, Tapia O, Melo A, de Aretxabala X, et al. (2005) [Frequency of K-ras mutation in biliary and pancreatic tumors]. *Rev. Med. Chil.* 133: 1434-1440.

[94] Saetta A, Lazaris AC, Davaris PS (1996) Detection of ras oncogene point mutations and simultaneous proliferative fraction estimation in gallbladder cancer. *Pathol Res. Pract.* 192: 532-540.

[95] Saetta AA, Papanastasiou P, Michalopoulos NV, Gigelou F, Korkolopoulou P, et al. (2004) Mutational analysis of BRAF in gallbladder carcinomas in association with K-ras and p53 mutations and microsatellite instability. *Virchows Arch* 445: 179-182.

[96] Li Q, Yang Z (2009) Expression of phospho-ERK1/2 and PI3-K in benign and malignant gallbladder lesions and its clinical and pathological correlations. *J. Exp. Clin. Cancer Res.* 28: 65.

[97] Kee SK, Lee JY, Kim MJ, Lee SM, Jung YW, et al. (2007) Hypermethylation of the Ras association domain family 1A (RASSF1A) gene in gallbladder cancer. *Mol. Cells* 24: 364-371.

[98] Ghosh M, Kamma H, Kawamoto T, Koike N, Miwa M, et al. (2005) MUC 1 core protein as a marker of gallbladder malignancy. *Eur. J. Surg. Oncol.* 31: 891-896.

[99] Kashiwagi H, Kijima H, Dowaki S, Ohtani Y, Tobita K, et al. (2001) MUC1 and MUC2 expression in human gallbladder carcinoma: a clinicopathological study and relationship with prognosis. *Oncol. Rep.* 8: 485-489.

[100] Yamato T, Sasaki M, Watanabe Y, Nakanuma Y (1999) Expression of MUC1 and MUC2 mucin core proteins and their messenger RNA in gall bladder carcinoma: an immunohistochemical and in situ hybridization study. *J. Pathol.* 188: 30-37.

[101] Miyahara N, Shoda J, Ishige K, Kawamoto T, Ueda T, et al. (2008) MUC4 interacts with ErbB2 in human gallbladder carcinoma: potential pathobiological implications. *Eur. J. Cancer* 44: 1048-1056.

[102] Finzi L, Barbu V, Burgel PR, Mergey M, Kirkwood KS, et al. (2006) MUC5AC, a gel-forming mucin accumulating in gallstone disease, is overproduced via an epidermal

growth factor receptor pathway in the human gallbladder. *Am. J. Pathol.* 169: 2031-2041.

[103] Sasaki M, Yamato T, Nakanuma Y, Ho SB, Kim YS (1999) Expression of MUC2, MUC5AC and MUC6 apomucins in carcinoma, dysplasia and non-dysplastic epithelia of the gallbladder. *Pathol Int* 49: 38-44.

[104] Wu XS, Akiyama Y, Igari T, Kawamura T, Hiranuma S, et al. (2005) Expression of homeodomain protein CDX2 in gallbladder carcinomas. *J. Cancer Res. Clin. Oncol.* 131: 271-278.

[105] Nomoto M, Izumi H, Ise T, Kato K, Takano H, et al. (1999) Structural basis for the regulation of UDP-N-acetyl-alpha-D-galactosamine: polypeptide N-acetylgalactosaminyl transferase-3 gene expression in adenocarcinoma cells. *Cancer Res.* 59: 6214-6222.

[106] Kornprat P, Rehak P, Lemmerer M, Gogg-Kamerer M, Langner C (2005) Analysis of trefoil factor family protein 1 (TFF1, pS2) expression in chronic cholecystitis and gallbladder carcinoma. *Virchows Arch.* 446: 505-510.

[107] Sanada T, Yokoi S, Arii S, Yasui K, Imoto I, et al. (2004) Skp2 overexpression is a p27Kip1-independent predictor of poor prognosis in patients with biliary tract cancers. *Cancer Sci.* 95: 969-976.

[108] Li SH, Li CF, Sung MT, Eng HL, Hsiung CY, et al. (2007) Skp2 is an independent prognosticator of gallbladder carcinoma among p27(Kip1)-interacting cell cycle regulators: an immunohistochemical study of 62 cases by tissue microarray. *Mod. Pathol.* 20: 497-507.

[109] Ma HB, Hu HT, Di ZL, Wang ZR, Shi JS, et al. (2005) Association of cyclin D1, p16 and retinoblastoma protein expressions with prognosis and metastasis of gallbladder carcinoma. *World J. Gastroenterol.* 11: 744-747.

[110] Legan M, Luzar B, Marolt VF, Cor A (2006) Expression of cyclooxygenase-2 is associated with p53 accumulation in premalignant and malignant gallbladder lesions. *World J. Gastroenterol.* 12: 3425-3429.

[111] Zhi YH, Liu RS, Song MM, Tian Y, Long J, et al. (2005) Cyclooxygenase-2 promotes angiogenesis by increasing vascular endothelial growth factor and predicts prognosis in gallbladder carcinoma. *World J. Gastroenterol.* 11: 3724-3728.

[112] Pai R, Soreghan B, Szabo IL, Pavelka M, Baatar D, et al. (2002) Prostaglandin E2 transactivates EGF receptor: a novel mechanism for promoting colon cancer growth and gastrointestinal hypertrophy. *Nat. Med.* 8: 289-293.

[113] Buchanan FG, Wang D, Bargiacchi F, DuBois RN (2003) Prostaglandin E2 regulates cell migration via the intracellular activation of the epidermal growth factor receptor. *J. Biol. Chem.* 278: 35451-35457.

[114] Yasumaru M, Tsuji S, Tsujii M, Irie T, Komori M, et al. (2003) Inhibition of angiotensin II activity enhanced the antitumor effect of cyclooxygenase-2 inhibitors via insulin-like growth factor I receptor pathway. *Cancer Res.* 63: 6726-6734.

[115] Husain SS, Szabo IL, Pai R, Soreghan B, Jones MK, et al. (2001) MAPK (ERK2) kinase--a key target for NSAIDs-induced inhibition of gastric cancer cell proliferation and growth. *Life Sci.* 69: 3045-3054.

[116] Quan ZW, Wu K, Wang J, Shi W, Zhang Z, et al. (2001) Association of p53, p16, and vascular endothelial growth factor protein expressions with the prognosis and metastasis of gallbladder cancer. *J. Am. Coll Surg.* 193: 380-383.

[117] Tian Y, Ding RY, Zhi YH, Guo RX, Wu SD (2006) Analysis of p53 and vascular endothelial growth factor expression in human gallbladder carcinoma for the determination of tumor vascularity. *World J. Gastroenterol.* 12: 415-419.

[118] Liu Z, Jiang L, Yang B, Liao D (2003) [The roles of VEGF and C-myc in occurrence, development and metastasis of gallbladder carcinoma]. Sheng Wu Yi Xue Gong Cheng Xue Za Zhi 20: 68-70.

[119] Yamamoto S, Kitadai Y, Tsuchida A, Sasaki T, Matsubara K, et al. (2000) Expression of platelet-derived endothelial cell growth factor/thymidine phosphorylase in human gallbladder lesions. *Eur. J. Cancer* 36: 257-263.

[120] Ishikawa F, Miyazono K, Hellman U, Drexler H, Wernstedt C, et al. (1989) Identification of angiogenic activity and the cloning and expression of platelet-derived endothelial cell growth factor. *Nature* 338: 557-562.

[121] Haraguchi M, Miyadera K, Uemura K, Sumizawa T, Furukawa T, et al. (1994) Angiogenic activity of enzymes. *Nature* 368: 198.

[122] Giatromanolaki A, Sivridis E, Simopoulos C, Polychronidis A, Gatter KC, et al. (2006) Hypoxia inducible factors 1alpha and 2alpha are associated with VEGF expression and angiogenesis in gallbladder carcinomas. *J. Surg. Oncol.* 94: 242-247.

[123] Wu W, Pan C, Yu H, Gong H, Wang Y (2008) Heparanase expression in gallbladder carcinoma and its correlation to prognosis. *J. Gastroenterol. Hepatol.* 23: 491-497.

[124] Xu LN, Zou SQ, Wang JM (2005) Action and mechanism of Fas and Fas ligand in immune escape of gallbladder carcinoma. *World J. Gastroenterol.* 11: 3719-3723.

[125] Zong H, Yin B, Chen J, Ma B, Cai D, et al. (2009) Over-expression of c-FLIP confers the resistance to TRAIL-induced apoptosis on gallbladder carcinoma. *Tohoku J. Exp. Med.* 217: 203-208.

[126] Roa JC, Vo Q, Araya JC, Villaseca M, Guzman P, et al. (2004) [Inactivation of CDKN2A gene (p16) in gallbladder carcinoma]. *Rev. Med. Chil.* 132: 1369-1376.

[127] Shi YZ, Hui AM, Li X, Takayama T, Makuuchi M (2000) Overexpression of retinoblastoma protein predicts decreased survival and correlates with loss of p16INK4 protein in gallbladder carcinomas. *Clin. Cancer Res.* 6: 4096-4100.

[128] Kim YT, Kim J, Jang YH, Lee WJ, Ryu JK, et al. (2001) Genetic alterations in gallbladder adenoma, dysplasia and carcinoma. *Cancer Lett* 169: 59-68.

[129] Wistuba, II, Gazdar AF, Roa I, Albores-Saavedra J (1996) p53 protein overexpression in gallbladder carcinoma and its precursor lesions: an immunohistochemical study. *Hum. Pathol.* 27: 360-365.

[130] Wistuba, II, Ashfaq R, Maitra A, Alvarez H, Riquelme E, et al. (2002) Fragile histidine triad gene abnormalities in the pathogenesis of gallbladder carcinoma. *Am. J. Pathol.* 160: 2073-2079.

[131] Shibata T, Kokubu A, Gotoh M, Ojima H, Ohta T, et al. (2008) Genetic alteration of Keap1 confers constitutive Nrf2 activation and resistance to chemotherapy in gallbladder cancer. *Gastroenterology* 135: 1358-1368, 1368 e1351-1354.

[132] Nakashima T, Kondoh S, Kitoh H, Ozawa H, Okita S, et al. (2003) Vascular endothelial growth factor-C expression in human gallbladder cancer and its relationship to lymph node metastasis. *Int. J. Mol. Med.* 11: 33-39.

[133] Wang JW, Peng SY, Li JT, Wang Y, Zhang ZP, et al. (2009) Identification of metastasis-associated proteins involved in gallbladder carcinoma metastasis by

proteomic analysis and functional exploration of chloride intracellular channel 1. *Cancer Lett.* 281: 71-81.

[134] Yue SQ, Yang YL, Zhou JS, Li KZ, Dou KF (2004) Relationship between urokinase-type plasminogen activator receptor and vascular endothelial growth factor expression and metastasis of gallbladder cancer. *World J. Gastroenterol.* 10: 2750-2752.

[135] Nemeth Z, Szasz AM, Tatrai P, Nemeth J, Gyorffy H, et al. (2009) Claudin-1, -2, -3, -4, -7, -8, and -10 protein expression in biliary tract cancers. *J. Histochem. Cytochem.* 57: 113-121.

[136] Prince S, Zeidman A, Dekel Y, Ram E, Koren R (2008) Expression of epithelial cell adhesion molecule in gallbladder carcinoma and its correlation with clinicopathologic variables. *Am. J. Clin. Pathol.* 129: 424-429.

[137] Varga M, Obrist P, Schneeberger S, Muhlmann G, Felgel-Farnholz C, et al. (2004) Overexpression of epithelial cell adhesion molecule antigen in gallbladder carcinoma is an independent marker for poor survival. *Clin. Cancer Res.* 10: 3131-3136.

[138] Puhalla H, Herberger B, Soleiman A, Filipits M, Laengle F, et al. (2005) E-cadherin and beta-catenin expression in normal, inflamed and cancerous gallbladder tissue. *AntiCancer Res.* 25: 4249-4254.

[139] Nemeth Z, Szasz AM, Somoracz A, Tatrai P, Nemeth J, et al. (2009) Zonula Occludens-1, Occludin, and E-cadherin Protein Expression in Biliary Tract Cancers. *Pathol. Oncol. Res.*

[140] Choi YL, Xuan YH, Shin YK, Chae SW, Kook MC, et al. (2004) An immunohistochemical study of the expression of adhesion molecules in gallbladder lesions. *J. Histochem. Cytochem.* 52: 591-601.

[141] Roa I, Ibacache G, Melo A, Morales E, Villaseca M, et al. (2002) [Subserous gallbladder carcinoma: expression of cadherine-catenine complex]. *Rev. Med. Chil.* 130: 1349-1357.

[142] Takahashi T, Shivapurkar N, Riquelme E, Shigematsu H, Reddy J, et al. (2004) Aberrant promoter hypermethylation of multiple genes in gallbladder carcinoma and chronic cholecystitis. *Clin. Cancer Res.* 10: 6126-6133.

[143] Sarrio D, Rodriguez-Pinilla SM, Hardisson D, Cano A, Moreno-Bueno G, et al. (2008) Epithelial-mesenchymal transition in breast cancer relates to the basal-like phenotype. *Cancer Res.* 68: 989-997.

[144] Adachi Y, Takeuchi T, Nagayama T, Ohtsuki Y, Furihata M (2009) Zeb1-mediated T-cadherin repression increases the invasive potential of gallbladder cancer. *FEBS Lett.* 583: 430-436.

[145] Okada K, Kijima H, Imaizumi T, Hirabayashi K, Matsuyama M, et al. (2009) Stromal laminin-5gamma2 chain expression is associated with the wall-invasion pattern of gallbladder adenocarcinoma. *Biomed. Res.* 30: 53-62.

[146] Chang XZ, Yu J, Zhang XH, Yin J, Wang T, et al. (2009) Enhanced expression of trophinin promotes invasive and metastatic potential of human gallbladder cancer cells. *J. Cancer Res. Clin. Oncol.* 135: 581-590.

[147] Oshikiri T, Hida Y, Miyamoto M, Hashida H, Katoh K, et al. (2001) RCAS1 as a tumour progression marker: an independent negative prognostic factor in gallbladder cancer. *Br. J. Cancer* 85: 1922-1927.

[148] Kim JH, Kim HN, Lee KT, Lee JK, Choi SH, et al. (2008) Gene expression profiles in gallbladder cancer: the close genetic similarity seen for early and advanced gallbladder cancers may explain the poor prognosis. *Tumour Biol.* 29: 41-49.

[149] Chang HJ, Yoo BC, Kim SW, Lee BL, Kim WH (2007) Significance of PML and p53 protein as molecular prognostic markers of gallbladder carcinomas. *Pathol. Oncol. Res.* 13: 326-335.

[150] Baylin SB (2005) DNA methylation and gene silencing in cancer. *Nat. Clin. Pract. Oncol.* 2 Suppl 1: S4-11.

[151] Garcia P, Manterola C, Araya JC, Villaseca M, Guzman P, et al. (2009) Promoter methylation profile in preneoplastic and neoplastic gallbladder lesions. *Mol. Carcinog.* 48: 79-89.

[152] Riquelme E, Tang M, Baez S, Diaz A, Pruyas M, et al. (2007) Frequent epigenetic inactivation of chromosome 3p candidate tumor suppressor genes in gallbladder carcinoma. *Cancer Lett.* 250: 100-106.

[153] Roa JC, Anabalon L, Roa I, Melo A, Araya JC, et al. (2006) Promoter methylation profile in gallbladder cancer. *J. Gastroenterol.* 41: 269-275.

[154] Bakos E, Hegedus T, Hollo Z, Welker E, Tusnady GE, et al. (1996) Membrane topology and glycosylation of the human multidrug resistance-associated protein. *J. Biol. Chem.* 271: 12322-12326.

[155] Kast C, Gros P (1997) Topology mapping of the amino-terminal half of multidrug resistance-associated protein by epitope insertion and immunofluorescence. *J. Biol. Chem.* 272: 26479-26487.

[156] Kast C, Gros P (1998) Epitope insertion favors a six transmembrane domain model for the carboxy-terminal portion of the multidrug resistance-associated protein. *Biochemistry* 37: 2305-2313.

[157] Pradeep R, Kaushik SP, Sikora SS, Bhattacharya BN, Pandey CM, et al. (1995) Predictors of survival in patients with carcinoma of the gallbladder. *Cancer* 76: 1145-1149.

[158] Potocnik U, Glavac MR, Golouh R, Glavac D (2001) The role of P-glycoprotein (MDR1) polymorphisms and mutations in colorectal cancer. *Pflugers Arch.* 442: R182-183.

[159] Yang X, Uziely B, Groshen S, Lukas J, Israel V, et al. (1999) MDR1 gene expression in primary and advanced breast cancer. *Lab. Invest.* 79: 271-280.

[160] Tokunaga Y, Hosogi H, Hoppou T, Nakagami M, Tokuka A, et al. (2001) Effects of MDR1/P-glycoprotein expression on prognosis in advanced colorectal cancer after surgery. *Oncol. Rep.* 8: 815-819.

[161] Schondorf T, Kurbacher CM, Gohring UJ, Benz C, Becker M, et al. (2002) Induction of MDR1-gene expression by antineoplastic agents in ovarian cancer cell lines. *AntiCancer Res.* 22: 2199-2203.

[162] Schneider J, Gonzalez-Roces S, Pollan M, Lucas R, Tejerina A, et al. (2001) Expression of LRP and MDR1 in locally advanced breast cancer predicts axillary node invasion at the time of rescue mastectomy after induction chemotherapy. *Breast Cancer Res.* 3: 183-191.

[163] Lu Z, Kleeff J, Shrikhande S, Zimmermann T, Korc M, et al. (2000) Expression of the multidrug-resistance 1 (MDR1) gene and prognosis in human pancreatic cancer. *Pancreas* 21: 240-247.

[164] Tada Y, Wada M, Kuroiwa K, Kinugawa N, Harada T, et al. (2000) MDR1 gene overexpression and altered degree of methylation at the promoter region in bladder cancer during chemotherapeutic treatment. *Clin. Cancer Res.* 6: 4618-4627.

[165] Bentires-Alj M, Barbu V, Fillet M, Chariot A, Relic B, et al. (2003) NF-kappaB transcription factor induces drug resistance through MDR1 expression in cancer cells. *Oncogene* 22: 90-97.

[166] Kool M, van der Linden M, de Haas M, Scheffer GL, de Vree JM, et al. (1999) MRP3, an organic anion transporter able to transport anti-cancer drugs. *Proc. Natl. Acad. Sci. USA* 96: 6914-6919.

[167] Zeng H, Bain LJ, Belinsky MG, Kruh GD (1999) Expression of multidrug resistance protein-3 (multispecific organic anion transporter-D) in human embryonic kidney 293 cells confers resistance to anticancer agents. *Cancer Res.* 59: 5964-5967.

[168] Young LC, Campling BG, Voskoglou-Nomikos T, Cole SP, Deeley RG, et al. (1999) Expression of multidrug resistance protein-related genes in lung cancer: correlation with drug response. *Clin. Cancer Res.* 5: 673-680.

[169] Cao L, Duchrow M, Windhovel U, Kujath P, Bruch HP, et al. (1998) Expression of MDR1 mRNA and encoding P-glycoprotein in archival formalin-fixed paraffin-embedded gall bladder cancer tissues. *Eur. J. Cancer* 34: 1612-1617.

[170] Fojo AT, Ueda K, Slamon DJ, Poplack DG, Gottesman MM, et al. (1987) Expression of a multidrug-resistance gene in human tumors and tissues. *Proc. Natl. Acad. Sci. USA* 84: 265-269.

[171] Yu LF, Wu YL (1998) Clinical relationship of study advances between multidrug gene and digestive tumor. *WCJD* 6: 915-916.

[172] Cao L, Peng S, Duchrow M (1999) [Expression of P-glycoprotein in benign and malignant gallbladder neoplasms]. Zhonghua Zhong Liu Za Zhi 21: 119-121.

[173] Wang J, Dou KF, Zhao R (2004) [Expression of P62 in gallbladder carcinoma tissues and its correlation with angiogenesis]. Xi Bao Yu Fen Zi Mian Yi Xue Za Zhi 20: 461-464.

[174] Tian Y, Zhu LL, Guo RX, Fan CF (2003) Correlation of P-glycoprotein expression with poor vascularization in human gallbladder carcinomas. *World J. Gastroenterol.* 9: 2817-2820.

[175] Dean, M., A. Rzhetsky, and R. Allikmets, The human ATP-binding cassette (ABC) transporter superfamily. Genome Res, 2001. **11**(7): p. 1156-66.

[176] Vasiliou, V., K. Vasiliou, and D.W. Nebert, Human ATP-binding cassette (ABC) transporter family. Hum Genomics, 2009. **3**(3): p. 281-90.

[177] Rost, D., et al., Expression and localization of the multidrug resistance proteins MRP2 and MRP3 in human gallbladder epithelia. Gastroenterology, 2001. 121(5): p. 1203-8.

[178] Aust, S., et al., Subcellular localization of the ABCG2 transporter in normal and malignant human gallbladder epithelium. Lab Invest, 2004. 84(8): p. 1024-36

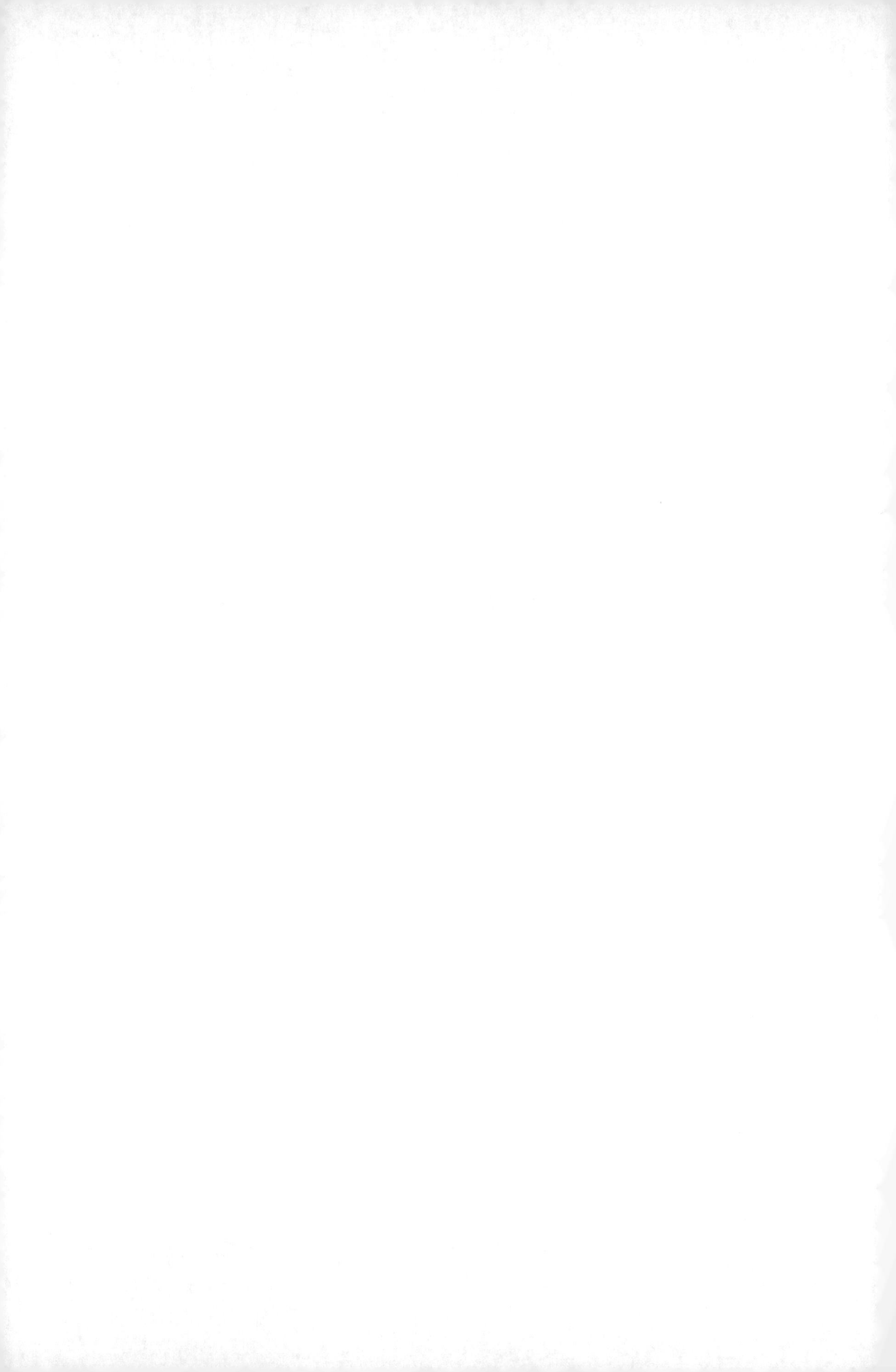

In: Field Cancerization: Basic Science and Clinical Applications ISBN 978-1-61761-006-6
Editor: Gabriel D. Dakubo

Chapter 14

Field Cancerization in Intraductal Papillary Mucinous Neoplasia of the Pancreas

Satoshi Tanno and Takeshi Obara

Abstract

Intraductal papillary mucinous neoplasm of the pancreas (IPMN) is increasingly recognized in clinical practice. They represent a unique clinicopathologic entity that is characterized by mucin production, cystic dilation of the pancreatic ducts, and intraductal papillary growth. Its characteristic biologic behavior includes a slow-growing and less aggressive nature with a favorable prognosis after patients undergo surgery compared with common pancreatic cancer. One of the important clinicopathologic and molecular features of IPMN is that multifocal occurrence of IPMN has been observed in the same pancreas and genetic heterogeneity in an individual IPMN has been reported. Furthermore, common pancreatic cancers are sometimes found distant from an IPMN. Recent molecular evidence supports the hypothesis that field cancerization or field defect exists in the pancreas with IPMN. Most of IPMNs are polyclonal and/or oligoclonal in origin, i.e., IPMNs may originate from molecularly distinct precursor lesions.

14.1. Introduction

The concept of field cancerization introduced by Slaughter et al. [1] has been invoked to explain the occurrence of multiple, independent, primary neoplasms. Molecular evidence for field cancerization and clonality has been studied extensively using a molecular marker, such as *p53* gene mutations, K-*ras* gene mutations, loss of heterozygosity, and X-chromosome inactivation (XCI) analysis in patients with head and neck carcinoma,[2,3,4] aerodigestive tract carcinoma,[5,6] breast carcinoma,[7] esophageal carcinoma,[8,9] bladder carcinoma [10], and pancreas [11,12].

Intraductal papillary-mucinous neoplasm of the pancreas (IPMN) is a relatively new tumor entity that is characterized as intraductal papillary growths of neoplastic and mucin-producing columnar cells [13,14,15,16,17,18,19,20]. In the past, they had been reported under various names, such as papillary carcinoma, ductectatic mucinous cystadenoma and mucin-producing tumor. The tumor shows variable degrees of mucin secretion, cystic dilatation and cytoarchitectural atypia. Compared with pancreatic ductal adenocarcinoma (pancreatic cancer), IPMN is a slow-growing tumor with a favorable prognosis after patients undergo surgery [16,18,19].

One of the important clinicopathologic and molecular features of IPMN is that multifocal occurrence of IPMNs has been observed in the same pancreas [21,22,23,24] and genetic heterogeneity in an individual IPMN has been reported [25]. These observations raise the questions of whether IPMNs may arise monoclonally from a single precursor cell with subsequent clonal expansion and metastasize or seed through pancreatic ducts to form secondary tumors in the same pancreas or whether there is a *field defect* that causes multiple primary neoplastic lesions.

This chapter describes recent findings of field cancerization in pancreatic tissues, especially focusing on IPMN, and sheds light on a significant role of field defects in the carcinogenesis in IPMN.

14.2. Multifocal Occurrence of Intraductal Papillary Mucinous Neoplasm of the Pancreas

Tumor multifocality of IPMN ranges from 9.8% to 32% (figure 14-1A, B) [21,22,23,24], and recurrences after surgical resection have been reported [22,23,24]. A study of IPMN treated with a total pancreatectomy showed multifocal discontinuous sites of dysplasia within the pancreatic ducts [26]. These facts may represent a *field defect* [10] in the multicentric, independent development of IPMNs.

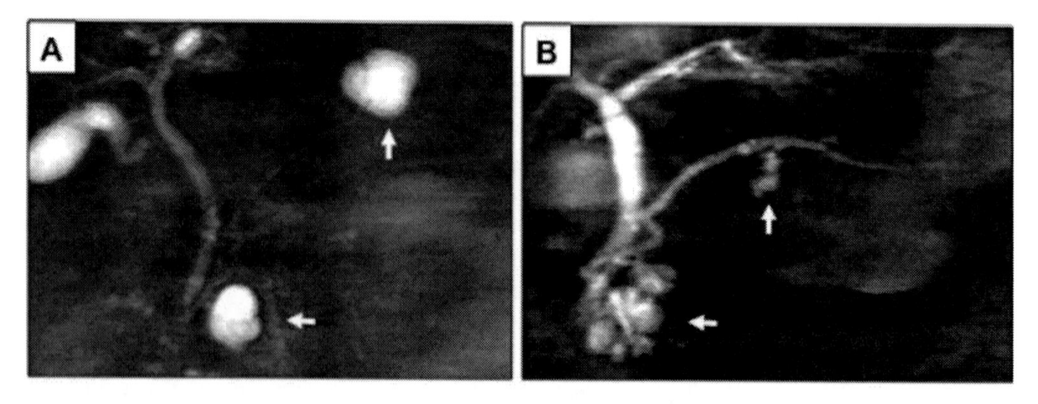

Figure 14.1. Multifocal occurrence of IPMN. Magnetic resonance cholangiopancreatography shows the multiplicity of IPMN in head and tail of the pancreas (A), and in head and body of the pancreas (B).

In addition, pancreatic cancers are sometimes found distant from an IPMN in about 3.3% to 9.2% of cases [27,28,29]. Conversely, small IPMNs have been detected incidentally in pancreata resected for pancreatic cancers [30]. There have also been reports of pancreatic cancers developing in the remnant pancreas several years after the resection of IPMN [27,31]. These observations may support the hypothesis that a *field defect* that causes multiple primary neoplastic lesions exists in pancreata harboring IPMN.

14.3. K-*ras* Codon 12 Mutations in Ductal Hyperplasia of the Pancreas with Intraductal Papillary Mucinous Neoplasm of the Pancreas

An assessment of field cancerization requires a good clonal marker to investigate and to qualify as a molecular marker: Such an alteration should 1) occur very early in the development of the lesion, 2) be maintained during progression of the lesion, 3) exhibit sufficient variability, and 4) be applicable in the majority of the lesions [32,33].

K-*ras* oncogene (chromosome 12p) is activated by point mutations in approximately 90% of pancreatic cancers, and these mutations involve codons 12 (most commonly), 13, and 61 [34]. K-*ras* codon 12 mutations occur frequently in approximately 13-83% of ductal hyperplasia [12,33,35,36,37,38,39,40,41]. Recent studies demonstrated a high prevalence of K-*ras* codon 12 mutations in ductal hyperplasia of patients with pancreatic cancers [12,42] and chronic pancreatitis [36]. Likewise, K-*ras* mutations are found frequently in 30-100% of IPMNs [35,36,37,38,39,40]. Because it is believed that K-*ras* mutation is a stable tumor marker throughout carcinogenesis [43,44], K-*ras* mutation is a good marker to investigate field cancerization of IPMN.

It has been reported that a stepwise increase in the frequency of K-*ras* codon 12 mutations are correlated with the stage of neoplastic evolution to carcinoma [33]. Furthermore, K-*ras* mutations of ductal hyperplasia were identified frequently in patients who had a disease- free pancreas [37,41]. Thus, K-*ras* mutations occur very early in ductal hyperplasia, which is regarded as a precursor lesion of pancreatic cancers [12,36,37,42,45]. Although K-*ras* mutations are found in ductal hyperplasias and probably play an important role in pancreatic carcinogenesis, it also has been suggested that K-*ras* mutations have a limited role and that only a small fraction of hyperplastic lesions with mutated K-*ras* progresses to cancer (< 1%) [37,42,46]. Nevertheless, K-*ras* mutation is an early key event leading to later genetic alterations, including inactivation of the *p16* tumor-suppressor gene [42,45].

14.4. Multiple, Distinct K-*ras* codon 12 Mutations in Intraductal Papillary Mucinous Neoplasm of the Pancreas

Because K-*ras* mutations are very early events in pancreatic ductal hyperplasia, a precursor lesion of IPMN, K-*ras* mutations can be used as a clonal markers to investigate field cancerization and clonality in the development of IPMNs as well as in pancreatic cancer. If multiple, different hyperplasias in the same pancreas have distinct K-*ras* mutation types, these hyperplasias are multicentric and independent lesions, which suggests field cancerization or field defect whereby carcinogenic insults result in the independent transformation of different epithelial cells [10].

Recent research indicated that multiple distinct K-*ras* codon 12 mutations were identified among different hyperplasias in 47-50% of patients with pancreatic cancer [12,42], and 6-12% of patients with pancreatic cancer had multiple, distinct mutations [42,47]. These data add the molecular support for field cancerization, which is compatible with multiple, independent, transforming events in each lesion occurring in the same pancreas.

Z'graggen et al. clearly demonstrated a stepwise increase in the incidence of K-*ras* mutations in the evolution of IPMN, suggesting a field defect [33]. In their study, multiple samples were microdissected from various lesions of different histologic grades. A recent study in which extensive multiple sampling from hyperplasia and IPMN was performed by Matsubayashi et al. demonstrated that *K-ras* mutations in hyperplasia were recognized in 11 of 12 patients with IPMNs (92%), and multiple *K-ras* mutations were identified in 5 of 11 patients with hyperplasia (45%) [12]. Izawa et al. reported that K-ras mutation is a very early event in a hyperplasia-adenoma-carcinoma sequence in the evolution of IPMN and that the incidence of K-ras mutations increases with pathologic atypia [11]. In their study, K-ras mutations were found in hyperplasia in 62% of patients with IPMNs, 65% of whom had multiple, distinct mutations in different hyperplasias. These studies demonstrate molecular evidence for field cancerization or field defect in the pancreas bearing IPMN, and suggest that patients with IPMN are at risk for synchronous and/or metachronous, multiple tumors before and after surgery, which may affect the current clinical approach [23,24,33].

14.5. Clonality and Field Cancerization of Intraductal Papillary Mucinous Neoplasm of the Pancreas

Tumor clonality is a fundamental issue directly relevant to tumorigenesis. Neoplastic tissues are believed to be comprised of a monoclonal cell population. However, some neoplasms, such as colon adenoma in patients with familial adenomatous polyposis [48], pancreatic endocrine tumors [49], and fibroadenoma of the breast [50], seem to be polyclonal in origin.

An assessment of clonality requires a good clonal maker based on genetic alterations [32,51]. The clonality of various tumors has been inferred using a polymerase chain reaction (PCR)-based assay for nonrandom X-chromosome inactivation (XCI) at the human androgen receptor gene locus (*HUMARA*) in female patients. The *HUMARA* assay, among other X-linked probes, has yielded superior results [52,53,54,55,56].

Clonal analyses of tumors yield conflicting results: Most indicate monoclonality, and some indicate polyclonality. Polyclonality is attributable either to contamination with stromal cells or to lesions comprised of more than one monoclonal, single tumor cell population [57,58]. In order to minimize contamination for clonality analysis, laser capture microdissection (LCM), a novel membrane-based microdissection technique, is useful [59,60]. Both a precise microdissection and a highly sensitive PCR technique enables analysis of multiple, different foci within each IPMN as well as epithelial cells from small ductal lesions.

Among the clonal markers applicable to IPMN, a combination of K-*ras* mutation analysis and the *HUMARA* assay has a greater impact on clonality analysis than either one used alone. Each method has some drawbacks: K-*ras* mutation analysis may underestimate the prevalence of different clones, because certain preferential mutation types occur at a relatively high frequency, resulting in the same mutation type in lesions that are probably of different clonal origin. The *HUMARA* assay is applicable only to female patients, and the results from approximately 10% female patients are uninformative.

If a given IPMN has multiple different mutations at K-*ras* codon 12, then the IPMN should be of polyclonal and/or oligoclonal origin, a mixture of daughter cells derived from two or more progenitor cells independently initiated by K-*ras* activation [61]. Izawa et al. have analyzed the clonality of IPMN using LCM with a combination of *HUMARA* assay and K-*ras* analysis [11]. In accordance with field cancerization in IPMN, most of IPMNs are polyclonal and/or oligoclonal, resulting from the fusion of separate lesions. The presence of intratumoral heterogeneity of K-*ras* mutations is evidentiary of polyclonal and/or oligoclonal origin rather than genetic heterogeneity occurring during tumor progression. *HUMARA* analysis of informative tumors showed that most of IPMNs were polyclonal and/or oligoclonal. Combining these data with the K-*ras* mutation status demonstrate that 80% of IPMNs are polyclonal and/or oligoclonal in origin. The evidence suggests that IPMNs are frequently polyclonal and/or oligoclonal. Most individual IPMNs can be considered a result of the fusion of two or more independent monoclonal cell populations that arose as a consequence of field cancerization.

Conclusion

Clonality analysis using a combination of K-*ras* codon 12 mutation and *HUMARA* analysis allows the identification of frequent, multiple, distinct mutations in different ductal hyperplasias from the same pancreas with IPMN. These data support the hypothesis that field cancerization or field defect exists in the pancreas with IPMN. Polyclonal and/or oligoclonal IPMN arises as a consequence of the fusion of two or more monoclonal neoplastic cell populations of independent origin.

References

[1] Slaughter DP, Southwick HW, Smejkal W (1953) Field cancerization in oral stratified squamous epithelium; clinical implications of multicentric origin. *Cancer* 6: 963-968.

[2] Kanjilal S, Strom SS, Clayman GL, Weber RS, el-Naggar AK, et al. (1995) p53 mutations in nonmelanoma skin cancer of the head and neck: molecular evidence for field cancerization. *Cancer Res.* 55: 3604-3609.

[3] Ren ZP, Hedrum A, Ponten F, Nister M, Ahmadian A, et al. (1996) Human epidermal cancer and accompanying precursors have identical p53 mutations different from p53

mutations in adjacent areas of clonally expanded non-neoplastic keratinocytes. *Oncogene* 12: 765-773.
[4] Lydiatt WM, Anderson PE, Bazzana T, Casale M, Hughes CJ, et al. (1998) Molecular support for field cancerization in the head and neck. *Cancer* 82: 1376-1380.
[5] Chung KY, Mukhopadhyay T, Kim J, Casson A, Ro JY, et al. (1993) Discordant p53 gene mutations in primary head and neck cancers and corresponding second primary cancers of the upper aerodigestive tract. *Cancer Res.* 53: 1676-1683.
[6] Sozzi G, Miozzo M, Pastorino U, Pilotti S, Donghi R, et al. (1995) Genetic evidence for an independent origin of multiple preneoplastic and neoplastic lung lesions. *Cancer Res.* 55: 135-140.
[7] Kuukasjarvi T, Karhu R, Tanner M, Kahkonen M, Schaffer A, et al. (1997) Genetic heterogeneity and clonal evolution underlying development of asynchronous metastasis in human breast cancer. *Cancer Res.* 57: 1597-1604.
[8] Wang LD, Zhou Q, Hong JY, Qiu SL, Yang CS (1996) p53 protein accumulation and gene mutations in multifocal esophageal precancerous lesions from symptom free subjects in a high incidence area for esophageal carcinoma in Henan, China. *Cancer* 77: 1244-1249.
[9] Tian D, Feng Z, Hanley NM, Setzer RW, Mumford JL, et al. (1998) Multifocal accumulation of p53 protein in esophageal carcinoma: evidence for field cancerization. *Int. J. Cancer* 78: 568-575.
[10] Sidransky D, Frost P, Von Eschenbach A, Oyasu R, Preisinger AC, et al. (1992) Clonal origin bladder cancer. *N. Engl. J. Med.* 326: 737-740.
[11] Izawa T, Obara T, Tanno S, Mizukami Y, Yanagawa N, et al. (2001) Clonality and field cancerization in intraductal papillary-mucinous tumors of the pancreas. *Cancer* 92: 1807-1817.
[12] Matsubayashi H, Watanabe H, Yamaguchi T, Ajioka Y, Nishikura K, et al. (1999) Multiple K-ras mutations in hyperplasia and carcinoma in cases of human pancreatic carcinoma. *Jpn J. Cancer Res.* 90: 841-848.
[13] Loftus EV, Jr., Olivares-Pakzad BA, Batts KP, Adkins MC, Stephens DH, et al. (1996) Intraductal papillary-mucinous tumors of the pancreas: clinicopathologic features, outcome, and nomenclature. Members of the Pancreas Clinic, and Pancreatic Surgeons of Mayo Clinic. *Gastroenterology* 110: 1909-1918.
[14] Azar C, Van de Stadt J, Rickaert F, Deviere M, Baize M, et al. (1996) Intraductal papillary mucinous tumours of the pancreas. Clinical and therapeutic issues in 32 patients. *Gut* 39: 457-464.
[15] Rivera JA, Fernandez-del Castillo C, Pins M, Compton CC, Lewandrowski KB, et al. (1997) Pancreatic mucinous ductal ectasia and intraductal papillary neoplasms. A single malignant clinicopathologic entity. *Ann. Surg.* 225: 637-644; discussion 644-636.
[16] Morohoshi T, Kanda M, Asanuma K, Kloppel G (1989) Intraductal papillary neoplasms of the pancreas. A clinicopathologic study of six patients. *Cancer* 64: 1329-1335.
[17] Rickaert F, Cremer M, Deviere J, Tavares L, Lambilliotte JP, et al. (1991) Intraductal mucin-hypersecreting neoplasms of the pancreas. A clinicopathologic study of eight patients. *Gastroenterology* 101: 512-519.
[18] Obara T, Maguchi H, Saitoh Y, Ura H, Koike Y, et al. (1991) Mucin-producing tumor of the pancreas: a unique clinical entity. *Am. J. Gastroenterol.* 86: 1619-1625.

[19] Yamada M, Kozuka S, Yamao K, Nakazawa S, Naitoh Y, et al. (1991) Mucin-producing tumor of the pancreas. *Cancer* 68: 159-168.

[20] Tanno S, Nakano Y, Nishikawa T, Nakamura K, Sasajima J, et al. (2008) Natural history of branch duct intraductal papillary-mucinous neoplasms of the pancreas without mural nodules: long-term follow-up results. *Gut* 57: 339-343.

[21] Rodriguez JR, Salvia R, Crippa S, Warshaw AL, Bassi C, et al. (2007) Branch-duct intraductal papillary mucinous neoplasms: observations in 145 patients who underwent resection. *Gastroenterology* 133: 72-79; quiz 309-310.

[22] Obara T, Saitoh Y, Maguchi H, Ura H, Kitazawa S, et al. (1992) Multicentric development of pancreatic intraductal carcinoma through atypical papillary hyperplasia. *Hum. Pathol.* 23: 82-85.

[23] Inagaki M, Maguchi M, Kino S, Obara M, Ishizaki A, et al. (1999) Mucin-producing tumors of the pancreas: clinicopathological features, surgical treatment, and outcome. *J. Hepatobiliary Pancreat Surg.* 6: 281-285.

[24] Fujii T, Obara T, Maguchi H, Tanno S, Ura H, et al. (1996) Clinicopathologic study of multiple muci-producing tumors of the pancreas: multicentric development of carcinoma through atypical hyperplasia. *J. Jpn Pancreat. Soc.* 11: 344-352.

[25] Fujii H, Inagaki M, Kasai S, Miyokawa N, Tokusashi Y, et al. (1997) Genetic progression and heterogeneity in intraductal papillary-mucinous neoplasms of the pancreas. *Am. J. Pathol.* 151: 1447-1454.

[26] Bendix Holme J, Jacobsen N, Rokkjaer M, Kruse A (2001) Total pancreatectomy in six patients with intraductal papillary mucinous tumour of the pancreas: the treatment of choice. *HPB* (Oxford) 3: 257-262.

[27] Sohn TA, Yeo CJ, Cameron JL, Iacobuzio-Donahue CA, Hruban RH, et al. (2001) Intraductal papillary mucinous neoplasms of the pancreas: an increasingly recognized clinicopathologic entity. *Ann. Surg.* 234: 313-321.

[28] Yamaguchi K, Ohuchida J, Ohtsuka T, Nakano K, Tanaka M (2002) Intraductal papillary-mucinous tumor of the pancreas concomitant with ductal carcinoma of the pancreas. *Pancreatology* 2: 484-490.

[29] Tada M, Kawabe T, Arizumi M, Togawa O, Matsubara S, et al. (2006) Pancreatic cancer in patients with pancreatic cystic lesions: a prospective study in 197 patients. *Clin. Gastroenterol Hepatol.* 4: 1265-1270.

[30] Adsay NV (2003) The "new kid on the block": Intraductal papillary mucinous neoplasms of the pancreas: current concepts and controversies. *Surgery* 133: 459-463.

[31] Komori T, Ishikawa O, Ohigashi H, Yamada T, Sasaki Y, et al. (2002) Invasive ductal adenocarcinoma of the remnant pancreatic body 9 years after resection of an intraductal papillary-mucinous carcinoma of the pancreatic head: a case report and comparison of DNA sequence in K-ras gene mutation. *Jpn J. Clin. Oncol.* 32: 146-151.

[32] van Oijen MG, Leppers Vd Straat FG, Tilanus MG, Slootweg PJ (2000) The origins of multiple squamous cell carcinomas in the aerodigestive tract. *Cancer* 88: 884-893.

[33] Z'Graggen K, Rivera JA, Compton CC, Pins M, Werner J, et al. (1997) Prevalence of activating K-ras mutations in the evolutionary stages of neoplasia in intraductal papillary mucinous tumors of the pancreas. *Ann. Surg.* 226: 491-498; discussion 498-500.

[34] Caldas C, Kern SE (1995) K-ras mutation and pancreatic adenocarcinoma. *Int. J. Pancreatol.* 18: 1-6.

[35] Yanagisawa A, Kato Y, Ohtake K, Kitagawa T, Ohashi K, et al. (1991) c-Ki-ras point mutations in ductectatic-type mucinous cystic neoplasms of the pancreas. *Jpn J. Cancer Res*. 82: 1057-1060.

[36] Yanagisawa A, Ohtake K, Ohashi K, Hori M, Kitagawa T, et al. (1993) Frequent c-Ki-ras oncogene activation in mucous cell hyperplasias of pancreas suffering from chronic inflammation. *Cancer Res*. 53: 953-956.

[37] Tada M, Ohashi M, Shiratori Y, Okudaira T, Komatsu Y, et al. (1996) Analysis of K-ras gene mutation in hyperplastic duct cells of the pancreas without pancreatic disease. *Gastroenterology* 110: 227-231.

[38] Tada M, Omata M, Ohto M (1991) Ras gene mutations in intraductal papillary neoplasms of the pancreas. Analysis in five cases. *Cancer* 67: 634-637.

[39] Sessa F, Solcia E, Capella C, Bonato M, Scarpa A, et al. (1994) Intraductal papillary-mucinous tumours represent a distinct group of pancreatic neoplasms: an investigation of tumour cell differentiation and K-ras, p53 and c-erbB-2 abnormalities in 26 patients. *Virchows Arch.* 425: 357-367.

[40] Hoshi T, Imai M, Ogawa K (1994) Frequent K-ras mutations and absence of p53 mutations in mucin-producing tumors of the pancreas. *J. Surg. Oncol.* 55: 84-91.

[41] Terhune PG, Phifer DM, Tosteson TD, Longnecker DS (1998) K-ras mutation in focal proliferative lesions of human pancreas. *Cancer Epidemiol. Biomarkers Prev.* 7: 515-521.

[42] Moskaluk CA, Hruban RH, Kern SE (1997) p16 and K-ras gene mutations in the intraductal precursors of human pancreatic adenocarcinoma. *Cancer Res*. 57: 2140-2143.

[43] Losi L, Benhattar J, Costa J (1992) Stability of K-ras mutations throughout the natural history of human colorectal cancer. *Eur. J. Cancer* 28A: 1115-1120.

[44] Luttges J, Schlehe B, Menke MA, Vogel I, Henne-Bruns D, et al. (1999) The K-ras mutation pattern in pancreatic ductal adenocarcinoma usually is identical to that in associated normal, hyperplastic, and metaplastic ductal epithelium. *Cancer* 85: 1703-1710.

[45] Wilentz RE, Geradts J, Maynard R, Offerhaus GJ, Kang M, et al. (1998) Inactivation of the p16 (INK4A) tumor-suppressor gene in pancreatic duct lesions: loss of intranuclear expression. *Cancer Res.* 58: 4740-4744.

[46] Luttges J, Reinecke-Luthge A, Mollmann B, Menke MA, Clemens A, et al. (1999) Duct changes and K-ras mutations in the disease-free pancreas: analysis of type, age relation and spatial distribution. *Virchows. Arch.* 435: 461-468.

[47] Motojima K, Urano T, Nagata Y, Shiku H, Tsurifune T, et al. (1993) Detection of point mutations in the Kirsten-ras oncogene provides evidence for the multicentricity of pancreatic carcinoma. *Ann. Surg.* 217: 138-143.

[48] Novelli MR, Williamson JA, Tomlinson IP, Elia G, Hodgson SV, et al. (1996) Polyclonal origin of colonic adenomas in an XO/XY patient with FAP. *Science* 272: 1187-1190.

[49] Perren A, Roth J, Muletta-Feurer S, Saremaslani P, Speel EJ, et al. (1998) Clonal analysis of sporadic pancreatic endocrine tumours. *J. Pathol.* 186: 363-371.

[50] Noguchi S, Motomura K, Inaji H, Imaoka S, Koyama H (1993) Clonal analysis of fibroadenoma and phyllodes tumor of the breast. *Cancer Res*. 53: 4071-4074.

[51] Wainscoat JS, Fey MF (1990) Assessment of clonality in human tumors: a review. *Cancer Res*. 50: 1355-1360.

[52] Allen RC, Zoghbi HY, Moseley AB, Rosenblatt HM, Belmont JW (1992) Methylation of HpaII and HhaI sites near the polymorphic CAG repeat in the human androgen-receptor gene correlates with X chromosome inactivation. *Am. J. Hum. Genet.* 51: 1229-1239.

[53] Busque L, Gilliland DG (1993) Clonal evolution in acute myeloid leukemia. *Blood* 82: 337-342.

[54] Willman CL, Busque L, Griffith BB, Favara BE, McClain KL, et al. (1994) Langerhans'-cell histiocytosis (histiocytosis X)--a clonal proliferative disease. *N. Engl. J. Med*. 331: 154-160.

[55] Nomura S, Kaminishi M, Sugiyama K, Oohara T, Esumi H (1996) Clonal analysis of isolated single fundic and pyloric gland of stomach using X-linked polymorphism. *Biochem. Biophys. Res. Commun.* 226: 385-390.

[56] Wu CD, Wickert RS, Williamson JE, Sun NC, Brynes RK, et al. (1999) Using fluorescence-based human androgen receptor gene assay to analyze the clonality of microdissected dendritic cell tumors. *Am. J. Clin. Pathol.* 111: 105-110.

[57] Farber E (1997) Monoclonal and polyclonal development of digestive tract tumors in chimeric mice. *Jpn J. Cancer Res.* 88: inside front cover.

[58] Garcia SB, Park HS, Novelli M, Wright NA (1999) Field cancerization, clonality, and epithelial stem cells: the spread of mutated clones in epithelial sheets. *J. Pathol.* 187: 61-81.

[59] Emmert-Buck MR, Bonner RF, Smith PD, Chuaqui RF, Zhuang Z, et al. (1996) Laser capture microdissection. *Science* 274: 998-1001.

[60] Sirivatanauksorn Y, Sirivatanauksorn V, Bhattacharya S, Davidson BR, Dhillon AP, et al. (1999) Evolution of genetic abnormalities in hepatocellular carcinomas demonstrated by DNA fingerprinting. *J. Pathol.* 189: 344-350.

[61] Enomoto T, Fujita M, Inoue M, Tanizawa O, Nomura T, et al. (1994) Analysis of clonality by amplification of short tandem repeats. Carcinomas of the female reproductive tract. *Diagn. Mol. Pathol.* 3: 292-297.

In: Field Cancerization: Basic Science and Clinical Applications ISBN 978-1-61761-006-6
Editor: Gabriel D. Dakubo

Chapter 15

Field Cancerization in Urothelial Carcinomas of the Upper Urinary Tract

Maximilian Burger and Arndt Hartmann

15.1. Introduction

The urinary tract is comprised of cavitary organs collecting, transporting and storing urine. The portion of the urinary tract from the renal calices to the bladder outlet is lined with urothelium. The upper urinary tract (i.e., the renal pelvis and the ureter) is lined with urothelium that demonstrate histological features similar to the urothelium of the urinary bladder. The upper urinary tract represents roughly 10% of the surface urinary tract.

Tumours of the upper urinary tract represent a minority of all urinary tract carcinomas. Histological resemblance and clinical patterns of tumor recurrence in the lower and the upper urinary tract suggest a relationship between the entities, while epidemiological relation with the hereditary non-polyposis colorectal cancer (HNPCC)-syndrome is unique to upper urinary tract neoplasia, suggesting upper urinary tract tumours do not merely comprise a subset of urothelial cancer. These observations have led to the detection of distinct molecular pathways in the tumorigenesis of upper versus lower tract neoplasms. In this chapter we review current evidence of field cancerization in urothelial carcinomas of the upper urinary tract and discuss clinical implications of these findings.

15.2. Urothelial Neoplasms of the Upper Urinary Tract

Malignant urothelial neoplasms of the upper urinary tract are relatively rare and account for approximately 8% of all urinary tract tumors [1]. These neoplasms derive from the urothelial lining of the ureter and renal pelvis and demonstrate histological features similar to urothelial cancer of the urinary bladder [2]. As has been observed in urothelial cancer of the bladder, smoking and occupational exposures to arylamines are important etiological factors accounting for more than half of the cases [3]. The fraction of tumors arising in the upper urinary tract of all urinary carcinomas is roughly equivalent to the fraction of the surface of the upper urinary tract with reference to the entire urinary tract. There is a certain lifetime risk of patients with cancer of the urinary bladder to develop neoplasms of the upper urinary tract and vice versa, although no consistent figures are given in the literature. Accordingly neoplasms of the upper urinary tract and the urinary bladder have long been viewed as one tumour entity.

15.3. Synchronous and Metachronous Tumours of the Upper Urinary Tract

Simultaneous (i.e., synchronous or metachronous) development of multifocal tumours within the urinary tract is an outstanding feature of this tumour entity, and one of the major clinical challenges in the management of this disease. Following surgical removal of one tumor in any location within the urinary tract, close and constant surveillance of the entire system is warranted. Not even radical removal of the bladder or one complete reno-ureteral unit defies development of novel urothelial cancers in the remaining parts [4,5]. Those subsequent tumours may feature identical or variable histological features [6,7].

The frequent cancer recurrences demonstrate a certain pattern, as patients with upper urinary tract tumors have a roughly 40% significant risk of developing subsequent bladder tumors following nephroureterectomy [8,9]. In contrast the same patients demonstrate a risk of tumor occurrence in the opposite reno-ureteral unit at a mere 2–6% rate [10,9]. In addition patients with initial tumors of the bladder subsequently develop upper urinary tract tumours in up to just 2% [11].

15.4. Mechanisms of Multifocal Urothelial Tumor Development: Importance of Both Monoclonality and Field Cancerization

The distinct nature of multifocal and frequently recurrent occurrence of cancers at spatially separated locations in the urinary tract has led to two hypothetical explanation of this phenomenon. On the one hand, secondary tumors are seen as originating from one clone, dubbed *monoclonality hypothesis*, while on the other hand, the continuous or perpetual action of oncogenic influences might spur de novo tumorigenesis at different locations and points in time, dubbed *field-cancerization hypothesis* [12]).

The former theory proposes all tumors to descend from one malignant cell that proliferate and spread to various locations to form subsequent neoplasias. This theory fits well with the observation of downstream secondary tumor formation following neoplasias in the upper urinary tract. Besides this, intraluminal migration within the urothelial lining is discussed as well [12]. The latter theory proposes secondary tumors to develop under the ongoing influence of various mutational agents effective throughout the urinary tract, such that subsequent tumors often are genetically different from the initial lesions. This theory fits well with the observation of tumors predominantly found at locations of prolonged exposure to urine, e.g. dilated upper urinary tracts, diverticula of the urinary bladder and in the lower half of the bladder.

Currently some recurrent tumors are found to be strictly monoclonal in analogy to the former theory, which is thought to be especially true for low grade and stage neoplasias, while especially high grade and stage tumors seem to be of heterogeneous clonal origin in analogy to the latter theory. It is noteworthy however, that those two basic mechanisms have been recognized to be present simultaneously, and that clones from one origin undergo further deteriorations under the perpetual influence of ongoing exposure to carcinogens [12].

In the course of this debate, it has been suggested by recent evidence that at least a portion of carcinomas of the upper urinary tract does not merely comprise a subunit of urothelial cancer. Epidemiological studies have shown that urothelial carcinomas of the upper urinary tract are part of the extracolonic tumor spectrum in patients with the HNPCC-syndrome. A variety of non-colonic cancers are found within this syndrome, e.g. up to 10% of patients are prone to develop endometrial malignancies. The relation of tumors of the upper urinary tract and the HNPCC-syndrome is quite remarkable, as the relative risk of urothelial carcinoma of the ureter and the renal pelvis is 21-fold and 14-fold elevated in HNPCC-patients, respectively. Furthermore the median age of onset has been reported to occur roughly 15 years earlier than in upper urinary tract cancers unrelated to the HNPCC-syndromes [13]. Among all tumors regarded as part of the HNPCC spectrum, urothelial carcinoma of the upper urinary tract rank third following colon and endometrial cancers [14,15]. This observation has given rise to the notion that a genetic defect may underlie the genesis of this tumor entity. Indeed colorectal tumors of the HNPCC type feature distinct molecular characteristics that are different from those of non-HNPCC colorectal carcinomas [16]. In the majority of patients with HNPCC, an alteration of mismatch repair (MMR) genes has been recognized as the genetic defect leading to the accumulation of mutations in short tandem repeat sequences, named microsatellites. The said phenomenon has been dubbed microsatellite instability accordingly [17,18,19,20].

According to the epidemiological data from recent studies that demonstrate more frequently molecular mechanisms that are specific to the HNPCC-syndrome, it raises the possibility that upper urinary tract tumors develop through different molecular mechanisms than tumors of the urinary bladder [21,22]. Genomic instability similar to HNPCC-related colonic cancers in urothelial carcinoma of the upper urinary tract was first reported by Takahash et al who described high rates of microsatellite instability in multifocal tumors of the upper and lower urinary tract [23]. These findings were not interpreted as suggesting a distinct molecular pathway in upper urinary tract neoplasia. Hartmann et al initially described prominent rates of microsatellite instability exceeding 20% of all tumors to be a distinct trait in the upper urinary tract [24, 25]. Catto and co-workers compared the rates of these parameters of genetic instability in the upper versus the lower urinary tract. This work was the first to focus on the so-called Bethesda panel established for the diagnosis of HNPCC syndrome in colonic tumors [21,26]. They found microsatellite instability to be present in 13% compared to just 1% of upper and lower urinary tract urothelial carcinomas, respectively. Despite the findings of lower rates in subsequent series reporting less than 10% and 5%, respectively, the tendency for microsatellite instability to be uniquely found in upper urothelial tract tumors as compared to bladder tumors is undisputed [27,28,29,22].

Taking the clinical evidence into account, both the field effect and the seeding effect seem to be relevant in the joint development of upper and lower urinary tract tumors. Later recurrences are often seen downstream from the initial tumor location and patients with upper urinary tract tumors frequently demonstrate subsequent tumors in downstream locations, while cancer of the urinary bladder is decisively less likely to be followed by neoplasm of the ureter and renal pelvis [30,31]. However many patients with upper urinary tract tumors never develop recurrence in the urinary bladder. Thus, molecular evidence supports field effect to be dominant. The work by Takahashi et al found simultaneous and consecutive urothelial carcinomas of the bladder and the upper urinary tract tumors that are derived from multiple clones to outnumber multifocal lesions stemming from one single clone [23].

Hafner and co-workers studied 94 synchronous or metachronous multifocal tumors from 19 patients with urothelial tumors in both the upper and lower urinary tract. Clonality of these multifocal tumors was determined by analysing loss of heterozygosity (LOH), a common methodology in bladder cancer research. Eight markers on chromosome 9 and one marker on 17p13 (*p53* locus) were used. In addition microsatellite instability was analysed by assessing six respective loci, and furthermore immunohistochemical protein expression of MSH2 was examined. In addition, the p53 gene was sequenced. The distinctive pattern of deletion showed monoclonality of multifocal tumors in nine of 19 patients studied. In contrast, four patients demonstrated at least two tumor clones with distinct genetic alterations in the ureter and renal pelvis. The authors thus concluded that some multifocal urothelial carcinomas are frequently monoclonal, whereas others are oligoclonal. Thus these data were the first to clearly suggest field cancerization to be relevant in addition to intraluminal tumor cell seeding [12].

In 2001 Takahashi and co-workers compared the genetic alteration pattern in 34 multifocal tumors in 15 patients with upper urinary tract and subsequent tumors occurring in the urinary bladder by analysing 21 microsatellite markers on chromosomes 2q, 4p, 4q, 8p, 9p, 9q, 11p and 17p. The resulting genetic variations suggested subsequent tumors in the lower urinary tract to stem from one single progenitor clone in 54% of patients. The authors concluded both mechanisms to be relevant, i.e. intraepithelial spread and development of subsequent tumors independently via field cancerization [77].

While these findings already marked both mechanisms as relevant, subsequent contributions put emphasis on either mechanisms of tumorigenesis. Jones and co-workers performed LOH assays for three microsatellite polymorphic markers on chromosomes 9p21 (IFNA and D9S171), p16, and 17p13 (TP53) in 58 tumors of the upper and lower urinary tract from 21 patients. In addition X-chromosome inactivation analysis was done on the specimens from 11 female patients. The authors report concordant allelic loss patterns in multifocal and simultaneous urothelial tumors in but 3 of 21 (14%) cases. A concordant pattern of non-random X-chromosome inactivation in coexisting neoplasia was seen in but 3 of 11 female patients. The authors thus report evidence for independent origin of tumours in the majority of coexisting urothelial carcinomas of the upper and lower urinary tract [33]. While this finding clearly supports the role of field effect, further data also suggest monoclonal origin to be relevant. Catto et al investigated 9 patients with 32 sequential tumors of the upper and lower urinary tract. Tumor clonality was assessed using microsatellite instability at 17 various loci. Furthermore epigenetic events were analysed by assessing methylation of 7 gene promoters. While the results demonstrated tumors to vary with regards to the initial tumour location, i.e. the upper versus the lower urinary tract, all alterations of the sequential tumors within each patient appeared related and thus were suggested to arise from a single clone [34].

Urologists have ever since discussed the clinical implications of these findings [22,35,36]. The current molecular evidence based on both intertwined mechanisms of field cancerization on the one hand and tumor seeding on the other finally offers explanation for the clinical phenomenon of frequent synchronous and metachronous recurrences at various locations throughout the urinary tract, and the differing characteristics of a considerable fraction of upper versus lower urinary tract tumors.

15.5. Clinical Relevance of Field Cancerization in Upper Urinary Tract

The urological community has embraced the need for thorough investigation of the entire urinary tract at diagnosis of any urothelial tumor at any location, and the need for continuous surveillance of the entire system regardless of the location of the initial lesion [5,4,37]. The insight into the meaning of field cancerization has led to the call for advising patients with bladder carcinoma to cease any exposure, i.e. smoking, to reduce the risk of subsequent tumors. The understanding of the meaning of seeding mechanisms has led to the call for radical removal of tumors without residue or spilling, as malignant cells persisting in the urinary tract spur subsequent recurrences [34,37]. It has been understood that on the one hand urothelial cancer of the upper and lower urinary tract share some distinct molecular characteristics of potential clinical meaning, e.g. the correlation of adverse cancer specific survival and the absence of mutation of FGFR3 (fibroblast-growth receptor type 3) [38,39,40], while on the other hand some characteristics relevant in the clinical assessment of urothelial cancer of the bladder are missing in the upper urinary tract, e.g. the relation of female and disadvantageous outcome in muscle-invasive disease [41]. Some characteristics are unique to urothelial cancer of the upper urinary tract, e.g. the relation of microsatellite instability and poor survival [42]. And it also has been understood that patients with initial tumors of the upper urinary tract need to be screened for HNPCC-syndrome related cancers and vice versa, HNPCC families require screening of the upper urinary tract [35,22].

References

[1] Lynch, C. F., Cohen, M. B.: Urinary system. *Cancer*, 75: 316–329, 1995.

[2] Eble JN, Sauter G, Epstein IJ, Sesterhenn IA (eds). WHO classification of tumours: Tumours of the urinary system and male genital organs. *World Health Organization*, Berlin, Springer, 2004.

[3] Tawfiek, E. R., Bagley, D. H.: Upper-tract transitional cell carcinoma. *Urology,* 50: 321–329, 1997.

[4] Stenzl A, Cowan NC, De Santis M, Jakse G, Kuczyk MA, Merseburger AS, Ribal MJ, Sherif A, Witjes JA. The updated EAU guidelines on muscle-invasive and metastatic bladder cancer. *Eur. Urol.* 2009 Apr;55(4):815-25.

[5] Babjuk M, Oosterlinck W, Sylvester R, Kaasinen E, Böhle A, Palou-Redorta J; European Association of Urology (EAU). EAU guidelines on non-muscle-invasive urothelial carcinoma of the bladder. *Eur. Urol.* 2008 Aug;54(2):303-14. Epub 2008
[6] Koss LG, Tiamson EM, Robbins MA. Mapping cancerous and pre- cancerous bladder changes. A study of the urotheliumintensurgicallyremoved bladders. *JAMA* 1974;227:281– 6.
[7] Epstein JI, Amin MB, Reuter VR, Mostofi FK, Bladder Consensus Conference Committee. The World Health Organization/International Society of Urological Pathology consensus classification of urothelial (transitional cell) neoplasms of the urinary bladder. Bladder Consensus Conference Committee. *Am. J. Surg. Pathol.* 1998;22:1435– 48.
[8] Kang CH, Yu TJ, Hsieh HH et al. The development of bladder tumours and contralateral upper urinary tract tumours after primary transitional cell carcinoma of the upper urinary tract. *Cancer* 2003; 98: 1620–6.
[9] Matsui Y, Utsunomiya N, Ichioka K et al. Risk factors for subsequent development of bladder cancer after primary transitional cell carcinoma of the upper urinary tract. *Urology* 2005; 65: 279–83.36
[10] Harris AL, Neal DE. Bladder cancer – field versus clonal origin. *N. Engl. J. Med.* 1992; 326: 759–61.
[11] Sidransky D, Frost P, Von Eschenbach A, Oyasu R, Preisinger AC, Vogelstein B. Clonal origin bladder cancer. *N. Engl. J. Med.* 1992; 326: 737–40. 39
[12] Hafner C, Knuechel R, Zanardo L, Dietmaier W, Blaszyk H, Cheville J, Hofstaedter F, Hartmann A. Evidence for oligoclonality and intraluminal seeding in multifocal urothelial carcinomas of the upper and lower urinary tract. *Oncogene* 2001;20:4910
[13] Watson, P., Lynch, H. T.: Extracolonic cancer in hereditary nonpolyposis colorectal cancer. *Cancer,* 71: 677–685, 1993.
[14] Roupret M, Catto J, Coulet F, et al. Microsatellite instability as indicator of MSH2 gene mutation in patients with upper urinary tract transitional cell carcinoma. *J. Med. Genet.* 2004;41:e91.
[15] Maul JS, Warner NR, Kuwada SK, Burt RW, Cannon-Albright LA. Extracolonic cancers associated with hereditary nonpolyposis colorectal cancer in the Utah Population Database. *Am. J. Gastroenterol.* 2006;101:1591-6.
[16] Ruschoff, J., Dietmaier, W., Luttges, J., Seitz, G., Bocker, T., Zirngibl, H., Schlegel,J., Schackert, H. K., Jauch, K. W., Hofstaedter, F.: Poorly differentiated colonicadenocarcinoma, medullary type: clinical, phenotypic, and molecular characteristics. *Am. J. Pathol.*, 150: 1815–1825, 1997.
[17] Bocker, T., Ruschoff, J., Fishel, R.: Molecular diagnostics of cancer predisposition: hereditary non-polyposis colorectal carcinoma and mismatch repair defects. *Biochim. Biophys. Acta*, 31: O1-O10, 1999.
[18] Loeb, L. A.: A mutator phenotype in cancer. *Cancer Res.*, 61: 3230–3239, 2001.
[19] Dietmaier, W., Wallinger, S., Bocker, T., Kullmann, F., Fishel, R., Ruschoff, J.: Diagnostic microsatellite instability: definition and correlation with mismatch repair protein expression. *Cancer Res.,* 57: 4749–4756, 1997.
[20] Peltomaki, P., Vasen, H. F.: Mutations predisposing to hereditary nonpolyposis colorectal cancer: database and results of a collaborative study. The International

Collaborative Group on Hereditary Nonpolyposis Colorectal Cancer. *Gastroenterology*, 113: 1146–1158, 1997.

[21] Catto, J. WF., Azzouzi, A.-R., Amira, N., Rehman, I., Feeley, K. M., Cross, S. S., Fromont, G., Sibony, M., Hamdy, F. C., Cussenot, O., Meuth, M.: Distinct patterns of microsatellite instability are seen in tumours of the urinary tract. *Oncogene*, 75: 8699–8706, 2003

[22] Rouprêt M, Yates DR, Comperat E, Cussenot O. Upper urinary tract urothelial cell carcinomas and other urological malignancies involved in the hereditary nonpolyposis colorectal cancer (lynch syndrome) tumour spectrum. *Eur. Urol.* 2008 Dec;54(6):1226-36.

[23] Takahashi T, Habuchi T, Kakehi Y, et al. Clonal and chronological genetic analysis of multifocal cancers of the bladder and upper urinary tract. *Cancer Res* 1998;58:5835-41.

[24] Hartmann A, Dietmaier W, Hofstadter F, et al. Urothelial carcinoma of the upper urinary tract: inverted growth pattern is predictive of microsatellite instability. *Hum. Pathol.* 2003;34:222-7.

[25] Hartmann A., Zanardo, L, Bocker-Edmonston, T., Blaszyk, H., Dietmaier, W., Stoehr, R., Cheville, J. C., Junker, K., Wieland, W., Knuechel, R. , Rueschoff, J., Hofstaedter, F., Fishel, R.: Frequent microsatellite instability in sporadic tumours of the upper urinary tract. *Cancer Research*, 62: 6796–6802, December 1, 2002

[26] Boland, C. R., Thibodeau, S. N., Hamilton, S. R., Sidransky, D., Eshleman, J. R., Burt, R. W., Meltzer, S. J., Rodriguez Bigas, M. A., Fodde, R., Ranzani, G. N., Srivastava, S. A.: National cancer institute workshop on microsatellite instability for cancer detection and familial predisposition: development of international criteria for the determination of microsatellite instability in colorectal cancer. *Cancer Res.*, 58: 5248–5257, 1998.

[27] Ericson KM, Isinger AP, Isfoss BL, Nilbert MC. Low frequency of defective mismatch repair in a population-based series of upper urothelial carcinoma. *BMC Cancer* 2005;5:23.

[28] Mongiat-Artus P, Miquel C, Van der Aa M, et al. Microsatellite instability and mutation analysis of candidate genes in urothelial cell carcinomas of upper urinary tract. *Oncogene* 2006;25:2113-8.

[29] Burger M, Burger SJ, Denzinger S, et al. Elevated microsatellite instability at selected tetranucleotide repeats does not correlate with clinicopathologic features of bladder cancer. *Eur. Urol* 2006;50:770-6.

[30] Kakizoe T, Fujita J, Murase T, Matsumoto K, Kishi K. Transitional cell carcinoma of the bladder in patients with renal pelvic and ureteral cancer. *J. Urol.* 1980;124: 17

[31] Koontz WW, Jr., Prout GR, Jr., Smith W, Frable WJ, Minnis JE. The use of int ravesical thio-tepa in the management of non-invasive carcinoma of the bladder. *J. Urol.* 1981;125:307

[32] Takahashi T, Kakehi Y, Mitsumori K et al. Distinct microsatellite alterations in upper urinary tract tumours and subsequent bladder tumours. *J. Urol.* 2001; 165: 672– 7.

[33] Jones TD, Eble JN, Wang M, MacLennan GT, Delahunt B, Brunelli M, Martignoni G, Lopez-Beltran A, Bonsib SM, Ulbright TM, Zhang S, Nigro K, Cheng L. Molecular genetic evidence for the independent origin of multifocal papillary tumours in patients with papillary renal cell carcinomas. *Clin. Cancer Res.* 2005 Oct 15;11(20):7226-33.

[34] Catto JW, Azzouzi AR, Rehman I, Feeley KM, Cross SS, Amira N, Fromont G, Sibony M, Cussenot O, Meuth M, Hamdy FC. Promoter hypermethylation is associated with tumor location, stage, and subsequent progression in transitional cell carcinoma. *J. Clin. Oncol. 2005* May 1;23(13):2903-10.

[35] Burger M. Editorial comment on: upper urinary tract urothelial cell carcinomas and other urological malignancies involved in the hereditary nonpolyposis colorectal cancer (Lynch syndrome) tumour spectrum. *Eur. Urol.* 2008 Dec;54(6):1236.

[36] Zigeuner R, Pummer K. Urothelial carcinoma of the upper urinary tract: surgical approach and prognostic factors. *Eur. Urol.* 2008 Apr;53(4):720-31.

[37] Zigeuner RE, Hutterer G, Chromecki T, Rehak P, Langner C. Bladder tumour development after urothelial carcinoma of the upper urinary tract is related to primary tumour location. *BJU Int.* 2006 Dec;98(6):1181-6.

[38] van Oers JM, Zwarthoff EC, Rehman I, Azzouzi AR, Cussenot O, Meuth M, Hamdy FC, Catto JW. FGFR3 mutations indicate better survival in invasive upper urinary tract and bladder tumours. *Eur. Urol.* 2009 Mar;55(3):650-7.

[39] Malats N, Real FX. Editorial comment on: FGFR3 mutations indicate better survival in invasive upper urinary tract and bladder tumours. *Eur. Urol.* 2009 Mar;55(3):658. Epub 2008 Jun 13.

[40] Burger M, Catto J, van Oers J, Zwarthoff E, Hamdy FC, Meuth M, Azzouri AR, Cussenot O, Wild PJ, Stoehr R, Hartmann A. [Mutation of the FGFR3 oncogene is an independent and favorable prognostic factor for tumor-specific survival in patients with urothelial carcinoma of the upper urinary tract]. *Verh. Dtsch. Ges. Pathol.* 2006;90:244-52.

[41] Fernández: Fernández MI, Shariat SF, Margulis V, Bolenz C, Montorsi F, Suardi N, Remzi M, Wood CG, Roscigno M, Kikuchi E, Oya M, Zigeuner R, Langner C, Weizer A, Lotan Y, Koppie TM, Raman JD, Karakiewizc P, Bensalah K, Schultz M, Bernier P. Evidence-based sex-related outcomes after radical nephroureterectomy for upper tract urothelial carcinoma: results of large multicenter study. *Urology*. 2009 Jan;73(1):142-6.

[42] Rouprêt M, Fromont G, Azzouzi AR, Catto JW, Vallancien G, Hamdy FC, Cussenot O. Microsatellite instability as predictor of survival in patients with invasive upper urinary tract transitional cell carcinoma. *Urology*. 2005 Jun;65(6):1233-7.

In: Field Cancerization: Basic Science and Clinical Applications ISBN 978-1-61761-006-6
Editor: Gabriel D. Dakubo

Chapter 16

Clonality of Multifocal Urothelial Cancer and Field Cancerization

Tomonori Habuchi and Tadao Kakizoe

Abstract

The simultaneous or metachronous development of multifocal tumors with identical or variable histological features in the urinary tract of a single patient is a well-known characteristic of urothelial cancer. To explain this phenomenon, two distinct concepts have been proposed: the "field cancerization" hypothesis, according to which urothelial cells in patients are primed to undergo transformation in multiclonal cells by previous carcinogenic insults, and the "single progenitor cell" hypothesis, which asserts that multifocal development is caused by the seeding or intraepithelial spread of transformed cells. On the other hand, there may be two kinds of field cancerization in urothelial carcinogenesis: one involving multiclonal neoplastic alterations by carcinogenic insults, and the other, clonal expansion and intraepithelial spread from a single progenitor transformed cell with a significant growth advantage. Recent molecular genetic and histological studies support the single progenitor cell hypothesis and indicate that the genetic and phenotypic diversity observed in multifocal urothelial tumors is a consequence of clonal evolution from a single transformed cell. Furthermore, the clonal expansion and spread of a preneoplastic or neoplastic progenitor cell with a growth advantage is the main mechanism of field cancerization in most urothelial cancer patients. The additional genetic alterations to these transformed cells would then give rise to a clinically evident tumor or multifocal tumors. Most metachronous multifocal tumors may arise from the *de novo* occurrence of the tumor from the cells in clonally expanded field cancerization or intraluminal seeding from evident tumor cells. An understanding of the mechanism of field cancerization and heterotopic recurrence of urothelial cancer may provide new prospects for early molecular detection and prevention of heterotopic recurrence of urothelial cancer.

16.1. Introduction

The simultaneous or metachronous development of multifocal tumors with identical or variable histological features in the urinary tract of a single patient is a well-known characteristic of urothelial cancer [1]. It is also common for urothelial cancer to be accompanied by surrounding abnormal urothelium ranging from dysplasia to carcinoma *in situ* [2, 3]. To explain this phenomenon, two distinct concepts have been proposed [4, 5]. The first, the "field cancerization" hypothesis, postulates that multiple cells become initiated or partially transformed as a result of carcinogenic insults and acquire independent genetic alterations. Therefore, multifocal tumors would arise synchronously or metachronously from distinct transformed cells. The second hypothesis proposes that the multifocal tumors are descendants of a single transformed cell, which proliferates and spreads by intraepithelial spread or intraluminal seeding. Intraepithelial spread may occur through the continuous migration and proliferation of transformed cells throughout the urothelium. Intraluminal seeding could occur through the release of tumor cells from the primary lesion followed by the implantation of the tumor cells at different sites of the urothelium. It should be noted that clonal expansion occurring by intraepithelial spread or intraluminal seeding might cause field cancerization. Therefore, there are two kinds of field cancerization in urothelium, one involving multiclonal neoplastic alterations in response to carcinogenic insults, and the other, a clonal expansion and intraepithelial spread from a single progenitor transformed cell.

Understanding the origin and mechanism of field cancerization and multifocality in urothelial cancer is important for the establishment of new strategies for the prevention and treatment of this cancer. Recent advances in molecular genetics have shed considerable light on the origin and mechanism of such field cancerization and multifocality in urothelial cancers. Importantly, recent extensive molecular histological studies have indicated that field cancerization in urothelial cancer patients is caused by clonal expansion and intraepithelial spread of a single premalignant transformed cell. In this chapter, current research delineating the mechanism behind the multifocality of urothelial cancer and field cancerization is reviewed and discussed.

16.2. Genetic and Histological Aspects of the Field in Urothelium of the Bladder, Ureter, and Renal Pelvis

Studies of chimeric animals and human tissue have shown that mucosal surface cells develop from the division of a limited number of stem cells to form a contiguous mono- or multilayered sheet consisting of cells with varying propensities for division, differentiation, and apoptosis [5]. A tendency of epithelial daughter cells to remain adjacent to each other due to coherent clonal growth results in variegation wherein the epithelium is composed of patches of monoclonal cells [5]. The size of the clonal patch on the epithelial surface may vary according to the tissue, ranging from 0.2–1.00 mm2 in the adult hair follicle to 100 mm2 in gastric epithelium [6]. This holds true for the urothelium of the renal pelvis, ureter, and bladder. Using a methylation-sensitive enzymatic polymerase chain reaction (PCR)–based X-chromosome inactivation analysis of urothelial cells microdissected from the female human bladder, Tsai et al. identified macroscopic urothelial patches of a monoclonal origin. According to their estimates, each patch was 120 mm2 in size and contained about 2×10^6 cells originating from a single stem cell [7]. Because the total internal surface area of the bladder is 300 cm2, only about 200–300 patches covered the large area of the bladder epithelium, suggesting that only 200–300 stem cells participated in the formation of bladder urothelium [7]. It was suggested that each stem cell may be predisposed by a random genetic event to be more susceptible to further genetic alterations caused by endogenous or exogenous factors that together would give rise to an overt tumor.

In support of this concept, Gimelbrant et al. recently showed widespread monoallelic expression of autosomal genes as well as X-chromosomal genes [8]. They examined allele-specific transcription of about 4000 human genes in clonal cell lines and found that more than 300 were subject to random monoallelic expression. For a majority of monoallelic genes, they also observed some clonal lines displaying biallelic expression. Conservative extrapolation from their data suggests that at least 1000 autosomal human genes are subject to random monoallelic expression [8]. This monoallelic expression can influence biological function by creating three distinct cell states for each given gene when the two alleles encode functionally different proteins. Monoallelic expression can contribute to cellular (or clonal) diversity even without polymorphism in genes of monoallelic expression, because of the differences in levels of gene expression. Widespread monoallelic expression suggests a mechanism that generates diversity in individual cells and their clonal descendants.

Taken together, these findings suggest that each urothelial cellular patch harbors varying degrees of genetic field defects that originated from a stem cell and are prevalent in daughter cells in the patch. If the patch is highly predisposed to undergo transformation, the result is the development of multiple cancer cell clones, providing the basis for field cancerization.

16.3. Clinical and Traditional Pathological Aspects of Multifocality of Urothelial Cancers of the Bladder, Urethra, Ureter, and Renal Pelvis

Urothelial cell carcinomas originate from the epithelial cells (also known as the transitional cell epithelium), which covers the luminal surface of nearly the entire urinary tract, extending from the renal pelvis, through the ureter and bladder, to the proximal urethra. About 70% of the tumors are papillary and confined to the urothelial mucosa or to the lamina propria; the remainder are mostly nonpapillary nodular or flat tumors that invade the muscle, perivesical fat, or surrounding organs [9]. The latter tumors are generally called "muscle invasive tumors" and are often associated with the lymph node and distant organ metastases, reflecting high malignant potential with a life-threatening risk. On the other hand, most papillary tumors are low grade, rarely progress, and are associated with a favorable prognosis, although such tumors often recur in the urinary tract after transurethral treatment.

The simultaneous or metachronous development of multifocal tumors with identical or variable histological features in the urothelial tract of a single patient is a well-known characteristic of urothelial cancer (figure 16-1) [1]. The following clinical and pathological characteristics of multifocality in urothelial cancer should be taken into account in deciding the treatment plan as well as in performing molecular genetic studies to determine the pathogenesis of the multifocal tumors.

1) It is common for urothelial cancer to be accompanied by surrounding abnormal urothelium ranging from dysplasia to carcinoma *in situ* [2, 3].
2) When superficial papillary urothelial carcinomas of the bladder are resected transurethrally (TUR), 50–80% of patients eventually have recurrent urothelial carcinomas of a similar biological nature in the normal-appearing bladder mucosa (figure 16-1A) [9].
3) When male patients are treated with cystoprostatectomy (i.e., removal of the bladder and prostate) for bladder cancer, there is still a 1.5-5% risk of urothelial carcinomas in the remaining urethra (figure 16-1B)[10]. Furthermore, while most primary cancers in the urethra are squamous cell carcinomas, almost all recurrent urethral tumors in patients with a history of bladder cancer are transitional cell carcinomas.
4) When simple nephrectomy, which leaves approximately one-third of the lower ureter intact, is performed for carcinomas of the upper urinary tract (i.e., the renal calyx, pelvis, and ureter), 20–50% of patients subsequently develop urothelial carcinomas in the remaining ureter [1]. Owing to these clinical findings, the standard surgery for renal pelvic or ureteral carcinomas at the present time is total nephroureterectomy, including removal of a small portion of the bladder with the ureteral orifice in the affected side.
5) Even when total nephroureterectomy is carried out for renal pelvic and ureteral carcinomas, 30–50% of patients exhibit subsequent carcinomas in the bladder (Figure 16-1C, right side) [11, 12].
6) On the other hand, patients with primary bladder cancers have only a 0.5–4% risk of subsequent upper urinary tract carcinomas (figure 16-1C, left side) [13]. However, the risk of subsequent upper urinary tract tumor is reported to rise to about 6-20% (15 to 22-fold greater risk!) if the patients have vesicoureteral reflux [14, 15].
7) Although rare, simultaneous carcinomas of the bilateral upper urinary tract are found in 1–5% of patients [11]. Approximately 2–3% of patients with unilateral upper urinary tract carcinoma experience subsequent contralateral upper urinary tract carcinoma (figure 16-1C) [16].

To explain these characteristics of multifocality, two distinct concepts have been proposed [4, 5]. The first is the field cancerization theory, proposed in 1953 by Slaughter et al, and it was based on observations of the multicentric development of cancers in the oral cavity, with the high impact of carcinogens and promoting agents being associated with some lifestyle factors [17]. According to this theory, multiple cells are partially transformed because of carcinogenic insults and acquire independent genetic alterations. Therefore, multifocal tumors arise synchronously or metachronously from distinct transformed cells. The second theory posits that the multifocal tumors are descendants of a single transformed cell, which proliferates and spreads by intraluminal seeding or intraepithelial spread. Intraluminal seeding could occur through the release of tumor cells from the primary lesion followed by the implantation of the tumor cells at different sites of the urothelium. Intraepithelial spread may occur through the continuous migration and proliferation of transformed cells throughout the urothelium. This theory is known as the single progenitor cell theory.

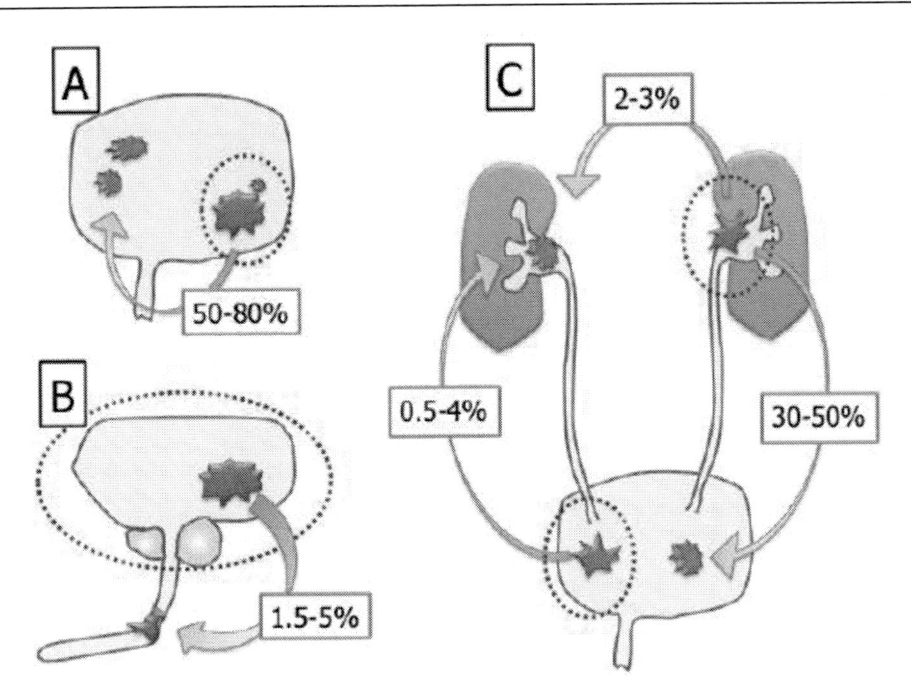

Figure 16.1. Importance of urinary flow in heterotopic recurrence of urothelial tumors of the urinary tract. When superficial papillary urothelial carcinomas of the bladder are resected endoscopically, 50–80% of patients eventually have recurrent urothelial carcinomas of a similar biological nature in the bladder mucosa (A). When male patients are treated with cystoprostatectomy (i.e., removal of the bladder and prostate) for bladder cancer, they still have a 1.5–5% risk of urothelial carcinomas in the remaining urethra (B). Patients with tumors of the upper urinary tract have about a 30–50 % risk of developing bladder cancer after nephroureterectomy, while such patients have an only a 2–3 % chance of developing tumors in the contralateral upper urinary tract (C). Patients with primary bladder cancers also have only a 0.5–4 % risk of subsequent upper urinary tract tumors (C). However, the risk of a subsequent upper urinary tract tumor is reported to rise to about 6–20% (15- to 22-fold greater risk) if the patients have vesicoureteral reflux.

Traditional clinical and pathological findings support both the multiclonal field cancerization theory and the single transformed cell theory. For example, the frequent presence of dysplasia and carcinoma *in situ* around or far from the primary tumor may be evidence of field cancerization [2, 3]. However, this observation may well be explained by the direct intraepithelial spread of a transformed preneoplastic cell around the primary tumor or tumor cell implantation via intraluminal dissemination, followed by attachment and regrowth at a distant site [4]. The phenomenon that heterotopic recurrences sometime arise many years after the eradication of the primary tumor favors the field cancerization theory. However, recent molecular analyses have indicated that the period of tumor dormancy or simply a clinically undetected state, or the period of multistep carcinogenesis, may be unexpectedly long (up to 9 years) in certain cases [18- 22]. Interestingly, as stated before, several clinical observations may be consistent with the single progenitor cell theory (figure 16-1A-C). These observations strongly suggest the importance of urinary flow in heterotopic recurrence, thus underscoring implantation or seeding from a transformed progenitor cell in the process of multifocality.

There may, however, be another theory to explain these phenomena. If a single transformed cell with significant growth advantage expands clonally and spreads intraepithelially with or without intraluminal seeding, clinically evident multifocal tumors may arise after acquiring additional genetic alterations. The presentation of metachronous multifocal urothelial tumors, which are often observed clinically, may well be explained by clonal field cancerization by a single transformed progenitor cell.

16.4. Genetic Aspects of Multifocal Tumors of the Bladder, Urethra, Ureter, and Renal Pelvis

Although many urologists and pathologists had favored the theory of field cancerization by multiclonal transformed cells to explain the multifocality in urothelial cancer, recent molecular genetic studies have provided strong evidence for a common clonal origin in most multifocal urothelial cancers.

16.4.1. X-Chromosome Inactivation Analysis

The first pioneering work in support of the single transformed cell theory came from analyses of X-chromosome inactivation in multifocal bladder tumors of 4 female patients [23]. In females, one of the two X-chromosomes is always maintained in an inactive state through DNA methylation at CpG sites, and the X-chromosome inactivation occurs early in development. Since the inactivation of either the paternal or maternal allele of the X-chromosome is determined randomly, the inactivated allele ought to be variable in each patient if multifocal urothelial tumors are derived from independent cells owing to field cancerization. If, instead, the multifocal tumors are derived from a single clone of transformed cells, the same X-chromosome ought to be inactivated in multifocal tumors in each patient. Sidransky et al. examined the origin (i.e., paternal or maternal) of the inactivated allele of the X-chromosome using a methylation-specific restriction enzyme and found that the same allele of the X-chromosome was inactivated in multiple tumors in each patient. Although the number of patients and tumors examined was small, the results strongly indicated that the multifocal bladder tumors were derived from clonally identical cells. More recently, using a PCR-based analysis along with methylation-specific restriction enzyme, Li et al. also showed that such multifocal tumors had the same X-chromosome inactivation pattern, supporting the view of an identical clonal origin in 35 synchronous and metachronous multifocal low-grade noninvasive urothelial cancers in 10 female patients [24]. These results strongly suggested that most, if not all, of the multifocal tumors in each patient derived from a common progenitor (transformed) cell, which might have progressed to overt tumors by the addition of further genetic or epigenetic alterations.

On the other hand, Jones et al. found that 1 of 10 female patients had a discordant pattern of nonrandom X-chromosome inactivation in multifocal urothelial cancers, indicating independent clonal origin in few cases [25]. (Although the authors claimed that another 6 cases in their study showed a random inactivation pattern, an apparent distinct inactivation pattern of the paternal or maternal allele was not observed in these 6 cases [25].) While performing and evaluating the X-chromosome inactivation analysis in tumor samples, we should be cautious regarding the following points: (a) contamination of normal tissues, (b) incomplete digestion of DNA samples, especially those prepared from formalin-fixed paraffin-embedded tissues, (c) abnormal hypermethylation or demethylation at tested DNA loci in the tumor genome, and (d) the presence of X-chromosome aneuploidy (deletion, trisomy, or higher number duplication). The pertinent interpretation of the results of the X-chromosome inactivation analysis may be hampered by these factors.

16.4.2. *p53* Mutational Genetic Fingerprint

The p53 gene (*p53*) is the most frequent target of somatic mutations found in human cancers. The location and patterns of *p53* mutations have been reported to be highly variable [26, 27]. Although certain carcinogens can cause specific mutation patterns, as evidenced by aflatoxin-induced *p53* mutations reported in a case of hepatocellular carcinoma, the *p53* mutation data bank reveals no significant carcinogen-specific hot spots for urothelial carcinomas [26, 27]. Therefore, *p53* mutations could be used as a "genetic fingerprint" to clarify clonal relationship between independent tumors.

Lunec et al have reported, as have we, cases of heterotopic synchronous or recurrent urothelial carcinomas of the bladder and upper urinary tract in which identical *p53* mutations were found in each patient [28, 29]. Similar findings of identical *p53* mutations in multifocal urothelial carcinomas have been reported by other groups [19, 22, 30, 31]. These results rather clearly showed that the tested multifocal tumors were derived from a common progenitor cell in each patient. On the other hand, some investigators found distinct *p53* mutations in multiple tumors in 1 patient and claimed that they presumably had a distinct cellular origin [32, 33]. However, importantly, because the *p53* alteration is not an early event in urothelial carcinogenesis, such divergent *p53* mutations might occur during the clonal evolution of malignant cells from a single transformed cell. Therefore, the different *p53* mutations might occur late in tumor development and characterize only heterogeneous subclones of one clonally derived tumor cell population [19, 22, 28, 29, 34, 35].

One caveat concerning use of a *p53* mutation pattern as a genetic fingerprint is that *p53* alterations in urothelial cancers are associated with aggressive type of tumors [29, 36]. Therefore, *p53* alterations might confer some advantage in terms of heterotopic spreading or seeding, and the same *p53* mutations found in multiple tumors might be caused by tumor aggressiveness or a highly malignant phenotype associated with the *p53* alteration. The finding in *p53* mutated tumors may therefore not apply to multifocal tumors without the *p53* mutation or tumors with low malignant potentials.

16.4.3. Loss of Heterozygosity and Microsatellite Alterations

Other genetic fingerprints for analyses of clonal origin of tumors are patterns of loss of heterozygosity (LOH) and microsatellite alterations. In general, in sporadic tumors, whether the maternal or paternal allele is deleted during the inactivation of tumor suppressor genes is determined randomly. Therefore, the chance that the same allele will be deleted in two tumors is 1/2, while that in the n tumors is (1/2) n–1. If there is a partial deletion of the chromosomal arm, the breakpoint in the chromosomal deletion can be used as a highly specific genetic fingerprint [20, 21]. To detect LOH in tumor cells, "microsatellite analyses" have been broadly used in many studies. Microsatellites are highly polymorphic short tandem DNA repeats (mostly 2–4 base pairs each) that are found throughout the human genome [37]. Two types of microsatellite alterations can be found in many cancers. One is LOH (allelic deletion), which is a hallmark of the inactivation of tumor suppressor genes and can be detected in exfoliated cancer cells in urine, as well as bladder tumor tissues [38-40]. The other is a somatic alteration of the microsatellite repeat length in cancer cells, which can be detected as a microsatellite shift, a new allele, or microsatellite instability [20, 38-40]. In the case of microsatellite shifts, a shift of alleles may occur throughout the genome, caused by the defect in the mismatch repair system (i.e., "microsatellite instability" in the strictest sense of the term). Since the pattern of microsatellite shift is highly variable and not related to tumor aggressiveness, the pattern can be used as a highly specific genetic fingerprint, which is unrelated to tumor grade or stage [38-40]. Using the LOH pattern and the microsatellite shift pattern, we analyzed the clonal relationship in 87 metachronous and synchronous multifocal tumors of the bladder and upper urinary tract in 29 patients [20]. Judging from the patterns of LOH, microsatellite shifts, and the breakpoint of subchromosomal deletion, multifocal tumors in at least 20 (80%) of 25 patients were considered to have developed from a common transformed progenitor cell [20]. Although the clonal relation or origin of the multifocal tumors in the remaining 5 (20%) patients remained unknown, the genetic heterogeneity found in multifocal tumors does not necessarily indicate that these tumors were derived from independent cells. The divergent genetic alterations may occur at a late stage in the progression during and after the clonal evolution from the single cells and heterotopic spreading. The extensive chronological analysis of recurrent multifocal urothelial tumors suggested the presence of considerable genetic diversity in heterogeneous subclones of one clonally derived tumor cell population [20, 21, 41]. Therefore, in regard to the clonal relationship, the results of patterns of LOH in multifocal tumors should be interpreted with caution. In summary, although distinct patterns in LOH, microsatellite shift, and subchromosomal deletion may be present in multifocal tumors, the results of published LOH and microsatellite studies are compatible with the theory that multifocal urothelial tumors are derived from a common progenitor cell.

16.4.4. DNA Methylation Profiles, mRNA Expression Profiles, Karyotyping, and Comparative Genomic Hybridization

New molecular markers such as epigenetic aberrant methylation patterns, alternate splicing patterns of mRNA, and mRNA expression patterns may also be used as a genetic fingerprint. However, because these genetic alterations are highly variable and unstable even in clonally identical cells, these genetic markers are not suitable for defining the clonal origin of multifocal tumors.

Although not definitive, recent studies of extensive cDNA expression profiling using a cDNA microarray provided interesting findings that may be compatible with the theory of intraepithelial spread and heterotopic seeding. Dyrskjot et al. found similar gene expression profile in superficial bladder carcinoma, distant carcinoma *in situ* lesions and histologically normal urothelium adjacent to these lesions [42]. Lindgren et al. found that similar expression profiles in multifocal bladder carcinomas in most patients and multifocal tumors in 18 of 22 patients were grouped adjacent to or in close vicinity of each other in the hierarchical cluster analysis [43]. They further found that the expression similarity was present even in multifocal tumors that were genetically heterogeneous [43].

Karyotyping by classical cytogenetic analysis of metaphase cells and comparative genomic hybridization (CGH) is also used for analyzing clonal relationship as a genetic fingerprint [34, 44, 45]. Although cytogenetic analyses cannot detect minor deletions or alterations, they provide a specific karyotypic pattern of chromosomal changes such as gains, deletions, translocations, inversions, and additional chromosomal fragments. The CGH pattern provides more precise detailed information on gains or losses at the subchromosomal level of each chromosome. Both methods can provide a global view of chromosomal and subchromosomal abnormalities in cancer cells. However, in contrast to the LOH analysis, neither technique can provide information regarding the alternate loss of the paternal or maternal allele.

16.5. Chronology of Clinical Tumor Presentation Does Not Correspond to Chronology of Genetic Alterations and Evolution

The genetic analysis of primary and recurrent urothelial tumors provides a good model for the chronological tracing of genetic alterations and evolution of human cancers. If the multifocal metachronous tumors are confirmed to derive from a single transformed cell by a marker genetic change (i.e., genetic fingerprint), the chronology of clinical tumor presentation can be compared with that of genetic evolution. Chronological analyses of multifocal tumors indicate that the time of clinical presentation of each tumor may not necessarily correlate with the order in which the genetic alterations occurred or with biological tumor development [19, 20, 41]. The results of molecular chronological analyses showed that the clinical chronology of evident tumors is distinct from the chronology of genetic alterations in urothelial tumors. For example, by analyzing LOH pattern in metachronous multifocal tumors, we found that the clinical chronology of evident lesions is distinct from the chronology of genetic alterations [20]. Thus, recurrent tumors with a greater number of genetic alterations could appear long before another recurrent tumor of the identical clonal origin with fewer genetic alterations. A similar observation was reported by van Tilborg et al., who also pointed out the frequent lack of correlation between the chronological appearance of overt tumors and genetic progression in multifocal metachronous tumors with an identical clonal origin [41]. A tumor with additional genetic alterations may develop earlier or later than a tumor without the alterations, even though the two tumors are shown to be derived from the same progenitor cell.

Furthermore, chronological genetic analyses indicated that urothelial tumors may have a significant dormant period even when the tumor cells have substantial genetic alterations and a highly malignant potential [18-22]. Representative cases with a long dormant period were reported in tumors with *p53* mutations. For example, a persistent but clinically dormant specific transformed cell with *p53* mutation in bladder urothelium was found 8–9 years prior to the onset of invasive bladder cancer [18, 19]. It should be noted, as later discussed, that the dormant period may be caused by the field cancerization by a clonally expanded preneoplastic transformed cell.

Furthermore, chronological genetic analyses may provide clues to the timing of each genetic alteration. Among the genetic alterations, the loss or deletion of chromosome 9 (9p or

9q, or both) was observed most commonly in multifocal tumors in each patient, supporting the view that the alteration of a putative gene(s) on chromosome 9 (p and q) may be one of the earliest genetic aberrations in the development of urothelial cancer [20, 23, 35, 46].

16.6. Histologic-Genetic Mapping of Multifocal Tumors and Nonmalignant Urothelium

As stated above, it is common for urothelial cancer to be accompanied by surrounding abnormal urothelium ranging from dysplasia to carcinoma *in situ*. It is quite reasonable to speculate that some genetic or epigenetic alterations are present in noncancerous urothelial cells with such pathological changes. Furthermore, such alterations may also be found in urothelial cells that appear morphologically and histopathologically normal in patients with urothelial cancer.

Using the CGH technique and LOH analyses on chromosomes 9p, 9q, and 17p, Obermann et al. showed that there was considerable genetic heterogeneity between papillary tumors and concomitant flat urothelial hyperplasia, indicating genetic evolution even in the early stage of tumorigenesis, or the distinct clonal origin between the two lesions. A clonal relationship between the two lesions seemed to be present in 5 of 10 cases, although it was not conclusive owing to the limited analytical methodology [47]. Chow et al. found LOH on chromosome 9q and other chromosomes in 8 of 15 (53%) papillary hyperplasias and none of 5 papillomas [48]. In 1 case, they found identical LOH patterns in papillary hyperplasia and recurrent carcinomas, suggesting that the papillary hyperplasia is the precursor of urothelial carcinomas and they are clonally related [48]. Hartman et al. analyzed microdissected dysplasia and carcinoma *in situ* by fluorescence in situ hybridization (FISH), LOH on chromosomes 9p, 9q, and 17, and TP53 mutational analysis in 31 patients [35]. They found similar rate of chromosome 9 deletions (86% and 75%), 17p deletions (84% and 53%), and TP53 mutations (72% and 67%) in carcinoma *in situ* and dysplasia. Among the 16 patients whose multifocal lesions were analyzed, there was considerable genetic heterogeneity between multifocal lesions in each patient, although similar genetic profiles were also found in some, suggesting that genetic evolution was at a rather early stage of dysplasia and carcinoma *in situ* [35]. The result suggested that although a common clonal origin is suggested in most cases of multifocal lesions of dysplasia or carcinoma *in situ*, multiple lesions originating from distinct clonal origins could not be ruled out [35]. Similarly, using FISH analysis on 5 chromosomes, Steidl et al. found the frequent presence of similar patterns of chromosomal aberrations in tumors and their associated urothelium, thus suggesting the same clonal origin [49].

Some researchers have attempted the genetic fine-mapping of cystectomized specimens to delineate the clonal relationship in multifocal bladder cancers and surrounding mucosal lesions [34, 44, 50-53]. Although cytogenetic analyses are not that specific and definitive, Simon et al. and Fadl-Elmula et al. showed that multifocal tumors presumably arising from a single clone have divergent genetic alterations due to clonal evolution [34, 44]. They both claimed that such multifocality was caused by intraepithelial spread or intraluminal seeding. Furthermore, by adding *p53* mutation analysis and *p53* immunohistochemical staining, Simon et al. found that clonally related genetic alterations detected in the normal-looking mucosa were mostly observed in the adjacent areas of evident tumors, rather than in distant areas [34]. They suggested that intraepithelial lateral migration is a more common mechanism than intraluminal seeding [34].

Similarly, Steidl et al showed that similar chromosomal aberrations detected by FISH were found in tumors and their adjacent normal-looking urothelium [49]. These results indicated that in most if not all cases, field cancerization in urothelial cancer is caused by intraepithelial spread of transformed cells since the normal urothelium and concurrent carcinomas showed identical genetic alterations. More recently, by analyzing LOH on chromosomes 8p, 9, and 17p in extensively micro-dissected tumor and histologically normal urothelial tissues using a genetic-mapping strategy, Stoehr et al. showed that the identical LOH found in tumor samples was also found in the surrounding histologically normal urothelial cells [54].

Interestingly, some markers showed LOH in almost all of the mapped areas, indicating extensive intraepithelial spread, whereas others were scattered and showed "focal islands" of LOH [55]. The results support the view that field cancerization in urothelial cancer may be caused by intraepithelial spread of transformed cells.

Studies involving fine *p53* mutation mapping of cystectomized specimens or samples obtained by random biopsies also showed that epithelial cells surrounding evident tumors often harbored the same *p53* mutation found in the evident tumors [31, 34, 35, 53]. Of interest, an identical *p53* mutation was found in surrounding histologically normal or preneoplastic urothelial areas as well as carcinoma *in situ* or dysplasia [31, 34, 35, 53, 56]. Remarkably, *p53* mutational genetic mapping has shown that urothelial cells with identical *p53* mutations or LOH on chromosome 9 covered almost the entire surface of the bladder in some cases [31, 55, 56].

These observations further support the premise that field cancerization is caused by insidious intraepithelial spread of genetically transformed preneoplastic cells that are morphologically normal looking. Finally, using LOH and aberrant methylation patterns at CpG sites as a genetic marker, Muto et al. showed that the same genetic alterations were found in normal-looking mucosa in some cystectomy specimens [51]. Interestingly, age-related hypermethylation at CpG sites may be present in histologically normal urothelium of non-cancer patients [57].

These data obtained by genetic fine-mapping of cystectomized bladder cancer specimens strongly suggest that cells with some genetic or epigenetic alterations generally spread into histologically normal-looking epithelium at the time of clinical presentation of overt urothelial cancer.

Therefore, field cancerization in urothelial cancer in most cases, if not all, is caused by insidious intraepithelial spread of genetically transformed cells that are morphologically normal looking. Since the genetically altered cells with identical genetic alterations are found in focal islands, intraluminal seeding may also contribute to the formation of field cancerization and multifocal tumors.

Finally, the fact that the results obtained by genetic fine-mapping were derived from cystectomy specimens means that the observation was derived from highly malignant tumors with invasive phenotype in most cases. Therefore, we should be prudent in extrapolating the findings to cases of low-grade papillary urothelial tumors.

16.7. From Field Cancerization Caused by Multiclonal Alterations to Field Cancerization by a Single Dominantly Transformed Clone: Hypothesis

As described above, the entire urothelium consists of patches of cells that have a common clonal origin. Each urothelial cellular patch harbors varying degrees of genetic field defects that originated from a stem cell and are prevalent in daughter cells in the patch (figures 16-2A and 16-3A). Some patches consist of cells that are highly susceptible to undergoing transformation, which may cause multiple tumors to develop, thereby providing the basis for field cancerization.

In addition, recent molecular studies have shown that the epigenetic alterations seen in urothelial cancer patients are often present even in the "normal" urothelium of control subjects [51, 57]. These epigenetic alterations are presumably preneoplastic changes that predispose the cells to further genetic alterations and malignant change. Therefore, although clinically evident tumors are presumably derived from a common cell, it is speculated that carcinogenic insult may cause multiclonal epigenetic or genetic alterations in a broad range of cells (figures 16-2B and 16-3B). However, in the early stages of carcinogenesis, most of these aberrant cells have no apparent growth advantage and multiple clones of cells that have some genetic or epigenetic defect may be present (figures 16-2B and 16-3B). At this very early stage of carcinogenesis, long before a tumor is clinically evident, field cancerization by multiclonal preneoplastic cells in minor transformed state is presumably present. These cells would be present in the polyclonal state; however, identifying the polyclonal transformed cells is difficult as they are not accompanied by any overt tumor and physicians have no chance to analyze such early stages of urothelial cells in the process of carcinogenesis. Furthermore, because the cells of each transformed clone are few and scattered, it is difficult to identify genetic alterations in these cells.

As a result of defense mechanisms, and because multiple genetic alterations are required for overt tumors to form, only a small proportion of cells or a single cell will progress to a further transformed state (figures 16-2C and 16-3C). Some transformed cells may have significant growth and biological advantages over surrounding normal epithelial cells; these cells will produce broad areas of preneoplastic change by intraepithelial spread or multifocal lesions by intraluminal seeding. During clonal expansion, additional genetic and epigenetic alterations will be acquired, thus presenting a heterogeneous phenotype (figures 16-2C and 16-3C). At this stage, urologists can clinically observe the spread of these lesions as carcinoma *in situ*, severe dysplasia, or multifocal tumors. More advanced tumors may derive from a dominant clone containing various genetic alterations that rendered a significant growth advantage over remaining clones (figures 16-2D and 16-3D). Multiple clones derived from an original transformed cell gradually evolve and acquire heterogeneous genotypes. In some cases, the heterogeneous multiple clones may be found clinically if these distinct clones have a similar growth rate and malignant potential (figures 16-2E and 16-3E). As mentioned above, some genetic heterogeneity, such as distinct *p53* alterations, may be present in multifocal tumors or distant areas of urothelium. However, the genetic heterogeneity presumably occurs as a result of clonal evolution from clonally expanded preneoplastic cells with a common clonal origin (figure 16-2E and 16-3E).

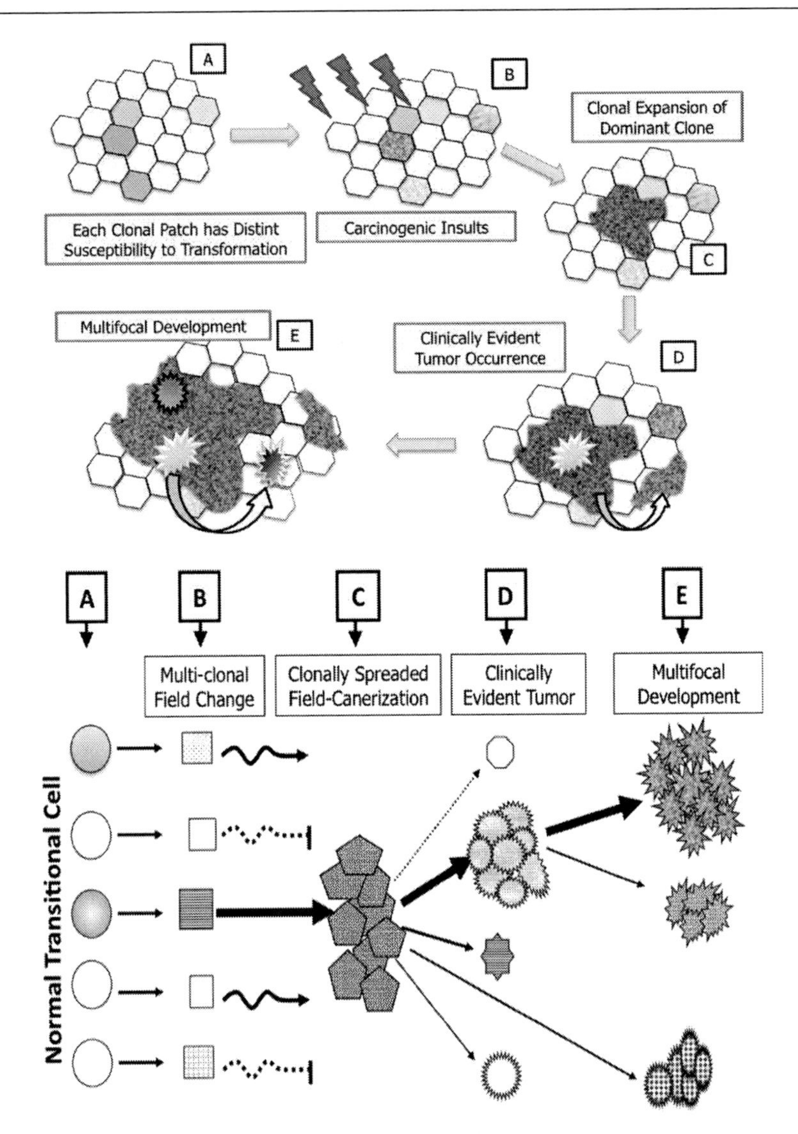

Figures 16.2. and 16.3. Possible pathway to field cancerization by clonally expanded spread and multifocal development of urothelial cancers. The entire urothelium consists of patches of cells having a common clonal origin. Each urothelial cellular patch harbors varying degrees of genetic field defects that originated from a stem cell and are prevalent in daughter cells in the patch. Some patches consist of cells that are highly susceptible to undergoing transformation, which may cause the development of multiple tumors, thus providing the basis of field cancerization (2A and 3A). Carcinogenic insults may cause multiclonal epigenetic or genetic alterations in a broad range of cells (2B and 3B). However, in the early stages of carcinogenesis, most of these aberrant cells have no apparent growth advantage, and multiple clones of cells that have some genetic or epigenetic defect may be present (2B and 3B). Because multiple genetic alterations are required for the formation of overt tumors, only a small proportion of cells or a single cell will progress to a further transformed state (2C and 3C). Some transformed cells may have significant growth and biological advantages over surrounding normal epithelial cells; these cells will produce broad areas of preneoplastic changes by intraepithelial spread or multifocal lesions by intraluminal seeding (2C and 3C). More advanced tumors may derive from a dominant clone containing various genetic alterations that render a significant growth advantage over remaining clones (2D and 3D). Multifocal metachronous tumors may arise from the *de novo* occurrence of a tumor that acquired further genetic alterations from cells that expanded clonally due to preneoplastic field change or by intraluminal seeding from evident tumor cells (2E and 3E).

In summary, urothelial carcinogenesis may be characterized by two kinds of field cancerization: one involving multiclonal neoplastic alterations resulting from carcinogenic insults, and the other, clonal expansion and intraepithelial spread from a single progenitor transformed cell. Most of the clinically evident field cancerization occurs by clonal expansion and intraepithelial spread. Multifocal metachronous tumors may arise from the *de novo* occurrence of a tumor that acquired further genetic alterations from cells that expanded clonally through preneoplastic field change or by intraluminal seeding from evident tumor cells (figures 16-2E and 16-3E).

16.8. Toward an Early Molecular Diagnosis and Prevention of Recurrence

Because most, if not all, recurrent multifocal tumors have the same clonal origin, recurrence can be monitored using urinary exfoliated cells by looking for the identical genetic alteration profiles observed in the original tumor [38-40]. If the recurrent tumors arise from distinct clones, this strategy for monitoring recurrence does not work. However, as shown by many molecular genetic studies, most recurrent tumors have some genetic markers that are identical to those of the original or former tumors. This holds true for detecting and monitoring the presence of field cancerization if the early genetic alterations are identified and can be monitored.

Among several recent molecular methodologies for the early detection of recurrent urothelial cancer, microsatellite analysis may be one of the most promising [38-40]. As mentioned before, two types of microsatellite alteration can be found in many cancers. One is LOH (allelic deletion) and the other is a somatic alteration of microsatellite repeats in cancer cells, which can be detected as microsatellite instability or a new allele. To detect microsatellite alterations in bladder cancer, DNA is extracted from exfoliated cells in urine and then subjected to PCR using DNA primers for a panel of known microsatellite markers. It has been reported that detection of microsatellite instability requires a ratio of tumor DNA to contaminating normal DNA of $>0.5\%$ [58], whereas the detection of LOH requires $\geq 20\%$ tumor DNA [59]. Generally, the more microsatellite markers used, the higher the sensitivity. Therefore, it is important to use a substantial number of microsatellite markers (15–20) at different loci. In several case-control studies involving the use of 15–20 microsatellite markers, the overall sensitivity and specificity of microsatellite analysis ranged from 72% to 97% and 80% to 100%, respectively [60]. Regarding follow-up of urothelial cancer patients, high sensitivity was also observed consistently in both primary and recurrent tumors [40, 61, 62]. These results strengthen the concept that the same transformed clone is the origin of heterotopic recurrence. Owing to the complexity of the detection procedures, the methodology is rather experimental at present, despite the excellent results demonstrated. A simpler, automated system to detect microsatellite alterations using urine sediment will be needed for routine clinical use.

Other genetic markers, such as *p53* mutation [18, 63], *ras* mutation [64], *FGFR3* mutation [65], or alternative splicing patterns [66], can be used in monitoring urothelial cancer recurrence in the urine sediment. Although detection of mutations in *de novo* tumors is difficult, once the location and pattern of the mutation are confirmed, it is not difficult technically to identify the presence of the same mutation in recurrent tumors. The mutation is screened in the primary tumor specimens, and subsequently, the same mutation can be monitored in the exfoliated cells in urine in the follow-up setting. However, again, because of the complicated procedures, this type of screening has not yet been used routinely in the clinical setting.

Because most cases of heterotopic recurrence of urothelial cancers are now recognized to occur as a result of intraluminal seeding or intraepithelial spread, it is important to prevent these steps in the course of treatment. Furthermore, the eradication of the cancerized field caused by clonally expanded intraepithelial spread may be an important step in preventing recurrences and progression.

It can be postulated with some confidence that surgical injury as a result of electrosurgical resection of bladder tumors may predispose tumor cells to adherence and growth, presumably owing to high concentrations of growth factors at the injury site as well as altered tissue structures [67, 68]. Furthermore, transurethral resection of the bladder tumor with loop electro-scissors, or surgical manipulation during nephroureterectomy, may disseminate a relatively large number of tumor cells. Therefore, to prevent early seeding after transurethral resection, the immediate instillation of chemotherapeutic agents may be effective. In fact, the benefit of an immediate single instillation therapy is well supported and confirmed by several randomized studies [69 - 72].

Another strategy is to give as many instillations of chemotherapeutic agents as possible because undetected preneoplastic or neoplastic cells can be assumed to have already spread broadly and distantly once the urothelial tumor is diagnosed. This may imply the eradication of field cancerization caused by clonal expansion and spread of a single transformed cell. However, because transurethral resection of the bladder tumor alone is adequate, treatment for many patients with bladder cancer, extensive adjuvant intravesical instillation therapy should be reserved for patients at high risk of recurrence [73, 74]. Although the efficacy of maintenance therapy using bacillus Calmette-Guérin (BCG) has been demonstrated in a large prospective study [75], some studies have not shown any benefit from therapy with BCG [76], doxorubicin [77], or epirubicin [78]. Some argue against maintenance therapy or an increase in the number of instillations based on the assertion that chemotherapeutic agents are mutagenic and potentially carcinogenic. However, it remains unknown whether maintenance intravesical chemotherapy increases the risk or incidence of subsequent bladder cancer [74].

Finally, chemoprevention of heterotopic recurrence in patients with urothelial cancer may be applied by focusing on the eradication of previously spread transformed preneoplastic cells or the *de novo* development of tumors from previously spread transformed cells. In this regard, chemoprevention of recurrence will be effective if the agent plays a significant role in preventing the further accumulation of genetic or epigenetic aberrations in transformed cells, for example by decreasing the availability of growth factors or vessel-promoting factors, or increasing other counteracting factors.

Conclusion

In most patients with urothelial cancers of the urinary tract, field cancerization in the urothelium is presumably caused by clonal expansion of transformed preneoplastic or neoplastic cells, which originate from a single transformed cell with a significant growth advantage. The growth advantage held by these preneoplastic or neoplastic cells would lead to extended intraepithelial spread and intraluminal seeding. Clinically evident tumor(s) may then arise after acquiring additional genetic alterations. Multifocal metachronous tumors may arise from the *de novo* occurrence of a tumor that acquired further genetic alterations from cells that had expanded through preneoplastic field change or by intraluminal seeding from evident tumor cells. Although the early stages of carcinogenesis occur long before there is clinical evidence of the tumor, field cancerization by multiclonal preneoplastic cells in insidious transformed state is presumably present. Therefore, in urothelial carcinogenesis, there may be two kinds of field cancerization in urothelium: one involving multiclonal neoplastic alterations by carcinogenic insults and the other, clonal expansion and intraepithelial spread from a single progenitor transformed cell. Eradication of clonally expanded field cancerization with the goal of preventing further heterotopic recurrence is a significant clinical task.

References

[1] Kakizoe, T. (2006). Development and progression of urothelial carcinoma. *Cancer Sci., 97*, 821-828.

[2] Mufti, G. R., and Singh, M. (1992). Value of random mucosal biopsies in the management of superficial bladder cancer. *Eur. Urol., 22*, 288-293.

[3] Cheng, L., Cheville, J. C., Neumann, R. M., and Bostwick, D. G. (1999). Natural history of urothelial dysplasia of the bladder. *Am. J. Surg. Pathol., 23*, 443-447.

[4] Harris, A. L., and Neal, D. E. (1992). Bladder cancer--field versus clonal origin. *N. Engl. J. Med., 326*, 759-761.

[5] Garcia, S. B., Park, H. S., Novelli, M., and Wright, N. A. (1999). Field cancerization, clonality, and epithelial stem cells: the spread of mutated clones in epithelial sheets. *J. Pathol., 187*, 61-81.

[6] Gartler, S. M., Gansini, E., Hutchison, H. T., Campbell, B., and Zechhi, G. (1971). Glucose-6-phosphate dehydrogenase mosaicism: ito;ozatopm om tje study of hair follicle variegation. *Ann. Hum. Genet., 35*, 1-7.

[7] Tsai, Y. C., Simoneau, A. R., Spruck, C. H., 3rd, Nichols, P. W., Steven, K., Buckley, J. D., and Jones, P. A. (1995). Mosaicism in human epithelium: macroscopic monoclonal patches cover the urothelium. *J. Urol., 153*, 1697-1700.

[8] Gimelbrant, A., Hutchinson, J. N., Thompson, B. R., and Chess, A. (2007). Widespread monoallelic expression on human autosomes. *Science, 318*, 1136-1140.

[9] Jones, JS; Campbell, SC. Non-muscle-invasive bladder cancer. In: Wein AJ, Kanoussi LR, Novick AC, Partin AW, Peters CA. Campbell-Walsh Urology: Ninth Ed. Philadelphia: Saunders Elsevier; 2007; 2447-2467.

[10] Hautmann, R. E., Volkmer, B. G., Schumacher, M. C., Gschwend, J. E., and Studer, U. E. (2006). Long-term results of standard procedures in urology: the ileal neobladder. *World J. Urol., 24*, 305-314.

[11] Kang, C. H., Yu, T. J., Hsieh, H. H., Yang, J. W., Shu, K., Huang, C. C., Chiang, P. H., and Shiue, Y. L. (2003). The development of bladder tumors and contralateral upper

urinary tract tumors after primary transitional cell carcinoma of the upper urinary tract. *Cancer, 98*, 1620-1626.

[12] Matsui, Y., Utsunomiya, N., Ichioka, K., Ueda, N., Yoshimura, K., Terai, A., and Arai, Y. (2005). Risk factors for subsequent development of bladder cancer after primary transitional cell carcinoma of the upper urinary tract. *Urology, 65*, 279-283.

[13] Kirkali, Z., and Tuzel, E. (2003). Transitional cell carcinoma of the ureter and renal pelvis. *Crit. Rev. Oncol. Hematol., 47*, 155-169.

[14] Amar, A. D., and Das, S. (1985). Upper urinary tract transitional cell carcinoma in patients with bladder carcinoma and associated vesicoureteral reflux. *J. Urol., 133*, 468-471.

[15] De Torres Mateos, J. A., Banus Gassol, J. M., Palou Redorta, J., and Morote Robles, J. (1987). Vesicorenal reflux and upper urinary tract transitional cell carcinoma after transurethral resection of recurrent superficial bladder carcinoma. *J. Urol., 138*, 49-51.

[16] Charbit, L., Gendreau, M. C., Mee, S., and Cukier, J. (1991). Tumors of the upper urinary tract: 10 years of experience. *J. Urol., 146*, 1243-1246.

[17] Slaughter, D. P., Southwick, H. W., and Smejkal, W. (1953). Field cancerization in oral stratified squamous epithelium; clinical implications of multicentric origin. *Cancer, 6*, 963-968.

[18] Hruban, R. H., van der Riet, P., Erozan, Y. S., and Sidransky, D. (1994). Brief report: molecular biology and the early detection of carcinoma of the bladder--the case of Hubert H. Humphrey. *N. Engl. J. Med., 330*, 1276-1278.

[19] Xu, X., Stower, M. J., Reid, I. N., Garner, R. C., and Burns, P. A. (1996). Molecular screening of multifocal transitional cell carcinoma of the bladder using p53 mutations as biomarkers. *Clin. Cancer Res, 2*, 1795-1800.

[20] Takahashi, T., Habuchi, T., Kakehi, Y., Mitsumori, K., Akao, T., Terachi, T., and Yoshida, O. (1998). Clonal and chronological genetic analysis of multifocal cancers of the bladder and upper urinary tract. *Cancer Res, 58*, 5835-5841.

[21] Takahashi, T., Habuchi, T., Kakehi, Y., Okuno, H., Terachi, T., Kato, T., and Ogawa, O. (2000). Molecular diagnosis of metastatic origin in a patient with metachronous multiple cancers of the renal pelvis and bladder. *Urology, 56*, 331.

[22] Vriesema, J. L., Aben, K. K., Witjes, J. A., Kiemeney, L. A., and Schalken, J. A. (2001). Superficial and metachronous invasive bladder carcinomas are clonally related. *Int. J. Cancer, 93*, 699-702.

[23] Sidransky, D., Frost, P., Von Eschenbach, A., Oyasu, R., Preisinger, A. C., and Vogelstein, B. (1992). Clonal origin bladder cancer. *N. Engl. J. Med., 326*, 737-740.

[24] Li, M., and Cannizzaro, L. A. (1999). Identical clonal origin of synchronous and metachronous low-grade, noninvasive papillary transitional cell carcinomas of the urinary tract. *Hum. Pathol., 30*, 1197-1200.

[25] Jones, T. D., Wang, M., Eble, J. N., MacLennan, G. T., Lopez-Beltran, A., Zhang, S., Cocco, A., and Cheng, L. (2005). Molecular evidence supporting field effect in urothelial carcinogenesis. *Clin. Cancer Res, 11*, 6512-6519.

[26] Hainaut, P., Hernandez, T., Robinson, A., Rodriguez-Tome, P., Flores, T., Hollstein, M., Harris, C. C., and Montesano, R. (1998). IARC Database of p53 gene mutations in human tumors and cell lines: updated compilation, revised formats and new visualisation tools. *Nucleic Acids Res, 26*, 205-213.

[27] Hollstein, M., Hergenhahn, M., Yang, Q., Bartsch, H., Wang, Z. Q., and Hainaut, P. (1999). New approaches to understanding p53 gene tumor mutation spectra. *Mutat. Res., 431*, 199-209.

[28] Lunec, J., Challen, C., Wright, C., Mellon, K., and Neal, D. E. (1992). c-erbB-2 amplification and identical p53 mutations in concomitant transitional carcinomas of renal pelvis and urinary bladder. *Lancet, 339*, 439-440.

[29] Habuchi, T., Takahashi, R., Yamada, H., Kakehi, Y., Sugiyama, T., and Yoshida, O. (1993). Metachronous multifocal development of urothelial cancers by intraluminal seeding. *Lancet, 342*, 1087-1088.

[30] Hafner, C., Knuechel, R., Zanardo, L., Dietmaier, W., Blaszyk, H., Cheville, J., Hofstaedter, F., and Hartmann, A. (2001). Evidence for oligoclonality and tumor spread by intraluminal seeding in multifocal urothelial carcinomas of the upper and lower urinary tract. *Oncogene, 20*, 4910-4915.

[31] Denzinger, S., Mohren, K., Knuechel, R., Wild, P. J., Burger, M., Wieland, W. F., Hartmann, A., and Stoehr, R. (2006). Improved clonality analysis of multifocal bladder tumors by combination of histopathologic organ mapping, loss of heterozygosity, fluorescence in situ hybridization, and p53 analyses. *Hum. Pathol., 37*, 143-151.

[32] Goto, K., Konomoto, T., Hayashi, K., Kinukawa, N., Naito, S., Kumazawa, J., and Tsuneyoshi, M. (1997). p53 mutations in multiple urothelial carcinomas: a molecular analysis of the development of multiple carcinomas. *Mod. Pathol., 10*, 428-437.

[33] Yamamoto, S., Tatematsu, M., Yamamoto, M., Fukami, H., and Fukushima, S. (1998). Clonal analysis of urothelial carcinomas in C3H/HeN<-->BALB/c chimeric mice treated with N-butyl-N-(4-hydroxybutyl)nitrosamine. *Carcinogenesis, 19*, 855-860.

[34] Simon, R., Eltze, E., Schafer, K. L., Burger, H., Semjonow, A., Hertle, L., Dockhorn-Dworniczak, B., Terpe, H. J., and Bocker, W. (2001). Cytogenetic analysis of multifocal bladder cancer supports a monoclonal origin and intraepithelial spread of tumor cells. *Cancer Res., 61*, 355-362.

[35] Hartmann, A., Schlake, G., Zaak, D., Hungerhuber, E., Hofstetter, A., Hofstaedter, F., and Knuechel, R. (2002). Occurrence of chromosome 9 and p53 alterations in multifocal dysplasia and carcinoma in situ of human urinary bladder. *Cancer Res., 62*, 809-818.

[36] Fujimoto, K., Yamada, Y., Okajima, E., Kakizoe, T., Sasaki, H., Sugimura, T., and Terada, M. (1992). Frequent association of p53 gene mutation in invasive bladder cancer. *Cancer Res, 52*(6), 1393-1398.

[37] Weber, J. L., and May, P. E. (1989). Abundant class of human DNA polymorphisms which can be typed using the polymerase chain reaction. *Am. J. Hum. Genet., 44*, 388-396.

[38] Mao, L., Lee, D. J., Tockman, M. S., Erozan, Y. S., Askin, F., and Sidransky, D. (1994). Microsatellite alterations as clonal markers for the detection of human cancer. *Proc. Natl. Acad. Sci. USA, 91*, 9871-9875.

[39] Mao, L., Schoenberg, M. P., Scicchitano, M., Erozan, Y. S., Merlo, A., Schwab, D., and Sidransky, D. (1996). Molecular detection of primary bladder cancer by microsatellite analysis. *Science, 271*, 659-662.

[40] Steiner, G., Schoenberg, M. P., Linn, J. F., Mao, L., and Sidransky, D. (1997). Detection of bladder cancer recurrence by microsatellite analysis of urine. *Nat. Med., 3*, 621-624.

[41] van Tilborg, A. A., de Vries, A., de Bont, M., Groenfeld, L. E., van der Kwast, T. H., and Zwarthoff, E. C. (2000). Molecular evolution of multiple recurrent cancers of the bladder. *Hum. Mol. Genet., 9*, 2973-2980.

[42] Dyrskjot, L., Kruhoffer, M., Thykjaer, T., Marcussen, N., Jensen, J. L., Moller, K., and Orntoft, T. F. (2004). Gene expression in the urinary bladder: a common carcinoma in situ gene expression signature exists disregarding histopathological classification. *Cancer Res., 64*, 4040-4048.

[43] Lindgren, D., Gudjonsson, S., Jee, K. J., Liedberg, F., Aits, S., Andersson, A., Chebil, G., Borg, A., Knuutila, S., Fioretos, T., Mansson, W., and Hoglund, M. (2008). Recurrent and multiple bladder tumors show conserved expression profiles. *BMC Cancer, 8*, 183.

[44] Fadl-Elmula, I., Gorunova, L., Mandahl, N., Elfving, P., Lundgren, R., Mitelman, F., and Heim, S. (1999). Cytogenetic monoclonality in multifocal uroepithelial carcinomas: evidence of intraluminal tumour seeding. *Br. J. Cancer, 81*, 6-12.

[45] Kawanishi, H., Takahashi, T., Ito, M., Matsui, Y., Watanabe, J., Ito, N., Kamoto, T., Kadowaki, T., Tsujimoto, G., Imoto, I., Inazawa, J., Nishiyama, H., and Ogawa, O. (2007). Genetic analysis of multifocal superficial urothelial cancers by array-based comparative genomic hybridisation. *Br. J. Cancer, 97*, 260-266.

[46] Knowles, M. A., Elder, P. A., Williamson, M., Cairns, J. P., Shaw, M. E., and Law, M. G. (1994). Allelotype of human bladder cancer. *Cancer Res., 54*, 531-538.

[47] Obermann, E. C., Junker, K., Stoehr, R., Dietmaier, W., Zaak, D., Schubert, J., Hofstaedter, F., Knuechel, R., and Hartmann, A. (2003). Frequent genetic alterations in flat urothelial hyperplasias and concomitant papillary bladder cancer as detected by CGH, LOH, and FISH analyses. *J. Pathol., 199*, 50-57.

[48] Chow, N. H., Cairns, P., Eisenberger, C. F., Schoenberg, M. P., Taylor, D. C., Epstein, J. I., and Sidransky, D. (2000). Papillary urothelial hyperplasia is a clonal precursor to papillary transitional cell bladder cancer. *Int. J. Cancer, 89*, 514-518.

[49] Steidl, C., Simon, R., Burger, H., Brinkschmidt, C., Hertle, L., Bocker, W., et al. (2002). Patterns of chromosomal aberrations in urinary bladder tumours and adjacent urothelium. *J. Pathol., 198*, 115-120.

[50] Louhelainen, J., Wijkstrom, H., and Hemminki, K. (2000). Allelic losses demonstrate monoclonality of multifocal bladder tumors. *Int. J. Cancer, 87*, 522-527.

[51] Muto, S., Horie, S., Takahashi, S., Tomita, K., and Kitamura, T. (2000). Genetic and epigenetic alterations in normal bladder epithelium in patients with metachronous bladder cancer. *Cancer Res., 60*, 4021-4025.

[52] Cianciulli, A. M., Leonardo, C., Guadagni, F., Marzano, R., Iori, F., De Nunzio, C., Franco, G., Merola, R., and Laurenti, C. (2003). Genetic instability in superficial bladder cancer and adjacent mucosa: an interphase cytogenetic study. *Hum. Pathol., 34*, 214-221.

[53] Stoehr, R., Knuechel, R., Boecker, J., Blaszyk, H., Schmitt, R., Filbeck, T., Hofstaedter, F., and Hartmann, A. (2002). Histologic-genetic mapping by allele-specific PCR reveals intraurothelial spread of p53 mutant tumor clones. *Lab. Invest., 82*, 1553-1561.

[54] Stoehr, R., Zietz, S., Burger, M., Filbeck, T., Denzinger, S., Obermann, E. C., Hammerschmied, C., Wieland, W. F., Knuechel, R., and Hartmann, A. (2005). Deletions of chromosomes 9 and 8p in histologically normal urothelium of patients with bladder cancer. *Eur. Urol., 47*, 58-63.

[55] Czerniak, B., Chaturvedi, V., Li, L., Hodges, S., Johnston, D., Roy, J. Y., Luthra, R., Logothetis, C., Von Eschenbach, A. C., Grossman, H. B., Benedict, W. F., and Batsakis, J. G. (1999). Superimposed histologic and genetic mapping of chromosome 9 in progression of human urinary bladder neoplasia: implications for a genetic model of multistep urothelial carcinogenesis and early detection of urinary bladder cancer. *Oncogene, 18*, 1185-1196.

[56] Chaturvedi, V., Li, L., Hodges, S., Johnston, D., Ro, J. Y., Logothetis, C., von Eschenbach, A. C., Batsakis, J. G., and Czerniak, B. (1997). Superimposed histologic and genetic mapping of chromosome 17 alterations in human urinary bladder neoplasia. *Oncogene, 14*, 2059-2070.

[57] Habuchi, T., Takahashi, T., Kakinuma, H., Wang, L., Tsuchiya, N., Satoh, S., Akao, T., Sato, K., Ogawa, O., Knowles, M. A., and Kato, T. (2001). Hypermethylation at 9q32-33 tumour suppressor region is age-related in normal urothelium and an early and frequent alteration in bladder cancer. *Oncogene, 20*, 531-537.

[58] Chen, X. Q., Stroun, M., Magnenat, J. L., Nicod, L. P., Kurt, A. M., Lyautey, J., Lederrey, C., and Anker, P. (1996). Microsatellite alterations in plasma DNA of small cell lung cancer patients. *Nat. Med., 2*, 1033-1035.

[59] Wang, Y., Hung, S. C., Linn, J. F., Steiner, G., Glazer, A. N., Sidransky, D., and Mathies, R. A. (1997). Microsatellite-based cancer detection using capillary array electrophoresis and energy-transfer fluorescent primers. *Electrophoresis, 18*, 1742-1749.

[60] Lokeshwar, V. B., Habuchi, T., Grossman, H. B., Murphy, W. M., Hautmann, S. H., Hemstreet, G. P., 3rd, Bono, A. V., Getzenberg, R. H., Goebell, P., Schmitz-Drager, B. J., Schalken, J. A., Fradet, Y., Marberger, M., Messing, E., and Droller, M. J. (2005). Bladder tumor markers beyond cytology: International Consensus Panel on bladder tumor markers. *Urology, 66*(6 Suppl 1), 35-63.

[61] Seripa, D., Parrella, P., Gallucci, M., Gravina, C., Papa, S., Fortunato, P., Alcini, A., Flammia, G., Lazzari, M., and Fazio, V. M. (2001). Sensitive detection of transitional cell carcinoma of the bladder by microsatellite analysis of cells exfoliated in urine. *Int. J. Cancer, 95*, 364-369.

[62] van Rhijn, B. W., Lurkin, I., Kirkels, W. J., van der Kwast, T. H., and Zwarthoff, E. C. (2001). Microsatellite analysis--DNA test in urine competes with cystoscopy in follow-up of superficial bladder carcinoma: a phase II trial. *Cancer, 92*, 768-775.

[63] Sidransky, D., Von Eschenbach, A., Tsai, Y. C., Jones, P., Summerhayes, I., Marshall, F., Paul, M., Green, P., Hamilton, S. R., Frost, P., and et al. (1991). Identification of p53 gene mutations in bladder cancers and urine samples. *Science, 252*, 706-709.

[64] Conejo, J. R., Parra, T., Cantero, M., Jimenez, A., Granizo, V., de Arriba, G., and Carballo, F. (1998). Detection of H-ras mutations in urine sediments by a mutant-enriched PCR technique. *Clin. Chem., 44*, 1570-1572.

[65] van Rhijn, B. W., Lurkin, I., Chopin, D. K., Kirkels, W. J., Thiery, J. P., van der Kwast, T. H., Radvanyi, F., and Zwarthoff, E. C. (2003). Combined microsatellite and FGFR3 mutation analysis enables a highly sensitive detection of urothelial cell carcinoma in voided urine. *Clin. Cancer Res., 9*, 257-263.

[66] Matsumura, Y., Hanbury, D., Smith, J., and Tarin, D. (1994). Non-invasive detection of malignancy by identification of unusual CD44 gene activity in exfoliated cancer cells. *Bmj, 308*(6929), 619-624.

[67] Soloway, M. S., and Masters, S. (1980). Urothelial susceptibility to tumor cell implantation: influence of cauterization. *Cancer, 46*, 1158-1163.
[68] See, W. A., Miller, J. S., and Williams, R. D. (1989). Pathophysiology of transitional tumor cell adherence to sites of urothelial injury in rats: mechanisms mediating intravesical recurrence due to implantation. *Cancer Res., 49*(, 5414-5418.
[69] Oosterlinck, W., Kurth, K. H., Schroder, F., Bultinck, J., Hammond, B., and Sylvester, R. (1993). A prospective European Organization for Research and Treatment of Cancer Genitourinary Group randomized trial comparing transurethral resection followed by a single intravesical instillation of epirubicin or water in single stage Ta, T1 papillary carcinoma of the bladder. *J. Urol., 149*, 749-752.
[70] Ali-el-Dein, B., Nabeeh, A., el-Baz, M., Shamaa, S., and Ashamallah, A. (1997). Single-dose versus multiple instillations of epirubicin as prophylaxis for recurrence after transurethral resection of pTa and pT1 transitional-cell bladder tumours: a prospective, randomized controlled study. *Br. J. Urol., 79*, 731-735.
[71] Okamura, K., Ono, Y., Kinukawa, T., Matsuura, O., Yamada, S., Ando, T., Fukatsu, T., Ohno, Y., and Ohshima, S. (2002). Randomized study of single early instillation of (2"R)-4'-O-tetrahydropyranyl-doxorubicin for a single superficial bladder carcinoma. *Cancer, 94*(9), 2363-2368.
[72] Gudjonsson, S., Adell, L., Merdasa, F., Olsson, R., Larsson, B., Davidsson, T., Richthoff, J., Hagberg, G., Grabe, M., Bendahl, P. O., Mansson, W., and Liedberg, F. (2009). Should All Patients with Non-Muscle-Invasive Bladder Cancer Receive Early Intravesical Chemotherapy after Transurethral Resection? The Results of a Prospective Randomised Multicentre Study. *Eur. Urol.*. In press.
[73] Rubben, H., Lutzeyer, W., Fischer, N., Deutz, F., Lagrange, W., and Giani, G. (1988). Natural history and treatment of low and high risk superficial bladder tumors. *J. Urol., 139*, 283-285.
[74] Sylvester, R. J., Oosterlinck, W., and Witjes, J. A. (2008). The schedule and duration of intravesical chemotherapy in patients with non-muscle-invasive bladder cancer: a systematic review of the published results of randomized clinical trials. *Eur. Urol., 53*, 709-719.
[75] Lamm, D. L., Blumenstein, B. A., Crissman, J. D., Montie, J. E., Gottesman, J. E., Lowe, B. A., Sarosdy, M. F., Bohl, R. D., Grossman, H. B., Beck, T. M., Leimert, J. T., and Crawford, E. D. (2000). Maintenance bacillus Calmette-Guerin immunotherapy for recurrent TA, T1 and carcinoma in situ transitional cell carcinoma of the bladder: a randomized Southwest Oncology Group Study. *J. Urol., 163*, 1124-1129.
[76] Badalament, R. A., Herr, H. W., Wong, G. Y., Gnecco, C., Pinsky, C. M., Whitmore, W. F., Jr., Fair, W. R., and Oettgen, H. F. (1987). A prospective randomized trial of maintenance versus nonmaintenance intravesical bacillus Calmette-Guerin therapy of superficial bladder cancer. *J. Clin. Oncol., 5*, 441-449.
[77] Flamm, J. (1990). Long-term versus short-term doxorubicin hydrochloride instillation after transurethral resection of superficial bladder cancer. *Eur. Urol., 17*, 119-124.
[78] Okamura, K., Kinukawa, T., Tsumura, Y., Otani, T., Itoh, H., Kobayashi, H., Matsuura, O., Kobayashi, M., Fukatsu, T., and Ohshima, S. (1998). A randomized study of short-versus long-term intravesical epirubicin instillation for superficial bladder cancer. Nagoya University Urological Oncology Group. *Eur. Urol., 33*, 285-288; discussion 289.

In: Field Cancerization: Basic Science and Clinical Applications ISBN 978-1-61761-006-6
Editor: Gabriel D. Dakubo

Chapter 17

Evidence of Skin Field Cancerization

J. Andrew Carlson, Michael Murphy, Andrzej Slominski and Vincent L. Wilson

Abstract

Skin cancer is the most common malignancy in humans, likely due to its location at the interface between internal and external environments and exposure to multiple carcinogens, mostly ultraviolet radiation (UVR) and human papillomaviruses (HPV). With increased longevity, changing patterns of sun exposure and greater UVR reaching the earth's surface due to ozone depletion, the incidence of skin cancer is steadily increasing worldwide. Moreover, skin cancer, mostly basal cell carcinoma (BCC) and squamous cell carcinoma (SCC) (collectively known as non-melanoma skin cancer (NMSC), is a substantial public health concern and one of the largest Medicare health expenditures. Individuals presenting with skin cancer are at high risk for synchronous and metachronous second primary skin cancers. This phenomenon is known as "field cancerization", where the entire cutaneous site affected is presumed to be mutagenized and is therefore at risk for multiple cancers. The recent application of molecular technologies to the examination of peri-lesional and more distant adjacent normal skin samples has demonstrated many of the genotypic aberrations found in cancer. These defects are the earliest changes of oncogenesis that occur in a stepwise, cumulative fashion culminating in metastatic cancer via initiation, promotion, selection, and clonal expansion. Moreover, these findings implicate two distinct levels of field cancerization: 1) molecular progression where histologically normal cells accumulate genomic damage; and 2) phenotypic progression denoted by evolution of histologically normal skin to precursors to in situ cancer that can be followed by invasion and ultimately metastatic disease. Phenotypic progression is also characterized by the expansion of genetically damaged tumor cells in the modified environment that facilitate tumor growth and suppress the host response. In this model, the cutaneous field develops a "tumor stem cell", which acquires a growth advantage and exhibits a "mutator phenotype" [i.e. genomic instability (GIS)] that enables it to expand beyond its histologically defined stem cell niche, form diverse clonal fields, and accrue further genetic alterations that eventuate into invasive cancer. GIS is manifested as single base mutations, gain or loss of whole or partial chromosomes, amplification of oncogenes, mismatch repair gene defects, and epigenetic alterations including hypermethylation of promoter DNA of key tumor suppressor genes, or genomic incorporation of the oncogenic HPV. The facilitating environment for tumor growth represents the local production of factors that allow the tumor cells to escape the immune system, to leave the tumor stem cell niche and expand into the surrounding environment. In this chapter, we review the epidemiologic evidence of field cancerization; etiologic factors that lead to genomic instability in the skin; the stem cell niche where cancer-causing genetic defects are most likely to be initiated, and from which the mutated clone must expand beyond; host factors that augment and accelerate the process such as immunosuppression; and the growing body of evidence that supports the concept of cutaneous field cancerization. Moreover, we discuss the potential utilization of field effect biomarkers in risk assessment, cancer prevention, margin control, and prognosis.

17.1. Introduction

The incidence and prevalence of skin cancer, specifically basal cell carcinoma (BCC) and squamous cell carcinoma (SCC), collectively known as non-melanoma skin cancer (NMSC), is greater than that of all other cancers combined, and is increasing worldwide in fair skinned individuals [1-6]. In addition, representing less than 7% of all skin cancers, melanoma (MM) is the most lethal cutaneous malignancy and accounts for about 75% of all deaths from skin tumors [7-9]. From 1992 to 2006 in the United States of America, NMSC has increased by 4.2% per year, and the estimated population of NMSC patients is 3,507,693, of whom 2,152,500 received treatment based on Medicare beneficiary data [4]. These figures may still be an underestimate as NMSC is not routinely reported to cancer registries because of the shear number of cases and their low mortality [10]. The incidence of MM is rising faster than any other malignancy and is therefore considered an epidemic cancer as it's incidence has increased 697% between 1950 and 2000 [3, 9, 11-13]. In the United States, the cost of treating this burden of skin cancer is one of the largest Medicare expenditures [14] and in 2004, it was estimated to be $2.4 billion [15]. Thus, primary prevention and early detection of skin cancer will have a significant impact on health expenditures, in addition to the wellbeing and longevity of those at risk for skin cancer [16].

Skin cancer patients often present with multiple synchronous primary tumors [4, 17-20] and are at substantial risk for additional metachronous second primary skin cancers with time [21-31]. Furthermore, these patients are at higher risk for second primary non-cutaneous malignancies, often those related to smoking or lymphoproliferative malignancies [21, 22, 24, 26, 27, 30, 32, 33]. The risk for second, non-cutaneous primaries is greatest for MM [24]. This high risk for multiple primary skin cancers implicates precancerous changes in the apparently normal skin surrounding the skin cancer; a process termed "field cancerization". Moreover, the development of non-cutaneous second primary cancers indicates the presence of genetic susceptibility (e.g., poor DNA repair mechanisms), depressed immunity, and/or systemic environmental exposures in skin cancer patients.

"Field cancerization" (a.k.a., field effect, field defect, or field cells) was first described by Slaughter et al. [34], who stated that all the epithelium of the upper aerodigestive tract had been mutagenized, presumably as a result of exposure to carcinogens such as tobacco smoke or nitrates, and therefore was at increased risk for multiple epithelial tumors. This pathogenic scheme is equally applicable to the skin. A growing body of evidence supports the concept of cutaneous field cancerization [35]. These studies have demonstrated the presence of some genotypic and phenotypic traits requisite for cancer [36] in histologically normal keratinocytes or melanocytes found in the proximity of a skin cancer, such as *TP53* hotspot mutations in normal keratinocytes [37], p53 protein expressing keratinocytic clones [38], and cyclin D1 gene amplifications [39]. In the setting of genotypically abnormal, but phenotypically (histologically) normal clones of keratinocytes or melanocytes, localized tumors are thought to emerge from these broad precancerous fields by a process of selection and clonal expansion of mutant cells [40, 41].

The high prevalence and external location of skin cancers provide an exceptional opportunity to study the events of field cancerization. In this review, most of the discussion will be restricted to the most common skin cancers: BCC, SCC, and MM. The topics that will be discussed include epidemiology of skin cancer; etiologic factors involved in skin cancer; clinical and histologic biomarkers that indicate the presence of field cancerization and impart a greater risk for skin cancer; the varied forms of genomic instability and their role in cutaneous carcinogenesis; the stem cell niche where cancer causing genetic defects are most likely initiated and from which the mutated clone must expand beyond; host factors that augment and accelerate the process, such as immunosuppression; and the growing body of evidence that supports the concept of cutaneous field cancerization. Lastly, we discuss the potential utilization of field effect biomarkers in prevention, margin control, and prognosis.

17.2. Skin Carcinogenesis

The accumulation of multiple DNA alterations through genomic instability (GIS) (i.e., “mutator cancer phenotype”), which affects crucial cell-cycle pathway genes controlling cell proliferation, differentiation and apoptosis are considered the hallmarks of cancer [36, 42-44]. Indeed, the recent genotype of the whole genome of a MM cell line has demonstrated evidence of widespread GIS. Numerous genetic aberrations were identified, most of which represented passenger gene mutations, but a minority consisted of driver gene mutations, which conferred the essential traits requisite for cancer cells [36, 45]. The 8 cardinal features of a cancer cell are (6 per Hanahan and Weinberg [36] and 2 supplemental to account for immunity and MM antigens [46]):

1. Self-sufficiency in growth signals
2. Insensitivity to anti-growth signals
3. Evasion of apoptosis
4. Limitless replication potential
5. Tissue invasion and metastasis
6. Angiogenesis
7. Escape from immune surveillance and production of immunosuppressive molecules
8. Altered melanocyte and keratinocyte differentiation/secretory molecules

The acquisition of these traits occurs through the progressive, stochastic accumulation of genetic defects via a process of initiation, promotion, selection, and clonal expansion [43, 47]. In the case of MM, BCC, and SCC, the phenotypic traits and genetic defects of cancer appear to occur in a sequential manner that correlate with specific clinical and histologic stages, supporting the prevailing theory of tumor progression [7, 43, 44, 48-51]. Listed below are prototypical pathways of skin carcinogenesis, each step of which is associated with the acquisition of one or more of the cardinal features of cancer. The number of stages appears to support the multi-hit hypothesis of cancer where 4-6 genetic hits are required for cancer to develop [52]. Also listed are the most common cell-cycle pathways altered during carcinogenesis. The precursors of SCC and MM, actinic keratoses (AK) and dysplastic melanocytic nevi, respectively, are also intermediate biomarkers of skin cancer, as they represent risk factors for the development of SCC, BCC and MM [53], and as well, harbor many overlapping genotypic alterations with SCC and MM, respectively [7, 54-57].

Basal Cell Carcinoma Progression

1. Normal follicular germinative/pluripotent keratinocyte stem cell
   No known precursors
2. BCC, low risk for local recurrence (Superficial > nodular patterns)
3. BCC, high risk for local recurrence (Infiltrative > morpheic patterns)
4. Metastatic BCC (rare occurrence)

Major pathway: activation of Sonic Hedgehog pathway (loss of *PTCH*); inactivation of *TP53*

Melanoma Progression UVR Related/Not Sun Related (Mucosal, Acral)

1. Normal melanocyte stem cell
2. Common nevus/melanotic macule
3. Dysplastic nevus/atypical lentiginous melanocytic hyperplasia
4. Radial growth phase (in situ/invasive, non-tumorgenic) MM
5. Vertical growth phase MM
6. Metastatic MM

Major pathway: activation of MAPKinase (RAS-RAF-MEK-ERK) and PTEN-PI3K-AKT; loss of CDKN2A ($p16^{INK4}/p14^{Arf}$); cyclin D gene amplification (acral MM); C-KIT mutation

Squamous Cell Carcinoma Progression, UVR Associated

1. Normal basal keratinocyte stem cell
2. Sun damaged skin (freckles, lentigines)
3. Actinic (solar) keratosis/squamous cell carcinoma in situ (SCCIS)
4. Invasive SCC
5. Metastatic SCC

Major pathway: Inactivation of *TP53*; aneuploidy; activation of Ras (MAPK pathway); reduced FasR (CD95-R)

Squamous Cell Carcinoma Progression, Chronic Fibrosing Inflammation Associated

1. Normal keratinocyte stem cell
2. Chronic fibro-inflammatory state with regenerative hyperplasia
3. Atypical keratinocytic hyperplasias
4. SCC
5. Metastatic SCC

Major pathway: Inactivation of *TP53*; aneuploidy

Squamous Cell Carcinoma Progression, High Risk HPV Associated

1. Normal keratinocyte
2. Anogenital or periungual warts
3. Squamous cell carcinoma in situ (? Use SCCIS..defined above)
4. SCC
5. Metastatic SCC

Major pathway: abrogation of *TP53* and Retinoblastoma proteins by high risk HPV E6 and E7 proteins

In all these schemes, it is commonly assumed that the first genomic hit/damage leads to the second step of cancer progression. Thus, much of the extant research to date has concentrated on skin cancer precursors and their associated cancers and metastases, and not on the detection of defects present in perilesional normal skin. Indeed, few studies have examined for the presence of signs of GIS such as driver and/or passenger (bystander) mutations in normal/structurally intact, perilesional skin. Moreover, even fewer studies have compared ostensibly, normal skin cells from the cancer field with normal cells from an unrelated, non-cancer field (e.g., sun exposed skin versus non-sun exposed skin). Considering that genomic aberrations are frequent in perilesional normal skin (NS) as documented in this review, the practice of using perilesional skin as normal controls is suspect.

As second primary tumors arise in these fields of perceived normal cells, genomic damage in regions affected by cancer must be clinically and histologically silent and will be detectable, in most cases only with highly sensitive tests. Considering that genomic analysis of human cancers has revealed a large number of genetic changes per cell and that the complexity of these changes differ from one type of cancer to another and even from patient to patient with the same type of cancer [44, 45, 58-60], the probability that apparently normal skin harbors cells with genomic aberrations, both relevant and irrelevant to carcinogenesis, is high.

In support of this supposition, skin fibroblasts from individuals in families with heritable forms of cancer, and from cancer-bearing individuals, show correlation with a significant increase in saturation density, as well as other neoplasia-related properties [58]. Thus, analysis of morphologically normal tissue, in this case, dermal fibroblasts by saturation density ("a field") revealed evidence of susceptibility to cancer that is regional and global in nature, likely reflecting local and systemic exposures to carcinogens and underlying germ cell genetic vulnerabilities.

These underlying, functional defects which predispose to cancer are not ostensibly those recognized as the hallmarks of cancer first proposed by Hanahan and Weinberg [36]. Recently, additional hallmarks for cancer have been proposed that describe existing structural rather than functional changes, which produce cancer susceptibility. These 5 additional hallmarks of cancer are related to the presence of cellular stress and produce a state of GIS:

1. DNA damage and replication stress
2. Oxidative stress
3. Metabolic stress
4. Mitotic stress
5. Proteotoxic stress

In effect, GIS is present at all stages of cancer, and the multistep model of field cancerization indicates two distinct levels of cancer progression: 1) *molecular progression* whereby histologically normal appearing cells undergo sequential cumulative acquisition of genomic damage; and 2) *phenotypic progression* whereby a neoplastic cell accumulates additional genetic aberrations that manifest as phenotype changes characteristic of cancer cells with progression from precursors to in situ cancer to invasive cancer, ultimately ending with metastatic disease [35].

17.3. Definition of the "Field" in Skin

A cutaneous "field" is a region of skin that has sustained genetic damage and developed clones of mutant cells (keratinocytes and/or melanocytes) due to repeated exposure to carcinogens such as UVR, chemicals, reactive oxygen species (ROS), and/or HPV. Therefore, the "field" is at increased risk for developing multiple skin cancers, simultaneously, and/or over time. This field defect can be normal appearing or bear clinical markers of field cancerization.

In most cases, the "field" will be sun-exposed skin with signs of solar damage (changes in pigmentation) and which, in more advanced cases, will exhibit precursors such as AK and solar lentigines. Other "fields" will be found at sites of chronic inflammation, scarring, or areas with numerous common melanocytic nevi or dysplastic melanocytic nevi.

In some "fields", the clones will be clinically and histologically silent; the genetic abnormalities that predispose to cancer will be detectable by genomic or proteomic assays such as gene mutation analysis or immunohistochemistry (IHC).

17.4. Cutaneous Stem Cells

Multiple stem or progenitor cell populations exist in the skin, which are involved in skin homeostasis and wound repair [61, 62]. Cutaneous stem cells are located in the basal layer of the epidermis, the bulge of the hair follicle, focally in the basal layer of the sebaceous gland, the follicular papillae, and the dermis in the connective tissue sheath of blood vessels and nerves. In addition, circulating hematopoietic stem cells can access the skin via blood vessels, particularly in response to injury and inflammation. The pluripotency of each stem cell increases with its deeper location in the dermis. In general, adult somatic stem cells retain pluripotency and self-renewal capabilities, while giving rise to progenitor, transient amplifying cells and terminally differentiated cells. Maintenance of self-renewal and pluripotency requires the stem cell to reside in a micro-environmental niche that provides a stable and resting environment necessary for maintenance of a stem cell phenotype. The niche environment act as a reservoir, by binding a large variety of cytokines and growth factors, which are slowly released and are essential to the continuation of the stem cell population [63, 64]. Also, adult stem cell DNA is hypermethylated (contains high levels of DNA 5-methyldeoxycytidine), which is most likely required for the silencing of multiple differentiation programs and maintenance of self-renewal and pluripotency capacity [65, 66]. A hallmark of stem cells, and likely cancer stem cells, is the expression of telomerase [67], which extends the number of cellular divisions these stem cells can undergo before reaching senescence.

17.5. Epidermal (Keratinocyte) Stem Cells

The human epidermis is organized into subunits, termed epidermal proliferative units (EPU), where each EPU is supported by one stem cell that undergoes asymmetric division producing transient amplifying cells and committed cells in a columnar pattern [68-70]. The EPU contains only one to ten basal cells per EPU and are distributed along the undulating basal layer, with no apparent bias for the site of origin of the EPU [70]. Slightly more stem cells occur along the flat regions of the basement membrane, but the stem cell numbers are relatively the same for the tip of rete ridges and overlying dermal papillae [70]. In addition to stem cells located along the basement membrane zone of interfollicular regions, keratinocyte stem cells are also found in the bulge of the hair follicle, which are involved in crucial developmental functions and serve as a reservoir for multipotent adult stem cells [69, 71]. For example, the bulge epithelial cells have been shown to express the essential melanocyte gene, microphthalmia transcription factor (Mitf) confirming that melanocyte precursors also reside in this niche [72, 73]. Epidermal stem cells express high levels of selective transcription factors such as beta1 integrin (74) and alpha6 integrin, and low levels of transferrin receptor [75], p63 [76], and an isoform of the stem cell antigen CD133 [77].

17.6. Melanocyte Stem Cells

Melanocytes are derived from neural crest cells, which migrate to the epidermis during embryogenesis. During this migration, melanocyte precursor cells progressively differentiate from a neural crest stem cell to melanoblasts which depending on their location in the skin can differentiate to terminally differentiated, dendritic, pigmented epidermal or follicular melanocytes [78, 79]. Each stage of development shows gradual lineage restriction dependent on Mitf expression and gain of expression of melanin-related proteins [80]. In the skin, melanocyte stem cells are located in the epidermis, the bulge of the hair follicle and the dermis, in association with nerve sheaths [81, 82]. Each of these stem cell niches is suspected of giving rise to phenotypically and genotypically distinct MM: epidermal melanocyte stem cells - superficial spreading MM; bulge melanocytes - lentigo maligna MM; and dermal melanocyte stem cells - nodular MM [83, 84]. This data indicates that each stem cell niche undergoes distinct genotoxic/environmental stresses.

17.7. Stem Cell Clonality and Development of Cancer Stem Cells

Each EPU and putative melanocyte proliferative unit represents a clone of cells, whose genotype will reflect that of its stem cell. As each unit is anatomically distinct, a mutant stem cell clone must expand beyond the confines of its proliferative unit and acquire further carcinogenic defects. Stem cells die if they suffer DNA damage rather than repair it, thus avoiding accumulation of replication errors [85]; thus, loss of stem cells due to genotoxic stress provides an opportunity for clonal expansion. Overcoming the restriction of mutant cell clones to one EPU would represent a breach of one rate-limiting step in the pathogenesis of skin cancer. These mutant cells grow exponentially and, thus, they can acquire additional errors of replication, some of which may confer a selective growth advantage, leading to expansion into adjacent EPU.

In the normal epidermis, UVR exposure results in low frequency point mutations in the TP53 gene that are fairly widely distributed [86, 87]. These epidermal p53 mutant clones were located mostly in the transient amplifying compartment only, or in both the stem cell and transiently amplifying compartment indicating that the target cells acquiring the p53 protein stabilizing mutation were either transient amplifying cells or stem cells, respectively (88; See figure 17-1). Most clones arise from transient amplifying cells as the epidermal p53 clones tend to regress [89]. These short-lived clones are shed as cornified squames, and never exceed or equal the size of the EPU, estimated to be about 35 basal cells in diameter in humans [90]; thus, they are not destined to progress to cancer. In order to produce a cancer field, there must be expansion into adjacent EPU by replacement of stem cells by early lineage, mutant daughter cells. Evidence of expansion of p53 clones beyond the confines of the EPU is demonstrated in chronically sun-damaged skin. Indeed, the size and number of epidermal p53 clones directly varies with the level of sun exposure [91] and increasing age [38]. In addition, they are more numerous and larger p53 keratinocyte clones adjacent to SCC than BCC and melanocytic nevi, linking these p53 clones to the pathogenesis of UVR related SCC [38]. Experimentally, the phenomenon of p53 clonal expansion has been demonstrated in mouse skin subjected to UVR [92]. Short term UVR exposures leads to the formation of epidermal p53 mutant stem cell clones that increase only in number, not exceeding an area of 16 ± 6 cells, the size of the EPU in murine dorsal skin. Chronic exposure of mouse skin to UVR leads to the expansion of these mutant clones to adjacent EPU (i.e., stem cell compartments).

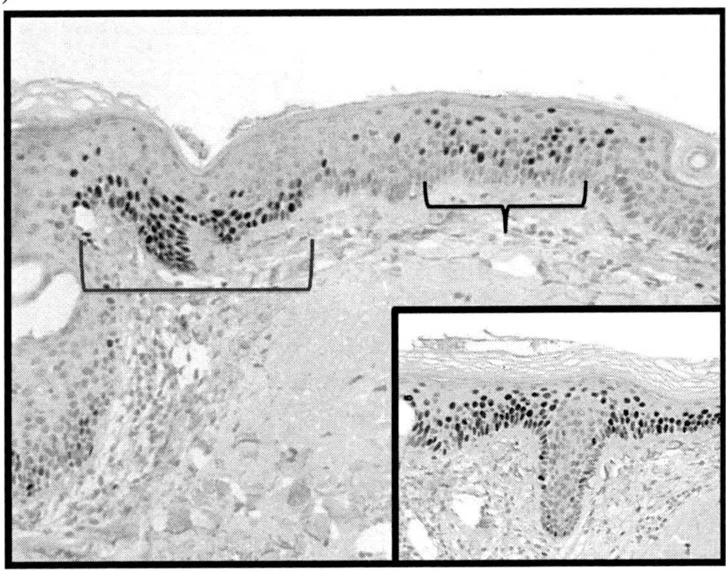

Figure 17.1. Tumor suppressor gene p53 protein mutant epidermal clones. Patterns of p53 protein expression correlate with mutational status: weak, scattered/dispersed nuclear expression correlates with wild type gene, whereas strong compact/continuous expression correlates with mutant p53 (4). Illustrated herein is putatively mutated stem cell given rise to mutant clone the size of epidermal proliferating units (EPU)(red bracket). In contrast, the black bracket shows suprabasal small patches of presumptively p53 mutated keratinocytes that likely represent transient amplifying cells. The insert shows a large mutant clone that replaces several EPUs, but spares central adnexal epithelium. The stem cells of the eccrine duct are not subjected to ultraviolet damage as they are located deeper in the dermis; thus, they are spared the mutagenic effect of UVR.

In this setting of chronic genotoxic stress, events of apoptosis as well as initiation and promotion (regenerative hyperplasia) occur, thereby producing GIS and clonal diversity. Clonal diversity is likely the strongest predictor for progression to invasive cancer [93].

17.8. Epidemiologic Evidence of Field Cancerization

The risk for skin cancer depends on genotype, phenotype and environmental exposures. In addition, it is a disease of old age as 80% of all NMSC occur in people aged 60 years or older [94]. Men have a higher incidence than women. Currently, a combination of prolonged/increased sun exposure, usage of tanning parlors, increased outdoor activities, changes in clothing style, increased longevity, and ozone depletion are contributing to the increasing incidence and prevalence of skin cancer, both NMSC and MM, which are the most common types of cancer in fair skinned populations [4-7]. In general, there is a ratio of 4:1

BCC to SCC, and 18-20:1 NMSC to MM [6]. Despite the rising incidence, these cancers are showing stable or decreasing mortality rates [6]. Other factors that influence skin cancer susceptibility are genetics that impact on skin phototype and DNA repair, and host level of immunity. A crucial factor affecting the susceptibility to UVR induced cancer is the level of skin pigmentation. In this context, melanin pigment acts not only as an optical filter absorbing UV energy, but also as a metabolically active bio-molecule that affects the functions of the cells to which the pigment was transferred [78, 95, 96]. It could be stated that no skin cancer patient ever has just one tumor. In fact, patients with skin cancer often present with multiple primaries and are at higher risk for second primary cutaneous tumors [4, 17-30]. For instance, NMSC patients present with a mean 1.63 NMSC per patient [4]; 30-40% of patients with BCC will develop one or more BCC within 10 years [97]; MM patients have a 32% higher risk of developing a second primary MM at any site compared to the general population [21]; and 57% of SCC patients are at risk for second primary SCC [24]. Thus, skin cancer is, itself, a risk factor for skin cancer implying that all skin or a region of skin (e.g. sun exposed) has been mutagenized, due to exposure to UVR or other carcinogens, and is at risk for multiple tumors ("the whole neighborhood is affected" [35]).

In the case of SCC, the fact that immunosuppressed patients such as organ transplant recipients (OTR) develop numerous and aggressive SCC attests to the presence of abundant "dormant" SCC precursors in the general population, which are controlled by normal immune functions [23, 55]. Furthermore, the risk of developing a subsequent skin cancer of a specific type depends on the type of prior NMSC. For example, the risk of developing a BCC in patients with a prior SCC is about equal to that risk among persons with a prior BCC, but the risk of developing an SCC in patients with a prior BCC is low (6%) [98]. This contrast in risk reflects underlying differences in genomic disruptions in the skin cancer fields, which give rise to BCC and SCC.

17.9. Clinical Risk Factors for Skin Cancer; Surrogate Markers of Field Cancerization

Table 17-1 lists the risk factors for skin cancer, which would also represent, in many cases, surrogate markers of field cancerization in sun-exposed sites. Sun exposure, UVR, and its effects on skin, which are dependent on skin type has the greatest impact on the development of BCC, SCC and MM [99]. In the case of MM, distinct genetic alterations have been identified at different anatomic sites and with different levels of sun exposure supporting epidemiologic studies that sun exposure is a factor in MM pathogenesis [83, 100]. For SCC, the cumulative dose of UVR is the strongest predictor for development of SCC [99]. In contrast, the risk of BCC is related to intensive UVR exposure during childhood and adolescence [6]. These correlations point to three distinct patterns of exposure to UVR and individual susceptibility to skin cancer: 1) intermittent sun exposure and propensity to develop multiple melanocytic nevi; 2) chronic sun exposed skin with solar lentigines and AK; and 3) multiple sun burns during childhood, sun sensitivity and freckling [94, 101, 102]. See figure 17-2.

Apart from a history of skin cancer, several other clinical phenotypes denote a high risk for skin cancer and represent intermediate biomarkers of skin cancer (53, 103). These biomarkers are AK, solar lentigines, and multiple melanocytic nevi and/or atypical (dysplastic) melanocytic nevi. For example, the number of nevi, either acquired or atypical, constitutes the best predictor of individual risk of MM, and the presence of large (i.e. >5 mm) or atypical nevi (i.e. large nevi with non-uniform color and irregular borders), independent of the number of smaller nevi, is associated with an elevated risk of MM (relative risk of 5.5 to 5.8) [101, 103]. If these latter patients also have a personal and family history of MM, their relative risk for melanoma is 444 [103].

Table 17.1. Risk factors for skin cancers and biomarkers of field cancerization

Biomarker	Skin cancer association	Reference
Clinical		
Age>50; male sex	SCC, BCC	[94, 102]
Red/blonde/light brown hair, blue eyes	MM, BCC	[94, 102, 103]
Fair skin, skin phototypes 1 and 2 (never/poorly tans, always/mostly burns)	BCC, MM, SCC	[94, 102, 103]
History of blistering sun burns	MM, BCC	[94, 102, 103]
Minimal erythema dose (MED)	All types	[123]
Sun damaged skin/large cumulative sun exposure	SCC, MM, BCC	[94, 102, 103]
Solar lentigines	MM, SCC	[94, 102, 103]
Actinic (Solar) keratoses (AK)	SCC	[94, 102, 103]
Melanocytic nevi, high counts or atypical (dysplastic)	MM	[94, 102, 103]
Chronic inflammatory and scarring disorders	SCC > > BCC and MM	[94, 102, 103]
Phototoxic drugs	SCC	[291]
Therapeutic exposure to PUVA, UVB, or ionizing radiation	SCC, BCC	[94, 102, 103]
Occupational exposures to coal tar, pitch, creosote, arsenic compounds, or radium	SCC, BCC	[94, 102, 103]
Exposure to tanning lamps	SCC, BCC, MM	[94, 102, 103]
Family history of skin cancer	MM, BCC, SCC	[94, 102, 103]
Geography (near equator/high altitude)	SCC	[94, 102]
HPV infection (warts, mostly anogenital and periungual)	SCC, BCC	[94, 102]
Histologic		
Seborrheic keratosis	All types (*FGFR3, PIK3CA*)	[110]
Focal acantholytic dyskeratosis*	All types (*ATP2A2*)*	[111]
Epidermolytic hyperkeratosis	All types (*KRT1, KRT10*)*	[111]
Hailey-Hailey-like acantholysis	All types (*ATP2C1*)*	[111]
Epidermodysplasia acanthoma	All types (*EVER 1, 2*)*	[112]
Actinic keratoses (AK)	SCC	[292]
Dysplastic melanocytic nevi	MM	[109]
Squamous cell carcinoma in situ (SCCIS; a.k.a Bowen's disease)	SCC, Merkel Cell carcinoma	[94, 102]
Sebaceous adenomas, keratoacanthomas with sebaceous differentiation	Sebaceous carcinoma (MMR gene defects)	[236]

*: Genes suspected to be affected, but not confirmed to date.

Chronically sun damaged skin in Caucasians is associated with skin wrinkling and dyspigmentation [101]. This mottled skin in the elderly is the result of extensive freckling, guttate hypomelanosis, solar lentigines, and seborrheic keratoses. Solar lentigines are a known risk factor for MM [104] and are the site of acquired atypical lentiginous melanocytic hyperplasias, putative precursors to MM (105, 106). AKs also occur in chronically sun damaged skin. How to identify if and when a specific AK will progress to SCC is unknown. The risk for progression of a single AK to SCC ranges from 0.25% to 20% per year. This risk is higher in patients with more than 5 lesions (94). Conversely, 82% of SCC arises in the background of AKs and 27% of SCC directly arises from an AK [107].

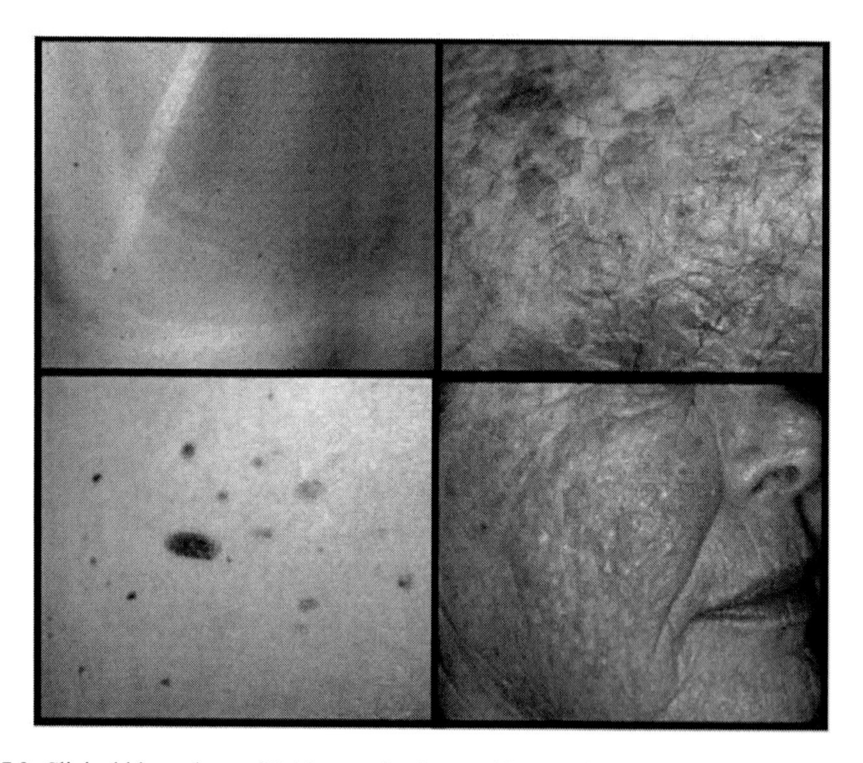

Figure 17.2. Clinical biomarkers of field cancerization are history of sunburns (top left panel); chronic sun damaged skin (mottled skin, the result of extensive freckling, guttate hypomelanosis, solar lentigines, wrinkling, and seborrheic keratoses (top right panel)); melanocytic nevi (bottom left panel); and actinic keratoses (AKs) (bottom right panel). The consequence of intermittent intense sun exposure and/or chronic sun exposure is the development of intermediate biomarkers of skin cancer: melanocytic nevi, both common and dysplastic or atypical (central nevus) and multiple AKS, respectively (bottom left and right panels); and over time BCC, MM, and/or SCC.

17.10. Histologic Markers of Field Cancerization

The first step in effective treatment is accurate diagnosis. AKs are scaly macules or papules that are often more easily recognized by palpation than visual inspection. Atypical melanocytic nevi often fulfill all the ABCDE (Asymmetry, irregular Border, two or more Colors, Diameter greater than 5mm, Enlarging, evolving) clinical criteria for MM. Conversely, benign tumors can mimic malignant tumors clinically.

Therefore, skin biopsy is required to confidently classify skin tumors suspected to be malignant or to confirm their benign nature [108]. Moreover, the identification of skin cancer precursors such as AK, squamous cell carcinoma in situ (SCCIS) (a.k.a. Bowen's disease) and atypical melanocytic nevi denotes the presence of field cancerization and high risk for skin cancer in that region.

In the case of melanocytic nevi, the grading of atypia correlates with risk of MM [109]. While up to 40% of MM are associated with a melanocytic nevus histologically, clinically, most MM arise de novo [103].

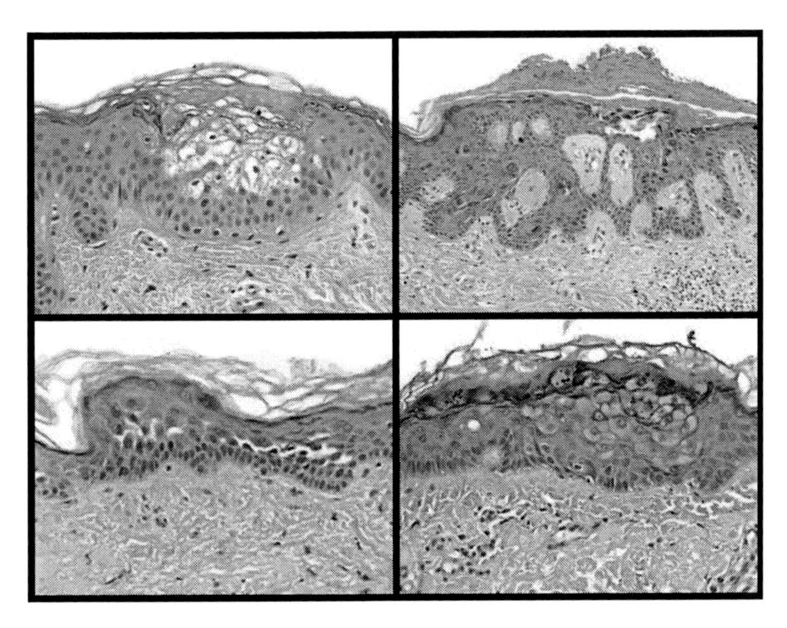

Figure 17.3. Incidental histologic epidermal markers of field cancerization: epidermolytic hyperkeratosis (top left panel); focal acantholytic dyskeratosis (top right panel); Hailey-Hailey-like acantholysis (bottom left panel) and focal beta-HPV (epidermodysplasia verruciformis) infection (bottom right panel) [1, 2]. Each of this epidermal histologic patterns correlates with a unique genodermatoses and germ-line mutation, but can also be seen as post-zygotic systematized (e.g. epidermal nevus) processes. As an incidental histologic finding, these patterns are seen significantly more frequently in the skin of elderly individuals adjacent to benign and malignant skin tumors (1). These incidental histologic findings could be considered passenger mutations, signifying wide spread genomic instability [3].

While it is accepted that the identification of precursors (like AK) and markers of risk (like atypical nevi) of skin cancer point to the presence of carcinogenic events that are directly involved in skin carcinogenesis, benign skin tumors and incidental histologic findings also point to co-existing genomic instability. However, these mutations appear to represent signs of background GIS (e.g. passenger mutations).

Seborrheic keratoses are benign skin tumors whose number increases with age and are found in higher frequency on sun-exposed skin [110]. Seborrheic keratoses frequently harbor activating mutations in Fibroblast Growth Factor Receptor 3 (FGFR3*)* and catalytic p110 subunit of class 1 phosphatidylinositol 3-kinase (PI3KCA) genes, which do not show UVR signature mutations [110]. Neither of these genes is involved in the pathogenesis of skin cancer, but they are found in a number of malignant tumors such as colon, breast, and bladder cancer. Thus, mutations in FGFR3 and PI3KCA may represent passenger mutations, collateral damage to underlying GIS.

Other specific histologic patterns also point to background GIS and can be seen incidentally, as small clonal events [111, 112]. See table 17-1 and figure 17-3. While none of these incidental findings have been shown to harbor mutations to date, each pattern is found in well-described genodermatoses due to specific germ line mutations, or as epidermal nevi (hamartomas) with post-zygotic mutations. These patterns are epidermolytic hyperkeratosis due to mutations in keratins 1 or 10 genes (*KRT1, KRT10*); focal acantholytic dyskeratosis found in Darier's disease due to mutation in the gene ATP2A2, which encodes the intracellular pump sarco/endoplasmic reticulum Ca(2+)-ATPase type 2 isoform (SERCA2); Hailey-Hailey disease or benign familial pemphigus acantholysis is due to mutation in *ATP2C1*, which encodes the human homolog of an ATP-powered pump that sequesters calcium into the Golgi in yeast; and epidermodysplasia verruciformis (EV) due to mutations of EVER 1 or 2 genes, which encode transmembrane channel-like (TMC) proteins that are postulated to function as ion channels or as signal transducers.

These incidental histologic patterns are found significantly more frequently in older individuals and adjacent to skin cancers [111], or in the case of focal acantholytic dyskeratosis, dysplastic melanocytic nevi [113]. These histologic patterns can also be found in small, benign keratoses, termed acanthomas, which may represent a clonal expansion of an incidental focus [114-117]. Unlike the first 3 patterns, the incidental EV phenotype represents a direct, not indirect, sign of neoplastic genetic damage to keratinocytes. Indeed, an increase risk for skin cancer exists for patients with detectable EV HPV DNA by PCR methods [118].

17.11. Etiologic Factors Producing Skin Field Cancerization

Multiple factors play a role in skin cancer including skin pigmentation (skin phototype), UVR, ionizing radiation, polycyclic aromatic hydrocarbons, arsenic, scars from burns and smallpox, chronic ulcers or sinus tracts (chronic inflammation), DNA repair capacity, specific genetic syndromes, and dysregulated melanogenesis. A long interval, decades exists between exposure (e.g., sunburn that results in initial DNA damage) and the onset of tumor formation. During this interval oncogenic processes must be active, but not observable clinically and/or histologically until tumor formation begins. The nature of these events that culminate in cancer is unknown.

17.11.1. Ultraviolet Light Radiation (UVR)

Over 80% of NMSC occur in sun-exposed sites, head and neck and back of hands, attesting to a role for UVR in carcinogenesis [6]. UVR is a spectrum of electromagnetic energy covering the wavelengths between 100 to 400 nm and includes vacuum UV, UVC, UVB and UVA [119]. The upper layers of the Earth's atmosphere filter out vaccum UV and UVC (200-290 nm). UVB (290-320 nm) and UVA (320-400 nm) reach the surface of the Earth and dependent on skin penetration, they can affect DNA integrity, cell and tissue homeostasis, induce mutations, affect the expression of a plethora of genes including oncogenes and tumor suppressor genes, modify the expression and activity of growth factors/cytokines and their receptors, and have local and systemic immunosuppressive effects [101, 120]. UVB causes direct damage to DNA and RNA by inducing covalent bond formation between adjacent pyrimidines, leading to the production of mutagenic photoproducts such as cyclobutane pyrimidine dimers (CPD) and pyrimidine-pyrimidine adducts [101, 121]. In addition to UVB, UVA is also an important risk factor of photocarcinogenesis, but acts through different mechanisms than UVB. UVA exposure leads to a photo-oxidative stress-mediated mechanism that results in the formation of reactive oxygen species (ROS) which interact with lipids, proteins and DNA to form adducts [101, 121]. In AK and SCC, UVA-signature mutations are located mostly in the basal layer of epidermis and UVB-signature mutations are found mostly within suprabasal keratinocytes [122]. This is in agreement with the depth of penetration of UVA and UVB into the skin. In Caucasians, 20-30 % of photons within the range of 290 – 320 nm reach keratinocytes, about 10 % penetrate the epidermis reaching the upper layers of the dermis and only 1% of UVR below 300 nm can enter the dermis. In contrast, UVA penetrates the dermis (50% of these photons in type I skin) [101].

UVB is about 1000-10000 more efficient than UVA in inducting DNA damage, erythema and cancers [101]. The mechanism of its action includes direct damage of DNA, since nucleic acids represent primary chromophores for UVB, producing pyrimidine (6-4) pyrimidone photoproducts (6-4PP) and CPD between adjacent pyrimidine sites (usually at TT, TC and CT sequences). 6-4PP and CPD represent 25% and 75% of adducts, respectively. Both types of photoproducts affect the structure of DNA with CPDs being more significant in UVR-induced carcinogenesis than 6-4PPs, because 6-4PPs adducts can be repaired with high efficiency, while CPD are removed slowly by transcription coupled repair [101]. CPDs are responsible for about 80% of UVB mutations in mammalian cells [101]. Lack of repair of the above photoadducts leads to mutations in several genes of which the most frequent are C to T and CC to TT transitions, termed UVB "fingerprint or signature mutations"[101]. Tandem CC to TT transitions, being the most specific mutation caused by UVR are rarely found in internal organs. The above DNA damage caused by UVB irradiation induces an inflammatory response that leads to cutaneous erythema. The minimal erythema dose, time per fixed amount of UVB exposure that causes erythema, could serve as a biomarker for exposure and internal dosage, thus risk for field cancerization [123].

Although UVA is less carcinogenic than UVB, it has a profound impact on photo-ageing, because of its deep penetration into the skin, in addition to playing a role in development of skin cancers [101, 121]. Although UVA is weakly absorbed by DNA, it is absorbed by other chromophores, and induces oxidative stress, generating ROS that damage DNA. The main target of ROS within DNA is guanine, with 8-oxo-7,8-dihydro-2'-guanine (8-oxoGua) being considered as the most prevalent presence of 8-oxoGua induces a T to G transversion, which is a UVA signature mutation [101]. Other common DNA changes induced by UVA are DNA strand breaks [124] and to a lesser degree than UVB, CPD [101, 121]. UVR-induced damage of DNA is a complex process that defies easy classification to UVB-induced dimers and UVA-induced oxidative damage [121].

Melanin, synthesized by epidermal melanocytes and transferred to keratinocytes, forms supranuclear caps that protect nuclear DNA from impinging UVR, thus reducing DNA damage. The amount and type of melanin (eumelanin > pheomelanin) represents the major photoprotective mechanism against UVR-induced DNA damage, and generally correlates inversely with the risk of skin cancer [78, 125]. The lack of melanin in oculocutaneous albinism is associated with a 50% incidence of SCC. However, this is not the case for patients with vitiligo, who also lack epidermal melanin [126]. Therefore, other co-existing mechanisms exist that produce genetic damage such as oxidative stress during melanogenesis and contributing to reduced DNA repair [78, 125, 127].

Robust and complex DNA repair mechanisms are required to prevent the harmful effects of UVR-induced DNA damage and such adduct formation [128, 129]. In addition, it appears that solar radiation early in life may result in persistent DNA damage such as DNA fragmentation and mitochondrial DNA deletions, and altered patterns of gene expression such as decreased RAD23 UVR excision repair and Growth Arrest and DNA Damage (GADD45) expression [130]. Thus, the capacity of the host to repair DNA damage is also a key factor in skin carcinogenesis.

17.11.2. DNA Repair Capacity

The most important DNA damage repair system is the nucleotide excision repair (NER) system,. This system can act in two pathways, e.g., faster transcription-coupled repair operating on transcribed strands of active genes, and slower global genome nucleotide excision repair removing lesions within the entire genome. Oxidative damage of DNA that is induced by UV radiation can be repaired by base excision repair, which partially overlap with transcription coupled repair system [101].

XP patients have more than 1000-fold increased incidence of skin cancer compared to the general population highlighting the importance of NER [101, 103]. Minor differences due to gene polymorphisms can also affect DNA repair capacity and result in increased susceptibility to skin cancer. Using the lymphocytic DNA repair capacity phenotype by the host-cell reactivation assay, Wang et al [129] detected a relative 16% reduction in DNA repair capacity in NMSC patients compared with controls. In addition, DNA repair capacity below the controls' median value was associated with significantly increased risk for BCC. However, patients with aggressive or multiple SCC tended to have a higher DNA repair capacity than those with nonaggressive or single SCC. Ageing is also associated with reduced DNA repair capacity [131].

17.11.3. Scarring and Inflammation and Its Persistence

Chronic inflammation and scarring are well-accepted risk factors for cancer [132, 133]. The longer inflammation persists, the higher the probability of developing cancer. In this setting, it is suspected that inflammatory mediators contribute to cancer by initiation, promotion and selection.

Persistent inflammation induces adaptive responses, resistance to apoptosis, and environmental changes such as stimulation of angiogenesis, which confer a survival advantage to a susceptible cell. DNA damage due to oxidative stress during the damage-regeneration cycle is suspected to be a major contributor to cancer development. Many examples of inflammation-promoted carcinogenesis exist and include non-healing ulcers, chronic scars (e.g., dystrophic epidermolysis bullosa), and sinus tracts [134].

Mostly, SCC occur in this setting, but MM, BCC and sarcomas can also complicate long standing wounds such as burn scars [135]. Another example is SCC arising in anogenital lichen sclerosus, a chronic fibro-inflammatory dermatosis characterized by dermal sclerosis, T cell cytotoxic response directed at basal keratinocytes, and activated macrophages with ROS production [136-139]. The epidermis overlying the sclerotic dermis of lichen sclerosus and scars shows a regenerative (proliferative) phenotype, which can promote carcinogenesis and produce a field effect [136, 140].

17.11.4. Human Papillomavirus: High Risk Genital Mucosal and Beta-Papillomavirus

HPV are found in a wide variety of clinical lesions of epithelial origin and normal skin. The number of known HPV genotypes is expanding rapidly with the application of highly sensitive detection methods [118, 141-143]. Phylogenetic tree analysis has shown that most human HPV can be classified into specific groups according to known tissue tropism and oncogenic potential [144]: cutaneous (CU), high- and low-risk genital-mucosal (GM), and epidermodysplasia verruciformis, now known as betapapillomavirus (betaPV) genotypes. GM-HPV infection is largely asymptomatic, short-lived and highly prevalent in young, sexually active populations, but decreases with advancing age after 24 years of age [145-148]. Non-genital skin studies of normal and immunosuppressed individuals have demonstrated a wide-spread prevalence of HPV, particularly the betaPV types, implicating host immune factors in the control of overt clinical disease and commensalisms [141-143]. High-risk GM-HPV types (e.g. HPV 16, 18, 33) have been identified as causal factors in SCC of the anogenital region (6). In addition, HPV are commonly identified in benign and malignant non-melanoma skin tumors from both immunocompetent and immunosuppressed patients [9-12]. Certain betaPV types (mostly 5, and 8, 14, 17, 20, 38 and 47) are strongly associated with NMSC where they interact with UVR [149, 150].

BetaPV may act as an epigenetic cofactor in cutaneous field cancerization [151, 152]. BetaPVs are prevalent and persistent infections of normal skin and are frequently detected in AK and SCC. Hypothetically, by preventing DNA repair and apoptosis caused by UVR-induced genotoxic damage, betaPV promote genomic instability, facilitating the creation of a pool of initiated keratinocytes at risk for progression to AK and SCC. A significantly higher number of betaPV types in perilesional compared to distant, normal skin supports the theory that betaPV contribute to field cancerization [152]. Hair follicles are considered reservoirs for betaPV infection; examination of plucked hairs can potentially act as a surrogate marker of betaPV burden and, thus, the risk for skin cancer.

17.11.5. Loss of Immune Surveillance (Local or Systemic Immune Suppression)

Abundant evidence exists of immune effects on human tumors [153], which include allografted (donor derived) tumors with immunosuppression and regression with cessation of immunosuppression [154], increased rate of BCC in acquired immunodeficiency syndrome [155], and specific metastatic spread to previously irradiated tissue [153]. In addition, aggressive BCC variants are associated with loss of host tumor immune response [48]. Organ transplant recipients (OTR) have early onset of NMSC, a high tumor burden, and aggressive SCC [19]. Generalized impaired host immune functions due to lymphomas are also associated with aggressive BCC and SCC [156-158]. In OTR, the risk for cancer is greater in sun-exposed skin compared to non sun-exposed skin [6], and the risk for NMSC is 49 times greater for OTR with skin cancer compared to those without, highlighting the presence of a field defect [23]. HPV infection may play a role in OTR SCC development, particularly beta-PV types 5 and 8 [159, 160].

UVR is a potent immunosuppressant [161] that stimulates local production of immunosuppressive molecules [162-164], and induces antigen-specific tolerance [165] as well as abrogating the effector phase of cell-mediated immunity [166]. UVR induced localized immune suppression may also contribute to field cancerization and the pathogenesis of skin cancer. Lymphedema and its inherent decrease in immune trafficking is another cause of localized immune suppression, which might contribute to field cancerization [167, 168]. Indeed, lymphatic vessels are reduced in sun-damaged skin supporting localized lymphedema as a cofactor in field cancerization [169]. For example, lymphedematous (phymatous) rosacea has a higher incidence of BCC than non-phymatous facial skin [170].

17.11.6. Genetic (Germ Cell) Factors That Increase the Risk for Skin Cancer

Table 17-2 lists genodermatoses that are associated with the development of skin cancer. These syndromes highlight the role of many of the etiologic factors that are involved in carcinogenesis, such as defective DNA repair, chromosome maintenance, HPV infection, immunity, lack of photo-protective melanin, loss of key tumor suppressor genes such *PTCH* and *CDKN2A*, and scarring.

17.11.7. Dysregulated Melanogenesis and Field Cancerization

Melanin pigment clearly protects against skin cancers including MM; however, the biosynthesis of melanin can affect cellular metabolism, because: a) it consists of a series of tightly coupled oxidoreduction reactions [78]; b) it generates several intermediates that can display cytotoxic, genotoxic or mutagenic activities [78, 171]; and c) because of the oxygen requirement imposed by active melanogenesis (which can lead to intracellular hypoxia), and melanin can act as a scavenger of free radicals, metal cations and many chemicals including cellular toxins [78, 96, 172]. In normal melanocytes, the process of melanin synthesis is highly controlled; since it takes place within the boundaries of specialized membrane bound organelles, the melanosomes (78), and therefore, protect melanocytes and surrounding cells from the harmful effect of solar radiation. In transformed melanocytes, this process could be dysregulated, which will affect the behavior of the cell, or its surrounding environment [78, 96, 120, 173].

Table 17.2. Genetic syndromes associated with increased risk for skin cancer and development of field cancerization

Syndrome (OMIM)	Inheritance	Genetic defect	Predominant skin cancer	Associated findings
Basal cell nevus (Gorlin) syndrome (#109400)	AD	PTCH1, 2 gene, SUFU gene	BCC	Developmental abnormalities, jaw cysts, falx calcifications
Bazex syndrome (Bazex-Dupre-Christol syndrome) (%301845)	XD	Gene map locus Xq24-q27	BCC	Follicular atrophoderma (ice-pick marks, dorsum of the hands), local anhidrosis and congenital hypotrichosis.
Dystrophic epidermolysis bullosa (#131750, #226600)	AD, AR	COL7A1	SCC in sites of scarring	Localized and generalized skin and mucosal blisters leading to scars, and dystrophic teeth and nails
Epidermodysplasia verruciformis (*605828, 605829)	AR	EVER1, 2 genes (affect cell mediated immunity)	SCC	In sun exposed regions, macules, pityriasis-like lesions, flat warts, plaques, and seborrheic keratoses that transform into SCC
Familial melanoma syndrome (%155600)	AD	CDKN2A (p16(INK4a); p14(ARF)), CDK4	MM	Multiple nevi, atypical nevi; pancreatic carcinoma, breast carcinoma and astrocytomas
KID syndrome (#148210)	AD	connexin-26 gene, GJB2	SCC	Keratitis, ichthyosis, deafness
Muir Torre Syndrome (%301845)	AD	DNA mismatch repair genes, MLH-1, MSH-2, MSH-6	Sebaceous neoplasms, keratoacanthoma	Other visceral cancers (genitourinary and gastrointestinal)
Oculocutaneous albinism (#203100, *611409)	AR	TYR gene (type 1); P gene (type 2)	SCC > BCC > MM	No pigment in skin, eyes, hair, nystagmus, impaired visual acuity
Rombo syndrome (180730)	AD	Unknown	BCC	Atrophoderma vermiculatum, trichoepitheliomas, hypotrichosis milia, and peripheral vasodilation with cyanosis.
Rothmund Thompson Syndrome (#268400)	AR	DNA helicase gene RECQL4	SCC	Poikiloderma including alopecia, dystrophic teeth and nails, cataracts
Werner Syndrome (#277700)	AR	DNA helicase RECQL2 gene	SCC	Early ageing with excess cancer risk, diabetes mellitus, atherosclerosis, cataracts, and osteoporosis
Xeroderma Pigmentosum (#278700-278810)	AR	XP genes, DNA repair	BCC, SCC, MM	Extreme sun sensitivity, early onset of sun damaged skin, eye abnormalities; neurologic degeneration

Adapted from Lee et al. (102) and Madan et al. (94).

AD: autosomal dominant. AR: autosomal recessive. OMIM: Online Mendelian Inheritance in Man. XD: X-linked dominant.

Specifically, dysregulated melanogenesis can modify cellular metabolism [96, 174, 175], and generate an oxidative and mutagenic environment [78, 172, 176]. Furthermore, intermediates of melanogenesis, when released into the environment in large amounts are immunosuppressive [172, 175]. Therefore, it has been proposed that uncontrolled melanogenesis should have a role, perhaps critical, in the progression of atypical melanotic melanocytic lesions, and, in the case of MM, may attenuate the beneficial effects of radio-, chemo-, photo-,immuno- and/or vaccine therapy [78, 175]. Thus, melanogenic metabolic activity, which protects normal melanocytes from different insults, can also make MM cells resistant to any type of therapy and allow them to escape the immune system response [78, 175, 177].

17.11.8. Evidence of Genomic Instability (GIS) in Histologically Normal Skin

GIS is accepted as the driving force of neoplasia and is the result of combination of several pathways: chromosomal instability (CIS), nucleotide instability (NIS), microsatellite instability (MSI), and epigenetic instability (EIS) [178-181]. However, there is little agreement on which form of GIS is most significant in carcinogenesis [44, 182, 183]. Recently, the whole genomes of several cancer types have been sequenced, including a MM cell line [44, 45, 59].

These efforts have demonstrated that the number of somatic mutations and rearrangements are large, with evidence that the majority are passengers. In the case of hereditary cancers, GIS results from mutations in DNA repair genes such as mismatch repair genes resulting in MSI, which drives cancer development [44]. However, for sporadic (non-hereditary) cancers, the molecular basis of GIS remains unclear. Recent high-throughput sequencing studies do not support a role for DNA repair gene inactivation, as they are infrequent before therapy [44].

In place of this pathway, more frequent mutations in tumor suppressor *TP53*, ataxia telangiectasia mutated (*ATM*) and cyclin-dependent kinase inhibitor 2A (*CDKN2A*: encodes p16INK4A and p14ARF) were identified. These trends support the hypothesis of oncogene-induced DNA replication stress, where derangements of *TP53*, *ATM* and *CDKN2A* allow for oncogene-induced DNA damage; all of which contribute to GIS [44].

Indeed, in the progression of AK to SCC, abnormalities in *CDK2NA* and *TP53* are common [184]. With respect to etiology of genomic events, in the case of MM, UVR signature mutations of *CDKN2A* and *TP53* are clearly involved in tumor development; however, ROS related mutations may also play a role in both early and late events in the progression of tumor evolution [45, 185].

The study of cutaneous field cancerization may well answer many questions regarding which type of GIS is earliest and most critical, marking the onset of irreversible damage and potential for evolution to skin cancer. These early field cancerization defects may also represent the core tumor stem cell defects that will persist throughout the natural history of the skin cancer [186].

Tables 17-3 to 17-6 list reports of NIS, CIS, MIS, EIS and gene expression abnormalities that have been identified in histologically normal skin (NS). While the data are few, these findings demonstrate that all types of GIS occur in histologically NS in the proximity of skin cancer. This review also underscores the value of comparing perilesional "NS" with anatomically matched NS not associated with skin cancer.

17.11.9. Nucleotide instability (NIS)

Table 17-3 lists events of NIS including non-synonymous mutations, deletions in mitochondrial DNA, and mutant clones in perilesional NS.

Table 17.3. Evidence of single base instability in histologically normal skin

Type of genomic aberration	Abnormality	Perilesional skin cancer	Reference
Non-synonymous mutations	TP53 mutations: UV signature mutations in 74% and 5% of sun-exposed and non-sun exposed NS from Australians in codons 245, 248 or 248. No mutants in non-sun exposed NS from France	None	[195]
	TP53 mutations NS: C>T transitions at dipyrimidine sequences (30%), T>C transitions (47%), and G>T transversions (12%)	NMSC	[196]
	TP53 mutations: no identical mutations found for NS p53 clones and adjacent AK or SCC	SCC	[197]
	TP53 mutations: p53 greater in chronically sun exposed NS than in covered NS. TP53 mutation frequency increases with age and is higher in patients with NMSC and its precursors than patients with benign skin tumors	BCC, SCC	[198]
	TP53 mutations: No mutations in non-exposed NS; multitude of mutations (missense and nonsense) in sun-exposed NS. Poor correlation between mutations and morphological phenotypes- p53 not determinant of phenotypes (early carcinogenic event)	BCC, SCC, XPC related	[199]
	TP53 mutations: 14 different mutations with UVR signature in 26 of 99 keratinocytes from sun exposed NS; both scattered keratinocytes and small cluster of p53-IHC+ keratinocytes (diameter of 10-15 basal cells)	None	[200]
	TP53 mutations: located in p53 exons 4-8, all missense, and 78% displayed a typical ultraviolet signature. Frequency of mutants similar for NS adjacent to BCC and SCC.	BCC, SCC	[201]
	TP53 and KRAS hotspot mutations: low frequency mutations found in genital NS of patients affected by kichen sclerosus (LS) and SCC. TP53 mutations and p53 clones* present in LS affected skin implicating selection and promotion of mutated NS keratinocytes	SCC, vulvar	[37]
Mutant clones*	p53 clones: accumulation in the chronically sun-exposed NS and clonal expansion of p53 mutant cells in NS adjacent to basal cell carcinoma.	BCC	[207]

Table 17.3 (Continued)

	p53 clones: larger and more frequent clones (60-3000cells) in sun-exposed versus sun-shielded NS	None	[91]
	p53 clones: progressive increasing mean p53 labeling index moving from non-sun-exposed NS to sun-exposed NS to NS adjacent AK skin to AK.	AK (SCC)	[208]
	p53 clones: estimated 1:15,000 prevalence of mutant stem cells producing clones in 70-80yr old Caucasian sun exposed NS at latitude 60° North	AK (SCC)	[87]
	p53 clones: present in NS adjacent to SCC and related to sun exposure	BCC, SCC	[209]
	p53 clones: common and larger in NS adjacent to BCC than controls. Labeling index low for ki-67 in p53 clones unlike pattern seen in AK and BCC	BCC	[210]
	p53 clones/labeling index: higher p53 expression in the non-sun exposed NS of OTR compared to immunocompetent control non-OTR non-sun exposed NS	None	[211]
	p53 clones: number and size increased with age in NS. p53 clones more numerous and greater in size in NS adjacent to SCC than NS adjacent to nevi and BCC, both of which showed similar number and size of NS p53 clones.	BCC, SCC	[38]
mtDNA mutations	mtDNA mutations: UV induced signatures in perilesional skin	BCC, SCC	[293]
Deletions; DNA fragmentation	mtDNA mutations: common deletion more frequent in sun-exposed NS than non-exposed NS and peripheral blood. Undescribed mtDNA mutation detected exclusively in NS.	None	[294]
	mtDNA deletions: abundant in margin tissue specimens from older patients; numbers correlated with the age; statistically significant difference between mtDNA deletions in tumors and margins- intact mtDNA in tumors more frequent	BCC, SCC	[204]
	mtDNA deletions and DNA fragmentation: NS adjacent to MM showed glutathione S-transferase M1 (GSTM1) null individuals with a sunburn history had increased levels of both DNA fragmentation by comet assays and mtDNA deletions relative to GSTM1 wild type patients with little or no sunburn history.	MM	[130]
DNA photoproducts	CPD: significantly more CPD in NS of BCC patients than normal controls after solar simulator radiation exposure with minimal erythema dose.	BCC	[212]

*: IHC expression patterns are a surrogate marker of p53 mutation [290, 295].

NIS is probably one of the earliest mechanisms at work in the development of skin cancers [42, 187]. Single base substitution mutations account for 85% or more of the activating and deactivating mutations in proto-oncogenes and tumor suppressor genes in human tissues [37, 188-191]. Although single base deletions and insertions are sometimes involved, single base substitutions represent the vast majority of these oncogenic errors [191-193]. This has been clearly demonstrated in human tissues for a number of proto-oncogenes and tumor suppressor genes, e.g. *BRAF, H-, K-,* and *N-RAS, RB* and *TP53* [50, 188, 189, 192-

194]. Missense single base substitution mutations alone comprise more than 75% of all identified disease-associated *TP53* mutations [193]. In histologically normal skin, mostly *TP53* and *KRAS* non-synonymous mutations have been identified in sun exposed NS and genital NS associated with lichen sclerosus [37, 195-201]. (? Tense in this sentence) Notably, these NS mutants are not concordant with most neighboring NMSC, but they were increased in size and number in patients with NMSC and showed similar mutational spectra [197, 200, 201]. In addition, in the setting of lichen sclerosus associated SCC, mutant p53 clones were larger than *KRAS* clones, implicating selective expansion of mutant clones [37]. For a limited number of oncogenic base sites tested (*KRAS* codon 12 and *TP53* codons 248 and 273), the prevalence of mutations were found to be generally greater than one mutant per 10^6 wild type cells in histologically genital NS [37]. This background prevalence of single base pair substitution mutations in genital NS is similar to sun-damaged NS [198] and for other normal tissues [191, 202, 203].

It is postulated that many of the identified genes with UVR-altered expression play no role in UVR-induced oncogenic processes, but may turn out to be useful as markers of underlying genomic instability and photo-ageing [204, 205]. NIS most likely plays an important role in the early development of cancer, by freeing the cell from inhibitory cell growth and division signals. Skin tumors express NIS, but it may be important as a potential prognostic biomarker. The expression of NIS in tumor stem cells may promote plasticity in response to local tissue environmental conditions and chemotherapeutic treatment. In addition, whole genome sequencing of MM cell-line COLO-829 (45) revealed 292 somatic mutations occurring in protein sequencing regions that compromised 187 non-synonymous substitutions leading to 172 missense and 15 nonsense changes and 105 synonymous (silent) mutations. The majority of the mutations were considered to be passenger mutations (not due to selection pressure) as the ratio of non-synonymous to synonymous substitutions was 1.74, which was not different than that expected by chance.

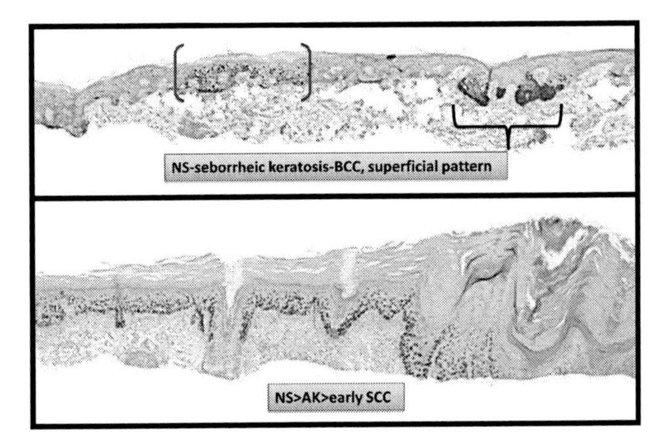

Figure 17.4. Multiple small clones and clonal expansion. Progression to cancer is denoted by an accumulation of genomic aberrations. P53 positive superficial BCC (top panel, right side) and seborrheic keratosis (top panel left middle) show mutant p53 expression pattern, but there are no intervening, overt mutant NS keratinocyte clones to implicate expansion of mutant *TP53* clone as a primary field cancer event. In contrast, wide spread p53 protein expression moving from normal skin to AK to SCC is found in the bottom panel implicating clonal expansion of p53 mutant commencing with a histologically normal keratinocyte and culminating with acquisition of further genomic aberrations to early invasive squamous cell carcinoma (right side, bottom panel).

As discussed above, *TP53* mutations appear to be a critical event in the formation of sporadic cancers [44]. In the skin, NMSC and MM arising in sun-damaged skin are associated with *TP53* mutations [185, 206]. In sun-damaged skin, clones of morphologically normal p53-expressing keratinocytes are present, whose size and number are directly proportional to the level of sun exposure and increasing age [38, 86, 87, 91, 207-211]. Approximately 60% of p53 clones in "normal" skin surrounding NMSC have missense *TP53* gene mutations (the vast majority of which are UVR-signature mutations), resulting in the translation of an altered protein [86]. While no firm link between epidermal p53 clones and synchronous tumors (including precursors like AK) has been identified, an association between these clones and skin cancer development exists ([86; See figure 17.4.)

In addition, from studies of MM and NMSC, it has been shown that both tumors and adjacent "normal" tissue contain: (i) identical UVR-induced homoplasmic mtDNA mutations and (ii) mtDNA deletions, with the perilesional skin containing different and/or more deletions in some cases [204, 205]. Therefore, MM and NMSC peritumoral NS may harbor expanded populations of cells (melanocytes and keratinocytes) with mutant mtDNA, as reported for p53 clones. Additional, but yet undefined, genetic alterations are required for subsequent progression to morphologically recognizable malignant skin cancer phenotypes [35, 86, 123, 130].

The number of CPD photoproducts produced in the skin after a fixed exposure to UVR (minimal erythema dose) differs between individuals with and without a history of BCC [212]. The induction and repair of photoproducts such as CPD could serve as a biomarker of risk for field cancerization [123].

17.11.10. Chromosomal Instability (CIS)

Table 17-4 lists events of CIS such as abnormal chromatin patterns by karyometry, aneusomy, oncogene amplification, and abnormal telomere lengths in histologically NS.

Aneuploidy and CIS characterize most human cancers. Several mechanisms allow for inaccurate chromosomal segregation during mitosis, including defective telomere metabolism, centrosome amplification, dysfunctional centromeres, and/or defective spindle checkpoint control [44, 213-215]. Two mechanisms that are thought to be the first step in CIS involve telomere length abnormalities, which result in telomere aggregation, breakage-bridge-fusion cycles, and centromere fragments and fusions. Aneuploidy, once present, autocatalytically contributes to greater CIS, thus GIS [216]. BCC, SCC and MM all show distinct, recurrent patterns of chromosomal gain, loss and gene amplification, highlighting the role of CIS in skin oncogenesis and how the dosage of specific genes impart specific cancer phenotypes [54, 83, 217-219].

Allelic Imbalance/Loss of Heterozygosity

Allelic imbalance, a deviation from the normal one to one ratio of alleles, or loss of heterozygosity is common to cancer and its precursors, but has also been demonstrated to exist in normal tissues such as normal mammary tissue adjacent to breast cancer [220]. Few studies have been performed where NS has been analyzed for allelic imbalance, with mixed results [197, 210, 221-223]. Loss of heterozygosity was detected in several NS samples at several chromosomal loci in perilesional skin associated with AK and SCC [222], and in MM perilesional skin, at the 8-oxoquanine DNA glycolase gene (hOGG1) [223]. Thus, allelic imbalance occurs in cutaneous skin cancer fields.

Table 17.4. Chromosomal (DNA content) instability in histologically normal skin

Type of genomic aberration	Abnormalities	Perilesional skin cancer	Reference
Allelic imbalance/ loss of heterozygosity	No LOH in p53 clones from NS in contrast to 11/30 LOH in AK and SCC	SCC	[197]
	No LOH for p53 gene or 9q22.3 in sun exposed NS, but LOH common for both SCCIS and SCC	SCC	[221]
	LOH of 9q (28.3%): higher in NS adjacent to BCC than NS adjacent to benign tumors	BCC	[210]
	LOH identified in 3 NS at D3S1923 (3q), D9S162 (9p), D9S160 (9q) and D13S170 (13q)	SCC, AK	[222]
	LOH of 8-oxoquanine DNA glycosylase 1 (*hOGG1*) gene in skin adjacent to melanoma in situ with melanocytic hyperplasia	MM	[223]
Karyometry (abnormal nuclei/chromatin patterns)	Nuclear chromatin abnormality: progression of nuclear chromatin abnormalities from NS to sun damaged NS to AK. Despite photoprotection for 3 months, additional damage accrued in sun exposed skin and AK	AK (SCC)	[226]
	Nuclear chromatin abnormality: in histopathologically NS, monotonically increasing damage for increased exposure to solar radiation (minimal exposed NS ~90 nuclei normal; sun exposed NS ~70-80% normal; individuals with AK: ~40% nuclei normal in sun exposed NS)	AK (SCC)	[227]
	Nuclear image analysis: no significant differences between sun and non-exposed NS, but higher values in sun exposed NS and greater variance	AK (SCC)	(228)
	Nuclear chromatin abnormality: sun exposure directly correlates with proportion of abnormal chromatin patterns in nuclei in NS. Notably, no differences identified between nuclei collected from early AK NS sites and AK	SCC	[224]
Aneuploidy/ Aneusomy/ Amplification	Amplification of 11q13.2 in normal melanocytes found in perilesional skin of acral MM	MM	[230]
	Aneusomy chromosome 17 in perilesional NS, not control NS	SCC, vulva	[49]
	Aneuploidy: DNA content index 1.12 ± 0.24/aneuploidy 30% in perilesional NS (n=10) vs. 1.14 ± 0.04/ 0 non-cancer related NS controls	SCC, vulvar	[50]
	Aneusomy chromosome 7 in 17% of nuclei scored in NS and NS safety margins	MM	[229]
	Amplification of 5p15 and 11q13 in histologically normal melanocytes found in perilesional NS of acral MM	MM	[39]
Telomere length/ dysfunction	Mean telomere length reduced in peri-BCC NS compared to dermis (mean difference 2.5 kb); however, similar results for non-cancer related NS. BCC showed increased mean telomere length in 13/20	BCC	(232)
	Age dependent loss: telomere reduction rates of 36 to 39 base per year	None	[231]

Karyometery

Karyometery provides an in situ method to measure nuclear abnormalities such as nuclear area, total optical density and chromatin distribution. These parameters have been shown to progressively increase with the evolution from normal to invasive and metastatic cancer [224]. The fact that the patterns of chromatin packaging are consistent with defined pathological subgroups may be considered as an indication of functional inter-relationships between nuclear structure and gene expression, suggesting that chromatin organization is under very tight cellular control and that chromatin phenotype impacts malignant potential [224, 225]. CIS and epigenetic mechanisms such as histone acetylation and methylation are likely to play a major role in determining chromatin pattern, (? Is this "and" required) and nuclear architecture, higher order chromatin organization and the topology of chromosomal territories in interphase cells, and result in chromatin phenotypes indicative of cancer. In the skin, several studies have documented monotonic progression and significant differences in nuclear chromatin abnormalities moving from sun shielded NS to sun-exposed NS to NS in a field of AK to AK-associated with SCC [224, 226-228]. In another study [228], DNA content was increased and showed larger variance in sun-exposed compared to sun-shielded NS. All of these results indicate the presence of aneuploidy, gene expression abnormalities and epigenetic derangements in histologically NS.

Aneusomy/Gene Amplification

Incomplete chromosomes and amplification of specific chromosome regions are common chromosomal abnormalities. Several FISH studies have demonstrated aneusomy for chromosome 17 in genital NS associated with lichen sclerosus and SCC [49], and aneusomy of chromosome 7 in MM perilesional NS [229]. Gene amplifications are a frequent chromosomal abnormality of acral MM [83]. Studies of acral MM perilesional skin utilizing FISH have revealed histologically normal melanocyte field cells with amplifications of 11q13.2 (locus of cyclin D1 gene) and 5p15 [39, 230]. See figure 17-5.

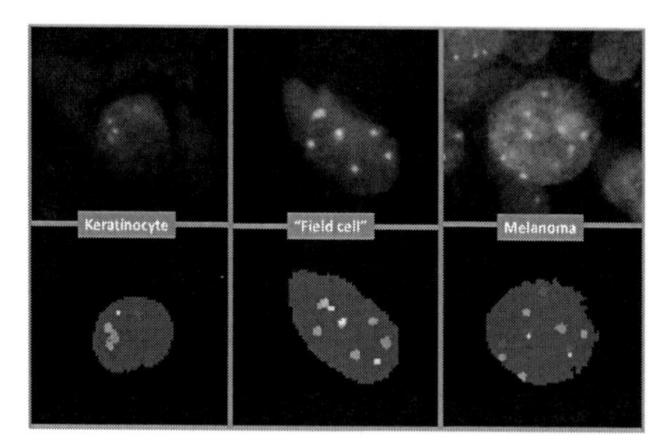

Figure 17.5. Melanocyte "field cell" with aneusomy in acral melanoma. Acral melanomas show clones of histologically normal appearing melanocytes with gene amplifications in perilesional skin [6]. Illustrated herein are cells taken from an acral melanoma and its perilesional skin examined using the UroVysionTMBladder Cancer Kit. (CEP® 3 SpectrumRedTM, CEP 7 SpectrumGreenTM, CEP 17 SpectrumAquaTm, and LSI® 9p21 SpectrumGold). The top fluorescent in situ hybridization images capture the red (chromosome 3), green (chromosome 7), and blue (chromosome 17) signals. The yellow 9p21 signal is not captured because of the high background it imparts. The lower computer generated images show all 4 probe signals. As the histologic sections do not include the whole nucleus, the lack of second signals is not interpreted as monosomy as seen in the normal keratinocyte nucleus for 9p21 and chromosomes 3 and 17. The middle melanocyte field cell shows aneusomy for chromosome 7 while the melanoma cell shows markedly abnormal chromatin pattern and gains of chromosomes 3 and 7. Note the preservation of 9p21, which is frequently lost with progression in melanoma.

Telomere Dysfunction

Telomeres are repetitive nucleoprotein complexes that cap and protect chromosomes from being recognized as double-stranded DNA breaks [215]. Dysfunctional telomeres are a driving force of GIS because of DNA degradation and recombination (breakage-bridge-fusion cycle). In humans, an age-dependent shortening of telomeres occurs [231]. In NS adjacent to BCC, mean telomere length was found to be reduced compared to dermal fibroblasts, but not site- and aged-matched non-cancer related NS [232]. Associated BCC showed either decreased or increased telomere length relative to the adjacent epidermis. As skin cancer is a disease predominately of the elderly, and telomeres shorten with age, it is likely that shortened telomeres in NS play a role in skin field cancerization, as is shown in the esophagus (see chapter 8).

17.11.11. Microsatellite Instability (MSI)

Table 17-5 lists MSI aberrations in normal skin. Microsatellites are repetitive DNA sequences spread throughout the genome, primarily in non-coding regions. Their length is an inherited trait, and they act as sites for recombination, promoters and binding sites for topoisomerases [178, 233, 234]. The most common microsatellite repeat is $(CA)_n$ The insertion or deletion of repeat units within a microsatellite may occur on rare occasions by slippage during DNA replication.

Disruption of mismatch repair (MMR) functions, which correct this replication error, leads to an increased variation in the lengths of microsatellites. The presence of microsatellite variants of different lengths in tumors, compared to normal tissue, is called microsatellite instability (MSI) and is a hallmark of MMR deficient familial and sporadic cancers. MSI is defined as the increased or decreased length of microsatellites, due to the insertion or deletion of one or more repeat units, in tumor tissue compared to normal tissue. Depending upon the number of microsatellite markers found to be altered, the tumor may be designated as MSI-L (low, infrequent instability) or MSI-H (high instability, ≥5 markers). At least two microsatellite markers should display altered lengths for a tumor to be designated as MSI positive. MSI positivity is frequently due to derangements of one or more genes of the MMR system: *hMSH2* (common), *hMLH1* (common), *hMSH3*, *hMSH6*, *hPMS1*, and *hPMS2*. Muir-Torre Syndrome (MTS), a phenotypic variant of hereditary nonpolyposis colorectal carcinoma syndrome is an autosomal dominant disorder caused by mutations in *hMSH2* and other MMR genes. Patients present with an internal malignancies, sebaceous neoplasms, and keratoacanthomas [234, 235].

Amongst skin cancers, the majority of MSI events reported occur in sebaceous neoplasms [178, 233]. Recently, IHC testing for loss of MMR protein expression for internal malignancy-associated sebaceous neoplasms has been proven to be a viable, practical approach for confirmation of a suspected inherited MMR gene defect, as well as an accurate method to distinguish between sporadic and Muir-Torre syndrome-associated sebaceous lesions [236, 237]. Notably, MM has been reported in association with hereditary nonpolyposis colorectal carcinoma [238]. However, MSI does not appear to be common event in the evolution of most NMSC and MM [184, 239-242]. With respect to NS, both high and low MSI instability was detected in 18% of vulvar perilesional NS samples associated with vulvar SCC at the DNA and protein levels (Wilson and Carlson, unpublished data). In addition, loss of MMR protein expression was identified in BCC perilesional NS [239]. Thus, MSI plays a minor role in the common skin cancers and is an early event found in histologically NS.

Table 17.5. Microsatellite and epigenetic aberrations in histologically normal skin

Marker	Abnormality	Perilesional skin cancer	Reference
Microsatellite instability	Perilesional NS: loss MLH1 expression in 2/2 BCC with complete loss of MLH1 expression. Basal layer keratinocytes express MLH1 and MSH2; rare scattered spinous keratinocyte positive cells.	BCC	[239]
	Perilesional NS (n=12): IHC expression loss of 8% MLH1, 17% MSH2, and 8% MSH6. Low/high MSI detected in 8%/8% at BAT 25, 8%/8% at BAT26, 0/8% at D10S208, and 17%/0 at D10S587	SCC, vulvar	Wilson and Carlson, unpublished data
Specific gene promoter methylation	E-cadherin promoter hypermethylation: 2/9 NS, not associated with cancer. Increasing frequency of methylation from AK to SCCIS to SCC	None	[252]
	Death associated protein kinase (DAPK) and p16 Tumor suppressor promoter methylation in 1/9 NS, not related to cancer	None	[253]
	NS, perilesional, 1 sample: no Ras association domain family 1 (RASSF1) gene methylation detected	MM	[254]
	Normal keratinocyte cultures: no methylthioadenosine phosphorylase (MTAP) gene methylation detected	None	[255]
	Normal melanocyte cell lines (HEM1/2): no promoter methylation in 20 tumor suppressor genes tested	None	[256]
	Normal human epidermal melanocyte cell lines (2): 1/2 promoter methylation of WAP four-disulfide core domain 1 (WFCD1) (1 gene out of 30 tested)	None	[250]
	Perilesional NS (n=15): 33% RASSF1A, 21% DAPK; 0 p16; 12% p15; 38% MGMT; 6% GSTP1. NS control (n=5): 0 p15; 0 p16; 0 GSTP1; and 40% MGMT	SCC, vulvar	Wilson and Carlson, unpublished data

17.11.12. Epigenetic Instability (EIS) in Histologically Normal Skin

Table 17-5 lists events of EIS in NS such as tumor suppressor gene methylation. Control of gene expression resides in the adjustability of local chromatin structure and binding sites for transcription machinery. Chromatin structure is modulated by covalent modifications of amino acids in the N-terminal tails of chromatin histones (e.g., histone acetylation). Transcription binding sites for repressors or initiators of transcription are also dependent upon DNA 5-methyldeoxy–cytidine (5mdC) patterns [243, 244]. These covalent DNA/chromatin markers do not alter the genetic code, as the DNA sequence is intact, yet they are consistently inherited by daughter cells. Thus, the combination of 5mdC patterns and histone modifications comprise the epigenetic component of the human genome. Disruption of these 5mdC and chromatin histone modification patterns is involved in numerous biological processes, including genomic imprinting, embryogenesis, differentiation, ageing, inflammation, and oncogenesis [244-247]. In addition, non-CpG methylation occurs in human stem cells [e.g., CpHpH and CpHpG (H represents either A, C, or T)] [65]. Whether driven by a carcinogen(s), selection pressure, or occur spontaneously, the 5mdC patterns and loci specific chromatin histone modifications are substantially altered during the development of cancer. This process is equated to the accumulation of mutations in the cancer cell, and changes in these epigenetic patterns are sometimes referred to as epimutations [247, 248]. Regardless of terminology, the accumulation of aberrant epigenetic changes is termed epigenetic instability (EIS). In fact, tumors can be classified according to their gene-specific methylation profile [247]. In NMSC and MM, numerous genes are affected by EIS, namely tumor suppressor gene promoter methylation [243, 249-251]. Very little data is presently available for changes in specific histone modification for skin cancers. However, this is a rapidly growing area of research and the identification of enzymes involved in target site(s) modification may be valuable for the development of new therapies such as inhibitors of histone deacetylase inhibitors, histone methyltransferase inhibitors, and demethylase inhibitors many of which are in currently in progress [243].

Gene Promoter Methylation

Reports of EIS, specifically gene promoter methylation testing, in NS are few and the samples tested are mostly non-cancer associated NS or normal epidermal melanocyte cultures (Wilson and Carlson unpublished data) [250, 252-256]. Genes found to be methylated included E-cadherin, Death associated protein kinase (DAPK), Ras associated domain family 1 (RASSF1), WAP four-disulfide core domain 1T (WFCD1), p15INK4b cyclin-dependent kinase inhibitor 2B (CDKN2B), p16Ink4a (CDKN2A), O-6-methylguanine-DNA methyltransferase (MGMT) and glutathione S-transferase pi 1 (GSTP1). The differences in gene methylation frequencies found between perilesional genital NS and non-cancer associated genital NS point to the involvement of EIS in field cancerization (Wilson and Carlson, unpublished data).

17.12. Biochemical Aberrations in Histologically Normal Skin

Table 17.6 list reports of abnormal telomerase expression in NS and comparisons of NS with tumor and precursor gene expression analyses.

17.12.1. Telomerase Expression in Histologically Normal Skin

Telomeric repeats are produced by telomerase, a ribonucleoprotein that works in combination with several other telomere-binding proteins to regulate telomere length. The activating, catalytic subunit of telomerase, human telomerase reverse transcriptase (hTERT) is a crucial factor in cellular immortalization and carcinogenesis [67]. For example, telomerase activity (TA) levels significantly increase with histologic MM progression [257]. Multiple studies, mostly of BCC and perilesional NS, have examined TA and hTERT expression [258-264]. In general, TA is elevated in sun-damaged and inflamed NS compared to non-exposed NS [258-260]. Compared to the associated skin cancer, TA or hTERT expression is either lower or less frequent in NS [258, 261, 263]. In some cases, hTERT expression in perilesional NS is as elevated as the associated tumor [263]. Remarkably, BCC safety (NS) margins expressing telomerase were associated with shorter relapse free survival [264]. These data demonstrate that hTERT expression and TA activity are not restricted to cancer, and that telomerase plays a role in cutaneous field cancerization, perhaps by conferring enhanced proliferative capacity to preneoplastic, but histologically normal keratinocytes or melanocytes.

17.12.2. Expressional Aberrations in Normal Skin

A number of studies have used cDNA/oligonucleotide microarray technology to investigate gene expression profiles in NMSC and "NS", perilesional in many cases (reviewed in [123])[51, 130, 228, 265-274]. Specific cell-cycle pathways and biological processes underlying MM, BCC and SCC pathogenesis were identified, and these gene expression profiles correlated with histologic stepwise models of progression, as anticipated.

Table 17.6. Expressional aberrations in histologically normal skin

Marker	Abnormality	Perilesional skin cancer	Reference
Telomerase activity (TA)/hTERT expression	TA extremely low in sun-protected skin; sun-damaged NS, psoriatic skin, and allergic contact dermatitis skin had increased TA, but < BCC, SCC, and MM	None	[258]
	21/39 sun exposed NS vs. 3/26 shielded NS telomerase +	BCC	[259]
	33% sun exposed NS telomerase + vs. 0% shielded NS	None	[260]
	TA in 26/30 (87%) BCC tissues and in 8/25 (32%) of the tumor-free surgical margin tissues. TA levels correlated significantly with p53 expression levels.	BCC	[261]
	hTERT expression similar in BCC as NS with basal cell expression; however NS shows extension to suprabasal cells	BCC	[262]
	hTERT: higher levels in BCC vs. perilesional NS; 2/11 NS elevated. TA: 75% BCC + vs. 17% NS +	BCC	[263]
	Telomerase positive tumor margin NS associated with shorter relapse free survival	BCC	[264]
Gene expression analysis	pRB abnormally expressed in 2/6 genital NS	SCC, vulvar	[296]
	High levels of expression of Ataxia Telangiectasia Mutated gene (*ATM*) in NS, compared to MM	MM	[267]
	Ki-67 and p53 labeling indices significantly greater in sun-exposed NS vs. shielded NS	AK (SCC)	[228]

	Examined expression of multiple genes in NS, nevi, MM in situ, MM, and metastatic MM	MM	[268]
	BCC vs. perilesional NS: 165 upregulated genes, 115 downregulated genes identified. Extracellular matrix, cell junctions, motility, metastasis, oncogenes, tumor suppressors, DNA repair, cell cycle, immune regulation and angiogenesis.	BCC	[269]
	NS from 5 OTR (pooled) showed minor differential expression of some genes compared to 5 non-OTR NS and slight overlap with AK	SCC	[270]
	NS, no cancer vs. BCC, varied types. NS clustered together, but BCC exhibited varied gene expression patterns, which overlapped with NS on condition tree distribution	None	[271]
	NS vs. AK vs. SCC: 10/14 genes dysregulated and showing a correlation with progression	None	[272]
	BCC cells express a transcript signature that is significantly different from perilesional NS basal keratinocytes: upregulation of the Wnt signaling pathway; BCC increased sensitivity to ROS and dysregulated genes involved in antigen presentation.	BCC	[273]
	NS, perilesional: 2/21 BCC on hierarchical analysis clustered with 8 NS	BCC	[274]
	NS, perilesional: microarray analysis: in NS of GSTM1-null individuals or those with history of sunburn- upregulation of DNA ligases and downregulation of RAD23 UV excision repair gene, and the Growth Arrest and DNA Damage gene (GADD45) in NS	MM	[130]
	Sun exposed compared to non-sun exposed NS shows onset/weak expression of differentially expressed genes found in AK and SCC	SCC	[51]
	Increased numbers of melanocytes in sun damaged NS with undifferentiated, TRPM1 mRNA negative phenotype	MM	[72]

As a function of the methodologies used (i.e., comparative strategies based on tumor and normal cDNA co-hybrization), many of these studies sought to determine and validate (with PCR and IHC) differentially expressed genes, and not common and aberrantly expressed transcripts and proteins.

However, comparisons of site-matched NS with and without adjacent skin cancer have not been undertaken, so field cancerization effects, by design, could not be detected. Nevertheless, a few tumor samples were found to segregate with NS control expression profiles, highlighting overlap in gene expression of histologically NS with tumor, and implying field cancerization [270, 271, 274].

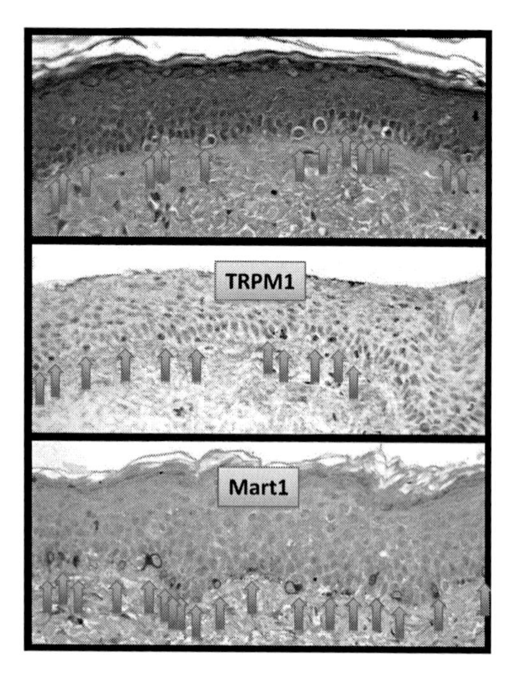

Figure 17.6. Expansion of "field" melanocytes in sun-damaged skin. Melanocyte TRPM1 mRNA expression is a marker of a fully differentiated melanocyte and loss of its expression is associated with melanoma progression (5). In sun-damaged skin, melanocyte hyperplasias are common (top panel). In this setting, expansion of MITF+MART1+TRPM1- occurs. These TRPM1- melanocytes could represent either normal melanocytes of reparative hyperplasia or mutant melanocyte clones, "field cells", which are presumptive precursors to melanoma.

In addition, gene expression patterns appear to reflect sunburn history. Of note, upregulation of DNA ligases and downregulation of RAD23 UV excision repair gene and the Growth Arrest and DNA Damage gene (GADD45) has been found in NS from patients with a history of sunburn compared to NS from patients without a history of sunburn [130].

By chromogenic in situ hybridization, TRPM1 mRNA expression has been shown to be specific for melanocytes and strongly associated with MITF and tyrosinase expression; the latter implicating (? implying) a mature melanocyte phenotype [72]. However, in normal skin, TRPM1 mRNA expression is dynamic, labels only a fraction of melanocytes, and changes according to its local environment.

Loss of TRPM1 mRNA expression relative to MITF was associated with a regenerative (melanoblast) phenotype overlying scars. This phenotype may also represent field cells as they are also found overlying solar elastosis (sun-damaged skin) and in the proximity of MM [72]. See figure 17-6.

17.13. Tumor-Extracellular Matrix Interactions: A Two-Way Street?

Conversion of melanocyte-keratinocyte and keratinocyte-keratinocyte to melanocyte-extracellular matrix (ECM) and keratinocyte-ECM interactions, respectively, is a crucial transition from a benign precursor to invasive and potentially metastatic tumor [48, 275].

Conversely, the stroma may also contribute to field cancerization [276]. Indeed, scars are associated with a change in epithelial and melanocyte phenotypes; specifically to a proliferative and activated phenotype [136, 140, 277]. Thus, the microenvironment, e.g., the associated tumor stroma, which acts as a non-healing wound [133], could determine the outcome of field cancerization, specifically the transition to an invasive phenotype [276]. In addition, the dermal milieu that supports the epidermis is also impacted by genetic cancer susceptibilities and exposures to carcinogens, which is reflected by the correlation of increased saturation density for dermal fibroblasts with individuals from families with heritable forms of cancer, and from cancer-bearing individuals [58]. See figure 17-7.

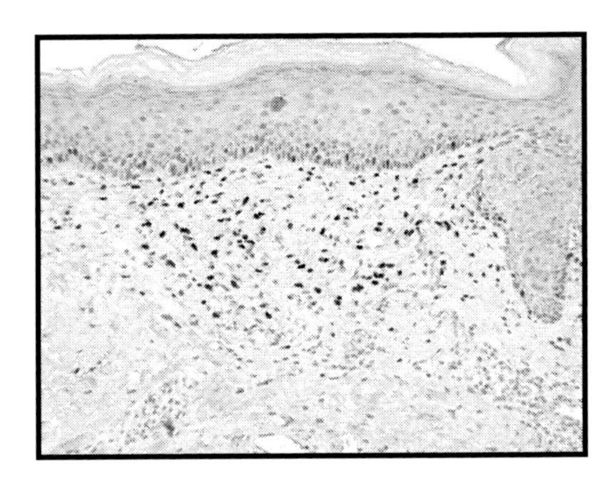

Figure 17.7. Presumptive mutant p53 dermal fibroblasts. Recently, it has been proposed that the saturation density of skin dermal fibroblasts could serve as a surrogate quantitative screening marker for human cancer susceptibility, including skin cancers (7). Illustrated herein is the rare phenomenon of a p53 patch of dermal fibroblasts attesting to underlying genomic instability of stromal cells, which themselves, may serve a role in cancer progression (8).

17.14. Clinical Implications of Field Cancerization

The concept of cutaneous field cancerization has possible utility in several areas of cutaneous oncology: more exact definition of surgical margins; identification of novel biomarkers of risk assessment for primary prevention and early cancer detection; and monitoring of tumor progress. Biomarkers that are strongly associated with risk of skin cancer development would be useful for identifying patients most likely to need care, which if started early could lead to decreased morbidity, mortality and costs by reducing the economic burden of late-stage disease. For example, if all elderly American patients with MM were diagnosed and effectively treated at an early stage, the annual costs for treating those aged 65 years or above would be US$ 99-161 (€ 72-117) million, which is 40-65% less than is currently being spent [16]. Based on the shear numbers of NMSC, primary prevention would likely have an even greater impact on health care expenditures as well as quality of life. Lastly, field cancerization biomarkers could also play a role in clinical trials to assess the efficacy of agents used for chemoprevention of skin cancer, or to monitor response to therapy in late-stage disease. With regard to the latter, the earliest carcinogenic changes that create field cancerization and clonal expansion may also represent the core defects of the cancer stem cell, which will persist throughout the natural history of the tumor. Indeed, a specific core of stable genetic cases was identified throughout disease progression and clonal evolution of MM [186]. Both targeting treatment against, and monitoring for, these core tumor stem cell dependent defects could greatly increase the efficacy of current MM management.

17.14.1 Margin Control and Minimal Residual Disease

Skin cancers frequently recur (locally persist) for years at, or in the proximity of, excision sites, despite wide safety margins and evidence of complete excision. The in situ detection of field cells, melanocytes or keratinocytes, in excision margins which harbor precursor genomic changes by FISH or IHC could aid in the rational planning of surgical margins, particularly in regions where function or cosmetic concerns could be compromised by standard surgical guidelines. For example, the application of standard wide excision ≥1cm margins for MM at acral sites (palm, sole, nail unit) could result in functional morbidity. As acral MM frequently harbor gene amplifications, FISH could be used to map margins of occult 'field cells' surrounding the MM. These have been detected up to an average 4.5-6.1mm from the primary MM, which is less than the 1 cm recommended excision margin for a melanoma of <2 mm in Breslow thickness, and 2 cm for melanoma of >2 mm in Breslow thickness [39]. Other oncogenic events such as clonal populations of mutant *TP53* keratinocytes in the marginal tissue of skin cancers may also be predictive of relapse/recurrence, and thereby, their absence could help define appropriate excision margins.

17.14.2. Chemoprevention of Skin Cancer

UVR is the complete carcinogen as it can both initiate and promote MM and NMSC. Despite efforts to educate the public about the importance of protecting skin from excessive ultraviolet light (primary prevention), as documented above, the incidence of skin cancer has continued to rise [1-9, 278]. Numerous agents, topical or oral, have been developed that are potentially efficacious for the inhibition or reversal of cancer development: retinoids; difluoromethylornithine; T4 endonuclease V; polyphenolic antioxidants like (-)-epigallocatechin gallate, which is found in green tea and grape seed extract; silymarin; isoflavone genestein; nonsteroidal anti-inflammatory drugs; curcumin; lycopene; vitamin E; beta-carotene; and selenium. Systemic retinoids have proven to be effective in preventing NMSC in individuals at high risk or who have numerous tumors [279]. To assess the efficacy of these agents, biomarkers of field cancerization can serve as endpoints to monitor the efficacy of these agents as precursors and molecular or proteomic signs of field cancerization are more common than frank cancer; utilization of these field markers could reduced sample size, length, and the cost of clinical trials [280]. For example, the reduction in the number of AK or dysplastic nevi could serve as potential targets for chemoprevention strategies. These variables could also be used in the testing of additional groups of promising preventive or therapeutic factors that include melatonin and its derivatives [281, 282] or vitamin D [283] and its novel derivatives [284, 285].

Conclusion

The classical concept of "field cancerization" emphasizes genetic events represented by point mutations, chromosomal aberrations, and incorporation of viral vectors. These events all correspond to the classic concept of initiation. The novel concept includes non-genetic changes in the local environment represented by the local production of factors that allow the initiated cells to leave the stem cell niche and expand into the surrounding proliferative units and escape immune surveillance. These latter events correlate with the classical concept of promotion and culminate in the production of a cancer field. Promoter activity could be signaled by growth factors, cytokines, immunosuppressive neuropeptides or glucocorticoids produced in the skin subjected to a stressful environment [162, 163], which also causes downregulation of local protective signaling systems [281, 282, 284, 286]. Alternative splicing of crucial regulatory genes may also play a role in this phenomenon [287-289].

Skin cancer, because of the sheer numbers and easy accessibility to observation, therapy, and sampling, provides an *in vivo* model to study the events of field cancerization and the impact of applied knowledge to its management. The studies reviewed herein report epidemiologic evidence of a high risk for second primary skin cancers in skin cancer fields, and the presence of molecular aberrations in histologically NS located adjacent to or some distance from skin cancers. These data provide direct support for skin field cancerization and highlight the occurrence of multiple types of GIS, including NIS, CIS, MIS and EIS occurring in morphologically NS. As skin cancer is the most frequent and one of the costliest cancers to manage, the development of effective strategies to identify those predisposed to cancer in order to implement preventive measures, coupled with efforts to increase the sensitivity and specificity of early detection efforts will have the (? Re-phrase) **greatest impact on decreasing** the burden of skin disease. As molecular biomarkers of cutaneous field cancerization may represent the crucial, core defects of cancer stem cells, they likely offer the greatest potential for early detection, accurate staging, and more effective therapy of skin cancer. Lastly, the skin can be considered a window into the health of the individual. Some of these field cancerization biomarkers may as well assess the individual's systemic risk for cancer.

References

[1] Miller DL, Weinstock MA. Nonmelanoma skin cancer in the United States: incidence. *J. Am. Acad. Dermatol.* 1994 May;30(5 Pt 1):774-8.

[2] Diepgen TL, Mahler V. The epidemiology of skin cancer. *Br. J. Dermatol.* 2002 Apr;146 Suppl 61:1-6.

[3] Jemal A, Siegel R, Ward E, Hao Y, Xu J, Thun MJ. Cancer statistics, 2009. CA Cancer *J. Clin.* 2009 Jul-Aug;59(4):225-49.

[4] Rogers HW, Weinstock MA, Harris AR, Hinckley MR, Feldman SR, Fleischer AB, et al. Incidence estimate of nonmelanoma skin cancer in the United States, 2006. *Arch. Dermatol.* 2010 Mar;146(3):283-7.

[5] Stern RS. Prevalence of a history of skin cancer in 2007: results of an incidence-based model. *Arch. Dermatol.* 2010 Mar;146(3):279-82.

[6] Leiter U, Garbe C. Epidemiology of melanoma and nonmelanoma skin cancer--the role of sunlight. *Adv. Exp. Med. Biol.* 2008;624:89-103.

[7] Carlson JA, Ross JS, Slominski AJ. New techniques in dermatopathology that help to diagnose and prognosticate melanoma. *Clin. Dermatol.* 2009 Jan-Feb;27(1):75-102.

[8] Rigel DS, Carucci JA. Malignant melanoma: prevention, early detection, and treatment in the 21st century. CA *Cancer J. Clin.* 2000 Jul-Aug;50(4):215-36; quiz 37-40.

[9] Beddingfield FC, 3rd. The melanoma epidemic: res ipsa loquitur. *Oncologist.* 2003;8(5):459-65.

[10] Eide MJ, Krajenta R, Johnson D, Long JJ, Jacobsen G, Asgari MM, et al. Identification of patients with nonmelanoma skin cancer using health maintenance organization claims data. *Am. J. Epidemiol.* 2010 Jan 1;171(1):123-8.

[11] Desmond RA, Soong SJ. Epidemiology of malignant melanoma. *Surg. Clin. North Am.* 2003 Feb;83(1):1-29.

[12] Thompson JF, Morton DL, Kroon BBE. *Textbook of Melanoma*. London: Martin Dunitz; 2004.

[13] Thompson JF, Scolyer RA, Kefford RF. Cutaneous melanoma. *Lancet.* 2005 Feb 19;365(9460):687-701.

[14] Housman TS, Feldman SR, Williford PM, Fleischer AB, Jr., Goldman ND, Acostamadiedo JM, et al. Skin cancer is among the most costly of all cancers to treat for the Medicare population. *J. Am. Acad. Dermatol.* 2003 Mar;48(3):425-9.

[15] Bickers DR, Lim HW, Margolis D, Weinstock MA, Goodman C, Faulkner E, et al. The burden of skin diseases: 2004 a joint project of the American Academy of Dermatology Association and the Society for Investigative Dermatology. *J. Am. Acad. Dermatol.* 2006 Sep;55(3):490-500.

[16] Seidler AM, Pennie ML, Veledar E, Culler SD, Chen SC. Economic Burden of Melanoma in the Elderly Population: Population-Based Analysis of the Surveillance, Epidemiology, and End Results (SEER)-Medicare Data. *Arch. Dermatol.* 2010 Mar;146(3):249-56.

[17] Martinez JC, Otley CC. Megasession: excision of numerous skin cancers in a single session. *Dermatol Surg.* 2005 Jul;31(7 Pt 1):757-61; discussion 61-2.

[18] Schinstine M, Goldman GD. Risk of synchronous and metachronous second nonmelanoma skin cancer when referred for Mohs micrographic surgery. *J. Am. Acad Dermatol.* 2001 Mar;44(3):497-9.

[19] Berg D, Otley CC. Skin cancer in organ transplant recipients: Epidemiology, pathogenesis, and management. *J. Am. Acad. Dermatol.* 2002 Jul;47(1):1-17; quiz 8-20.

[20] Veness MJ, Quinn DI, Ong CS, Keogh AM, Macdonald PS, Cooper SG, et al. Aggressive cutaneous malignancies following cardiothoracic transplantation: the Australian experience. *Cancer.* 1999 Apr 15;85(8):1758-64.

[21] Spanogle JP, Clarke CA, Aroner S, Swetter SM. Risk of second primary malignancies following cutaneous melanoma diagnosis: A population-based study. *J. Am. Acad. Dermatol.* 2010 Mar 9.

[22] Bradford PT, Freedman DM, Goldstein AM, Tucker MA. Increased risk of second primary cancers after a diagnosis of melanoma. *Arch. Dermatol.* 2010 Mar;146(3):265-72.

[23] Tessari G, Naldi L, Boschiero L, Nacchia F, Fior F, Forni A, et al. Incidence and clinical predictors of a subsequent nonmelanoma skin cancer in solid organ transplant

recipients with a first nonmelanoma skin cancer: a multicenter cohort study. *Arch Dermatol.* 2010 Mar;146(3):294-9.

[24] Cantwell MM, Murray LJ, Catney D, Donnelly D, Autier P, Boniol M, et al. Second primary cancers in patients with skin cancer: a population-based study in Northern Ireland. *Br. J. Cancer*. 2009 Jan 13;100(1):174-7.

[25] McCaul KA, Fritschi L, Baade P, Coory M. The incidence of second primary invasive melanoma in Queensland, 1982-2003. *Cancer Causes Control.* 2008 Jun;19(5):451-8.

[26] Maitra SK, Gallo H, Rowland-Payne C, Robinson D, Moller H. Second primary cancers in patients with squamous cell carcinoma of the skin. *Br. J. Cancer.* 2005 Feb 14;92(3):570-1.

[27] Crocetti E, Carli P. Risk of second primary cancers, other than melanoma, in an Italian population-based cohort of cutaneous malignant melanoma patients. *Eur. J. Cancer Prev.* 2004 Feb;13(1):33-7.

[28] Savoia P, Quaglino P, Verrone A, Bernengo MG. Multiple primary melanomas: analysis of 49 cases. *Melanoma Res.* 1998 Aug;8(4):361-6.

[29] Goggins WB, Tsao H. A population-based analysis of risk factors for a second primary cutaneous melanoma among melanoma survivors. *Cancer*. 2003 Feb 1;97(3):639-43.

[30] Wassberg C, Thorn M, Yuen J, Ringborg U, Hakulinen T. Second primary cancers in patients with squamous cell carcinoma of the skin: a population-based study in Sweden. *Int. J. Cancer*. 1999 Feb 9;80(4):511-5.

[31] Bangash SJ, Green WH, Dolson DJ, Cognetta AB, Jr. Eruptive postoperative squamous cell carcinomas exhibiting a pathergy-like reaction around surgical wound sites. *J. Am. Acad Dermatol.* 2009 Nov;61(5):892-7.

[32] Nugent Z, Demers AA, Wiseman MC, Mihalcioiu C, Kliewer EV. Risk of second primary cancer and death following a diagnosis of nonmelanoma skin cancer. *Cancer Epidemiol Biomarkers Prev.* 2005 Nov;14(11 Pt 1):2584-90.

[33] Rosenberg CA, Greenland P, Khandekar J, Loar A, Ascensao J, Lopez AM. Association of nonmelanoma skin cancer with second malignancy. *Cancer*. 2004 Jan 1;100(1):130-8.

[34] Slaughter DP, Southwick HW, Smejkal W. Field cancerization in oral stratified squamous epithelium; clinical implications of multicentric origin. *Cancer.* 1953 Sep;6(5):963-8.

[35] Dakubo GD, Jakupciak JP, Birch-Machin MA, Parr RL. Clinical implications and utility of field cancerization. *Cancer Cell Int*. 2007;7:2.

[36] Hanahan D, Weinberg RA. The hallmarks of cancer. *Cell.* 2000 Jan 7;100(1):57-70.

[37] Tapp RA, Feng J, Jones JW, Carlson JA, Wilson VL. Single base instability is promoted in vulvar lichen sclerosus. *J. Invest Dermatol.* 2007 Nov;127(11):2563-76.

[38] Backvall H, Wolf O, Hermelin H, Weitzberg E, Ponten F. The density of epidermal p53 clones is higher adjacent to squamous cell carcinoma in comparison with basal cell carcinoma. *Br.J. Dermatol.* 2004 Feb;150(2):259-66.

[39] North JP, Kageshita T, Pinkel D, LeBoit PE, Bastian BC. Distribution and significance of occult intraepidermal tumor cells surrounding primary melanoma. *J. Invest Dermatol.* 2008 Aug;128(8):2024-30.

[40] Braakhuis BJ, Tabor MP, Kummer JA, Leemans CR, Brakenhoff RH. A genetic explanation of Slaughter's concept of field cancerization: evidence and clinical implications. *Cancer Res*. 2003 Apr 15;63(8):1727-30.

[41] Hittelman WN. Genetic instability in epithelial tissues at risk for cancer. *Ann. N Y Acad Sci.* 2001 Dec;952:1-12.
[42] Bielas JH, Loeb LA. Mutator phenotype in cancer: timing and perspectives. *Environ. Mol. Mutagen.* 2005 Mar-Apr;45(2-3):206-13.
[43] Nowell PC. Tumor progression: a brief historical perspective. *Semin. Cancer Biol.* 2002 Aug;12(4):261-6.
[44] Negrini S, Gorgoulis VG, Halazonetis TD. Genomic instability--an evolving hallmark of cancer. *Nat. Rev. Mol. Cell Biol.* 2010 Mar;11(3):220-8.
[45] Pleasance ED, Cheetham RK, Stephens PJ, McBride DJ, Humphray SJ, Greenman CD, et al. A comprehensive catalogue of somatic mutations from a human cancer genome. *Nature.* 2010 Jan 14;463(7278):191-6.
[46] Gould Rothberg BE, Bracken MB, Rimm DL. Tissue biomarkers for prognosis in cutaneous melanoma: a systematic review and meta-analysis. *J. Natl. Cancer Inst.* 2009 Apr 1;101(7):452-74.
[47] Loeb LA, Bielas JH, Beckman RA. Cancers exhibit a mutator phenotype: clinical implications. *Cancer Res.* 2008 May 15;68(10):3551-7; discussion 7.
[48] Kaur P, Mulvaney M, Carlson JA. Basal cell carcinoma progression correlates with host immune response and stromal alterations: a histologic analysis. *Am. J. Dermatopathol.* 2006 Aug;28(4):293-307.
[49] Carlson JA, Healy K, Tran TA, Malfetano J, Wilson VL, Rohwedder A, et al. Chromosome 17 aneusomy detected by fluorescence in situ hybridization in vulvar squamous cell carcinomas and synchronous vulvar skin. *Am. J. Pathol.* 2000 Sep;157(3):973-83.
[50] Carlson JA, Amin S, Malfetano J, Tien AT, Selkin B, Hou J, et al. Concordant p53 and mdm-2 protein expression in vulvar squamous cell carcinoma and adjacent lichen sclerosus. *Appl. Immunohistochem Mol. Morphol.* 2001 Jun;9(2):150-63.
[51] Padilla RS, Sebastian S, Jiang Z, Nindl I, Larson R. Gene expression patterns of normal human skin, actinic keratosis, and squamous cell carcinoma: a spectrum of disease progression. *Arch. Dermatol.* 2010 Mar;146(3):288-93.
[52] Armitage P, Doll R. The age distribution of cancer and a multi-stage theory of carcinogenesis. *Br. J. Cancer.* 1954 Mar;8(1):1-12.
[53] Dore JF, Pedeux R, Boniol M, Chignol MC, Autier P. Intermediate-effect biomarkers in prevention of skin cancer. *IARC Sci Publ.* 2001;154:81-91.
[54] Ashton KJ, Carless MA, Griffiths LR. Cytogenetic alterations in nonmelanoma skin cancer: a review. *Genes Chromosomes Cancer. 2005* Jul;43(3):239-48.
[55] Boukamp P. Non-melanoma skin cancer: what drives tumor development and progression? *Carcinogenesis.* 2005 Oct;26(10):1657-67.
[56] Blokx WA, van Dijk MC, Ruiter DJ. Molecular cytogenetics of cutaneous melanocytic lesions - diagnostic, prognostic and therapeutic aspects. *Histopathology.* 2010 Jan;56(1):121-32.
[57] Dadzie OE, Yang S, Emley A, Keady M, Bhawan J, Mahalingam M. RAS and RAF mutations in banal melanocytic aggregates contiguous with primary cutaneous melanoma: clues to melanomagenesis. *Br. J. Dermatol.* 2009 Feb;160(2):368-75.
[58] Rubin H. Saturation density of skin fibroblasts as a quantitative screen for human cancer susceptibility. *Cancer Epidemiol Biomarkers Prev.* 2009 Sep;18(9):2366-72.

[59] Pleasance ED, Stephens PJ, O'Meara S, McBride DJ, Meynert A, Jones D, et al. A small-cell lung cancer genome with complex signatures of tobacco exposure. *Nature.* 2010 Jan 14;463(7278):184-90.

[60] Boland CR, Ricciardiello L. How many mutations does it take to make a tumor? *Proc. Natl. Acad. Sci. USA.* 1999 Dec 21;96(26):14675-7.

[61] Benitah SA. Epidermal stem cells in skin homeostasis and cutaneous carcinomas. *Clin. Transl Oncol.* 2007 Dec;9(12):760-6.

[62] Lau K, Paus R, Tiede S, Day P, Bayat A. Exploring the role of stem cells in cutaneous wound healing. *Exp. Dermatol.* 2009 Nov;18(11):921-33.

[63] LeBleu VS, Macdonald B, Kalluri R. Structure and function of basement membranes. *Exp Biol. Med.* (Maywood). 2007 Oct;232(9):1121-9.

[64] Iozzo RV. Basement membrane proteoglycans: from cellar to ceiling. *Nat. Rev. Mol. Cell Biol.* 2005 Aug;6(8):646-56.

[65] Lister R, Pelizzola M, Dowen RH, Hawkins RD, Hon G, Tonti-Filippini J, et al. Human DNA methylomes at base resolution show widespread epigenomic differences. *Nature.* 2009 Nov 19;462(7271):315-22.

[66] Broske AM, Vockentanz L, Kharazi S, Huska MR, Mancini E, Scheller M, et al. DNA methylation protects hematopoietic stem cell multipotency from myeloerythroid restriction. *Nature genetics.* 2009 Nov;41(11):1207-15.

[67] Harley CB. Telomerase and cancer therapeutics. *Nat. Rev. Cancer.* 2008 Mar;8(3):167-79.

[68] Parkinson EK. Epidermal keratinocyte stem cells: their maintenance and regulation. *Seminars in cell biology.* 1992 Dec;3(6):435-44.

[69] Potten CS, Booth C. Keratinocyte stem cells: a commentary. *J. Invest Dermatol.* 2002 Oct;119(4):888-99.

[70] Ghazizadeh S, Taichman LB. Organization of stem cells and their progeny in human epidermis. *J. Invest Dermatol.* 2005 Feb;124(2):367-72.

[71] Lippens S, Hoste E, Vandenabeele P, Agostinis P, Declercq W. Cell death in the skin. *Apoptosis.* 2009 Apr;14(4):549-69.

[72] Lu S, Slominski A, Yang S-E, Sheehan C, Ross J, Carlson JA. The correlation of TRPM1 (Melastatin) mRNA expression with microphthalmia-associated transcription factor (MITF) and other melanogenesis-related proteins in normal and pathological skin, hair follicles and melanocytic nevi. *J. Cutan Pathol.* 2010;37(Suppl. 1):26–40.

[73] Gleason BC, Crum CP, Murphy GF. Expression patterns of MITF during human cutaneous embryogenesis: evidence for bulge epithelial expression and persistence of dermal melanoblasts. *J. Cutan. Pathol.* 2008;35:615-22.

[74] Jones PH, Harper S, Watt FM. Stem cell patterning and fate in human epidermis. *Cell.* 1995 Jan 13;80(1):83-93.

[75] Li A, Simmons PJ, Kaur P. Identification and isolation of candidate human keratinocyte stem cells based on cell surface phenotype. *Proc. Natl. Acad. Sci. USA.* 1998 Mar 31;95(7):3902-7.

[76] Pellegrini G, Dellambra E, Golisano O, Martinelli E, Fantozzi I, Bondanza S, et al. p63 identifies keratinocyte stem cells. *Proc. Natl. Acad. Sci. USA.* 2001 Mar 13;98(6):3156-61.

[77] Yu Y, Flint A, Dvorin EL, Bischoff J. AC133-2, a novel isoform of human AC133 stem cell antigen. *J. Biol. Chem.* 2002 Jun 7;277(23):20711-6.

[78] Slominski A, Tobin DJ, Shibahara S, Wortsman J. Melanin pigmentation in mammalian skin and its hormonal regulation. *Physiol Rev*. 2004 Oct;84(4):1155-228.
[79] Slominski A, Wortsman J, Plonka PM, Schallreuter KU, Paus R, Tobin DJ. Hair follicle pigmentation. *J. Invest Dermatol.* 2005 Jan;124(1):13-21.
[80] White RM, Zon LI. Melanocytes in development, regeneration, and cancer. *Cell Stem Cell.* 2008 Sep 11;3(3):242-52.
[81] Grichnik JM. Melanoma, nevogenesis, and stem cell biology. *J. Invest Dermatol.* 2008 Oct;128(10):2365-80.
[82] Cramer SF. Stem cells for epidermal melanocytes--a challenge for students of dermatopathology. *Am. J. Dermatopathol.* 2009 Jun;31(4):331-41.
[83] Curtin JA, Fridlyand J, Kageshita T, Patel HN, Busam KJ, Kutzner H, et al. Distinct sets of genetic alterations in melanoma. *N. Engl J. Med.* 2005 Nov 17;353(20):2135-47.
[84] Zalaudek I, Marghoob AA, Scope A, Leinweber B, Ferrara G, Hofmann-Wellenhof R, et al. Three roots of melanoma. *Arch. Dermatol.* 2008 Oct;144(10):1375-9.
[85] Cairns J. Somatic stem cells and the kinetics of mutagenesis and carcinogenesis. *Proc. Natl. Acad. Sci. USA.* 2002 Aug 6;99(16):10567-70.
[86] Backvall H, Asplund A, Gustafsson A, Sivertsson A, Lundeberg J, Ponten F. Genetic tumor archeology: microdissection and genetic heterogeneity in squamous and basal cell carcinoma. *Mutat Res.* 2005 Apr 1;571(1-2):65-79.
[87] Ren Z, Ponten F, Nister M, Ponten J. Reconstruction of the two-dimensional distribution of p53 positive patches in sun-exposed skin morphologically normal skin. *Inter J. Oncol.* 1997;11:111-5.
[88] Brash DE, Ponten J. Skin precancer. *Cancer Surv*. 1998;32:69-113.
[89] Berg RJ, van Kranen HJ, Rebel HG, de Vries A, van Vloten WA, Van Kreijl CF, et al. Early p53 alterations in mouse skin carcinogenesis by UVB radiation: immunohistochemical detection of mutant p53 protein in clusters of preneoplastic epidermal cells. *Proc. Natl .Acad. Sci .USA.* 1996 Jan 9;93(1):274-8.
[90] Asplund A, Guo Z, Hu X, Wassberg C, Ponten F. Mosaic pattern of maternal and paternal keratinocyte clones in normal human epidermis revealed by analysis of X-chromosome inactivation. *J. Invest Dermatol.* 2001 Jul;117(1):128-31.
[91] Jonason AS, Kunala S, Price GJ, Restifo RJ, Spinelli HM, Persing JA, et al. Frequent clones of p53-mutated keratinocytes in normal human skin. *Proc. Natl. Acad. Sci. USA.* 1996 Nov 26;93(24):14025-9.
[92] Zhang W, Remenyik E, Zelterman D, Brash DE, Wikonkal NM. Escaping the stem cell compartment: sustained UVB exposure allows p53-mutant keratinocytes to colonize adjacent epidermal proliferating units without incurring additional mutations. *Proc. Natl. Acad. Sci. USA*. 2001 Nov 20;98(24):13948-53.
[93] Merlo LM, Pepper JW, Reid BJ, Maley CC. Cancer as an evolutionary and ecological process. *Nat. Rev. Cancer.* 2006 Dec;6(12):924-35.
[94] Madan V, Lear JT, Szeimies RM. Non-melanoma skin cancer. *Lancet.* 2010 Feb 20;375(9715):673-85.
[95] Wood JM, Jimbow K, Boissy RE, Slominski A, Plonka PM, Slawinski J, et al. What's the use of generating melanin? *Exp. Dermatol.* 1999 Apr;8(2):153-64.
[96] Slominski A, Paus R, Schanderdorf D. Melanocytes as sensory and regulatory cells in the epidermis. *J. Theor. Biol.* 1993;164:103-20.

[97] Hoy WE. Nonmelanoma skin carcinoma in Albuquerque, New Mexico: experience of a major health care provider. *Cancer.* 1996 Jun 15;77(12):2489-95.

[98] Marcil I, Stern RS. Risk of developing a subsequent nonmelanoma skin cancer in patients with a history of nonmelanoma skin cancer: a critical review of the literature and meta-analysis. *Arch Dermatol.* 2000 Dec;136(12):1524-30.

[99] Armstrong BK, Kricker A. The epidemiology of UV induced skin cancer. *J. Photochem. Photobiol. B.* 2001 Oct;63(1-3):8-18.

[100] Curtin JA, Busam K, Pinkel D, Bastian BC. Somatic activation of KIT in distinct subtypes of melanoma. *J. Clin. Oncol.* 2006 Sep 10;24(26):4340-6.

[101] Brozyna A, Zbytek B, Granese J, Carlson JA, Ross J, Slominski A. Mechanism of UV-related carcinogenesis and its contribution to nevi/melanoma. *Expert. Rev. Dermatol.* 2007;2(4):451-69.

[102] Lee DA, Miller SJ. Nonmelanoma skin cancer. *Facial Plast Surg Clin. North Am.* 2009 Aug;17(3):309-24.

[103] Carlson JA, Slominski A, Linette GP, Mihm MC, Jr., Ross JS. Biomarkers in melanoma: predisposition, screening and diagnosis. *Expert Rev. Mol. Diagn.* 2003 Mar;3(2):163-84.

[104] Naldi L, Altieri A, Imberti GL, Gallus S, Bosetti C, La Vecchia C. Sun exposure, phenotypic characteristics, and cutaneous malignant melanoma. An analysis according to different clinico-pathological variants and anatomic locations (Italy). *Cancer Causes Control.* 2005 Oct;16(8):893-9.

[105] Andersen WK, Labadie RR, Bhawan J. Histopathology of solar lentigines of the face: a quantitative study. *J. Am. Acad. Dermatol.* 1997 Mar;36(3 Pt 1):444-7.

[106] Kossard S. Atypical lentiginous junctional naevi of the elderly and melanoma. *Australas J. Dermatol.* 2002 May;43(2):93-101.

[107] Mittelbronn MA, Mullins DL, Ramos-Caro FA, Flowers FP. Frequency of pre-existing actinic keratosis in cutaneous squamous cell carcinoma. *Int J Dermatol.* 1998 Sep;37(9):677-81.

[108] Olson R, Jones DM, Carlson JA. The role of dermatopathology in clinical dermatology. *Journal of Malaysian Dermatology.* 2007;19(August):5-17.

[109] Arumi-Uria M, McNutt NS, Finnerty B. Grading of atypia in nevi: correlation with melanoma risk. *Mod Pathol.* 2003 Aug;16(8):764-71.

[110] Hafner C, Vogt T. Seborrheic keratosis. *J. Dtsch Dermatol. Ges.* 2008 Aug;6(8):664-77.

[111] Carlson JA, Scott D, Wharton J, Sell S. Incidental histopathologic patterns: possible evidence of 'field cancerization' surrounding skin tumors. *Am. J. Dermatopathol.* 2001 Oct;23(5):494-6.

[112] Rohwedder A, Foong H, Tyring SK, Rady P, Carlson JA. Incidental epidermodysplasia verruciformis human papillomavirus infection (EV acanthoma): evidence for 'field cancerization' and a putative cofactor in seborrheic keratosis. *J. Cutan Pathol.* 2008 Dec;35(12):1151-5.

[113] Hutcheson AC, Nietert PJ, Maize JC. Incidental epidermolytic hyperkeratosis and focal acantholytic dyskeratosis in common acquired melanocytic nevi and atypical melanocytic lesions. *J. Am. Acad. Dermatol.* 2004 Mar;50(3):388-90.

[114] Brownstein MH. Acantholytic acanthoma. *J. Am. Acad. Dermatol.* 1988 Nov;19(5 Pt 1):783-6.

[115] Roten SV, Bhawan J. Isolated dyskeratotic acanthoma. A variant of isolated epidermolytic acanthoma. *Am. J. Dermatopathol.* 1995 Feb;17(1):63-6.
[116] Ko CJ, Iftner T, Barr RJ, Binder SW. Changes of epidermodysplasia verruciformis in benign skin lesions: the EV acanthoma. *J. Cutan Pathol.* 2007 Jan;34(1):44-8.
[117] Ko CJ, Barr RJ, Subtil A, McNiff JM. Acantholytic dyskeratotic acanthoma: a variant of a benign keratosis. *J. Cutan Pathol.* 2008 Mar;35(3):298-301.
[118] Harwood CA, Surentheran T, Sasieni P, Proby CM, Bordea C, Leigh IM, et al. Increased risk of skin cancer associated with the presence of epidermodysplasia verruciformis human papillomavirus types in normal skin. *Br. J. Dermatol.* 2004 May;150(5):949-57.
[119] Bjorn LM. Photobiology: *The Science of Life and Light.* Second ed. New York: Springer; 2008.
[120] Slominski A, Pawelek J. Animals under the sun: effects of ultraviolet radiation on mammalian skin. *Clin. Dermatol.* 1998 Jul-Aug;16(4):503-15.
[121] Runger TM. How different wavelengths of the ultraviolet spectrum contribute to skin carcinogenesis: the role of cellular damage responses. *J. Invest Dermatol.* 2007 Sep;127(9):2103-5.
[122] Agar NS, Halliday GM, Barnetson RS, Ananthaswamy HN, Wheeler M, Jones AM. The basal layer in human squamous tumors harbors more UVA than UVB fingerprint mutations: a role for UVA in human skin carcinogenesis. *Proc. Natl. Acad. Sci. USA.* 2004 Apr 6;101(14):4954-9.
[123] Greinert R. Skin cancer: new markers for better prevention. *Pathobiology.* 2009;76(2):64-81.
[124] Kielbassa C, Roza L, Epe B. Wavelength dependence of oxidative DNA damage induced by UV and visible light. *Carcinogenesis.* 1997 Apr;18(4):811-6.
[125] Abdel-Malek ZA, Kadekaro AL, Swope VB. Stepping up melanocytes to the challenge of UV exposure. *Pigment Cell Melanoma Res.* 2010 Feb 1.
[126] Nordlund JJ. Nonmelanoma skin cancer in vitiligo patients. *J. Am. Acad Dermatol.* 2009 Dec;61(6):1080-1.
[127] Smit NP, van Nieuwpoort FA, Marrot L, Out C, Poorthuis B, van Pelt H, et al. Increased melanogenesis is a risk factor for oxidative DNA damage--study on cultured melanocytes and atypical nevus cells. *Photochem Photobiol.* 2008 May-Jun;84(3):550-5.
[128] Lear JT, Smith AG, Strange RC, Fryer AA. Detoxifying enzyme genotypes and susceptibility to cutaneous malignancy. *Br. J. Dermatol.* 2000 Jan;142(1):8-15.
[129] Wang LE, Li C, Strom SS, Goldberg LH, Brewster A, Guo Z, et al. Repair capacity for UV light induced DNA damage associated with risk of nonmelanoma skin cancer and tumor progression. *Clin. Cancer Res.* 2007 Nov 1;13(21):6532-9.
[130] Steinberg ML, Hubbard K, Utti C, Clas B, Hwang BJ, Hill HZ, et al. Patterns of persistent DNA damage associated with sun exposure and the glutathione S-transferase M1 genotype in melanoma patients. *Photochem Photobiol.* 2009 Jan-Feb;85(1):379-86.
[131] Takahashi Y, Moriwaki S, Sugiyama Y, Endo Y, Yamazaki K, Mori T, et al. Decreased gene expression responsible for post-ultraviolet DNA repair synthesis in aging: a possible mechanism of age-related reduction in DNA repair capacity. *J. Invest Dermatol.* 2005 Feb;124(2):435-42.

[132] Moore MM, Chua W, Charles KA, Clarke SJ. Inflammation and cancer: causes and consequences. *Clin. Pharmacol Ther*. 2010 Apr;87(4):504-8.

[133] Dvorak HF. Tumors: wounds that do not heal. Similarities between tumor stroma generation and wound healing. N. *Engl J. Med*. 1986 Dec 25;315(26):1650-9.

[134] Cruikshank AH, McConnell EM, Miller DG. Malignancy in scars, chronic ulcers and sinuses. *J Clin Pathol*. 1963;16:573-80.

[135] Kowal-Vern A, Criswell BK. Burn scar neoplasms: a literature review and statistical analysis. *Burns*. 2005 Jun;31(4):403-13.

[136] Carlson JA, Ambros R, Malfetano J, Ross J, Grabowski R, Lamb P, et al. Vulvar lichen sclerosus and squamous cell carcinoma: a cohort, case control, and investigational study with historical perspective; implications for chronic inflammation and sclerosis in the development of neoplasia. *Hum Pathol*. 1998 Sep;29(9):932-48.

[137] Carli P, De Magnis A, Mannone F, Botti E, Taddei G, Cattaneo A. Vulvar carcinoma associated with lichen sclerosus. Experience at the Florence, Italy, Vulvar Clinic. *J. Reprod Med*. 2003 May;48(5):313-8.

[138] Carlson JA, Grabowski R, Chichester P, Paunovich E, Malfetano J. Comparative immunophenotypic study of lichen sclerosus: epidermotropic CD57+ lymphocytes are numerous--implications for pathogenesis. *Am. J. Dermatopathol*. 2000 Feb;22(1):7-16.

[139] Sander CS, Ali I, Dean D, Thiele JJ, Wojnarowska F. Oxidative stress is implicated in the pathogenesis of lichen sclerosus. *Br. J. Dermatol.* 2004 Sep;151(3):627-35.

[140] Smoller BR, Krueger J, McNutt NS, Hsu A. "Activated" keratinocyte phenotype is unifying feature in conditions which predispose to squamous cell carcinoma of the skin. *Mod Pathol*. 1990;3(2):171-5.

[141] Antonsson A, Erfurt C, Hazard K, Holmgren V, Simon M, Kataoka A, et al. Prevalence and type spectrum of human papillomaviruses in healthy skin samples collected in three continents. *J. Gen. Virol.* 2003 Jul;84(Pt 7):1881-6.

[142] Antonsson A, Forslund O, Ekberg H, Sterner G, Hansson BG. The ubiquity and impressive genomic diversity of human skin papillomaviruses suggest a commensalic nature of these viruses. *J. Virol*. 2000 Dec;74(24):11636-41.

[143] Antonsson A, Karanfilovska S, Lindqvist PG, Hansson BG. General acquisition of human papillomavirus infections of skin occurs in early infancy. *J. Clin. Microbiol.* 2003 Jun;41(6):2509-14.

[144] Chan SY, Delius H, Halpern AL, Bernard HU. Analysis of genomic sequences of 95 papillomavirus types: uniting typing, phylogeny, and taxonomy. *J. Virol.* 1995;69(5):3074-83.

[145] Chan JK, Monk BJ, Brewer C, Keefe KA, Osann K, McMeekin S, et al. HPV infection and number of lifetime sexual partners are strong predictors for 'natural' regression of CIN 2 and 3. *Br. J. Cancer*. 2003 Sep 15;89(6):1062-6.

[146] Franco EL, Villa LL, Sobrinho JP, Prado JM, Rousseau MC, Desy M, et al. Epidemiology of acquisition and clearance of cervical human papillomavirus infection in women from a high-risk area for cervical cancer. *J. Infect Dis*. 1999 Nov;180(5):1415-23.

[147] Koutsky L. Epidemiology of genital human papillomavirus infection. *Am. J. Med.* 1997;102(5A):3-8.

[148] Dunne EF, Unger ER, Sternberg M, McQuillan G, Swan DC, Patel SS, et al. Prevalence of HPV infection among females in the United States. *JAMA*. 2007 Feb 28;297(8):813-9.

[149] Orth G. Human papillomaviruses associated with epidermodysplasia verruciformis in non-melanoma skin cancers: guilty or innocent? *J. Invest Dermatol.* 2005 Jul;125(1):xii-xiii.

[150] Caldeira S, Zehbe I, Accardi R, Malanchi I, Dong W, Giarre M, et al. The E6 and E7 proteins of the cutaneous human papillomavirus type 38 display transforming properties. *J. Virol.* 2003 Feb;77(3):2195-206.

[151] Plasmeijer EI, Neale RE, de Koning MN, Quint WG, McBride P, Feltkamp MC, et al. Persistence of betapapillomavirus infections as a risk factor for actinic keratoses, precursor to cutaneous squamous cell carcinoma. *Cancer Res*. 2009 Dec 1;69(23):8926-31.

[152] Plasmeijer EI, Neale RE, Buettner PG, de Koning MN, Ter Schegget J, Quint WG, et al. Betapapillomavirus infection profiles in tissue sets from cutaneous squamous cell-carcinoma patients. *Int. J. Cancer*. 2009 Oct 23;126(11):2614-21.

[153] Zhang HG, Grizzle WE. Aging, immunity, and tumor susceptibility. *Immunol Allergy Clin. North Am*. 2003 Feb;23(1):83-102, vi.

[154] Wilson RE, Hager EB, Hampers CL, Corson JM, Merrill JP, Murray JE. Immunologic rejection of human cancer transplanted with a renal allograft. *N. Engl. J. Med*. 1968 Feb 29;278(9):479-83.

[155] Franceschi S, Dal Maso L, Arniani S, Crosignani P, Vercelli M, Simonato L, et al. Risk of cancer other than Kaposi's sarcoma and non-Hodgkin's lymphoma in persons with AIDS in Italy. Cancer and AIDS Registry Linkage Study. *Br. J. Cancer*. 1998 Oct;78(7):966-70.

[156] Oram Y, Orengo I, Griego RD, Rosen T, Thornby J. Histologic patterns of basal cell carcinoma based upon patient immunostatus. *Dermatol Surg*. 1995 Jul;21(7):611-4.

[157] Mehrany K, Byrd DR, Roenigk RK, Weenig RH, Phillips PK, Nguyen TH, et al. Lymphocytic infiltrates and subclinical epithelial tumor extension in patients with chronic leukemia and solid-organ transplantation. *Dermatol Surg*. 2003 Feb;29(2):129-34.

[158] Weimar VM, Ceilley RI, Goeken JA. Aggressive biologic behavior of basal- and squamous-cell cancers in patients with chronic lymphocytic leukemia or chronic lymphocytic lymphoma. *J Derm Surg Oncol*. 1979 Aug;5(8):609-14.

[159] Casabonne D, Lally A, Mitchell L, Michael KM, Waterboer T, Pawlita M, et al. A case-control study of cutaneous squamous cell carcinoma among Caucasian organ transplant recipients: the role of antibodies against human papillomavirus and other risk factors. *Int. J. Cancer*. 2009 Oct 15;125(8):1935-45.

[160] Stockfleth E, Nindl I, Sterry W, Ulrich C, Schmook T, Meyer T. Human papillomaviruses in transplant-associated skin cancers. *Dermatol. Surg.* 2004 May;30(4 Pt 2):604-9.

[161] Kripke ML. Ultraviolet radiation and immunology: something new under the sun--presidential address. *Cancer Res*. 1994 Dec 1;54(23):6102-5.

[162] Slominski A. A nervous breakdown in the skin: stress and the epidermal barrier. *J. Clin. Invest*. 2007 Nov;117(11):3166-9.

[163] Slominski A, Wortsman J. Neuroendocrinology of the skin. *Endocr. Rev.* 2000 Oct;21(5):457-87.

[164] Slominski A, Wortsman J, Luger T, Paus R, Solomon S. Corticotropin releasing hormone and proopiomelanocortin involvement in the cutaneous response to stress. *Physiol. Rev.* 2000 Jul;80(3):979-1020.

[165] Schwarz T. Ultraviolet radiation-induced tolerance. *Allergy.* 1999 Dec;54(12):1252-61.

[166] Schwarz A, Maeda A, Wild MK, Kernebeck K, Gross N, Aragane Y, et al. Ultraviolet radiation-induced regulatory T cells not only inhibit the induction but can suppress the effector phase of contact hypersensitivity. *J. Immunol.* 2004 Jan 15;172(2):1036-43.

[167] Ruocco E, Puca RV, Brunetti G, Schwartz RA, Ruocco V. Lymphedematous areas: privileged sites for tumors, infections, and immune disorders. *Int J Dermatol* 2007 Jun;46(6):662.

[168] Benson PM, Pessoa CM, Lupton GP, Winton GB. Basal cell carcinomas arising in chronic lymphedema. *J. Dermatol. Surg. Oncol.* 1988 Jul;14(7):781-3.

[169] Kajiya K, Kunstfeld R, Detmar M, Chung JH. Reduction of lymphatic vessels in photodamaged human skin. *J. Dermatol. Sci.* 2007 Sep;47(3):241-3.

[170] Acker DW, Helwig EB. Rhinophyma with carcinoma. *Arch. Dermatol.* 1967 Mar;95(3):250-4.

[171] Meyskens FL, Jr., Farmer PJ, Yang S, Anton-Culver H. New perspectives on melanoma pathogenesis and chemoprevention. *Recent Results Cancer Res.* 2007;174:191-5.

[172] Slominski A, Zbytek B, Slominski R. Inhibitors of melanogenesis increase toxicity of cyclophosphamide and lymphocytes against melanoma cells. *Int. J. Cancer.* 2009 Mar 15;124(6):1470-7.

[173] Urbanska K, Romanowska-Dixon B, Elas M, Pajak S, Paziewski E, Bryk J, et al. Experimental ruthenium plaque therapy of amelanotic and melanotic melanomas in the hamster eye. *Melanoma Res.* 2000 Feb;10(1):26-35.

[174] Slominski A, Paus R. Towards defining receptors for L-tyrosine and L-dopa. *Mol. Cell Endocrinol.* 1994 Mar;99(2):C7-11.

[175] Slominski A, Paus R, Mihm M. Inhibition of melanogenesis as an adjuvant strategy in the treatment of melanotic melanomas: selective review and hypothesis. *Anticancer Res.* 1998;18:3709-16.

[176] Fruehauf JP, Meyskens FL, Jr. Reactive oxygen species: a breath of life or death? *Clin Cancer Res.* 2007 Feb 1;13(3):789-94.

[177] Slominski A. Neuroendocrine activity of the melanocyte. *Exp. Dermatol.* 2009 Sep;18(9):760-3.

[178] Hussein MR, Wood GS. Microsatellite instability and its relevance to cutaneous tumorigenesis. *J. Cutan Pathol.* 2002 May;29(5):257-67.

[179] Cahill DP, Kinzler KW, Vogelstein B, Lengauer C. Genetic instability and darwinian selection in tumours. *Trends Cell Biol.* 1999 Dec;9(12):M57-60.

[180] Ushijima T. Epigenetic field for cancerization. *J. Biochem. Mol. Biol.* 2007 Mar 31;40(2):142-50.

[181] Lengauer C, Kinzler KW, Vogelstein B. Genetic instabilities in human cancers. *Nature.* 1998 Dec 17;396(6712):643-9.

[182] Duesberg PH. Are cancers dependent on oncogenes or on aneuploidy? *Cancer Genet Cytogenet.* 2003 May;143(1):89-91.

[183] Michor F, Iwasa Y, Vogelstein B, Lengauer C, Nowak MA. Can chromosomal instability initiate tumorigenesis? *Semin. Cancer Biol.* 2005 Feb;15(1):43-9.
[184] Kanellou P, Zaravinos A, Zioga M, Stratigos A, Baritaki S, Soufla G, et al. Genomic instability, mutations and expression analysis of the tumour suppressor genes p14(ARF), p15(INK4b), p16(INK4a) and p53 in actinic keratosis. *Cancer Lett.* 2008 Jun 8;264(1):145-61.
[185] Hocker T, Tsao H. Ultraviolet radiation and melanoma: a systematic review and analysis of reported sequence variants. *Hum. Mutat.* 2007 Feb 12.
[186] Sabatino M, Zhao Y, Voiculescu S, Monaco A, Robbins P, Karai L, et al. Conservation of genetic alterations in recurrent melanoma supports the melanoma stem cell hypothesis. *Cancer Res.* 2008 Jan 1;68(1):122-31.
[187] Beckman RA, Loeb LA. Efficiency of carcinogenesis with and without a mutator mutation. *Proc. Natl. Acad Sci USA.* 2006 Sep 19;103(38):14140-5.
[188] Blanquet V, Turleau C, Gross-Morand MS, Senamaud-Beaufort C, Doz F, Besmond C. Spectrum of germline mutations in the RB1 gene: a study of 232 patients with hereditary and non hereditary retinoblastoma. *Hum. Mol. Genet.* 1995 Mar;4(3):383-8.
[189] Hussain SP, Harris CC. Molecular epidemiology of human cancer: contribution of mutation spectra studies of tumor suppressor genes. *Cancer Res.* 1998 Sep 15;58(18):4023-37.
[190] Fearon ER, Vogelstein B. A genetic model for colorectal tumorigenesis. *Cell.* 1990 Jun 1;61(5):759-67.
[191] Wilson VL. Detecting rare mutations associated with cancer risk. *Am. J. Pharmacogenomics*. 2001;1(4):283-93.
[192] Stenson PD, Mort M, Ball EV, Howells K, Phillips AD, Thomas NS, et al. The Human Gene Mutation Database: 2008 update. *Genome Med.* 2009 Jan 22;1(1):13.
[193] Petitjean A, Mathe E, Kato S, Ishioka C, Tavtigian SV, Hainaut P, et al. Impact of mutant p53 functional properties on TP53 mutation patterns and tumor phenotype: lessons from recent developments in the IARC TP53 database. *Hum. Mutat.* 2007 Jun;28(6):622-9.
[194] Kumar R, Angelini S, Hemminki K. Activating BRAF and N-Ras mutations in sporadic primary melanomas: an inverse association with allelic loss on chromosome 9. *Oncogene.* 2003 Dec 18;22(58):9217-24.
[195] Nakazawa H, English D, Randell PL, Nakazawa K, Martel N, Armstrong BK, et al. UV and skin cancer: specific p53 gene mutation in normal skin as a biologically relevant exposure measurement. *Proc. Natl. Acad. Sci. USA.* 1994 Jan 4;91(1):360-4.
[196] Kanjilal S, Strom SS, Clayman GL, Weber RS, el-Naggar AK, Kapur V, et al. p53 mutations in nonmelanoma skin cancer of the head and neck: molecular evidence for field cancerization. *Cancer Res.* 1995 Aug 15;55(16):3604-9.
[197] Ren ZP, Ahmadian A, Ponten F, Nister M, Berg C, Lundeberg J, et al. Benign clonal keratinocyte patches with p53 mutations show no genetic link to synchronous squamous cell precancer or cancer in human skin. *Am. J. Pathol.* 1997 May;150(5):1791-803.
[198] Ouhtit A, Ueda M, Nakazawa H, Ichihashi M, Dumaz N, Sarasin A, et al. Quantitative detection of ultraviolet-specific p53 mutations in normal skin from Japanese patients. *Cancer Epidemiol Biomarkers Prev.* 1997 Jun;6(6):433-8.
[199] Williams C, Ponten F, Ahmadian A, Ren ZP, Ling G, Rollman O, et al. Clones of normal keratinocytes and a variety of simultaneously present epidermal neoplastic

lesions contain a multitude of p53 gene mutations in a xeroderma pigmentosum patient. *Cancer Res*. 1998 Jun 1;58(11):2449-55.

[200] Ling G, Persson A, Berne B, Uhlen M, Lundeberg J, Ponten F. Persistent p53 mutations in single cells from normal human skin. *Am. J Pathol*. 2001 Oct;159(4):1247-53.

[201] Backvall H, Stromberg S, Gustafsson A, Asplund A, Sivertsson A, Lundeberg J, et al. Mutation spectra of epidermal p53 clones adjacent to basal cell carcinoma and squamous cell carcinoma. *Exp. Dermatol*. 2004 Oct;13(10):643-50.

[202] Aguilar F, Harris CC, Sun T, Hollstein M, Cerutti P. Geographic variation of p53 mutational profile in nonmalignant human liver. *Science*. 1994 May 27;264(5163):1317-9.

[203] Wilson VL, Yin X, Thompson B, Wade KR, Watkins JP, Wei Q, et al. Oncogenic base substitution mutations in circulating leukocytes of normal individuals. *Cancer Res*. 2000 Apr 1;60(7):1830-4.

[204] Eshaghian A, Vleugels RA, Canter JA, McDonald MA, Stasko T, Sligh JE. Mitochondrial DNA deletions serve as biomarkers of aging in the skin, but are typically absent in nonmelanoma skin cancers. *J. Invest Dermatol*. 2006 Feb;126(2):336-44.

[205] Hubbard K, Steinberg ML, Hill H, Orlow I. Mitochondrial DNA deletions in skin from melanoma patients. *Ethn. Dis*. 2008 Spring;18(2 Suppl 2):S2-38-43.

[206] Giglia-Mari G, Sarasin A. TP53 mutations in human skin cancers. *Hum Mutat*. 2003 Mar;21(3):217-28.

[207] Urano Y, Asano T, Yoshimoto K, Iwahana H, Kubo Y, Kato S, et al. Frequent p53 accumulation in the chronically sun-exposed epidermis and clonal expansion of p53 mutant cells in the epidermis adjacent to basal cell carcinoma. *J. Invest Dermatol*. 1995 Jun;104(6):928-32.

[208] Einspahr J, Alberts DS, Aickin M, Welch K, Bozzo P, Grogan T, et al. Expression of p53 protein in actinic keratosis, adjacent, normal-appearing, and non-sun-exposed human skin. *Cancer Epidemiol Biomarkers Prev*. 1997 Aug;6(8):583-7.

[209] Liang SB, Ohtsuki Y, Furihata M, Takeuchi T, Iwata J, Chen BK, et al. Sun-exposure- and aging-dependent p53 protein accumulation results in growth advantage for tumour cells in carcinogenesis of nonmelanocytic skin cancer. *Virchows Arch*. 1999 Mar;434(3):193-9.

[210] Tabata H, Nagano T, Ray AJ, Flanagan N, Birch-MacHin MA, Rees JL. Low frequency of genetic change in p53 immunopositive clones in human epidermis. *J. Invest Dermatol*. 1999 Dec;113(6):972-6.

[211] Hudson AR, Antley CM, Kohler S, Smoller BR. Increased p53 staining in normal skin of posttransplant, immunocompromised patients and implications for carcinogenesis. *Am. J. Dermatopathol*. 1999 Oct;21(5):442-5.

[212] Mabruk MJ, Toh LK, Murphy M, Leader M, Kay E, Murphy GM. Investigation of the effect of UV irradiation on DNA damage: comparison between skin cancer patients and normal volunteers. *J. Cutan Pathol*. 2009 Jul;36(7):760-5.

[213] Cahill DP, Lengauer C, Yu J, Riggins GJ, Willson JK, Markowitz SD, et al. Mutations of mitotic checkpoint genes in human cancers. *Nature*. 1998 Mar 19;392(6673):300-3.

[214] Lengauer C. Aneuploidy and genetic instability in cancer. *Semin. Cancer Biol*. 2005 Feb;15(1):1.

[215] Silva AG, Graves HA, Guffei A, Ricca TI, Mortara RA, Jasiulionis MG, et al. Telomere-centromere-driven genomic instability contributes to karyotype evolution in a mouse model of melanoma. *Neoplasia.* 2010 Jan;12(1):11-9.

[216] Fabarius A, Hehlmann R, Duesberg PH. Instability of chromosome structure in cancer cells increases exponentially with degrees of aneuploidy. *Cancer Genet Cytogenet.* 2003 May;143(1):59-72.

[217] Quinn AG, Sikkink S, Rees JL. Basal cell carcinomas and squamous cell carcinomas of human skin show distinct patterns of chromosome loss. *Cancer Res.* 1994 Sep 1;54(17):4756-9.

[218] Bastian BC, LeBoit PE, Hamm H, Brocker EB, Pinkel D. Chromosomal gains and losses in primary cutaneous melanomas detected by comparative genomic hybridization. *Cancer Res.* 1998 May 15;58(10):2170-5.

[219] Carless MA, Griffiths LR. Cytogenetics of melanoma and nonmelanoma skin cancer. *Adv. Exp. Med. Biol.* 2008;624:227-40.

[220] Heaphy CM, Bisoffi M, Fordyce CA, Haaland CM, Hines WC, Joste NE, et al. Telomere DNA content and allelic imbalance demonstrate field cancerization in histologically normal tissue adjacent to breast tumors. *Int. J. Cancer.* 2006 Jul 1;119(1):108-16.

[221] Ahmadian A, Ren ZP, Williams C, Ponten F, Odeberg J, Ponten J, et al. Genetic instability in the 9q22.3 region is a late event in the development of squamous cell carcinoma. *Oncogene.* 1998 Oct 8;17(14):1837-43.

[222] Kushida Y, Miki H, Ohmori M. Loss of heterozygosity in actinic keratosis, squamous cell carcinoma and sun-exposed normal-appearing skin in Japanese: difference between Japanese and Caucasians. *Cancer Lett.* 1999 Jun 1;140(1-2):169-75.

[223] Pashaei S, Li L, Zhang H, Spencer HJ, Schichman SA, Fan CY, et al. Concordant loss of heterozygosity of DNA repair gene, hOGG1, in melanoma in situ and atypical melanocytic hyperplasia. *J. Cutan. Pathol.* 2008 Jun;35(6):525-31.

[224] Krouse RS, Alberts DS, Prasad AR, Yozwiak M, Bartels HG, Liu Y, et al. Progression of skin lesions from normal skin to squamous cell carcinoma. *Anal. Quant Cytol. Histol.* 2009 Feb;31(1):17-25.

[225] Cremer T, Cremer C. Chromosome territories, nuclear architecture and gene regulation in mammalian cells. *Nat. Rev. Genet.* 2001 Apr;2(4):292-301.

[226] Ranger-Moore J, Bartels PH, Bozzo P, Einspahr J, Liu Y, Saboda K, et al. Karyometric analysis of actinic damage in unexposed and sun-exposed skin and in actinic keratoses in untreated individuals. *Anal. Quant Cytol. Histol.* 2004 Jun;26(3):155-65.

[227] Bartels PH, Krouse RS, Prasad AR, Yozwiak M, Liu Y, Bartels HG, et al. Actinic damage in histopathologically normal skin. *Anal Quant Cytol Histol.* 2008 Dec;30(6):316-22.

[228] Carpenter PM, Linden KG, McLaren CE, Li KT, Arain S, Barr RJ, et al. Nuclear morphometry and molecular biomarkers of actinic keratosis, sun-damaged, and nonexposed skin. *Cancer Epidemiol Biomarkers Prev.* 2004 Dec;13(12):1996-2002.

[229] Udart M, Utikal J, Krahn GM, Peter RU. Chromosome 7 aneusomy. A marker for metastatic melanoma? Expression of the epidermal growth factor receptor gene and chromosome 7 aneusomy in nevi, primary malignant melanomas and metastases. *Neoplasia.* 2001 May-Jun;3(3):245-54.

[230] Bastian BC, Kashani-Sabet M, Hamm H, Godfrey T, Moore DH, 2nd, Brocker EB, et al. Gene amplifications characterize acral melanoma and permit the detection of occult tumor cells in the surrounding skin. *Cancer Res*. 2000 Apr 1;60(7):1968-73.

[231] Nakamura K, Izumiyama-Shimomura N, Sawabe M, Arai T, Aoyagi Y, Fujiwara M, et al. Comparative analysis of telomere lengths and erosion with age in human epidermis and lingual epithelium. *J. Invest Dermatol.* 2002 Nov;119(5):1014-9.

[232] Wainwright LJ, Middleton PG, Rees JL. Changes in mean telomere length in basal cell carcinomas of the skin. *Genes Chromosomes Cancer*. 1995 Jan;12(1):45-9.

[233] Hussein MR, Wood GS. Microsatellite instability in human melanocytic skin tumors: an incidental finding or a pathogenetic mechanism? *J. Cutan Pathol.* 2002 Jan;29(1):1-4.

[234] Thibodeau SN, French AJ, Roche PC, Cunningham JM, Tester DJ, Lindor NM, et al. Altered expression of hMSH2 and hMLH1 in tumors with microsatellite instability and genetic alterations in mismatch repair genes. *Cancer Res*. 1996 Nov 1;56(21):4836-40.

[235] Mangold E, Pagenstecher C, Leister M, Mathiak M, Rutten A, Friedl W, et al. A genotype-phenotype correlation in HNPCC: strong predominance of msh2 mutations in 41 patients with Muir-Torre syndrome. *J. Med. Genet*. 2004 Jul;41(7):567-72.

[236] Abbas O, Mahalingam M. Cutaneous sebaceous neoplasms as markers of Muir-Torre syndrome: a diagnostic algorithm. *J. Cutan Pathol*. 2009 Jun;36(6):613-9.

[237] Morales-Burgos A, Sanchez JL, Figueroa LD, De Jesus-Monge WE, Cruz-Correa MR, Gonzalez-Keelan C, et al. MSH-2 and MLH-1 protein expression in Muir Torre syndrome-related and sporadic sebaceous neoplasms. *P R Health Sci J.* 2008 Dec;27(4):322-7.

[238] Ponti G, Losi L, Pellacani G, Wannesson L, Cesinaro AM, Venesio T, et al. Malignant melanoma in patients with hereditary nonpolyposis colorectal cancer. *Br. J. Dermatol.* 2008 Jul;159(1):162-8.

[239] Saetta AA, Aroni K, Stamatelli A, Lazaris AC, Patsouris E. Expression of mismatch repair enzymes, hMLH1 and hMSH2 is not associated with microsatellite instability and P53 protein accumulation in basal cell carcinoma. *Arch. Dermatol Res*. 2005 Sep;297(3):99-107.

[240] Young LC, Listgarten J, Trotter MJ, Andrew SE, Tron VA. Evidence that dysregulated DNA mismatch repair characterizes human nonmelanoma skin cancer. *Br. J. Dermatol.* 2008 Jan;158(1):59-69.

[241] Uribe P, Wistuba, II, Gonzalez S. Allelotyping, microsatellite instability, and BRAF mutation analyses in common and atypical melanocytic nevi and primary cutaneous melanomas. *Am. J. Dermatopathol*. 2009 Jun;31(4):354-63.

[242] Hussein MR, Sun M, Tuthill RJ, Roggero E, Monti JA, Sudilovsky EC, et al. Comprehensive analysis of 112 melanocytic skin lesions demonstrates microsatellite instability in melanomas and dysplastic nevi, but not in benign nevi. *J. Cutan. Pathol.* 2001 Aug;28(7):343-50.

[243] Howell PM, Jr., Liu S, Ren S, Behlen C, Fodstad O, Riker AI. Epigenetics in human melanoma. *Cancer Control.* 2009 Jul;16(3):200-18.

[244] Jones PA, Liang G. Rethinking how DNA methylation patterns are maintained. *Nat. Rev Genet.* 2009 Nov;10(11):805-11.

[245] Sharma S, Kelly TK, Jones PA. Epigenetics in cancer. *Carcinogenesis.* 2010 Jan;31(1):27-36.

[246] Bartolomei MS. Genomic imprinting: employing and avoiding epigenetic processes. *Genes Dev*. 2009 Sep 15;23(18):2124-33.

[247] Esteller M. Epigenetics in cancer. *N. Engl J. Med.* 2008 Mar 13;358(11):1148-59.

[248] Sharma S, Kelly TK, Jones PA. Epigenetics in cancer. *Carcinogenesis*. Jan;31(1):27-36.

[249] van Doorn R, Gruis NA, Willemze R, van der Velden PA, Tensen CP. Aberrant DNA methylation in cutaneous malignancies. *Semin. Oncol.* 2005 Oct;32(5):479-87.

[250] Liu S, Ren S, Howell P, Fodstad O, Riker AI. Identification of novel epigenetically modified genes in human melanoma via promoter methylation gene profiling. *Pigment Cell Melanoma Res.* 2008 Oct;21(5):545-58.

[251] Patino WD, Susa J. Epigenetics of cutaneous melanoma. *Adv. Dermatol.* 2008;24:59-70.

[252] Chiles MC, Ai L, Zuo C, Fan CY, Smoller BR. E-cadherin promoter hypermethylation in preneoplastic and neoplastic skin lesions. *Mod Pathol.* 2003 Oct;16(10):1014-8.

[253] Tyler LN, Ai L, Zuo C, Fan CY, Smoller BR. Analysis of promoter hypermethylation of death-associated protein kinase and p16 tumor suppressor genes in actinic keratoses and squamous cell carcinomas of the skin. *Mod. Pathol.* 2003 Jul;16(7):660-4.

[254] Spugnardi M, Tommasi S, Dammann R, Pfeifer GP, Hoon DS. Epigenetic inactivation of RAS association domain family protein 1 (RASSF1A) in malignant cutaneous melanoma. *Cancer Res.* 2003 Apr 1;63(7):1639-43.

[255] Behrmann I, Wallner S, Komyod W, Heinrich PC, Schuierer M, Buettner R, et al. Characterization of methylthioadenosin phosphorylase (MTAP) expression in malignant melanoma. *Am. J. Pathol.* 2003 Aug;163(2):683-90.

[256] Furuta J, Umebayashi Y, Miyamoto K, Kikuchi K, Otsuka F, Sugimura T, et al. Promoter methylation profiling of 30 genes in human malignant melanoma. *Cancer Sci.* 2004 Dec;95(12):962-8.

[257] Miracco C, Pacenti L, Santopietro R, Laurini L, Biagioli M, Luzi P. Evaluation of telomerase activity in cutaneous melanocytic proliferations. *Hum. Pathol.* 2000 Sep;31(9):1018-21.

[258] Taylor RS, Ramirez RD, Ogoshi M, Chaffins M, Piatyszek MA, Shay JW. Detection of telomerase activity in malignant and nonmalignant skin conditions. *J. Invest Dermatol.* 1996 Apr;106(4):759-65.

[259] Ueda M, Ouhtit A, Bito T, Nakazawa K, Lubbe J, Ichihashi M, et al. Evidence for UV-associated activation of telomerase in human skin. *Cancer Res.* 1997 Feb 1;57(3):370-4.

[260] Wu A, Ichihashi M, Ueda M. Correlation of the expression of human telomerase subunits with telomerase activity in normal skin and skin tumors. *Cancer.* 1999 Nov 15;86(10):2038-44.

[261] Fabricius EM, Bezeluk A, Kruse-Boitschenko U, Wildner GP, Klein M. Clinical significance of telomerase activity in basal cell carcinomas and in tumour-free surgical margins. *Int J Oncol.* 2003 Nov;23(5):1389-99.

[262] Burnworth B, Arendt S, Muffler S, Steinkraus V, Brocker EB, Birek C, et al. The multi-step process of human skin carcinogenesis: a role for p53, cyclin D1, hTERT, p16, and TSP-1. *Eur. J. Cell Biol.* 2007 Dec;86(11-12):763-80.

[263] Saleh S, King-Yin Lam A, Gertraud Buettner P, Glasby M, Raasch B, Ho YH. Telomerase activity of basal cell carcinoma in patients living in North Queensland, Australia. *Hum. Pathol.* 2007 Jul;38(7):1023-9.

[264] Fabricius EM, Kruse-Boitschenko U, Khoury R, Wildner GP, Raguse JD, Klein M, et al. Localization of telomerase hTERT protein in frozen sections of basal cell carcinomas (BCC) and tumor margin tissues. *Int. J. Oncol.* 2009 Dec;35(6):1377-94.

[265] Bonifas JM, Pennypacker S, Chuang PT, McMahon AP, Williams M, Rosenthal A, et al. Activation of expression of hedgehog target genes in basal cell carcinomas. *J. Invest Dermatol.* 2001 May;116(5):739-42.

[266] Serewko MM, Popa C, Dahler AL, Smith L, Strutton GM, Coman W, et al. Alterations in gene expression and activity during squamous cell carcinoma development. *Cancer Res.* 2002 Jul 1;62(13):3759-65.

[267] Smith AP, Weeraratna AT, Spears JR, Meltzer PS, Becker D. SAGE identification and fluorescence imaging analysis of genes and transcripts in melanomas and precursor lesions. *Cancer Biol Ther.* 2004 Jan;3(1):104-9.

[268] Smith AP, Hoek K, Becker D. Whole-genome expression profiling of the melanoma progression pathway reveals marked molecular differences between nevi/melanoma in situ and advanced-stage melanomas. *Cancer Biol Ther.* 2005 Sep;4(9):1018-29.

[269] Howell BG, Solish N, Lu C, Watanabe H, Mamelak AJ, Freed I, et al. Microarray profiles of human basal cell carcinoma: insights into tumor growth and behavior. *J. Dermatol Sci.* 2005 Jul;39(1):39-51.

[270] Nindl I, Dang C, Forschner T, Kuban RJ, Meyer T, Sterry W, et al. Identification of differentially expressed genes in cutaneous squamous cell carcinoma by microarray expression profiling. *Mol. Cancer.* 2006;5:30.

[271] O'Driscoll L, McMorrow J, Doolan P, McKiernan E, Mehta JP, Ryan E, et al. Investigation of the molecular profile of basal cell carcinoma using whole genome microarrays. *Mol. Cancer.* 2006;5:74.

[272] Dang C, Gottschling M, Manning K, O'Currain E, Schneider S, Sterry W, et al. Identification of dysregulated genes in cutaneous squamous cell carcinoma. *Oncol. Rep.* 2006 Sep;16(3):513-9.

[273] Asplund A, Gry Bjorklund M, Sundquist C, Stromberg S, Edlund K, Ostman A, et al. Expression profiling of microdissected cell populations selected from basal cells in normal epidermis and basal cell carcinoma. *Br. J. Dermatol.* 2008 Mar;158(3):527-38.

[274] Yu M, Zloty D, Cowan B, Shapiro J, Haegert A, Bell RH, et al. Superficial, nodular, and morpheiform basal-cell carcinomas exhibit distinct gene expression profiles. *J. Invest Dermatol.* 2008 Jul;128(7):1797-805.

[275] Carlson JA, Linette GP, Aplin A, Ng B, Slominski A. Melanocyte receptors: clinical implications and therapeutic relevance. *Dermatol Clin.* 2007 Oct;25(4):541-57, viii-ix.

[276] Ge L, Meng W, Zhou H, Bhowmick N. Could stroma contribute to field cancerization? *Med. Hypotheses.* 2010 Feb 8.

[277] Carlson JA, Mu XC, Slominski A, Weismann K, Crowson AN, Malfetano J, et al. Melanocytic proliferations associated with lichen sclerosus. *Arch. Dermatol.* 2002 Jan;138(1):77-87.

[278] Wright TI, Spencer JM, Flowers FP. Chemoprevention of nonmelanoma skin cancer. *J. Am. Acad. Dermatol.* 2006 Jun;54(6):933-46; quiz 47-50.

[279] Otley CC, Stasko T, Tope WD, Lebwohl M. Chemoprevention of nonmelanoma skin cancer with systemic retinoids: practical dosing and management of adverse effects. *Dermatol Surg*. 2006 Apr;32(4):562-8.

[280] Einspahr JG, Stratton SP, Bowden GT, Alberts DS. Chemoprevention of human skin cancer. *Crit. Rev. Oncol. Hematol.* 2002 Mar;41(3):269-85.

[281] Slominski A, Tobin DJ, Zmijewski MA, Wortsman J, Paus R. Melatonin in the skin: synthesis, metabolism and functions. *Trends Endocrinol. Metabol.*:. 2008 Jan-Feb;19(1):17-24.

[282] Slominski A, Wortsman J, Tobin DJ. The cutaneous serotoninergic/melatoninergic system: securing a place under the sun. *Faseb J.* 2005 Feb;19(2):176-94.

[283] Bikle DD, Oda Y, Xie Z. Vitamin D and skin cancer: a problem in gene regulation. The *J Steroid Biochem Molec Biol*. 2005 Oct;97(1-2):83-91.

[284] Slominski A. Are suberythemal doses of ultraviolet B good for your skin? *Pigment Cell Melanoma Res*. 2009 Apr;22(2):154-5.

[285] Slominski AT, Janjetovic Z, Fuller BE, Zmijewski MA, Tuckey RC, Nguyen MN, et al. Products of Vitamin D3 or 7-Dehydrocholesterol Metabolism by Cytochrome P450scc Show Anti-Leukemia Effects, Having Low or Absent Calcemic Activity. *PLoS One*. 2010;5(3):e9907.

[286] Bikle DD. Vitamin D receptor, UVR, and skin cancer: a potential protective mechanism. *J. Invest Dermatol*. 2008 Oct;128(10):2357-61.

[287] Zmijewski MA, Slominski AT. CRF1 receptor splicing in epidermal keratinocytes: potential biological role and environmental regulations. *J. Cell Physiol*. 2009 Mar;218(3):593-602.

[288] Slominski A, Zbytek B, Zmijewski M, Slominski RM, Kauser S, Wortsman J, et al. Corticotropin releasing hormone and the skin. *Front Biosci*. 2006;11:2230-48.

[289] Slominski A, Wortsman J, Pisarchik A, Zbytek B, Linton EA, Mazurkiewicz JE, et al. Cutaneous expression of corticotropin-releasing hormone (CRH), urocortin, and CRH receptors. *FASEB J.* 2001 Aug;15(10):1678-93.

[290] Ren ZP, Ponten F, Nister M, Ponten J. Two distinct p53 immunohistochemical patterns in human squamous-cell skin cancer, precursors and normal epidermis. *Int. J. Cancer*. 1996 Jun 21;69(3):174-9.

[291] Turner ML. Sun, drugs, and skin cancer: a continuing saga. *Arch. Dermatol*. 2010 Mar;146(3):329-31.

[292] Roewert-Huber J, Stockfleth E, Kerl H. Pathology and pathobiology of actinic (solar) keratosis - an update. *Br. J. Dermatol*. 2007 Dec;157 Suppl 2:18-20.

[293] Durham SE, Krishnan KJ, Betts J, Birch-Machin MA. Mitochondrial DNA damage in non-melanoma skin cancer. *Br. J. Cancer*. 2003 Jan 13;88(1):90-5.

[294] Berneburg M, Gattermann N, Stege H, Grewe M, Vogelsang K, Ruzicka T, et al. Chronically ultraviolet-exposed human skin shows a higher mutation frequency of mitochondrial DNA as compared to unexposed skin and the hematopoietic system. *Photochem. Photobiol*. 1997 Aug;66(2):271-5.

[295] Ren ZP, Hedrum A, Ponten F, Nister M, Ahmadian A, Lundeberg J, et al. Human epidermal cancer and accompanying precursors have identical p53 mutations different from p53 mutations in adjacent areas of clonally expanded non-neoplastic keratinocytes. *Oncogene*. 1996 Feb 15;12(4):765-73.
[296] Rolfe KJ, Crow JC, Benjamin E, Reid WM, Maclean AB, Perrett CW. Cyclin D1 and retinoblastoma protein in vulvar cancer and adjacent lesions. *Int. J. Gynecol Cancer.* 2001 Sep-Oct;11(5):381-6.

In: Field Cancerization: Basic Science and Clinical Applications ISBN 978-1-61761-006-6
Editor: Gabriel D. Dakubo

Chapter 18

Management of Field Cancerization: The Case of Actinic Keratosis

Kave Shams and Girish Gupta

Abstract

The aim of this chapter is to illustrate how field cancerization is treated using actinic keratosis (AK) as an example. Being skin lesions, AKs provide an excellent example for our purposes as they are common and are readily seen, making it easy to demonstrate the effects of treatment. This chapter will initially familiarize the reader with AKs. It will outline the current definition of AKs, including their epidemiology, clinical features, pathogenesis, recent controversies regarding their classification and their natural history. Choosing the type of treatment to employ is a challenging pursuit. Basic principles underlying this treatment choice will therefore be discussed. Current treatments for AKs and the associated field cancerization are numerous and varied. The remainder of the chapter is dedicated to presenting and discussing the nature of the different treatment modalities available, the evidence base for their efficacy, common and alternative application regimes and comparisons with other treatment types.

18.1. Introduction

Actinic keratosis (AK) is a clinical term for areas of focal abnormal keratinocyte proliferation in the epidermis. Risk factors for the development of AKs include sun exposure, increasing age, fair hair, organ transplantation and the subsequent immunosuppression and PUVA-therapy [1, 2, 3]. The most important risk factor however is cumulative exposure to ultraviolet (UV) radiation [1]. Although the use of sun beds may be a risk factor, day-to-day sun-exposure alone is sufficient for AKs to arise in susceptible individuals [4, 5, 6]. It thus follows that AKs are commonly encountered on photo-exposed body parts, such as the face, scalp, neck, ears and arms [7].

Actinic keratoses are very common. Epidemiological studies in the United Kingdom show a prevalence of 15% in men and 6% in women, with rates increasing to 34% and 18%

respectively in those above 70 years of age [8]. Studies in Japan show a substantially lower prevalence rate at 0.4% (diagnosed histologically), illustrating significant global variation, likely due to environmental as well as genetic factors [9]. Not surprisingly, there are high prevalence rates in Australia, at up to 60% in some studies [10]. The epidemiology of AK highlights the relative importance of UV-exposure and skin-type in its pathogenesis.

Lesions are typically macules and/or papules with rough surfaces, and with a variable degree of inflammation [3]. They are commonly multiple, and the abnormal keratinocytes may produce rough scales, which can be very thick in some cases (figure 18-1) [7]. The diagnosis tends to be on clinical grounds, and biopsies are rarely undertaken unless there is doubt about the diagnosis. Histologically, there are abnormal keratinocytes in the epidermis, with increased number of mitoses, acanthosis and hyperkeratosis [1]. There is typically a sharp boundary between affected and normal epithelium histologically, and there may be mild dysplasia through to severe dysplasia in AKs, which may be difficult to distinguish from squamous cell carcinoma (SCC) *in situ* (Bowen's disease) [7].

18.2. Field Cancerization

"Cancer does not arise as an isolated cellular phenomenon but rather as an anaplastic tendency involving many cells at once" [11].

The concept of field cancerization was introduced in 1953 by Slaughter *et al.* in order to explain the occurrence of multiple adjacent cancers and recurrent cancers [11, 12]. There has been increasing molecular evidence for field cancerization since, with fields of genetically abnormal cells being described in tissues of e.g., the head and neck, gastrointestinal tract, breast and also in skin [13].

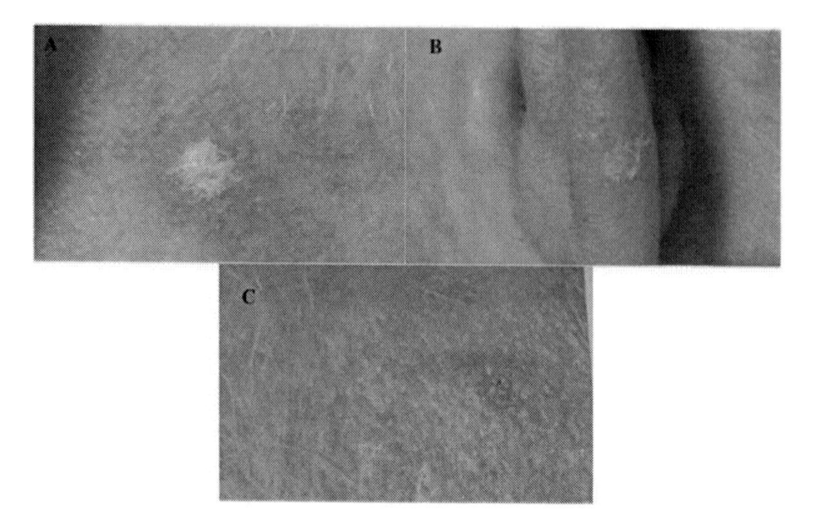

Figure 18.1. Actinic keratoses on photodamaged skin in elderly Caucasian male: (A) neck; thick yellow crust on erythematous base, (B) ear; thin white crust and (C) forehead; faint erythema and subtle scale. This variant is often more easily palpated than it is seen. (*Images provided by Dr E. Hamill*).

Carcinogens may cause multiple genetic abnormalities in different cells within a field (polycloncal model) or give rise to a single genetic abnormality within a field, with subsequent expansion of the abnormal cell population (clonal expansion model) [14]. The 'multiple genetic hit model of cancer' suggests that such pre-cancerous, genetically abnormal cells, within the skin require further mutations prior to becoming cancerous [15]. Increasing amounts of data are available regarding the nature of the genetic aberrations that underlie AKs. UV-radiation is the principal aetiological factor in AK development, and UVB (wavelength 290-320 nm) causes thymidine dimer formation and thus DNA and RNA damage in cells [3].

Mutations in the p53 gene are particularly common in AKs and are proportional to the amount of sun exposure [15]. Several types of p53 mutations have been found, which may possibly vary depending on the type of carcinogen. p53 mutations have also been found in apparently normal skin adjacent to skin cancers, giving further evidence of the concept of field cancerization, beyond clinically evident disease [16]. p53 monitors DNA damage and regulates cell apoptosis [17]. Mutations in the gene encoding p53 can render it non-functional, thus enabling further mutations within the genome to occur more readily without cells being induced to undergo apoptosis [3]. Normal keratinocytes also express CD95, which like p53 regulates apoptosis and thereby plays a part in UV-induced cell death. CD95 is upregulated with chronic sun exposure, but importantly is significantly downregulated in proportion to the degree of dysplasia in AKs and squamous cell carcinomas (SCCs) [18]. Other molecular changes in AKs include loss of heterozygosity at several loci, down regulation of the TRAIL receptor, and increased expression of tenascin-C with large splice variants in AK and SCC [19, 20, 21, 22].

There are several chromosomal abnormalities that are shared between AKs and SCCs, including losses at chromosome 3p, 8q, 9p, 13q, 11p, 17p, and 18p [23]. However, there are molecular differences between them. Squamous cell carcinomas for instance tend to have more complex karyotypes [24]. Another tumor suppressor gene, the *p16(INK4a)* is significantly more likely to be inactivated in SCCs than in AKs, and it is proposed that this inactivation may be an important step in the alterations that drive progression towards invasive malignancy [25]. This may provide a molecular means by which these two conditions can be distinguished.

The concept of field cancerization provides an explanation for multiple tumors and tumor recurrence. Patients with AKs typically have multiple lesions, and there is a high level of recurrence after treatment. It has been previously suggested that AK should be regarded as a field abnormality of the skin, extending beyond the visible borders of the individual lesion [7]. There is molecular evidence for field cancerization in the AK lesion and in the adjacent apparently normal skin. Hence, there is a strong case to treat not only the visible AK lesion, but also the field in which it is encountered so as to reduce recurrence, disease progression and new tumor formation.

18.3. Controversy Surrounding Nomenclature

"Classification schemes are human constructs imposed on nature that enable us to better understand the seemingly limitless complexity of the natural world" [26].

Actinic keratoses were probably first described in a form recognised today at the turn of the last century, as was their tendency to progress to malignancy [27]. They are generally considered to be premalignant, and as being an entity along a point on a continuum from normal epithelium to squamous cell carcinoma [28, 29]. It is in this context, that several classification schemes have been suggested, to take into account the fact that there appears to be variation in terms of degree of epithelial abnormality in AKs. One example is the 'keratinocyte intraepithelial neoplasia' (KIN) system, which is analogous to the cervical intraepithelial neoplasia (CIN) system for cervical dysplasia [30]. However, others as far back as in 1938 have suggested that they are in fact malignant [31]. The controversy surrounding the nature of AKs is thus not a new one, but has received renewed attention of late. Some argue that AKs are not premalignant but are instead a form of thin squamous cell carcinoma. The proponents argue that AKs are cancerous already, based on their histological features, their ability to cause mortality and since AKs do not commonly resolve spontaneously [32].

There has been opposition to such a change in nomenclature. Some assert that there is a histological continuum between AK and cancer [29], that there is little evidence of mortality and that AKs have indeed been shown to regress in significant numbers. Ultimately it can be argued that changing the nomenclature such that we define AK as cancer, is unhelpful to the clinician and the patient alike, and is unlikely to alter our treatment of AKs significantly [33]. The debate is presently ongoing.

18.4. The Case for No Treatment

"The vast majority of professors do not become deans, but the vast majority of deans were once professors" [34].

Reported progression rates of AK to SCC are fairly variable. Studies in Australia have shown that the incidence of SCC in those with AKs is quite low at 0.24% per annum [35]. Low progression rates from AK to SCC of 0.1% have been found in other studies, whilst demonstrating that most SCCs that did occur arose from pre-existing AKs [36]. It would appear logical that a greater number of AKs entails a greater risk of malignant transformation. Mathematical models do for instance predict that an individual with 7.7 AKs would have a 10-year risk of malignant transformation of 10% [37]. It follows that the need to treat AKs needs to be tailored to the individual based on the risk in that person. Studies in the UK have furthermore shown that 21% of AKs may resolve spontaneously over a one-year period [38]. It is however important to make a distinction between histological/molecular resolution, and improvement in cosmetic appearance of an AK.

A study has looked into the use of sunscreens as a lone measure (Sun Protection Factor (SPF) 17) in patients with AKs. It found that there was a significant reduction in AK numbers with sunscreen use, whilst use of the placebo cream led to an increase in the number of AKs [39]. Another study randomised its 1621 subjects to regular (daily) use of SPF-16 versus discretionary use. It also found a significant reduction in the incidence of new AKs with regular sunscreen use, at a rate equivalent to one new AK per two-year period [40].

Overall, the above data suggest that very few AKs progress to cause significant mortality, and a proportion do in fact regress. Furthermore, it also highlights the importance of secondary prevention in the form of sunscreen use. High recurrence rates of treated AKs also underlines the importance of regular follow-up after treatment, and patient education, so that new lesions are promptly identified. Current clinical guidelines suggest that no treatment may be an option in certain circumstances [41]. However, whilst it is accepted that most AKs cause little morbidity or mortality, we at present lack the means to predict which untreated lesions may cause problems. It is perhaps for this reason that there is a general consensus that most patients with AKs should be treated.

18.5 Principles of Treatment

"... I shall eradicate the lesion tenderly without too much disruption to the patient's life" [33].

There are a multitude of treatment options available, broadly divided into topical drugs or destructive therapies. They vary considerably in efficacy, in terms of side effects, cost and availability. Choosing to treat and choosing the means by which to treat is a complex decision making process, and some factors influencing this decision are discussed below.

18.5.1. The Accuracy of Diagnosis

Actinic keratoses are generally diagnosed on clinical grounds, and treatment commenced thereafter. Clinical diagnostic accuracy has however been questioned, and in a study where clinicians diagnosed AKs clinically, the correct diagnosis was reached in only 74% of cases [42]. It is important that biopsies are undertaken should there be significant diagnostic doubt, prior to commencing treatment.

18.5.2. To Treat the Lesion, the Field or the Entire Patient?

The concept of field cancerization in AK has already been mentioned and there is evidence for pre-malignant changes, which extend into apparently normal skin surrounding the AK. It has thus been advocated that treatment should encompass the entire field, although what constitutes this 'field' is still vaguely defined [14]. Some would also advocate that AK treatment should include at least a survey of the patient's entire skin. This is because AK in one location is a marker of excessive sun exposure, which rarely befalls a single body part [33].

Treatments such as creams/gels and photodynamic therapy lend themselves better to be applied over larger surface areas. Other modes of treatment, such as cryosurgery, are perhaps better suited to treat more discrete areas. The development of the concept of field cancerization has profoundly affected the choice of treatment, and over what area it is applied.

18.5.3. What Are We Treating?

There has been controversy as to whether AKs are a point along a path of progression from normal epithelium to cancer, or a cancer already [32]. For the individual in the community, the word 'cancer' will inevitably have certain connotations, usually not positive ones. If we subscribe to AK being cancer, and explain it as such to our patients, we may in so doing increase patients' expectations to receive aggressive and extensive treatment in all cases.

18.5.4. Absolute and Relative Risk

Most epidemiological studies show low progression rates of AKs to malignancy [35, 36]. However, the lifetime risk of one AK in an elderly patient is very different to the risk of multiple AKs in a young adult. The increased risk of the latter patient will at least in part relate to field cancerization, and more aggressive treatment will be warranted in such patients with a high absolute risk of malignancy over a lifetime.

18.5.5. Patient Preferences

Adverse effects vary between the treatments. Imiquimod and 5-fluorouracil can induce marked skin inflammation and topical diclofenac possibly less so. Photodynamic therapy, laser, chemical peels and dermabrasion may be painful, whilst healing in the latter three may be protracted. Treatments such as cryosurgery and laser therapy are associated with a significant risk of scarring, which is particularly relevant when treatment is administered over a large surface area.

18.5.6. Clinician Preferences and Local Resources

Treatment modalities such as cryosurgery and laser therapy are highly operator dependent, and it is likely that the choice of treatment is governed in part by the clinician's experience and preferences. Treatments such as photodynamic therapy, dermabrasion and laser therapy will furthermore need specialist equipment. Topical treatments in contrast are more widely available, and additionally can be applied by the patient at home.

18.5.7. Financial Considerations

Treatments vary significantly in terms of cost, and whilst data are available on relative costs of treatments, less is known about cost-effectiveness. Due to the high prevalence of AKs, the generation of such data will be essential for guiding treatment choice.

18.6. Treatment Options

Efficacy of the different treatment options is a pivotal part of treatment selection. However, there is poor correlation between existing trials in terms of outcome measures. Some studies assess improvement in the appearance of AKs, some measure the reduction in absolute numbers of AKs whereas others report complete clearance rates. The latter could be clinical or histological. Very few assess histological/molecular markers of field cancerization before or after treatment.

Studies are generally small, and follow-up periods relatively short. Treatment regimes often differ between the studies in terms of dosage or treatment duration, making direct comparisons challenging. In addition, treatment modalities are often combined in the clinical setting (e.g., cryosurgery followed by topical pharmacological treatment) despite the lack of study data that are only beginning to emerge.

18.6.1. Imiquimod

Imiquimod is a toll-like receptor agonist that upregulates the expression of pro-inflammatory genes [43]. Specifically, it induces translocation of several transcription factors, most importantly NFκB, to the nucleus that activates expression of a multitude of pro-inflammatory genes. Ultimately there is generation of for instance TNFα, IFNα, interleukins and chemokines [44]. It also upregulates the pro-apoptotic CD95 receptor that is known to be downregulated in AKs and SCCs [45]. Imiquimod has been licensed for the treatment of genital warts, and more recently basal cell carcinomas and AKs [46]. Studies in skin affected with AKs show an increase in lymphocytes and activated dendritic cells after topical treatment with imiquimod [47]. One can speculate that the enhanced immuno-surveillance by imiquimod-activated leukocytes facilitates the recognition of the abnormal keratinocytes present in and around AKs. It is also possible that imiquimod has anti-angiogenic effects in addition to its immuno-regulatory role, which may contribute to its clinical efficacy [48]. It is applied topically, and is suitable for field treatment.

A randomised controlled study of 36 patients with histologically confirmed AKs showed clinical and histological clearance in 84% of the subjects, when imiquimod was applied 3 times per week for a minimum of 12 weeks. The treatment was well tolerated with erythema, ulcers and scabbing being among the side effects observed. The recurrence rate in this study was 10% at one year [49], and up to 20% at two years with no subjects developing SCCs [50]. Two larger studies with 492 and 286 patients in each, where imiquimod was again applied 3 times per week but for 16 weeks, showed a response rate of 48.3% [51] (complete or partial clinical clearance) and 57.1% [52] (complete histological clearance) respectively. Erythema and scabbing/crusting were common side effects, being noted in approximately one-third of patients [52]. Long-term studies have assessed recurrence of AKs at 16 months post-treatment with imiquimod, applied 3 times per week versus 2 times per week for a total of 16 weeks. Recurrence rates were significantly higher in those applying the treatment 2 times per week as opposed to 3 (42.6% versus 24.7%) [53].

Imiquimod often induces significant inflammation. A less intensive application regime was evaluated in a small study with 20 patients, where imiquimod was applied once per week for 24 weeks. This showed an improvement in 46.7% of patients [54]. Side effects may be possibly milder with this regime, but the sample size was small, long-term data are lacking and results thus far suggest a diminished clinical response. Other alternative dosage regimes have shown good efficacy. A study of 829 patients with AKs of the head, showed a clearance rate of 68.9% when imiquimod was applied once a day, 3 days a week for 4 weeks. This was followed by a second course if AKs remained [55]. However, long-term follow up in a trial with a similar dosage regime to this (complete clearance rates of 53.7% overall) shows a recurrence rate of 39% at one year after treatment with imiquimod and 57% with placebo [56]. There is thus scope to achieve similar clearance rates with shorter courses, extended according to need, but at the cost of possibly higher recurrence rates.

Overall, 5% imiquimod cream applied 3 times per week for 16 weeks has been the most common regime used, due to higher clearance rates demonstrated in the larger trials [55], although the practice has been modified to include shorter treatment periods of 6 weeks, which may be repeated as needed.

There are several studies directly comparing imiquimod to other treatments. One study of 49 patients compared 3% diclofenac gel to imiquimod applied 3 times per week for 12 weeks, and showed a similar response rate for both [57].

Another study compared the use of imiquimod with cryosurgery and 5-Fluorouracil, and found that the clearance rate was significantly higher with imiquimod at 73% (versus 32% for cryotherapy and 67% for 5-Fluorouracil). The clearance rate was sustained in this study with imiquimod at one year, with higher recurrence rates being noted with the other forms of treatment [58].

Despite good clearance rates, imiquimod remains one of the more costly treatment options for AKs [59], and is considerably more expensive than 5-Fluorouracil [41]. Thus, it is unclear whether it is more cost-effective compared to other treatments available, and further comparative studies will be needed.

18.6.2. 5-Fluorouracil

5-Fluorouracil (5-FU) is believed to act through inhibition of DNA synthesis and possibly RNA function [60], and has been relatively well studied as a topical treatment for AKs over several decades. Studies tend to be small and dosage regimes varied, which makes comparisons difficult.

In a small study, patients with AKs of the hands applied topical 5-FU twice daily for 3 weeks, or received a single course of photodynamic therapy (PDT). The lesional area was found to reduce by 70% with 5-FU, and 73% with PDT, and adverse effects included pain and erythema with both forms of treatment [61]. A study into the treatment of AKs on the face compared the application of 5% 5-FU again twice daily for three weeks with trichloroacetic acid (TCA) peel. This showed a reduction of the number of AKs with either treatment, which was sustained for a year [62].

Overall, a systematic review suggests that half of patients treated with 5-FU will achieve complete clearance of AKs. Long-term data however, indicate that recurrence occurs in two-thirds of those treated at one year after treatment with 5-FU [63], which compares poorly with current data for imiquimod.

Less intensive regimes have been suggested and a small study used a once-twice weekly pulsed treatment with 5-FU for an average of 6.7 weeks, where 98% of lesions were cleared on average. Erythema was noted, but irritation was minimal [64]. Similar small-scale studies have however shown disappointing results with little or no improvement in most subjects [65]. In fact, more intensive inflammation may be associated with increased clearance of AKs.

A newer formulation of 0.5% fluorouracil is available, and systemic absorption may be four times lower than with the use of the 5% preparation [66]. In a single-blind study, patients were treated for 4 weeks, applying 0.5% fluorouracil once daily, or 5% fluorouracil twice daily.

Total clearance was comparable for both regimes at 43%, and patients overall felt the 0.5% preparation was more tolerable [67]. A systematic review suggests at least as good response rates with the 0.5% preparation as compared to the 5% preparation (86.1% reduction in number of AKs versus 79.5% respectively) [63]. Study qualities are variable, often poor and further larger-scale studies will be needed.

18.6.3. Diclofenac

The use of 3% diclofenac sodium in 2.5% hyaluronic acid gel is now well established, although the mode by which non-steroidal anti-inflammatory drugs (NSAIDs) exert their anti-tumorigenic effect is unknown. Breakdown products of arachidonic acid are believed to play part in tumorigenesis, and it may be that inhibition of COX-enzymes by NSAIDs explains their beneficial effect in the treatment of AKs [68]. Indeed, a study of 1621 patients has shown that regularly ingested NSAIDs for prolonged periods, is associated with a lower number of AKs and a lower SCC risk [69].

A trial of 195 patients where topical diclofenac was used twice daily for 60 days showed a clearance rate of 33% 30-days post-treatment. It was generally well tolerated [70]. Another study extended the above treatment regime to 90 days in 96 subjects, with an increase in AK clearance rate to 50% [71]. Histological clearance was achieved in 23.1% of patients after the use of topical diclofenac for 3 months in one study, and a significant down-grading of the AK was observed, with a reduced number of mitoses [72]. Diclofenac also has a role as an adjunct to cryosurgery, where cryosurgery is used to treat the visible lesion, and diclofenac used for field treatment. Cryosurgery alone for AK yielded a clearance rate of 21%, whilst this was increased significantly to 46% when diclofenac was applied for 90 days post cryosurgery, in a study of 714 patients [73].

Longer-term data are still relatively scarce after treatment with diclofenac, and further studies with longer follow-up will be needed in order to compare efficacy with the other topical treatments available.

18.6.4. Retinoids

Retinoids act on cellular transcription factors to mediate an anti-proliferative effect [74] and increase the number of Langerhan's cells in the skin [75]. Early studies have evaluated etretinate in AKs, showing an 84% complete or partial lesion clearance [76]. A mean decrease in number of AKs of 37.8% and 30.3% has been achieved with the use of arotinoid methyl sulfone and tretinoin respectively [77]. However, a retrospective study where retinaldehyde had been applied for 6-12 months did not appear to confer any protective effect on the development of AKs [78]. The use of topical tretinoin has furthermore been evaluated as an adjunct before and after trichloroacetic peels for the treatment of photodamaged skin, but no difference in outcome was found with the addition of topical retinoids [79].

Systemic retinoids (20mg acitretin daily for 12 months) have been studied in renal transplant patients with AKs. The treatment appears to have been well tolerated and led to an improvement of AKs after 12 months treatment [75]. However, it is questionable whether this potentially toxic treatment is cost-effective, safe or yields any long-term benefit in terms of morbidity and mortality.

Response rates with retinoids compared to other topical treatments are comparatively poor and studies tend to be small with little long-term data. Retinoids are therefore rarely used in clinical practice to treat AKs.

18.6.5. Photodynamic Therapy

Photodynamic therapy (PDT) is relatively well studied in the treatment of AKs, Bowen's disease and basal cell carcinomas [80]. A topical treatment is applied to the area affected, commonly methyl aminolevulinate (MAL) or 5-aminolevulonic acid (ALA), leading to increased porphyrins in the tissue. Phototoxicity will then occur upon illumination with light of specific wavelengths. Such an approach lends itself well to field directed treatment.

A study evaluating MAL-PDT versus placebo in 80 patients showed a complete clearance rate of 89% with good cosmetic results at 3-month follow-up post-treatment, after patients were treated twice [81]. 5-aminolevulonic acid-PDT application has been shown to induce complete clearance of AKs in 78% at 12 months [82]. Direct comparison between MAL-PDT and ALA-PDT for AKs of the scalp in a small study, showed similar efficacy with either option [83]. Studies into a single application of MAL-PDT versus two treatments concluded that clearance rates were similar in both groups. However, better clearance rates were achieved for thicker AK lesions with two treatments versus one [84]. A study comparing the use of MAL-PDT with cryotherapy on AKs of the extremities showed the latter to be superior in terms of efficacy [85]. Although pain is reported to be a common complaint with PDT, it was nonetheless well tolerated and preferred by patients over cryotherapy in this study [86]. A study into ALA-PDT versus cryosurgery did show comparable results in AK clearance (69% and 75% respectively), but with higher level of patient satisfaction and better cosmetic outcomes with PDT [87]. Comparisons between ALA-PDT and imiquimod in a small study showed clearance of 65% and 56% of AK lesions respectively, again with patient preference for PDT [88]. Studies specifically evaluating patient perception of PDT showed better recovery time and equivalent or higher preference for PDT in the treatment of AKs [89]. Photodynamic therapy also compared favourably to other treatments for AK in pharmacoeconomic analyses, where PDT is the least expensive option compared to diclofenac and 5-FU [59]. It is thus an attractive option, but is time-consuming and will require specialist equipment unlike creams/gels.

18.6.6. Cryosurgery

The histological abnormality in AKs lies in the epidermis and hence treatments destroying the epidermal layer make intuitive sense. There is a preponderance of destructive therapies used in the United States where such a procedure was undertaken in 78% of visits for AKs [90] and more money has been spent on destructive therapies than on pharmacological treatments [91]. Cryosurgery, where liquid nitrogen is utilised to destroy abnormal epithelial cells, is well established in the treatment of individual AK lesions. As discussed above, it compares well with PDT in terms of clearance [87].

Cryosurgery is by its nature less practical for larger number of lesions due in part to pain and the risk of blistering/scarring. However, in a study of 373 patients, more extensive cryosurgery (so called 'cryopeeling') was employed to treat both AKs and surrounding skin. This extensive form of cryosurgery was found to be effective in treating lesions, preventing recurrent AKs and reduced the likelihood of the development of SCCs [92]. However, its potential side effects renders 'cryopeeling' an unlikely form of field treatment in practice.

Cryosurgery is often used together with a topical agent, where the former is used to treat the visible lesion and the latter is used to treat the field. Trials have shown that the addition of diclofenac can more than double clearance rates [73]. Cryosurgery has the advantage of being relatively readily available and rapid to administer, but there is a high degree of operator variability and a risk of ulceration, scarring and pigmentary changes. With an increasing move to administer 'field treatment' it may be that cryosurgery becomes relevant mainly as an adjunct to other treatment modalities, rather than a stand-alone therapy.

18.6.7. Laser Therapy

The use of laser, which can destroy epithelial tissue through the delivery of high-energy pulses of light, is well established in dermatological practice and is also employed in the treatment of AKs. The principle of treatment is akin to cryosurgery, with the difference that laser resurfacing is more commonly used than extensive cryosurgery.

A study in which 29 patients with AKs were treated with an Er:YAG laser, a complete clearance rate of 90% was shown [93]. Field-directed treatment with laser can be less practical and more time consuming, but a small study evaluating the use of the Er:YAG laser for skin resurfacing under local anaesthetic, demonstrated decreased solar elastosis 3 months after treatment, and few adverse effects [94].

A retrospective review of 24 patients evaluated full-face Er:YAG and carbon dioxide laser treatment, and demonstrated clearance of AKs in most patients (94% total reduction in AK numbers), with 58.3% of patients developing no new lesions at 2-years. Side effects did however include pigmentary abnormalities, scarring and infection [95]. Long-term data from other studies into full-face carbon dioxide laser resurfacing showed a long average AK free period of 27.4 months [96]. Laser therapy may thus yield good long-term results with a single treatment. A small study compared the efficacy of carbon dioxide laser resurfacing with trichloroacetic acid peel and 5-FU cream (applied twice daily for 3 weeks) and showed 83% to 92% reduction in AKs, with no significant differences between the groups [97]. More comparative studies are however needed to delineate the role of laser resurfacing better in the treatment of AKs.

As with many destructive therapies, the use of laser is highly operator dependent, equipment is costly and treatment often less practical for multiple lesions. The use of laser has several potential side effects, including scarring, which (although quite rare) may be an unacceptable risk to some patients. With the advent of effective topical treatments, the risks associated with laser treatment may be increasingly difficult to justify. Despite some promising data, studies often are retrospective and are highly variable in their outcome measures and further prospective larger scale studies will be needed.

18.6.8. Dermabrasion, Chemical Peels, Curettage and Surgery

Dermabrasion, where the epidermal layer is removed, has been evaluated in a small study, showing a complete clearance rate of 96% at one year, and 54% at 5 years in the 23 subjects [98]. It may also be effective in the treatment of AKs of the scalp [99], but studies into the use of dermabrasion for AKs are scarce, despite its capability of field directed treatment.

Chemical peels are the better studied of the above destructive therapies, and can successfully treat AKs and larger surface areas [62]. A small study comparing 5-FU with 35% trichloroacetic acid showed AKs reduced by 75% with an improvement in histological atypia with both treatments [100].

Shave excision of the abnormal lesion in AK and surgical excision can both be employed, but mainly for individual lesions [101]. They do have the advantage of allowing histological analysis, and may be of particular value where the diagnosis is in doubt. They are not suitable for extensive lesions, due to scarring and pigmentary changes, which may follow. The procedures are not suitable for field treatment for the same reason. Generally, there are few trials evaluating surgical treatments for AKs, and it is likely that their use will remain confined to cases where histological analysis is required.

Conclusion

Actinic keratoses are areas of abnormal keratinocytes in the epithelium, mostly as a result of cumulative UV-exposure. They are common, especially in the Caucasian population. We may regard AKs as part of a continuum in the development of SCC or as a cancer already. In either case, AKs are unlikely to cause significant harm to the patient. We lack, at present, the means to ascertain which lesions will remain static/resolve spontaneously and which may indeed cause problems. Most clinicians thus tend to treat AKs.

Treatment options are numerous and the one to choose depends on a multitude of factors. Adverse effects, ease of application, availability, cost, efficacy and suitability to treat larger areas is highly variable between treatment types. The choice will depend on the specific circumstances of the individual patient in question and on what the aim of treatment is.

Evidence suggests that molecular abnormalities predisposing to the development of malignancy, recurrent or new AKs, reside not only in the clinical lesion, but also in the surrounding apparently normal skin. Actinic keratosis is thus an example of field cancerization of the skin.

There is an increasing trend towards treating not only the apparent lesion, but also the area of field cancerization surrounding it. This is often done through topical treatment (such as imiquimod, 5-fluorouracil, diclofenac, PDT), or more rarely through employing a physically destructive treatment (such as laser resurfacing, dermabrasion, or chemical peels). Little is known about how the boundaries of this 'field' should be defined. Future studies will need to take into account how this field is outlined, and how its definition and treatment may (or indeed may not) affect treatment outcome.

A great deal of research is currently undertaken to better understand AKs. In the future, it is conceivable that as new molecular treatment targets are found, new therapies will be subsequently developed. In the interim larger, higher quality, long-term trials of existing treatments are needed.

References

[1] Hensen P, Müller ML, Haschemi R *et al.* Predisposing factors of actinic keratosis in a North-West German population. *Eur. J. Dermatol.* 2009 Jul-Aug;19(4):345-54.

[2] Ulrich C, Christophers E, Sterry W *et al.* [Skin diseases in organ transplant patients] *Hautarzt*. 2002 Aug;53(8):524-33.

[3] Roewert-Huber J, Stockfleth E, Kerl H. Pathology and pathobiology of actinic (solar) keratosis - an update. *Br. J. Dermatol.* 2007 Dec;157 Suppl 2:18-20.

[4] Speight EL, Dahl MG, Farr PM. Actinic keratosis induced by use of sunbed. *BMJ.* 1994 Feb 5;308(6925):415.

[5] Cox NH. Actinic keratosis induced by a sunbed. *BMJ.* 1994 Apr 9;308(6934):977-8.

[6] Salasche SJ. Epidemiology of actinic keratoses and squamous cell carcinoma. *J. Am. Acad. Dermatol.* 2000 Jan;42(1 Pt 2):4-7.

[7] MacKie RM, Quinn AG. Non-melanoma skin cancer and other epidermal tumours. In: Rook's Textbook of Dermatology (Burns T, Breathnach SM, Cox HN, Griffiths CEM, eds), 7th edn. Oxford: Blackwell Publishing, 2004; 36.1-36.50

[8] Memon AA, Tomenson JA, Bothwell J *et al.* Prevalence of solar damage and actinic keratosis in a Merseyside population. *Br. J. Dermatol.* 2000 Jun;142(6):1154-9.

[9] Naruse K, Ueda M, Nagano T *et al.* Prevalence of actinic keratosis in Japan. *J Dermatol Sci.* 1997 Sep;15(3):183-7.

[10] Frost CA, Green AC. Epidemiology of solar keratoses. *Br. J. Dermatol.* 1994 Oct;131(4):455-64.

[11] Slaughter DP. The multiplicity of origin of malignant tumours: colletive review, *Int. Abstr. Surg.*; 79: 89-98.

[12] Slaugher DP, Southwick HW, Smejkal W. Field cancerization in oral stratified squamous epithelium; clinical implications of multicentric origin. *Cancer.* 1953 Sep;6(5):963-8.

[13] Braakhuis BJ, Tabor MP, Kummer JA *et al.* A genetic explanation of Slaughter's concept of field cancerization: evidence and clinical implications. *Cancer Res.* 2003 Apr 15;63(8):1727-30.

[14] Vatve M, Ortonne JP, Birch-Machin MA *et al.* Management of field change in actinic keratosis. *Br. J. Dermatol.* 2007 Dec;157 Suppl 2:21-4.

[15] Jonason AS, Kunala S, Price GJ *et al.* Frequent clones of p53-mutated keratinocytes in normal human skin. *Proc. Natl. Acad. Sci. USA.* 1996 Nov 26;93(24):14025-9.

[16] Kanjilal S, Strom SS, Clayman GL *et al.* p53 mutations in nonmelanoma skin cancer of the head and neck: molecular evidence for field cancerization. *Cancer Res.* 1995 Aug 15;55(16):3604-9.

[17] Stubbert LJ, Smith JM, Hamill JD *et al.* The anti-apoptotic role for p53 following exposure to ultraviolet light does not involve DDB2. *Mutat Res.* 2009 Apr 26;663(1-2):69-76.

[18] Filipowicz E, Adegboyega P, Sanchez RL *et al.* Expression of CD95 (Fas) in sun-exposed human skin and cutaneous carcinomas. *Cancer.* 2002 Feb 1;94(3):814-9.

[19] Kushida Y, Miki H, Ohmori M. Loss of heterozygosity in actinic keratosis, squamous cell carcinoma and sun-exposed normal-appearing skin in Japanese: difference between Japanese and Caucasians. *Cancer Lett.* 1999 Jun 1;140(1-2):169-75.

[20] Rehman I, Takata M, Wu YY *et al.* Genetic change in actinic keratoses. *Oncogene.* 1996 Jun 20;12(12):2483-90.

[21] Bachmann F, Buechner SA, Wernli M *et al.* Ultraviolet light downregulates CD95 ligand and TRAIL receptor expression facilitating actinic keratosis and squamous cell carcinoma formation. *J. Invest. Dermatol.* 2001 Jul;117(1):59-66.

[22] Dang C, Gottschling M, Roewert J *et al.* Tenascin-C patterns and splice variants in actinic keratosis and cutaneous squamous cell carcinoma. *Br. J. Dermatol.* 2006 Oct;155(4):763-70.

[23] Ashton KJ, Weinstein SR, Maguire DJ *et al.* Chromosomal aberrations in squamous cell carcinoma and solar keratoses revealed by comparative genomic hybridization. *Arch. Dermatol.* 2003 Jul;139(7):876-82.

[24] Jin Y, Jin C, Salemark L, Wennerberg J *et al.* Clonal chromosome abnormalities in premalignant lesions of the skin. *Cancer Genet Cytogenet* 2002 Jul 1;136(1):48-52.

[25] Mortier L, Marchetti P, Delaporte E *et al.* Progression of actinic keratosis to squamous cell carcinoma of the skin correlates with deletion of the 9p21 region encoding the p16(INK4a) tumor suppressor. *Cancer Lett.* 2002 Feb 25;176(2):205-14.

[26] Spencer JM. On the nature of actinic keratosis and matters that transcend it. C*osmet Dermatol.* 2004;17:418.

[27] Dubreuilh WA. Des hyperkeratoses circonscrites (1). *Ann. Dermatol. Venereol.* 1896;27:1158-204.

[28] Jorizzo JL, Carney PS, Ko WT *et al.* Treatment options in the management of actinic keratosis. *Cutis.* 2004 Dec;74(6 Suppl):9-17.

[29] Epstein E. Quantifying actinic keratosis: assessing the evidence. *Am. J. Clin. Dermatol.* 2004;5(3):141-4.

[30] Fu W, Cockerell CJ. The actinic (solar) keratosis: a 21st-century perspective. *Arch Dermatol.* 2003 Jan;139(1):66-70.

[31] Sutton RL. Early epidermal neoplasia: description and interpretations – the theory of mutation in the origin of cancer. *Arch. Derm. Syphil.* 1938;37:737-80.

[32] Ackerman AB, Mones JM. Solar (actinic) keratosis is squamous cell carcinoma. *Br. J. Dermatol.* 2006 Jul;155(1):9-22.

[33] Marks R. Who benefits from calling a solar keratosis a squamous cell carcinoma? *Br. J. Dermatol.* 2006 Jul;155(1):23-6.

[34] Person JR. An actinic keratosis is neither malignant nor premalignant: it is an initiated tumor. *J. Am. Acad. Dermatol.* 2003 Apr;48(4):637-8.

[35] Marks R, Foley P, Goodman G *et al.* Spontaneous remission of solar keratoses: the case for conservative management. *Br. J. Dermatol.* 1986 Dec;115(6):649-55.

[36] Marks R, Rennie G, Selwood TS. Malignant transformation of solar keratoses to squamous cell carcinoma. *Lancet* 1988 Apr 9;1(8589):795-7.

[37] Dodson JM, DeSpain J, Hewett JE *et al.* Malignant potential of actinic keratoses and the controversy over treatment. A patient-oriented perspective. *Arch. Dermatol.* 1991 Jul;127(7):1029-31.

[38] Harvey I, Frankel S, Marks R *et al.* Non-melanoma skin cancer and solar keratoses. I. Methods and descriptive results of the South Wales Skin Cancer Study. *Br. J. Cancer.* 1996 Oct;74(8):1302-7.

[39] Thompson SC, Jolley D, Marks R. Reduction of solar keratoses by regular sunscreen use. *N. Engl. J. Med.* 1993 Oct 14;329(16):1147-51.

[40] Darlington S, Williams G, Neale R *et al.* A randomized controlled trial to assess sunscreen application and beta carotene supplementation in the prevention of solar keratoses. *Arch. Dermatol.* 2003 Apr;139(4):451-5.

[41] de Berker D, McGregor JM, Hughes BR *et al.* Guidelines for the management of actinic keratoses. *Br. J. Dermatol.* 2007 Feb;156(2):222-30.

[42] Venna SS, Lee D, Stadecker MJ *et al.* Clinical recognition of actinic keratoses in a high-risk population: how good are we? *Arch. Dermatol.* 2005 Apr;141(4):507-9.

[43] Meyer T, Stockfleth E. Clinical investigations of Toll-like receptor agonists. *Expert Opin. Investig. Drugs*. 2008 Jul;17(7):1051-65.

[44] Schön MP, Schön M. Imiquimod: mode of action. *Br. J. Dermatol.* 2007 Dec;157 Suppl 2:8-13.

[45] Berman B, Sullivan T, De Araujo T *et al.* Expression of Fas-receptor on basal cell carcinomas after treatment with imiquimod 5% cream or vehicle. *Br. J. Dermatol.* 2003 Nov;149 Suppl 66:59-61.

[46] A Gaspari A, Tyring SK, Rosen T. Beyond a decade of 5% imiquimod topical therapy. *J. Drugs Dermatol.* 2009 May;8(5):467-74.

[47] Ooi T, Barnetson RS, Zhuang L *et al.* Imiquimod-induced regression of actinic keratosis is associated with infiltration by T lymphocytes and dendritic cells: a randomized controlled trial. *Br. J. Dermatol.* 2006 Jan;154(1):72-8.

[48] Li VW, Li WW, Talcott KE *et al.* Imiquimod as an antiangiogenic agent. *J. Drugs Dermatol.* 2005 Nov-Dec;4(6):708-17.

[49] Stockfleth E, Meyer T, Benninghoff B *et al.* A randomized, double-blind, vehicle-controlled study to assess 5% imiquimod cream for the treatment of multiple actinic keratoses. *Arch. Dermatol.* 2002 Nov;138(11):1498-502.

[50] Stockfleth E, Christophers E, Benninghoff B *et al.* Low incidence of new actinic keratoses after topical 5% imiquimod cream treatment: a long-term follow-up study. *Arch. Dermatol.* 2004 Dec;140(12):1542.

[51] Korman N, Moy R, Ling M *et al.* Dosing with 5% imiquimod cream 3 times per week for the treatment of actinic keratosis: results of two phase 3, randomized, double-blind, parallel-group, vehicle-controlled trials. *Arch. Dermatol.* 2005 Apr;141(4):467-73.

[52] Szeimies RM, Gerritsen MJ, Gupta G *et al.* Imiquimod 5% cream for the treatment of actinic keratosis: results from a phase III, randomized, double-blind, vehicle-controlled, clinical trial with histology. *J. Am. Acad. Dermatol.* 2004 Oct;51(4):547-55.
[53] Lee PK, Harwell WB, Loven KH *et al.* Long-term clinical outcomes following treatment of actinic keratosis with imiquimod 5% cream. *Dermatol. Surg.* 2005 Jun;31(6):659-64.
[54] Zeichner JA, Stern DW, Uliasz A *et al.* Placebo-controlled, double-blind, randomized pilot study of imiquimod 5% cream applied once per week for 6 months for the treatment of actinic keratoses. *J. Am. Acad. Dermatol.* 2009 Jan;60(1):59-62. Epub 2008 Oct 19.
[55] Stockfleth E, Sterry W, Carey-Yard M *et al.* Multicentre, open-label study using imiquimod 5% cream in one or two 4-week courses of treatment for multiple actinic keratoses on the head. *Br. J. Dermatol.* 2007 Dec;157 Suppl 2:41-6.
[56] Jorizzo J, Dinehart S, Matheson R *et al.* Vehicle-controlled, double-blind, randomized study of imiquimod 5% cream applied 3 days per week in one or two courses of treatment for actinic keratoses on the head. *J. Am. Acad. Dermatol.* 2007 Aug;57(2):265-8.
[57] Kose O, Koc E, Erbil AH *et al.* Comparison of the efficacy and tolerability of 3% diclofenac sodium gel and 5% imiquimod cream in the treatment of actinic keratosis. *J. Dermatolog. Treat.* 2008;19(3):159-63.
[58] Krawtchenko N, Roewert-Huber J, Ulrich M *et al.* A randomised study of topical 5% imiquimod vs. topical 5-fluorouracil vs. cryosurgery in immunocompetent patients with actinic keratoses: a comparison of clinical and histological outcomes including 1-year follow-up. *Br. J. Dermatol.* 2007 Dec;157 Suppl 2:34-40.
[59] Gold MH. Pharmacoeconomic analysis of the treatment of multiple actinic keratoses. *J. Drugs Dermatol.* 2008 Jan;7(1):23-5.
[60] Eaglstein WH, Weinstein GD, Frost P. Fluorouracil: mechanism of action in human skin and actinic keratoses. I. Effect on DNA synthesis in vivo. *Arch. Dermatol.* 1970 Feb;101(2):132-9.
[61] Kurwa HA, Yong-Gee SA, Seed PT *et al.* A randomized paired comparison of photodynamic therapy and topical 5-fluorouracil in the treatment of actinic keratoses. *J. Am. Acad. Dermatol.* 1999 Sep;41(3 Pt 1):414-8.
[62] Witheiler DD, Lawrence N, Cox SE *et al.* Long-term efficacy and safety of Jessner's solution and 35% trichloroacetic acid vs 5% fluorouracil in the treatment of widespread facial actinic keratoses. *Dermatol. Surg.* 1997 Mar;23(3):191-6.
[63] Askew DA, Mickan SM, Soyer HP *et al.* Effectiveness of 5-fluorouracil treatment for actinic keratosis--a systematic review of randomized controlled trials. *Int. J. Dermatol.* 2009 May;48(5):453-63.
[64] Pearlman DL. Weekly pulse dosing: effective and comfortable topical 5-fluorouracil treatment of multiple facial actinic keratoses. *J. Am. Acad. Dermatol.* 1991 Oct;25(4):665-7.
[65] Epstein E. Does intermittent "pulse" topical 5-fluorouracil therapy allow destruction of actinic keratoses without significant inflammation? *J. Am. Acad. Dermatol.* 1998 Jan;38(1):77-80.
[66] Kaur RR, Alikhan A, Maibach HI. Comparison of topical 5-fluorouracil formulations in actinic keratosis treatment. *J. Dermatolog. Treat.* 2009 Nov 1. [Epub ahead of print].

[67] Loven K, Stein L, Furst K *et al.* Evaluation of the efficacy and tolerability of 0.5% fluorouracil cream and 5% fluorouracil cream applied to each side of the face in patients with actinic keratosis. *Clin. Ther.* 2002 Jun;24(6):990-1000.

[68] Patel MJ, Stockfleth E. Does progression from actinic keratosis and Bowen's disease end with treatment: diclofenac 3% gel, an old drug in a new environment? *Br. J. Dermatol.* 2007 May;156 Suppl 3:53-6.

[69] Butler GJ, Neale R, Green AC *et al.* Nonsteroidal anti-inflammatory drugs and the risk of actinic keratoses and squamous cell cancers of the skin. *J. Am. Acad. Dermatol.* 2005 Dec;53(6):966-72.

[70] Rivers JK, Arlette J, Shear N *et al.* Topical treatment of actinic keratoses with 3.0% diclofenac in 2.5% hyaluronan gel. *Br. J. Dermatol.* 2002 Jan;146(1):94-100.

[71] Wolf JE Jr, Taylor JR, Tschen E *et al.* Topical 3.0% diclofenac in 2.5% hyaluronan gel in the treatment of actinic keratoses. *Int. J. Dermatol.* 2001 Nov;40(11):709-13.

[72] Dirschka T, Bierhoff E, Pflugfelder A *et al.* Topical 3.0% diclofenac in 2.5% hyaluronic acid gel induces regression of cancerous transformation in actinic keratoses. *J. Eur. Acad. Dermatol. Venereol.* 2009 Aug 26. [Epub ahead of print].

[73] Wolf JE Jr, Taylor JR, Tschen E *et al.* Topical 3.0% diclofenac in 2.5% hyaluronan gel in the treatment of actinic keratoses. *Int. J. Dermatol.* 2001 Nov;40(11):709-13.

[74] Dawson MI. Synthetic retinoids and their nuclear receptors. *Curr. Med. Chem. Anticancer Agents*. 2004 May;4(3):199-230.

[75] Carneiro RV, Sotto MN, Azevedo LS *et al.* Acitretin and skin cancer in kidney transplanted patients. Clinical and histological evaluation and immunohistochemical analysis of lymphocytes, natural killer cells and Langerhans' cells in sun exposed and sun protected skin. *Clin. Transplant*. 2005 Feb;19(1):115-21.

[76] Moriarty M, Dunn J, Darragh A *et al.* Etretinate in treatment of actinic keratosis. A double-blind crossover study. *Lancet* 1982 Feb 13;1(8268):364-5.

[77] Misiewicz J, Sendagorta E, Golebiowska A *et al.* Topical treatment of multiple actinic keratoses of the face with arotinoid methyl sulfone (Ro 14-9706) cream versus tretinoin cream: a double-blind, comparative study. *J. Am. Acad. Dermatol.* 1991 Mar;24(3):448-51.

[78] Campanelli A, Naldi L. A retrospective study of the effect of long-term topical application of retinaldehyde (0.05%) on the development of actinic keratosis. *Dermatology*. 2002;205(2):146-52.

[79] Humphreys TR, Werth V, Dzubow L *et al.* Treatment of photodamaged skin with trichloroacetic acid and topical tretinoin. *J. Am. Acad. Dermatol.* 1996 Apr;34(4):638-44.

[80] Braathen LR, Szeimies RM, Basset-Seguin N *et al.* Guidelines on the use of photodynamic therapy for nonmelanoma skin cancer: an international consensus. International Society for Photodynamic Therapy in Dermatology, 2005. *J. Am. Acad. Dermatol.* 2007 Jan;56(1):125-43.

[81] Pariser DM, Lowe NJ, Stewart DM *et al.* Photodynamic therapy with topical methyl aminolevulinate for actinic keratosis: results of a prospective randomized multicenter trial. *J. Am. Acad. Dermatol.* 2003 Feb;48(2):227-32.

[82] Tschen EH, Wong DS, Pariser DM *et al.* Photodynamic therapy using aminolaevulinic acid for patients with nonhyperkeratotic actinic keratoses of the face and scalp: phase

IV multicentre clinical trial with 12-month follow up. *Br. J. Dermatol.* 2006 Dec;155(6):1262-9.

[83] Moloney FJ, Collins P. Randomized, double-blind, prospective study to compare topical 5-aminolaevulinic acid methylester with topical 5-aminolaevulinic acid photodynamic therapy for extensive scalp actinic keratosis. *Br. J. Dermatol.* 2007 Jul;157(1):87-91.

[84] Tarstedt M, Rosdahl I, Berne B *et al.* A randomized multicenter study to compare two treatment regimens of topical methyl aminolevulinate (Metvix)-PDT in actinic keratosis of the face and scalp. *Acta. Derm. Venereol.* 2005;85(5):424-8.

[85] Kaufmann R, Spelman L, Weightman W *et al.* Multicentre intraindividual randomized trial of topical methyl aminolaevulinate-photodynamic therapy vs. cryotherapy for multiple actinic keratoses on the extremities. *Br. J. Dermatol.* 2008 May;158(5):994-9.

[86] Smits T, Moor AC. New aspects in photodynamic therapy of actinic keratoses. *J. Photochem. Photobiol.* B. 2009 Sep 4;96(3):159-69.

[87] Szeimies RM, Karrer S *et al.* Photodynamic therapy using topical methyl 5-aminolevulinate compared with cryotherapy for actinic keratosis: A prospective, randomized study. *J. Am. Acad. Dermatol.* 2002 Aug;47(2):258-62.

[88] Sotiriou E, Apalla Z, Maliamani F *et al.* Intraindividual, right-left comparison of topical 5-aminolevulinic acid photodynamic therapy vs. 5% imiquimod cream for actinic keratoses on the upper extremities. *J. Eur. Acad. Dermatol. Venereol.* 2009 Sep;23(9):1061-5.

[89] Tierney EP, Eide MJ, Jacobsen G *et al.* Photodynamic therapy for actinic keratoses: survey of patient perceptions of treatment satisfaction and outcomes. *J. Cosmet Laser Ther.* 2008 Jun;10(2):81-6.

[90] Feldman SR, Fleischer AB Jr, Williford PM *et al.* Destructive procedures are the standard of care for treatment of actinic keratoses. *J. Am. Acad. Dermatol.* 1999 Jan;40(1):43-7.

[91] Warino L, Tusa M, Camacho F *et al.* Frequency and cost of actinic keratosis treatment. *Dermatol. Surg.* 2006 Aug;32(8):1045-9.

[92] Chiarello SE. Cryopeeling (extensive cryosurgery) for treatment of actinic keratoses: an update and comparison. *Dermatol. Surg.* 2000 Aug;26(8):728-32.

[93] Wollina U, Konrad H, Karamfilov T. Treatment of common warts and actinic keratoses by Er:YAG laser. *J. Cutan Laser Ther.* 2001 Jun;3(2):63-6.

[94] Jiang SB, Levine VJ, Nehal KS *et al.* Er:YAG laser for the treatment of actinic keratoses. *Dermatol Surg.* 2000 May;26(5):437-40.

[95] Iyer S, Friedli A, Bowes L *et al.* Full face laser resurfacing: therapy and prophylaxis for actinic keratoses and non-melanoma skin cancer. *Lasers Surg. Med.* 2004;34(2):114-9.

[96] Sherry SD, Miles BA, Finn RA. Long-term efficacy of carbon dioxide laser resurfacing for facial actinic keratosis. *J. Oral. Maxillofac. Surg.* 2007 Jun;65(6):1135-9.

[97] Hantash BM, Stewart DB, Cooper ZA *et al.* Facial resurfacing for nonmelanoma skin cancer prophylaxis. *Arch. Dermatol.* 2006 Aug;142(8):976-82.

[98] Coleman WP 3rd, Yarborough JM, Mandy SH. Dermabrasion for prophylaxis and treatment of actinic keratoses. *Dermatol. Surg.* 1996 Jan;22(1):17-21.

[99] Winton GB, Salasche SJ. Dermabrasion of the scalp as a treatment for actinic damage. *J. Am. Acad. Dermatol.* 1986 Apr;14(4):661-8.

[100] Lawrence N, Cox SE, Cockerell CJ *et al.* A comparison of the efficacy and safety of Jessner's solution and 35% trichloroacetic acid vs 5% fluorouracil in the treatment of widespread facial actinic keratoses. *Arch. Dermatol.* 1995 Feb;131(2):176-81.
[101] Emmett AJ, Broadbent GD. Shave excision of superficial solar skin lesions. *Plast Reconstr Surg*. 1987 Jul;80(1):47-54.

In: Field Cancerization: Basic Science and Clinical Applications ISBN 978-1-61761-006-6
Editor: Gabriel D. Dakubo

Chapter 19

Field Cancerization in Endometrial Carcinoma

Tracy Tipton, Jinping Li, Juan Ren, Russell Broaddus, Yi Lisa Hwa, Donald Gallup and Shi-Wen Jiang

Abstract

As increasing amounts of data highlighting the importance of the cancer "field" in regard to tumorigenesis begin to surface, efforts to understand the interchanges between tumors and their microenvironments have amplified. It is well documented that interactions between epithelial and stromal components are critical for normal tissue function as well as malignant transformation. Through paracrine/autocrine mechanisms, stromal cells affect epithelial gene expression and proliferation. The uterine endometrium is subject to tight hormonal control, and the synchronized action of glandular epithelial and stromal cells is required for menstrual cycling, fertility, and menopausal adaptation. Endometrial carcinoma (EC) is the most prevalent gynecologic malignancy, and the fourth most common cancer in women. Several studies on EC pathogenesis have concentrated on the stromal milieu surrounding hyperplastic/malignant cells. Here, we describe the cancer field associated with endometrial carcinoma and discuss the nature and role of major field factors involved in EC tumorigenesis and metastasis, including inflammation, angiogenesis, hormonal regulation, obesity/diabetes, and epigenetics. Knowledge of EC fields and their cancerizing alterations will help our understanding of EC pathogenesis, which may lead to improved management of endometrial cancer patients.

19.1. Introduction

Endometrial carcinoma (EC) is the most widespread gynecologic cancer, and the fourth most common malignancy in women, following breast, lung and colorectal cancers [1]. The American Cancer Society estimates that there will be 42,160 new cases of EC in 2009, along with 7,470 associated deaths in the United States alone [2]. From 2006-2009, a considerable increase in both the number of new cases (7.9%, increase) and deaths (5.1% increase) was documented. While the exact cause of this finding is unknown, obesity, diabetes and hypertension are all recognized etiological factors for EC, and their rise may contribute to the trend.

Endometrial carcinoma arises from glandular epithelial cells that are buried in a rich stromal milieu. Although most studies on EC pathogenesis concentrate on the malignant cells themselves, extra-epithelial factors, including the stromal and vascular components and paracrine mechanisms, have drawn increasing attention. The term "field cancerization", which collectively refers to the involvement of these factors, was originally coined in 1953 by Slaughter and colleagues [3]. The concept describes a process by which tumors arise and progress upon induction of a "defect" (or histological anomaly) in the tumor "field", which includes the primary tumor as well as the surrounding environment. The concept emphasizes the constant physical and functional interactions among the numerous factors present in the tumor microenvironment. In this chapter, we provide an overview on the "field" alterations associated with the development of endometrial carcinoma. We attempt to explain the pathogenesis of the malignancy using the concept of "field cancerization". Potential applications of the concept in risk assessment and early detection of EC is also discussed.

19.2. The Different Background and Risk Factors for Type I and II Endometrial Carcinoma

Although the majority of EC patients are diagnosed early and benefit from a relatively favorable survival rate, those with later stage malignancies have a high propensity for recurrence and a poor prognosis [1]. Type I EC is an estrogen-dependent malignancy that typically carries a good prognosis. Type II EC, independent of estrogen, is the more aggressive subtype with less favorable prognosis [4]. Type II EC account for only about 10% of total EC cases, although they cause the most deaths. Risk factors for Type I EC include obesity, diabetes, hypertension, anovulation, early menarche, nulliparity, unopposed estrogen exposure, polycystic ovarian syndrome, and heavy menstruation. Conversely, no significant link has been established between these factors and risk of developing Type II EC. Moreover, Type I EC is generally detected during the perimenopausal stage, while Type II detection tends to be diagnosed in late postmenopausal women[5, 6].

Examination of clinicopathological characteristics in EC reveals a stark contrast between the two subtypes. Many Type I ECs exhibit microsatellite instability (MSI) and promoter hypermethylation of MLH1. Microsatellite instability and MLH1 silencing are less frequently observed in Type II ECs. Type II tumors also tend to be less differentiated, more deeply invasive to myometrium, and more prone toward lymph node metastasis [5, 6]. Several genes have been identified that are commonly mutated in either subtype. Tumor suppressor genes such as PTEN and MMR, and oncogenes K-RAS, E-cadherin and beta-catenin, are preferentially mutated in Type I tumors. Type II ECs, in contrast, tend to contain mutations in p53 and CDC4, as well as oncogenes Her-2/neu, c-fms, c-myc, c-jun and hTERT [5, 7]. It is also characteristic of Type II tumors to over-express epidermal growth factor receptor (EGF-R) and insulin-like growth factor receptor (IGF-R) [5]. The p53 tumor suppressor gene mutation in EC is significant in that it is very rare in Type I EC, even in advanced-stage, whereas it is found in 80-90% of Type II tumors including early stage cases [5]. Thus, p53 mutation is considered a relatively reliable marker EC subtype marker. Further distinguishing the two EC subtypes is the fact that Type I and II EC generally develop from a different "field": Type I tumors commonly develop in a background of atypical complex hyperplasia, whereas Type II EC appears to arise in a background of atrophic endometrium [4, 5].

19.3. Monoclonal Verses Polyclonal Interpretation of Multifocal Primary Tumors

Whether a particular neoplasm has a monoclonal or polyclonal origin has been debated for years with regards to various cancer types. A wealth of evidence supporting both hypotheses has been published over the past couple of decades, although a clear mechanism has yet to be established. The general observation that sparks the debate is the presence of multiple primary tumors at different sites within a patient. According to monoclonal origin, the multifocal malignancy develops from a single precursor cell that multiplies and spreads to different loci. Simon et al. showed evidence for a monoclonal origin of multifocal bladder tumors based on cytogenetic analysis of tumor specimens from patients with multifocal bladder cancer. Identical chromosomal aberrations were found between tumors of a specific case, as well as identical mutations in the tumor suppressor gene TP53 in two cases, suggesting a monoclonal source. However, it should be noted that this study was conducted on cystectomy samples of late-stage tumors of advanced histology [7]. Genomic characterization of a more representative sample of multifocal bladder tumors is necessary for the application of these data to bladder cancer in general. Moreover, the presence of identical chromosomal aberrations, and ubiquitous specific mutations in a set of primary tumors found in a particular patient does not automatically restrict the interpretation to a monoclonal initiation. All cells of a specific tissue may have some degree of chromosomal similarity to begin with. Considering also that these same cells experience similar carcinogenic and/or risk factors (i.e. alcohol, cigarette smoke, pollution, diethylstilbestrol, etc.) by virtue of residing within the same human body, these data alone cannot rule out the possibility for polyclonality.

Polyclonal tumor origination, on the other hand, attempts to explain the presence of multifocal malignancies through the concept of field cancerization (although the concept can also be applied to multifocal tumors of monoclonal origin). Slaughter et al. first used the term field cancerization in 1953 in reference to their work with malignant, oral stratified-squamous epithelium. The researchers found significant abnormalities in the surgical margins of excised tumors, which included histologically "normal' or noncancerous cells [3]. The abnormalities included marked hyperplasia, atrophy, and/or atypia, all of which are hallmarks of a precancerous lesion [4]. This helped to explain the high propensity of recurrence of malignancy after surgical excision of the tumor. The study concluded that it is possible that exposure to a carcinogen for a variable period of time may lead to the development of a defective "field" of cells. The defect would leave a group of cells hyper-susceptible to the development of multiple precancerous lesions, and the subsequent progression to multifocal tumors [3]. Of course, a mixed monoclonal/polyclonal etiology is certainly plausible, and therefore the real question to consider is which of these mechanisms contributes most significantly to tumorigenesis.

A considerable amount of evidence for field cancerization has been gathered in the past decade. Cancers of the head and neck provide a classic example of the phenomenon. A field size of 7 cm has been measured in patients with head and neck squamous cell carcinoma (HNSCC). Mucosal protein profiling of 73 healthy individuals, 113 HNSCC patients, 99 tumor-distant samples, and 18 tumor-adjacent samples showed that 27.3 % of tumor-distant and 72 % of tumor-adjacent specimens contained aberrant protein profiles, suggesting a field cancerization effect [8]. The clonal nature of multifocal HNSCC tumors is still being debated as supportive data based on comparative genomic hybridization and/or loss of heterozygosity analysis for both polyclonality and monoclonality has continued to gather [8-10].

Only relatively recently has the concept of field cancerization been applied to endometrial neoplasms. Moinfar and colleagues examined endometrial stromal sarcoma (ESS) tumors and benign endometrial stromal nodules (ESN) for loss of heterozygosity (LOH) and microsatellite instability (MSI). Twenty-three ESS samples (20 low grade and 3 high grade sarcomas), 4 ESN samples, and several noncancerous myometrial and endometrial tissues adjacent to and distant from the tumors were collected. Normal cervical epithelial and stromal cells were also collected and examined. Fifteen (55.5%) ESS cases exhibited LOH with respect to at least one polymorphic marker. In 10 of 15 stromal tumors, noncancerous and histologically normal endometrial or myometrial tissues displayed LOH. Moreover, observed genetic aberrations were often present in different tissue components (normal myometrium, normal cervical stroma, endometrial stromal sarcoma, etc.) within a given case, indicative of an independent acquisition of the genetic alteration(s) in the multifocal loci. The lack of MSI identification in any of the specimens suggests that the pathogenesis of ESS proceeds by pathways other than through an alteration of MLH1-mediated DNA mismatch-repair deficiencies, as is observed in EC [11].

19.4. The Role of the Tumor Microenvironment in Endometrial Carcinoma Development

The observation that different tumors of a given cancer type and grade often differ drastically in the rate of progression and degree of malignancy suggests that the process of tumorigenesis is significantly more complex than some might initially imagine. Current studies in the fields of epigenetics, proteomics, autocrine/paracrine mechanisms, inflammation, angiogenesis, obesity, and several more have already highlighted this idea. An interesting area that has been frequently studied in many cancer types is the importance of stromal-epithelial interactions to the progression of malignancy. Epithelial tissue development, maturation and remodeling, as well as maintenance of homeostasis, are all dependent on interactions with stromal elements. Accordingly, disturbance of this partnership often results in disruption of cell function and occasionally carcinogenesis. Several authors have proposed that the acquisition of mesenchymal features by epithelial cells is a key facilitator for the invasion and metastasis of many cancers [12-14]. Xie and colleagues, in a study of the S100A4 calcium-binding protein, provide strong evidence for such an epithelial to mesenchymal transition (EMT) in EC. Although the biological role of S100A4 is largely unknown, its over-expression in numerous malignancies, particularly those at advanced-stages with aggressive phenotypes, is well documented [15-23]. The data revealed differential expression of S100A4 in stromal cells of benign endometrium and grade 1 carcinomas; and in tumor epithelial cells of grade 3 endometrioid carcinomas, uterine papillary serous carcinoma, and malignant mixed müllerian tumors. These findings provide support for the presence of EMT, a process during which epithelial cells down-regulate adhesion proteins, lose their polarity, and acquire an enhanced invasive/migratory capacity [13] [15]. Moreover, several EMT-promoting transcription factors were also recently shown to be expressed in EC, including Twist, ZEB1, and HOXA10 [15, 24-26]. Interestingly, many parallels can be drawn between the stromal response associated with tumorigenesis and the stromal environment characteristic of a wound. Key features of both stromal milieus include transdifferentiation and proliferation of fibroblasts, initiation of the inflammatory and angiogenesis processes, and extracellular remodeling [27]. The malignant transformation is thus crucially dependent on the stromal response, which may help to explain why some cancers progress slowly and even go through periods of dormancy, while others advance and metastasize rapidly. It could be that different stromal environments have varying degrees of resistance/susceptibility to carcinogenesis. Traditionally, studies of epithelial cancer pathogenesis have primarily focused on the actual malignant, epithelial cells. Recent research, however, has placed more emphasis on how the whole tissue/tumor microenvironment influences carcinogenesis [27]. The observation by Moinfar et al. that LOH is present in both noncancerous stromal and primary breast tumors of a given case suggests that genetic anomalies in stromal cells might play a role in or even propel the process of carcinogenesis [11, 27].

The estrogenic pathway is a primary moderator of the tumor-stromal interaction in breast and endometrial cancers. Matsumoto et al. transfected reporter cells with a green fluorescent protein (GFP) tagged estrogen response element (ERE) gene and incubated these with EC stromal cells to determine whether the stromal cells could activate the ERE. Aromatase is a crucial enzyme in this process in that it catalyses the conversion of androgens into estrogens. Addition of aromatase inhibitors (AIs) to the EC stroma down-regulated GFP, whereas supplementation of testosterone, a substrate for aromatase, enhanced the expression of GFP. The principal implication of these findings is that the stromal environment plays a key role in the regulation of ERE in EC, and therefore directly influences the pathogenesis of EC. Moreover, the results suggest that this particular paracrine, tumor-stromal interaction is partially mediated through the aromatase enzyme. Interestingly, of the 18 cases that Mitsuyo and colleagues analyzed, one case showed high GFP expression even before the addition of testosterone, and this effect was not reversed with addition of AIs [28]. This finding highlights a key feature of endometrial cancer, the variability of hormone dependency. There are obviously mechanisms other than estrogen receptor (ER) stimulation by estrogen itself that can lead to the transcription of ERE and its subsequent carcinogenesis-promoting effect. Ligand-independent activation of ER by growth factors via activation of MAPK and phosphorylation of ER have been documented [29]. It would be interesting to see if the effects of EC stromal cells on EC pathogenesis are also dependent on stromal growth factor concentration. More effective therapeutic modalities for the treatment of EC are likely dependent on the identification of such factors, particularly for patients suffering from estrogen-independent malignancies. Although Type I, estrogen-dependent ECs tend to have a good prognosis, these patients may further respond to aromatase inhibitors and benefit from new treatments targeting autocrine pathways [28].

Further evidence for the impact of stromal-epithelial interactions on EC pathogenesis comes from a study assessing the effect of aging on carcinogenesis. Rinehart and colleagues incubated endometrial epithelial cells with endometrial stromal fibroblasts (ESFs) of varying ages. They found that young adult ESFs inhibit certain behaviors that promote tumorigenesis, such as anchorage independent proliferation and colony outgrowth by EC cells. These ESFs were also shown to stimulate formation of normal tissue structure by endometrial tumors. As the ESFs age, their anti-malignant activities progressively decrease, leading to a stromal environment that is more conducive to tumorigenesis. The expression of one gene in ESFs in particular, that encoding the cytokine interleukine-1α (IL-1α), increased directly with age. Treatment with IL-1α accelerated the age-related changes of ESFs while treatment with IL-1 receptor antagonists helped to maintain the phenotype associated with young adult ESFs. It should be noted that additional age-related factors associated with the precancerous/cancerous epithelial cells also play roles in malignant transformation, such as compromised DNA repair and immune systems, and increased time for exposure to carcinogens. Nevertheless, Rinehart et al. show that the tissue microenvironment influences age-related endometrial cancer susceptibility [30].

Insight into the precise mechanisms by which the tumor microenvironment affects malignant transformation requires a molecular classification of each cell type within a given field [31]. Allinen and colleagues purified distinctive human breast cells (epithelial, myoepithelial, endothelial, myofibroblasts, fibroblasts, and leukocytes) using cell type-specific surface markers and magnetic beads. Serial analysis of gene expression (SAGE) was then employed for molecular characterization of these cell types in normal human breast tissue, ductal carcinoma in situ (DCIS), and invasive ductal carcinoma (IDC). The results revealed stark contrasts in gene expression profiles for the different cell types throughout malignant progression, with the most noticeable difference being detected between normal and DCIS tissue, suggestive of an early influence of a stromal field on tumorigenesis [31, 32].

Recently, Polyak et al. presented an interesting comparison between the tumorigenic process and the evolution of ecosystems. Firstly, survival of the fittest is evident in regard to the continuous selection of proliferatively-advantageous tumor cells [33]. Secondly, primary tumor and adjacent stromal cells are constantly placing selective pressures on each other through paracrine mechanisms, thereby generating an altered "ecosystem" [33, 34]. Further, metastatic tumor cells represent those "organisms" that have adapted such that they are able to migrate and proliferate in a new environment, thus placing additional selective pressures on prior occupiers of the new milieu. Additionally, exogenous selective stress is introduced upon treatment with therapeutic agents, and those pre-neoplastic and tumor cells that have acquired resistance to such agents will remain viable [33]. The authors carry the analogy even further by mentioning ongoing efforts to use a combination of molecular techniques and mathematical formulas in describing the progression of malignancies, similar to methods currently used in evaluating and predicting patterns of evolution [34]. Anderson and colleagues recently presented a mathematical model for tumor invasion that factors in the selective effects conferred by primary-cellular and micro-environmental conditions, such as hypoxia and heterogeneous extracellular matrix [35]. The model, supported by experimental data, suggests that such effects provide significant selective pressure for tumor evolution and metastatic progression [33] [35]. Similar to measuring ecological variables and using mathematical equations to predict, identify, and quantify evolution, it would be encouraging to see if such a mathematical model describing carcinogenesis can be as prolific. Several hurdles need to be cleared before that is realized. Firstly, few experts agree on the best way to represent even the simplest of molecular pathways [35]. Secondly, the abundance and diversity of tumorigenic molecules make a comprehensive, all-inclusive model difficult to construct. Thirdly, individualization of such a model, which would require the inclusion of such factors as diet, lifestyle, carcinogenic exposure, age, weight, genetic predisposition, etc...for each patient, would add further complexity. Fourthly, any model coming reasonably close to including all such factors would likely require computational power that either does not exist or is too expensive to be economically feasible [35]. Lastly, the effects of a change in a single molecular variable are difficult to predict and need to be determined experimentally [35]. Despite the formidable obstacles, a mathematical model for tumorigenesis bears strong implications for the diagnosis, prognosis and treatment of cancer.

19.5. Angiogenesis as a Factor for Endometrial Carcinoma Microenvironment

The endometrial field of a woman during her reproductive years is unique in that it changes cyclically with the menstrual cycle. An important implication of this continual sequence of endometrial breakdown and re-growth is the recurrent need for angiogenesis. Given the obvious malignancy-favoring effects that blood vessel formation has on pre-neoplastic cells, it's worth exploring how aberrant angiogenic regulation influences tumorigenesis [36]. The cyclically dynamic angiogenesis characteristic of the endometrium may help to explain the high prevalence of EC. Indeed, given enough time, Murphy's Law in relation to endometrial carcinogenesis is bound to prove true, especially in the presence of additional risk factors such as obesity, estrogen exposure, diabetes, aging, etc. Although the exact mechanism by which endometrial angiogenesis occurs is not completely understood, it is generally accepted that hormonal regulation is paramount to the process. Evidence for estrogen as an angiogenesis promoter is well documented. This regulation appears to affect both the endometrial epithelia and the surrounding stroma. For example, estrogen receptor ERα and ERβ are both expressed in endometrial vascular smooth muscle [36, 37]. Likewise, ERβ was expressed in the endometrial endothelia [38]. In vitro, estradiol increased endometrial endothelial proliferation within 48 hours, along with the establishment of capillary formation and branching within 8 days [39]. In addition, estradiol enhanced the proliferative reaction of endothelial cells to vascular endothelial growth factor (VEGF), suggesting a synergistic relationship between estrogen and VEGF [40]. Studies have also identified progesterone as an angiogenesis promoter, although the mechanism appears to be different than that of estrogen. Estrogen, for example, stimulates angiogenesis with concomitant vasodilation, whereas progesterone does not [41, 42]. Relaxin peptide, like progesterone, is secreted by the corpus luteum and is initially detected during the late secretory phase of the menstrual cycle [43]. Relaxin has angiogenesis-stimulating effects on the endometrium through induction of VEGF expression by endometrial cells [44]. Adrenomedullin is another peptide hormone that presumably plays a role in the establishment of angiogenic patterns. Numerous tissue types express this factor and its effects are enacted through paracrine, autocrine, and perhaps even endocrine mechanisms. These effects include cell cycle and differentiation regulation, as well as vasodilation and angiogenesis [41, 45].

Endometrial endothelial cells express the peptide both in vitro and in vivo [46]. Adrenomedullin also up-regulates cyclic-adenosine monophosphate (cAMP) in endometrial epithelia in vitro, thereby showing some properties of an autocrine peptide hormone [46].

The angiogenic effects of the forementioned factors are primarily mediated through VEGF, a potent vasculo/angio-genesis promoting cell mitogen [36]. Myometrial microvascular endothelial cell tube formation was increased by 65% upon transfection with human recombinant VEGF compared with control cells in a study by Albrecht and colleagues. Comparable increases were observed when these cells were co-cultured with endometrial epithelia. Additional angiogenic augmentation was detected when the endothelial cells were co-cultured with epithelial cells and estrogen. Tube formation in endothelial cells co-cultured with endometrial stromal cells was similar to that seen in media alone, regardless of estrogen presence [47]. Taken together these data suggest that myometrial endothelial vascularization is related to VEGF production by endometrial epithelia, which is enhanced in the presence of estrogen [36, 47]. In a mouse xenograft model, progesterone up-regulated expression of VEGF and its receptor (VEGFR-2). Such induction, though significant, was quite slow compared to the quick effects of estrogen on angiogenesis. Moreover, the mRNA up-regulation was predominantly detected in the endometrial stroma as opposed to epithelia [36] [42, 48]. One factor that complicates the characterization of VEGF's role in endometrial vascularization is the diversity of endometrial VEGF-A splice variants (VEGF121, VEGF145, VEGF165, VEGF189, and VEGF206) [49-51]. The isoforms differ substantially in various properties, such as receptor relations, anticoagulant binding affinity, extracellular matrix (ECM) interactions, and solubility [52]. To illustrate, while the VEGF189 isoform remains thoroughly sequestered in the ECM, the VEGF121 gene product is freely diffusible. Such diversity may afford cells with a locally dense population of site-specific VEGF's, thereby optimizing vascular control and response to angiogenic factors [36, 52].

Ueda et al. recently performed a study assessing how various angiogenic factors, including the different members of the VEGF family (VEGF-A, -B, -C, and -D), affect tumor cell migration and invasion capacities by detecting mRNA expression levels of such factors in 16 human gynecological cancer cell lines [53]. The authors found a significant statistical correlation between expression of VEGF-C and cell migration and invasion levels as evaluated by haptotactic migration and invasion assay. Further, there was a considerable correlation between VEGF-C and matrix metalloproteinase-2 (MMP-2) expression levels, suggesting that the enhanced migratory and invasive potential afforded to cancer cells expressing relatively high levels of VEGF-C partially arises through an increased capacity to digest through tissue barriers [53].

VEGF-C may further contribute to tumor aggression by facilitating lymph-node metastasis. Indeed, VEGF-C's receptor, VEGFR-3, is primarily expressed in lymphatic endothelia [54]. Moreover, Studies of VEGF-C-transgenic mice reveal a connection between VEGF-C expression and lymphatic endothelial hyperplasia [53, 55]. Such findings are crucial to understanding EC progression and metastasis as lymph node involvement is an important route for EC spreading. Mariani et al. performed a study on 82 EC patients analyzing various phenotypic and molecular variables upon preoperative curettage in relation to prediction of lymph node metastasis. Their results suggested that unfavorable levels of p53, bcl-2, and/or detection of a non-endometrioid histology reliably predicted positive lymph node status in EC [56]. Hirai and colleagues performed a similar study investigating VEGF-A and VEGF-C expression in 228 cases of uterine EC from postmenopausal women in regard to conventional

EC risk factors, vascular invasion, depth of invasion, lymphatic invasion, and lymph node metastasis [57]. VEGF-A was the first characterized member of the VEGF family, and its involvement in both recurrent angiogenesis during the menstrual cycle as well as pathological angiogenesis associated with benign and malignant diseases of the endometrium has been thoroughly investigated [57, 58]. Regulation of VEGF-A expression is hormone cycle dependent, with estrogen being a potent stimulator of VEGF-A expression [57-60]. Hirai et al. found that VEGF-A expression is associated with vascular invasion, depth of invasion, and disease-free five and ten year survival (DF5YRS and DF10YRS, respectively); while VEGF-C expression was closely related to lymphatic vessel invasion, lymph node metastasis, and DF5YRS and DF10YRS. In fact, multivariate analysis revealed that VEGF-C expression is the third most important factor in predicting DF5YRS and DF10YRS for women with EC, next to lymph node metastasis and serosal/parametrial invasion, both independent risk factors for surgically treated EC's [57].

Hormonal induction of VEGF expression and subsequent vascularization, though an important promoter of angiogenesis, is not the only factor in this process. Since endothelium of blood vessels physically contacts adjacent tissues throughout vascular development, reciprocal signaling between endothelial vessel cells and surrounding tissues is highly possible [61]. Although much research is necessary for the elucidation of a comprehensive, integrated mechanism for vascularization, recent studies have identified several factors that are involved in endometrial angiogenesis. The expression of the angiogenic factor thymidine phosphorylase (TP), for example, is associated with increased microvessel density in EC [62]. Thymidine phosphorylase expression is also connected with the unfavorable prognostic features presented in Type II tumors (i.e. deep myometrial invasion, lymph node metastasis, and advanced staging) [5, 63]. Ribatti et al. recently highlighted the importance of mast cell (MC) influence on angiogenesis and neovascularization in endometrial carcinogenesis by associating MC count with EC staging. The authors employed murine monoclonal antibodies for endothelial cell marker CD31 and MC marker tryptase to distinguish the two cell types and found that MC profusion is directly correlated with EC progression and microvessel abundance [64]. Another study showed that mice lacking MC's exhibited protracted angiogenesis, which was normalized upon MC introduction [65]. Given the various cytokines and VEGF, as well as an assortment of other angiogenic factors expressed by MC, MC induction of vascularization is likely multifaceted [64]. Tryptase, another product of MC, deserves special attention for its role in endothelial angiogenesis. Introduction of tryptase alone induces capillary expansion in a dose dependent manner. The growth is restrained by specific tryptase inhibitors. Moreover, several studies have revealed an association between tryptase-positive MC and a poor prognosis in melanoma and multiple myeloma [65, 66]. It would be interesting to see how tryptase inhibitors affect pathogenesis of EC and other malignancies. While the findings presented in this section primarily concern angiogenesis, they also highlight the tumor-promoting effects imposed by changes in the tissue field.

19.6. Epigenetics and Field Cancerization

Aberrant DNA methylation represents an early event in the process of carcinogenesis for many different cancers [1, 67, 68]. Indeed, one of the hallmarks of cancer is the combination of global hypomethylation with regional, promoter hypermethylation, the former leading to increased chromosomal instability and LOH and the latter responsible for gene silencing [15, 69-71]. DNA methylation is achieved by addition of a methyl group to the 5' position of the pyrimidine ring of deoxycytidines in CpG dinucleotides [72]. Based on its preference for non-methylated DNA substrates, DNA-methytransferase-3B (DNMT3B) putatively assumes the primary role in de novo DNA methylation [73, 74]. Histone deacetylation by histone deactylase enzyme (HDAC) represents another chromosomal alteration associated with transcription silencing [73]. How HDAC and DNMT3B function together to regulate gene expression is not fully understood. Some studies show that a DNA methylation event can trigger histone acetylation modification, whereas other data provide evidence for the reciprocal—DNA methylation modification resulting from alteration of histone acetylation [75-82]. In regard to EC, Jin and colleagues found that DNMT3B is over-expressed in Grade I and Grade III endometrioid carcinomas compared to normal controls. Additionally, the authors showed that the well-differentiated Ishikawa cell line expressed low levels of DNMT3B in comparison with the poorly differentiated KLE cell line, the latter of which expressed DNMT3B at levels similar to those found in carcinomas. These results indicate a correlation between DNMT3B over-expression and EC development and progression [73]. Accordingly, the potential value of DNMT3B inhibitors in EC treatment warrants attention. The DNMT inhibitor 5-Aza-2'-deoxycytidine (ADC) covalently apprehends DNMT upon metabolic integration into genomic DNA, thereby promoting DNA demethylation [83, 84]. Likewise, HDAC inhibitors facilitate gene transcription by inducing hyperacetylation of histones H3 and H4 [83, 85, 86]. Moreover, the synergistic reactivation of methylation-silenced genes accomplished by concomitant administration of ADC and HDAC inhibitors has been well documented [83, 87-89]. Xiong et al. observed that HDAC inhibitors down-regulate DNMT3B expression. The authors employed quantitative real-time PCR and Western blot techniques and found that TSA suppresses DNMT3B mRNA and protein expression in human EC cells. Consequently, de novo methylation was considerably diminished. Subsequent studies showed that, following TSA treatment, DNMT3B mRNA stability was reduced and its half-life was shortened from 4 hours to 2.5 hours. These results suggested that TSA activates a DNMT3B-targeting RNase(s) or inhibits the function of other proteins that are required for DNMT3B stabilization [83, 90-93]. More recently, Silanes et al found that HuR, an mRNA stabilizing factor, is able to bind to the 3'-UTR of DNMT3B transcripts and modulate mRNA stability, thereby providing a potential mechanism by which HDAC inhibitors may regulate DNMT3B activity [94]. Identification of such factors will need to be explored further for a more complete understanding of the mechanism by which TSA and other HDAC inhibitors alter DNMT3B stability and expression [83]. Dowdy and colleagues also highlighted the anticancer effects of HDAC inhibitors in a recent study in which they show that TSA can act synergistically with the chemotherapy agent paclitaxel to affect microtubule stabilization and apoptosis in papillary serous endometrial cancer cells [95]. Similarly, Jiang et al. recently published findings that depict HDAC inhibitors as potent inducers of apoptosis in both Type I and Type II endometrial cancer cells [96]. Such findings point to the promise of HDAC inhibitors for the treatment of EC and other cancers [83, 96].

The inclusion of epigenetic considerations in the study of field cancerization is rare, although several research projects have made strides in addressing the issue. One study assessing methylation statuses of various promoters from lung tissues of former and current smokers revealed a high correlation (94%) between p16 promoter methylation status of bronchial epithelium from non-cancerous lung lobes and primary cancer tissues from the same patient. Accordingly, the researchers reasoned that aberrant promoter methylation may induce a field defect that promotes further genetic and epigenetic alterations and favors progression to lung cancer [1, 97]. Aberrant DNA methylation of genes from endometrial cancer/stromal cells has also been indentified and characterized. Genes epigenetically silenced in EC include MGMT [98], PTEN [99, 100], PR [75, 101, 102], HOXA11, THBS2 [103], PEG3 [104], and GSTP1 [105].

Microsatellite instability (MSI) is partially caused by the epigenetic silencing of DNA repair gene hMLH1 [106, 107]. Methylation of hMLH1 is reportedly associated with 7% of endometrial hyperplasia, predominantly those characterized by atypical complex hyperplastic morphology. This particular histological subtype is believed to directly preclude EC [108-110]. Aberrant methylation of S100A4, a gene up-regulated in several (particularly aggressive) carcinomas, has also been extensively investigated. Specifically, Xie et al. employed methylation-specific PCR techniques and found that S100A4 over-expression in advanced EC cases is correlated with hypomethylation of S100A4 within the first intron [15]. Future studies will be required to obtain a more extensive promoter EC-specific methylation panel, which could be used for EC screening and staging.

Importantly, epigenetic alterations are not restricted to the malignant cells themselves. Epigenetic modifications and associated changes in gene expression in tumor-adjacent stromal cells is well characterized [33]. Hu and colleagues analyzed methylation patterns of different cell types (epithelial and myoepithelial cells, and stromal fibroblasts) from normal human breast tissue, ductal carcinoma in situ (DCIS), and invasive breast cancer tissue using methylation-specific digital karyotyping (MSDK) techniques. The researchers found significant differences in the methylation patterns in stromal cells from each tissue type. Moreover, the most profound difference was seen between stromal cells of normal and invasive breast cancer tissue, suggestive of a tumor stage specific alteration of methylation regulation [33, 111] [32].

Differential DNA methylation patterns in normal vs. tumor-associated stromal cells were also detected in two independent studies assessing the methylation status of particular genes in HER2+ breast and prostate tumors [33, 112-114]. Moreover, Jiang et al. recently examined methylation profiles of short-term primary cultured myofibroblasts from gastric cancers using methylation-sensitive single nucleotide polymorphism (MSNP) and found global hypomethylation and regional hypermethylation of selected genes in tumor-associated myofibroblasts [33, 115].

Such findings hint at the potential therapeutic efficacy of epigenetic modification reagents not only for pre-malignant and primary tumor cells, but also for tumor-associated stromal cells [115]. In addition to acquiring aberrant methylation patterns, stromal cells can also influence epigenetic alterations in neighboring cancer cells. Lin and colleagues co-cultured human breast cancer cell line MCF10A with fibroblasts isolated from breast cancer or normal breast tissues. The authors found that primary fibroblasts from breast cancer patients trigger epigenetic silencing of the Cystatin M (CST6) tumor suppressor gene in breast epithelial cells through hyper-activation of the AKT-signaling pathway. This finding supports the general idea that the tumor-microenvironment influences tumor-progression; and more specifically, that such influences can take effect through epigenetic aberrations [116].

19.7. Inflammation and Endometrial Carcinoma Tumorigenesis

Inflammation is another factor that makes the tissue microenvironment more susceptible to neoplastic developments. Rudolf Virchow first proposed the connection between inflammation and tumorigenesis in 1863 after detecting numerous leukocytes in neoplastic tissues. Multiple studies have since lent support to this hypothesis, and 25% of all cancers are related to chronic infection and inflammation. The overproduction of reactive oxygen/nitrogen species (ROS/RNS, respectively) during the inflammatory response is thought to play an important role. The DNA damage inflicted by ROS and RNS is well documented and includes DNA base modifications, strand breaks, and cross-links contributing to replication errors and genomic instability [117, 118]. Inflammation has also been linked with non-genomic epimutations through alteration of DNA methylation and histone modification patterns [119]. Furthermore, high concentrations of ROS/RNS have been implicated in the modification of normal protein functions. Nitric oxide, for instance, is known to cause hyperphosphorylation and inactivation of tumor suppressor protein Rb in human colon cancer cells, thus potentiating tumorigenesis.

Persistent inflammation can also generate a field defect through the creation of a malignancy-favoring, signaling environment. The pro-inflammatory cytokines TNF-α and IL-6, over-expressed in inflammatory, hyperplastic tissues, have both been shown to stimulate proliferation, although high concentrations of TNF-α cause necrosis. TNF-α may promote tumorigenesis in certain cancers. For example, TNF-α and TNF-α-receptor knockout mice are resistant to skin cancer. Pro-inflammatory cytokines, in general, are also thought to promote angiogenesis through up-regulation of angiogenic factors, such as VEGF, VEGFR, IL-8, NO, ICAM-1 and VCAM-1[117, 118]. Chemokines, soluble cytokines that localize via chemotaxis, along with their receptors, have been shown to induce malignant transformation in different tumor types. Chemokines afford cells with metastatic capabilities by up-regulating matrix-metalloproteinases (MMPs) [117]. COX-2, a modified form of cyclooxygenase, can be induced by pro-inflammatory cytokines and ROS. COX-2 maintains the inflammatory state by catalyzing the synthesis of lipid intermediaries of inflammation, inducing proliferation, and inhibiting apoptosis [117]. One study showed that COX-2 knockout mice and mice treated with COX-2 inhibitors exhibited resistance to tumorigenesis [120, 121]. Prostaglandins, especially PGE2, are also apoptosis-inhibitors and proliferation-promoters and are up-regulated by COX-2 [117]. PGE2 has also been implicated in the recruitment and activation of pro-angiogenic factors [122]. Additionally, the transcription factor NF-κB is activated in response to inflammatory signals, which can promote tumorigenesis through regulation of other pro-inflammatory factors, cell-cycle regulatory and apoptotic genes, and angiogenic factors [117, 118]. The malignant-favoring effects of inflammation were further highlighted in a recent xenograft model of human ductal carcinoma in situ, in which inflammatory fibroblasts from rheumatoid arthritis patients more effectively augmented malignant growth and invasion than did tumor-associated fibroblasts [33, 123].

The role of inflammation in EC pathogenesis is not fully understood, but it is undoubtedly significant. Modugno et al. suggest that the effect of the menstrual cycle on the endometrium is analogous to a state of chronic inflammation caused by tissue damage [118].

The endometrium incurs such damage during the late secretory phase of the menstrual cycle when acid hydrolases are released as a result of lysosomal degradation [124]. The ensuing inflammatory responses include platelet accumulation, cytokine/prostaglandin secretion, and thrombosis [125]. Endometrial vasodilation-induced hypoxia causes the activation of NF-κB, which results in production and release of COX-2 [118, 126], prostaglandin, and pro-inflammatory cytokines. This series of events later leads to menstruation, after which the remaining endometrial epithelia begin the "healing" process through cell migration, proliferation, and angiogenesis [118, 127]. Modugno and colleagues also point out the fact that many EC risk factors (i.e. unopposed estrogen exposure, anovulation, heavy menstruation, late menopause, early menarche, obesity, diabetes, polycystic ovary syndrome, aging, etc.) may also be sources of inflammation [118]. Serum concentrations of inflammatory cytokines IL-6 and TNF-α, for example, increase with age and body mass index (BMI) [128]. TNF-α is also elevated in women with polycystic ovarian syndrome [129]. Similarly, there is considerable evidence for cytokine activation and chronic inflammation associated with insulin-independent diabetes [130].

19.8. Estrogen and Progesterone Effect on Endometrial Carcinoma Cancer Field

Estrogen and progesterone can induce and inhibit inflammatory cytokine production, respectively [118]. Specifically, estrogen mediates the synthesis of several pro-inflammatory cytokines and growth factors, along with their receptors, in a menstrual stage-specific manner [131]. Conversely, progesterone induces the expression of prostaglandin dehydrogenase, leading to the decomposition of prostaglandins [132]. Further, cytokine-mediated expression of COX-2 is also hindered by progestins [133]. Progesterone and its receptor (PR) are able to inhibit the pro-inflammatory actions of NF-κB [134]. Mice lacking a specific PR exhibited intense uterine inflammation according to one study [135]. While estrogen positively influences cytokine production, evidence reveals that the reciprocal may also occur. Specifically, IL-6 and TNF-α synergistically augment the actions of aromatase, 17β-hydroxysteroid dehydrogenase (17β-HSD), and estrone sulfatase, the three key enzymes for the production of estrogen [118, 136-138]. Aggressive EC stage-advancement seen in some patients might be related to this reciprocal positive-feedback between inflammatory cytokines and estrogen. Such findings suggest that administration of anti-inflammatory medications, along with concomitant maintenance of a healthy estrogen/progesterone balance, may prove beneficial for women at high risk for developing EC as well as those currently diagnosed with the malignancy.

The observation that the pro-inflammatory and anti-inflammatory actions of estrogen and progesterone (respectively) influence both the endometrial epithelia and the surrounding stromal and perivascular cells points to the significance of the microenvironment field in EC pathogenesis [139]. The impact of the field is correspondingly highlighted in endometriosis, a condition characterized by the migration and subsequent implantation of endometrial cells into an area outside of the uterine cavity. The response by stromal cells of normal, eutopic endometrium to progesterone is the production of water-soluble factors that activate 17β-hydroxysteroid dehydrogenase type 2 (17β-HSD2) in epithelial cells. This enzyme is responsible for converting biologically active estradiol to the inactive estrone. Cheng et al. showed that endometriotic stromal cells fail to produce and secrete those factors responsible for the paracrine activation of 17β-HSD2, consequently resulting in an excess of biologically active estrogen [140].

Long-term exposure to unopposed estrogen is a well-documented etiological factor for breast and endometrial cancers. Estrogen secretion by maturing Graafian follicles is necessary for the proliferative phase of the menstrual cycle, during which the endometrial lining thickens [141]. The positive effect on cell growth afforded to cells by estrogen is predominantly mediated through up-regulation of insulin-like growth factor 1 (IGF-1) in stromal cells [142]. Thus, estrogen affords endometrial cells with increased proliferative potential. Elevated estrogen concentration and the associated transcriptional modifications in stromal cells appear to be an important catalyst in the initiation of a field defect. Not surprisingly, exogenous estrogens administered to women during the proliferative phase prolong the phase and cause increased endometrial growth [141]. Progestins, in addition to their role in the induction of maturation of the endometrial glands and stroma, function in an anti-estrogenic fashion through activation of 17β-HSD2 [141, 143], thus hampering growth of the endometrial layer. Moreover, progesterone induces up-regulation of the IGF-1 binding protein (IGFBP-1), which effectively binds and sequesters IGF-1. These observations provide a rational at the molecular level for the use of progesterone in estrogen replacement therapy. Concomitant administration of both hormones leaves the endometrium shallower and slightly atrophic, with inactive and narrow glands [141].

Tamoxifen is an estrogen-like, triphenylethylene compound that was approved by the Food and Drug Administration for the treatment of breast cancer in 1978 [141, 144]. Its primary effect is accomplished through competition with estrogen for ER binding, thus acting as an anti-estrogen in breast cells. Significant evidence, however, suggests that tamoxifen exerts an estrogenic effect in other tissues, most notably the endometrium [144]. Tamoxifen has been shown to promote proliferative behavior and induce hyperplasia in the endometrium of breast cancer patients. Moreover, it has also been implicated in the development of multifocal, benign endometrial polyps [141]. ER-negative human endometrial cancer cells transplanted into mice grew at a similar pace compared to controls regardless of treatment with tamoxifen or estrogen. Conversely, ER-positive EC cells treated with either tamoxifen or estrogen experienced significantly accelerated proliferation-rates compared to controls. Progesterone receptors were also up-regulated in tamoxifen treated xenograft models, lending additional evidence to tamoxifen's presumed estrogenic role in endometrial cells [144].

19.9. Obesity and Diabetes as Additional Endometrial Cancerization Risk Factors

Obesity, nulliparity, infertility, estrogen replacement therapy, hypertension, diabetes mellitus, and a general lack of physical exercise have all been implicated in EC development [143, 145]. According to statistics from 2007 gathered by the Center for Disease Control, approximately 35.3 percent of adult women in the U.S. are obese (BMI $\geq$ 30) [146]. Indeed, EC prevalence has been shown to be nearly 10 times greater in industrialized countries compared with Asia or rural Africa where obesity is less prevalent. Data also show that, for a given geographic area, EC risk is lower prior to modernization and elevated shortly thereafter. Moreover, threat of developing EC increases after moving from a low-risk area to a high-risk, Westernized area, suggesting that there are more contributing factors to the development of this disease than genetics alone [143].

Obesity and type 2, insulin-independent diabetes are both associated with insulin resistance. Insulin resistance results in persistently elevated plasma insulin concentrations. Chronically elevated plasma insulin levels, in turn, alter the expression of IGF-1, IGFBP-1, and IGFBP-2. Specifically, IGF-1 is up-regulated while the IGF binding proteins are down-regulated, thus favoring cell growth [143]. Studies have shown that elevated insulin concentrations, through over-expression of IGF-1, also down-regulate sex hormone-binding globulin (SHBG), a protein responsible for binding sex hormones, especially testosterone and estradiol. Thus, obesity/diabetes-related insulin resistance, in addition to promoting cell growth via the IGF/IGFBP system, also increases the concentration of bioavailable estrogens [143, 147]. Moreover, obesity promotes peripheral aromatization of androgens to estrogens in adipose tissue [143].

Results from a study by Serin and colleagues indicate that obesity plays a larger role in the thickening of the endometrial lining in postmenopausal women than does hypertension, although evidence suggests that each has an independent connection to EC [145, 148]. Fifty-eight obese women, 40 hypertensive obese women, 28 hypertensive non-obese women, and 56 non-obese healthy women were examined by Papanicolaou cervical smear. Endometrial thickness was significantly elevated in obese women compared to healthy controls, regardless of the presence of hypertension, whereas endometrial thickness of non-obese hypertensive patients was not significantly different from healthy controls [145]. Additional studies will be required to assess the mechanism by which hypertension affords women with greater EC risks, although the condition has been implicated in insulin resistance, thus connecting hypertension with IGF-1, a potent stimulator of cell growth and inhibitor of apoptosis[149, 150].

Conclusion

Although cancer cells originate from epithelial cells, malignant transformation is more likely a concerted process involving both epithelial and stromal cells. Extra-epithelial components undergo dramatic changes during cancer development. If diagnosed early, most EC can be successfully treated with relatively favorable prognosis. Better understanding of epithelial-stromal interactions can potentially lead to the development of new diagnostic and therapeutic modalities. Based on the above discussion, biomarkers produced by stromal cells associated with EC may prove useful for early diagnosis or postsurgical surveillance for recurrence. It is also possible to develop new chemo- or immuno-therapeutic strategies targeting stromal cell processes. Indeed, combined application of traditional therapeutic regimens with anti-inflammatory and stromal-directed reagents, thereby suppressing the effects of the cancer field, may be explored for better treatment of advanced stage endometrial carcinoma.

Acknowledgments

Shi-Wen Jiang is the Distinguished Cancer Scholar supported by the Georgia Cancer Coalition (GCC). This work is partially funded by the research grants from National Institute of Health (NIH/R01 HD41577, Shi-Wen Jiang); NIH/National Cancer Institute MD Anderson Uterine Cancer SPORE (Jinping Li, Russell Broaddus, Shi-Wen Jiang), Gynecologic Cancer Foundation (GCF, Shi-Wen Jiang), and research supplement from the Mayo Medical College (Yi Lisa Hwa, Shi-Wen Jiang, Jinping Li), and Mercer University School of Medicine (Shi-Wen Jiang, Jinping Li, Tracy Tipton). Corespondence should be addressed to Shi-Wen Jiang, M.D.

References

[1] Jiang, S.W., J. Li, K. Podratz, and S. Dowdy, Application of DNA methylation biomarkers for endometrial cancer management. *Expert Rev. Mol. Diagn*, 2008. 8(5): p. 607-16.

[2] NCI, Http://www.cancer.gov/cancertopics/types/endometrial.

[3] Slaughter, D.P., H.W. Southwick, and W. Smejkal, Field cancerization in oral stratified squamous epithelium; clinical implications of multicentric origin. *Cancer,* 1953. 6(5): p. 963-8.

[4] Brown, L., Pathology of uterine malignancies. Clin Oncol (R Coll Radiol), 2008. 20(6): p. 433-47.

[5] Berstein, L.M., Santen, Richard J. , Innovative Endocrinology of Cancer. *Book Chapter*, 2008: p. 166-188.

[6] Emons, G., G. Fleckenstein, B. Hinney, A. Huschmand, and W. Heyl, Hormonal interactions in endometrial cancer. *Endocr. Relat. Cancer*, 2000. 7(4): p. 227-42.

[7] Simon, R., E. Eltze, K.L. Schafer, et al., Cytogenetic analysis of multifocal bladder cancer supports a monoclonal origin and intraepithelial spread of tumor cells. *Cancer Res.*, 2001. 61(1): p. 355-62.

[8] Dakubo, G.D., J.P. Jakupciak, M.A. Birch-Machin, and R.L. Parr, Clinical implications and utility of field cancerization. *Cancer Cell Int.*, 2007. 7: p. 2.

[9] Scholes, A.G., J.A. Woolgar, M.A. Boyle, et al., Synchronous oral carcinomas: independent or common clonal origin? *Cancer Res.,* 1998. 58(9): p. 2003-6.

[10] van Oijen, M.G. and P.J. Slootweg, Oral field cancerization: carcinogen-induced independent events or micrometastatic deposits? *Cancer Epidemiol. Biomarkers Prev.*, 2000. 9(3): p. 249-56.

[11] Moinfar, F., M.L. Kremser, Y.G. Man, et al., Allelic imbalances in endometrial stromal neoplasms: frequent genetic alterations in the nontumorous normal-appearing endometrial and myometrial tissues. *Gynecol. Oncol.*, 2004. 95(3): p. 662-71.

[12] Thiery, J.P., Epithelial-mesenchymal transitions in tumour progression. *Nat. Rev. Cancer*, 2002. 2(6): p. 442-54.

[13] Kang, Y. and J. Massague, Epithelial-mesenchymal transitions: twist in development and metastasis. *Cell*, 2004. 118(3): p. 277-9.

[14] Gotzmann, J., M. Mikula, A. Eger, et al., Molecular aspects of epithelial cell plasticity: implications for local tumor invasion and metastasis. *Mutat. Res.,* 2004. 566(1): p. 9-20.

[15] Xie, R., D.S. Loose, G.L. Shipley, et al., Hypomethylation-induced expression of S100A4 in endometrial carcinoma. *Mod. Pathol.*, 2007. 20(10): p. 1045-54.

[16] Gongoll, S., G. Peters, M. Mengel, et al., Prognostic significance of calcium-binding protein S100A4 in colorectal cancer. *Gastroenterology*, 2002. 123(5): p. 1478-84.

[17] Nakamura, T., T. Ajiki, S. Murao, et al., Prognostic significance of S100A4 expression in gallbladder cancer. *Int. J. Oncol.*, 2002. 20(5): p. 937-41.

[18] Sato, N., N. Fukushima, A. Maitra, et al., Gene expression profiling identifies genes associated with invasive intraductal papillary mucinous neoplasms of the pancreas. *Am. J. Pathol.*, 2004. 164(3): p. 903-14.

[19] Davies, B.R., M. O'Donnell, G.C. Durkan, et al., Expression of S100A4 protein is associated with metastasis and reduced survival in human bladder cancer. *J. Pathol.,* 2002. 196(3): p. 292-9.

[20] Cho, Y.G., S.W. Nam, T.Y. Kim, et al., Overexpression of S100A4 is closely related to the aggressiveness of gastric cancer. *Apmis*, 2003. 111(5): p. 539-45.

[21] Albertazzi, E., F. Cajone, B.E. Leone, et al., Expression of metastasis-associated genes h-mts1 (S100A4) and nm23 in carcinoma of breast is related to disease progression. *DNA Cell Biol.*, 1998. 17(4): p. 335-42.

[22] Kimura, K., Y. Endo, Y. Yonemura, et al., Clinical significance of S100A4 and E-cadherin-related adhesion molecules in non-small cell lung cancer. *Int. J. Oncol.*, 2000. 16(6): p. 1125-31.

[23] Gupta, S., T. Hussain, G.T. MacLennan, et al., Differential expression of S100A2 and S100A4 during progression of human prostate adenocarcinoma. *J. Clin. Oncol.*, 2003. 21(1): p. 106-12.

[24] Spoelstra, N.S., N.G. Manning, Y. Higashi, et al., The transcription factor ZEB1 is aberrantly expressed in aggressive uterine cancers. *Cancer Res.*, 2006. 66(7): p. 3893-902.

[25] Kyo, S., J. Sakaguchi, S. Ohno, et al., High Twist expression is involved in infiltrative endometrial cancer and affects patient survival. *Hum. Pathol.*, 2006. 37(4): p. 431-8.

[26] Yoshida, H., R. Broaddus, W. Cheng, S. Xie, and H. Naora, Deregulation of the HOXA10 homeobox gene in endometrial carcinoma: role in epithelial-mesenchymal transition. *Cancer Res.*, 2006. 66(2): p. 889-97.

[27] Weaver, V.M. and P. Gilbert, Watch thy neighbor: cancer is a communal affair. *J. Cell Sci.*, 2004. 117(Pt 8): p. 1287-90.

[28] Matsumoto, M., Y. Yamaguchi, Y. Seino, et al., Estrogen signaling ability in human endometrial cancer through the cancer-stromal interaction. *Endocr. Relat. Cancer*, 2008. 15(2): p. 451-63.

[29] Font de Mora, J. and M. Brown, AIB1 is a conduit for kinase-mediated growth factor signaling to the estrogen receptor. *Mol. Cell Biol.*, 2000. 20(14): p. 5041-7.

[30] Rinehart, C.A., J.M. Watson, V.R. Torti, and D. Palmieri, The role of interleukin-1 in interactive senescence and age-related human endometrial cancer. *Exp. Cell Res.*, 1999. 248(2): p. 599-607.

[31] Hu, M. and K. Polyak, Molecular characterisation of the tumour microenvironment in breast cancer. *Eur. J. Cancer*, 2008. 44(18): p. 2760-5.

[32] Allinen, M., R. Beroukhim, L. Cai, et al., Molecular characterization of the tumor microenvironment in breast cancer. *Cancer Cell*, 2004. 6(1): p. 17-32.
[33] Polyak, K., I. Haviv, and I.G. Campbell, Co-evolution of tumor cells and their microenvironment. *Trends Genet.*, 2009. 25(1): p. 30-8.
[34] Merlo, L.M., J.W. Pepper, B.J. Reid, and C.C. Maley, Cancer as an evolutionary and ecological process. *Nat. Rev. Cancer*, 2006. 6(12): p. 924-35.
[35] Anderson, A.R., A.M. Weaver, P.T. Cummings, and V. Quaranta, Tumor morphology and phenotypic evolution driven by selective pressure from the microenvironment. *Cell*, 2006. 127(5): p. 905-15.
[36] Girling, J.E. and P.A. Rogers, Recent advances in endometrial angiogenesis research. *Angiogenesis*, 2005. 8(2): p. 89-99.
[37] Lecce, G., G. Meduri, M. Ancelin, C. Bergeron, and M. Perrot-Applanat, Presence of estrogen receptor beta in the human endometrium through the cycle: expression in glandular, stromal, and vascular cells. *J. Clin. Endocrinol. Metab.*, 2001. 86(3): p. 1379-86.
[38] Krikun, G., F. Schatz, R. Taylor, et al., Endometrial endothelial cell steroid receptor expression and steroid effects on gene expression. *J. Clin. Endocrinol. Metab.*, 2005. 90(3): p. 1812-8.
[39] Kayisli, U.A., J. Luk, O. Guzeloglu-Kayisli, et al., Regulation of angiogenic activity of human endometrial endothelial cells in culture by ovarian steroids. *J. Clin. Endocrinol. Metab.*, 2004. 89(11): p. 5794-802.
[40] Iruela-Arispe, M.L., J.C. Rodriguez-Manzaneque, and G. Abu-Jawdeh, Endometrial endothelial cells express estrogen and progesterone receptors and exhibit a tissue specific response to angiogenic growth factors. *Microcirculation*, 1999. 6(2): p. 127-40.
[41] Gerrard, J.M. and J.G. White, Prostaglandins and thromboxanes: "middlemen" modulating platelet function in hemostasis and thrombosis. *Prog. Hemost. Thromb.*, 1978. 4: p. 87-125.
[42] Ma, W., J. Tan, H. Matsumoto, et al., Adult tissue angiogenesis: evidence for negative regulation by estrogen in the uterus. *Mol. Endocrinol.*, 2001. 15(11): p. 1983-92.
[43] Ivell, R., Endocrinology. This hormone has been relaxin' too long! *Science*, 2002. 295(5555): p. 637-8.
[44] Unemori, E.N., M.E. Erikson, S.E. Rocco, et al., Relaxin stimulates expression of vascular endothelial growth factor in normal human endometrial cells in vitro and is associated with menometrorrhagia in women. *Hum. Reprod.*, 1999. 14(3): p. 800-6.
[45] Zhao, Y., S. Hague, S. Manek, et al., PCR display identifies tamoxifen induction of the novel angiogenic factor adrenomedullin by a non estrogenic mechanism in the human endometrium. *Oncogene*, 1998. 16(3): p. 409-15.
[46] Nikitenko, L.L., I.Z. MacKenzie, M.C. Rees, and R. Bicknell, Adrenomedullin is an autocrine regulator of endothelial growth in human endometrium. *Mol. Hum. Reprod.*, 2000. 6(9): p. 811-9.
[47] Albrecht, E.D., J.S. Babischkin, Y. Lidor, et al., Effect of estrogen on angiogenesis in co-cultures of human endometrial cells and microvascular endothelial cells. *Hum. Reprod.*, 2003. 18(10): p. 2039-47.
[48] Hyder, S.M., J.C. Huang, Z. Nawaz, et al., Regulation of vascular endothelial growth factor expression by estrogens and progestins. *Environ. Health Perspect*, 2000. 108 Suppl 5: p. 785-90.

[49] Charnock-Jones, D.S., A.M. Sharkey, J. Rajput-Williams, et al., Identification and localization of alternately spliced mRNAs for vascular endothelial growth factor in human uterus and estrogen regulation in endometrial carcinoma cell lines. *Biol. Reprod.,* 1993. 48(5): p. 1120-8.

[50] Torry, D.S., V.J. Holt, J.A. Keenan, et al., Vascular endothelial growth factor expression in cycling human endometrium. *Fertil. Steril.*, 1996. 66(1): p. 72-80.

[51] Bausero, P., F. Cavaille, G. Meduri, S. Freitas, and M. Perrot-Applanat, Paracrine action of vascular endothelial growth factor in the human endometrium: production and target sites, and hormonal regulation. *Angiogenesis*, 1998. 2(2): p. 167-82.

[52] Ferrara, N., Vascular endothelial growth factor: basic science and clinical progress. *Endocr. Rev.*, 2004. 25(4): p. 581-611.

[53] Ueda, M., Y. Terai, K. Kumagai, et al., Vascular endothelial growth factor C gene expression is closely related to invasion phenotype in gynecological tumor cells. *Gynecol. Oncol.*, 2001. 82(1): p. 162-6.

[54] Joukov, V., K. Pajusola, A. Kaipainen, et al., A novel vascular endothelial growth factor, VEGF-C, is a ligand for the Flt4 (VEGFR-3) and KDR (VEGFR-2) receptor tyrosine kinases. *Embo J.*, 1996. 15(7): p. 1751.

[55] Jeltsch, M., A. Kaipainen, V. Joukov, et al., Hyperplasia of lymphatic vessels in VEGF-C transgenic mice. *Science*, 1997. 276(5317): p. 1423-5.

[56] Mariani, A., T.J. Sebo, J.A. Katzmann, et al., Endometrial cancer: can nodal status be predicted with curettage? *Gynecol. Oncol.*, 2005. 96(3): p. 594-600.

[57] Hirai, M., A. Nakagawara, T. Oosaki, et al., Expression of vascular endothelial growth factors (VEGF-A/VEGF-1 and VEGF-C/VEGF-2) in postmenopausal uterine endometrial carcinoma. *Gynecol. Oncol.*, 2001. 80(2): p. 181-8.

[58] Folkman, J., Seminars in Medicine of the Beth Israel Hospital, Boston. Clinical applications of research on angiogenesis. *N. Engl. J. Med.*, 1995. 333(26): p. 1757-63.

[59] Shweiki, D., A. Itin, G. Neufeld, H. Gitay-Goren, and E. Keshet, Patterns of expression of vascular endothelial growth factor (VEGF) and VEGF receptors in mice suggest a role in hormonally regulated angiogenesis. *J. Clin. Invest.*, 1993. 91(5): p. 2235-43.

[60] Cullinan-Bove, K. and R.D. Koos, Vascular endothelial growth factor/vascular permeability factor expression in the rat uterus: rapid stimulation by estrogen correlates with estrogen-induced increases in uterine capillary permeability and growth. *Endocrinology*, 1993. 133(2): p. 829-37.

[61] Cleaver, O. and D.A. Melton, Endothelial signaling during development. *Nat. Med.,* 2003. 9(6): p. 661-8.

[62] Mazurek, A., P. Kuc, S. Terlikowski, and T. Laudanski, Evaluation of tumor angiogenesis and thymidine phosphorylase tissue expression in patients with endometrial cancer. *Neoplasma*, 2006. 53(3): p. 242-6.

[63] Sivridis, E., Angiogenesis and endometrial cancer. *Anticancer Res.*, 2001. 21(6B): p. 4383-8.

[64] Ribatti, D., N. Finato, E. Crivellato, et al., Neovascularization and mast cells with tryptase activity increase simultaneously with pathologic progression in human endometrial cancer. *Am. J. Obstet. Gynecol.*, 2005. 193(6): p. 1961-5.

[65] Starkey, J.R., P.K. Crowle, and S. Taubenberger, Mast-cell-deficient W/Wv mice exhibit a decreased rate of tumor angiogenesis. *Int. J. Cancer*, 1988. 42(1): p. 48-52.

[66] Ribatti, D., M.G. Ennas, A. Vacca, et al., Tumor vascularity and tryptase-positive mast cells correlate with a poor prognosis in melanoma. *Eur. J. Clin. Invest.*, 2003. 33(5): p. 420-5.

[67] Umbricht, C.B., E. Evron, E. Gabrielson, et al., Hypermethylation of 14-3-3 sigma (stratifin) is an early event in breast cancer. *Oncogene*, 2001. 20(26): p. 3348-53.

[68] Ibanez de Caceres, I., C. Battagli, M. Esteller, et al., Tumor cell-specific BRCA1 and RASSF1A hypermethylation in serum, plasma, and peritoneal fluid from ovarian cancer patients. *Cancer Res.*, 2004. 64(18): p. 6476-81.

[69] Zhou, X.C., S.C. Dowdy, K.C. Podratz, and S.W. Jiang, Epigenetic considerations for endometrial cancer prevention, diagnosis and treatment. *Gynecol. Oncol.*, 2007. 107(1): p. 143-53.

[70] Gaudet, F., J.G. Hodgson, A. Eden, et al., Induction of tumors in mice by genomic hypomethylation. *Science*, 2003. 300(5618): p. 489-92.

[71] Das, P.M. and R. Singal, DNA methylation and cancer. *J. Clin. Oncol.*, 2004. 22(22): p. 4632-42.

[72] Jeltsch, A., Beyond Watson and Crick: DNA methylation and molecular enzymology of DNA methyltransferases. *Chembiochem,* 2002. 3(4): p. 274-93.

[73] Jin, F., S.C. Dowdy, Y. Xiong, et al., Up-regulation of DNA methyltransferase 3B expression in endometrial cancers. *Gynecol. Oncol.*, 2005. 96(2): p. 531-8.

[74] Hsieh, C.L., In vivo activity of murine de novo methyltransferases, Dnmt3a and Dnmt3b. *Mol. Cell Biol.*, 1999. 19(12): p. 8211-8.

[75] Xiong, Y., S.C. Dowdy, J. Gonzalez Bosquet, et al., Epigenetic-mediated upregulation of progesterone receptor B gene in endometrial cancer cell lines. *Gynecol. Oncol.,* 2005. 99(1): p. 135-41.

[76] Esteller, M. and J.G. Herman, Cancer as an epigenetic disease: DNA methylation and chromatin alterations in human tumours. *J. Pathol.*, 2002. 196(1): p. 1-7.

[77] Eden, S., T. Hashimshony, I. Keshet, H. Cedar, and A.W. Thorne, DNA methylation models histone acetylation. *Nature,* 1998. 394(6696): p. 842.

[78] Nan, X., H.H. Ng, C.A. Johnson, et al., Transcriptional repression by the methyl-CpG-binding protein MeCP2 involves a histone deacetylase complex. *Nature*, 1998. 393(6683): p. 386-9.

[79] Selker, E.U., Trichostatin A causes selective loss of DNA methylation in Neurospora. *Proc. Natl. Acad. Sci. USA*, 1998. 95(16): p. 9430-5.

[80] Szyf, M., L. Eliasson, V. Mann, G. Klein, and A. Razin, Cellular and viral DNA hypomethylation associated with induction of Epstein-Barr virus lytic cycle. *Proc. Natl. Acad. Sci. USA*, 1985. 82(23): p. 8090-4.

[81] Cervoni, N. and M. Szyf, Demethylase activity is directed by histone acetylation. *J. Biol. Chem.*, 2001. 276(44): p. 40778-87.

[82] Baylin, S.B., M. Esteller, M.R. Rountree, et al., Aberrant patterns of DNA methylation, chromatin formation and gene expression in cancer. *Hum. Mol. Genet.*, 2001. 10(7): p. 687-92.

[83] Xiong, Y., S.C. Dowdy, K.C. Podratz, et al., Histone deacetylase inhibitors decrease DNA methyltransferase-3B messenger RNA stability and down-regulate de novo DNA methyltransferase activity in human endometrial cells. *Cancer Res.*, 2005. 65(7): p. 2684-9.

[84] Santi, D.V., A. Norment, and C.E. Garrett, Covalent bond formation between a DNA-cytosine methyltransferase and DNA containing 5-azacytosine. *Proc. Natl. Acad. Sci. USA*, 1984. 81(22): p. 6993-7.

[85] Yoshida, M., M. Kijima, M. Akita, and T. Beppu, Potent and specific inhibition of mammalian histone deacetylase both in vivo and in vitro by trichostatin A. *J. Biol. Chem.,* 1990. 265(28): p. 17174-9.

[86] Boffa, L.C., G. Vidali, R.S. Mann, and V.G. Allfrey, Suppression of histone deacetylation in vivo and in vitro by sodium butyrate. *J. Biol. Chem.*, 1978. 253(10): p. 3364-6.

[87] Yang, X., D.L. Phillips, A.T. Ferguson, et al., Synergistic activation of functional estrogen receptor (ER)-alpha by DNA methyltransferase and histone deacetylase inhibition in human ER-alpha-negative breast cancer cells. *Cancer Res.*, 2001. 61(19): p. 7025-9.

[88] Bovenzi, V. and R.L. Momparler, Antineoplastic action of 5-aza-2'-deoxycytidine and histone deacetylase inhibitor and their effect on the expression of retinoic acid receptor beta and estrogen receptor alpha genes in breast carcinoma cells. *Cancer Chemother. Pharmacol.*, 2001. 48(1): p. 71-6.

[89] Ghoshal, K., J. Datta, S. Majumder, et al., Inhibitors of histone deacetylase and DNA methyltransferase synergistically activate the methylated metallothionein I promoter by activating the transcription factor MTF-1 and forming an open chromatin structure. *Mol Cell Biol,* 2002. 22(23): p. 8302-19.

[90] Ross, J., Control of messenger RNA stability in higher eukaryotes. *Trends Genet.*, 1996. 12(5): p. 171-5.

[91] Wennborg, A., B. Sohlberg, D. Angerer, G. Klein, and A. von Gabain, A human RNase E-like activity that cleaves RNA sequences involved in mRNA stability control. *Proc. Natl. Acad. Sci. USA*, 1995. 92(16): p. 7322-6.

[92] Joseph, B., M. Orlian, and H. Furneaux, p21(wafl) mRNA contains a conserved element in its 3'-untranslated region that is bound by the Elav-like mRNA-stabilizing proteins. *J. Biol. Chem.*, 1998. 273(32): p. 20511-6.

[93] Sela-Brown, A., J. Silver, G. Brewer, and T. Naveh-Many, Identification of AUF1 as a parathyroid hormone mRNA 3'-untranslated region-binding protein that determines parathyroid hormone mRNA stability. *J. Biol. Chem.*, 2000. 275(10): p. 7424-9.

[94] de Silanes, I.L., M. Gorospe, H. Taniguchi, et al., The RNA-binding protein HuR regulates DNA methylation through stabilization of DNMT3b mRNA. *Nucleic Acids Res*, 2009. 37(8): p. 2658-71.

[95] Dowdy, S.C., S. Jiang, X.C. Zhou, et al., Histone deacetylase inhibitors and paclitaxel cause synergistic effects on apoptosis and microtubule stabilization in papillary serous endometrial cancer cells. *Mol. Cancer Ther.,* 2006. 5(11): p. 2767-76.

[96] Jiang, S., S.C. Dowdy, X.W. Meng, et al., Histone deacetylase inhibitors induce apoptosis in both Type I and Type II endometrial cancer cells. *Gynecol. Oncol.*, 2007. 105(2): p. 493-500.

[97] Belinsky, S.A., W.A. Palmisano, F.D. Gilliland, et al., Aberrant promoter methylation in bronchial epithelium and sputum from current and former smokers. *Cancer Res.,* 2002. 62(8): p. 2370-7.

[98] Furlan, D., I. Carnevali, B. Marcomini, et al., The high frequency of de novo promoter methylation in synchronous primary endometrial and ovarian carcinomas. *Clin. Cancer Res.*, 2006. 12(11 Pt 1): p. 3329-36.

[99] Macdonald, N.D., H.B. Salvesen, A. Ryan, et al., Molecular differences between RER+ and RER- sporadic endometrial carcinomas in a large population-based series. *Int. J. Gynecol. Cancer,* 2004. 14(5): p. 957-65.

[100] Salvesen, H.B., N. MacDonald, A. Ryan, et al., PTEN methylation is associated with advanced stage and microsatellite instability in endometrial carcinoma. *Int. J. Cancer*, 2001. 91(1): p. 22-6.

[101] Ehrlich, C.E., P.C. Young, F.B. Stehman, G.P. Sutton, and W.M. Alford, Steroid receptors and clinical outcome in patients with adenocarcinoma of the endometrium. *Am. J. Obstet. Gynecol.*, 1988. 158(4): p. 796-807.

[102] Sasaki, M., A. Dharia, B.R. Oh, et al., Progesterone receptor B gene inactivation and CpG hypermethylation in human uterine endometrial cancer. *Cancer Res.,* 2001. 61(1): p. 97-102.

[103] Whitcomb, B.P., D.G. Mutch, T.J. Herzog, et al., Frequent HOXA11 and THBS2 promoter methylation, and a methylator phenotype in endometrial adenocarcinoma. *Clin. Cancer Res.*, 2003. 9(6): p. 2277-87.

[104] Dowdy, S.C., B.S. Gostout, V. Shridhar, et al., Biallelic methylation and silencing of paternally expressed gene 3 (PEG3) in gynecologic cancer cell lines. *Gynecol. Oncol.,* 2005. 99(1): p. 126-34.

[105] Chan, Q.K., U.S. Khoo, K.Y. Chan, et al., Promoter methylation and differential expression of pi-class glutathione S-transferase in endometrial carcinoma. *J. Mol. Diagn,* 2005. 7(1): p. 8-16.

[106] Esteller, M., Epigenetic lesions causing genetic lesions in human cancer: promoter hypermethylation of DNA repair genes. *Eur. J. Cancer*, 2000. 36(18): p. 2294-300.

[107] Herman, J.G., A. Umar, K. Polyak, et al., Incidence and functional consequences of hMLH1 promoter hypermethylation in colorectal carcinoma. *Proc. Natl. Acad. Sci. USA*, 1998. 95(12): p. 6870-5.

[108] Norris, H.J., M.P. Connor, and R.J. Kurman, Preinvasive lesions of the endometrium. *Clin. Obstet. Gynaecol*, 1986. 13(4): p. 725-38.

[109] Fox, H. and C.H. Buckley, The endometrial hyperplasias and their relationship to endometrial neoplasia. *Histopathology*, 1982. 6(5): p. 493-510.

[110] Nasir, A., D. Boulware, H.E. Kaiser, et al., Cyclooxygenase-2 (COX-2) expression in human endometrial carcinoma and precursor lesions and its possible use in cancer chemoprevention and therapy. *In Vivo*, 2007. 21(1): p. 35-43.

[111] Hu, M., J. Yao, L. Cai, et al., Distinct epigenetic changes in the stromal cells of breast cancers. *Nat. Genet.*, 2005. 37(8): p. 899-905.

[112] Fiegl, H., S. Millinger, G. Goebel, et al., Breast cancer DNA methylation profiles in cancer cells and tumor stroma: association with HER-2/neu status in primary breast cancer. *Cancer Res.*, 2006. 66(1): p. 29-33.

[113] Hanson, J.A., J.W. Gillespie, A. Grover, et al., Gene promoter methylation in prostate tumor-associated stromal cells. *J. Natl. Cancer Inst.,* 2006. 98(4): p. 255-61.

[114] Cairns, P., Gene methylation and early detection of genitourinary cancer: the road ahead. *Nat. Rev. Cancer*, 2007. 7(7): p. 531-43.

[115] Jiang, L., T.A. Gonda, M.V. Gamble, et al., Global hypomethylation of genomic DNA in cancer-associated myofibroblasts. *Cancer Res.*, 2008. 68(23): p. 9900-8.

[116] Lin, H.J., T. Zuo, C.H. Lin, et al., Breast cancer-associated fibroblasts confer AKT1-mediated epigenetic silencing of Cystatin M in epithelial cells. *Cancer Res.*, 2008. 68(24): p. 10257-66.

[117] Kundu, J.K. and Y.J. Surh, Inflammation: gearing the journey to cancer. *Mutat. Res*, 2008. 659(1-2): p. 15-30.

[118] Modugno, F., R.B. Ness, C. Chen, and N.S. Weiss, Inflammation and endometrial cancer: a hypothesis. *Cancer Epidemiol. Biomarkers Prev.*, 2005. 14(12): p. 2840-7.

[119] Hussain, S.P. and C.C. Harris, Inflammation and cancer: an ancient link with novel potentials. *Int. J. Cancer*, 2007. 121(11): p. 2373-80.

[120] Jacoby, R.F., K. Seibert, C.E. Cole, G. Kelloff, and R.A. Lubet, The cyclooxygenase-2 inhibitor celecoxib is a potent preventive and therapeutic agent in the min mouse model of adenomatous polyposis. *Cancer Res.*, 2000. 60(18): p. 5040-4.

[121] Peluffo, G.D., I. Stillitani, V.A. Rodriguez, M.J. Diament, and S.M. Klein, Reduction of tumor progression and paraneoplastic syndrome development in murine lung adenocarcinoma by nonsteroidal antiinflammatory drugs. *Int. J. Cancer*, 2004. 110(6): p. 825-30.

[122] Mann, J.R. and R.N. DuBois, Cyclooxygenase-2 and gastrointestinal cancer. *Cancer J.*, 2004. 10(3): p. 145-52.

[123] Hu, M., J. Yao, D.K. Carroll, et al., Regulation of in situ to invasive breast carcinoma transition. *Cancer Cell*, 2008. 13(5): p. 394-406.

[124] Epifanova, O., Effects of hormones on the cell cycle. In: Baserga R, editor. The cell cycle and Cancer. New York: M. Deckker, 1971. : p. 145.

[125] Srivastava, K., Prostaglandins and platelet function. *S. Fri. J. Sci.*, 1978. 74: p. 290.

[126] Kelly, R.W., A.E. King, and H.O. Critchley, Cytokine control in human endometrium. *Reproduction*, 2001. 121(1): p. 3-19.

[127] Sugino, N., A. Karube-Harada, T. Taketani, A. Sakata, and Y. Nakamura, Withdrawal of ovarian steroids stimulates prostaglandin F2alpha production through nuclear factor-kappaB activation via oxygen radicals in human endometrial stromal cells: potential relevance to menstruation. *J. Reprod. Dev.*, 2004. 50(2): p. 215-25.

[128] Wei, J., H. Xu, J.L. Davies, and G.P. Hemmings, Increase of plasma IL-6 concentration with age in healthy subjects. *Life Sci.*, 1992. 51(25): p. 1953-6.

[129] Gonzalez, F., K. Thusu, E. Abdel-Rahman, et al., Elevated serum levels of tumor necrosis factor alpha in normal-weight women with polycystic ovary syndrome. *Metabolism,* 1999. 48(4): p. 437-41.

[130] Li, Z.Z., J.B. Liu, L. Li, L. Jiao, and L. Chen, Intensive therapy for diabetes through influence on innate immune system. *Med. Hypotheses*, 2009. 72(6): p. 675-6.

[131] Tabibzadeh, S., Cytokines and the hypothalamic-pituitary-ovarian-endometrial axis. *Hum. Reprod.*, 1994. 9(5): p. 947-67.

[132] van der Burg, B. and P.T. van der Saag, Nuclear factor-kappa-B/steroid hormone receptor interactions as a functional basis of anti-inflammatory action of steroids in reproductive organs. *Mol. Hum. Reprod.*, 1996. 2(6): p. 433-8.

[133] Ishihara, O., K. Matsuoka, K. Kinoshita, M.H. Sullivan, and M.G. Elder, Interleukin-1 beta-stimulated PGE2 production from early first trimester human decidual cells is inhibited by dexamethasone and progesterone. *Prostaglandins*, 1995. 49(1): p. 15-26.

[134] Davies, S., D. Dai, I. Feldman, G. Pickett, and K.K. Leslie, Identification of a novel mechanism of NF-kappaB inactivation by progesterone through progesterone receptors in Hec50co poorly differentiated endometrial cancer cells: induction of A20 and ABIN-2. *Gynecol. Oncol.*, 2004. 94(2): p. 463-70.
[135] Lydon, J.P., F.J. DeMayo, C.R. Funk, et al., Mice lacking progesterone receptor exhibit pleiotropic reproductive abnormalities. *Genes. Dev.*, 1995. 9(18): p. 2266-78.
[136] Macdiarmid, F., D. Wang, L.J. Duncan, et al., Stimulation of aromatase activity in breast fibroblasts by tumor necrosis factor alpha. *Mol. Cell Endocrinol.*, 1994. 106(1-2): p. 17-21.
[137] Adams, E.F., B. Rafferty, and M.C. White, Interleukin 6 is secreted by breast fibroblasts and stimulates 17 beta-oestradiol oxidoreductase activity of MCF-7 cells: possible paracrine regulation of breast 17 beta-oestradiol levels. *Int. J. Cancer*, 1991. 49(1): p. 118-21.
[138] Purohit, A., Duncan LJ, Wang DY, Coldham NG, Ghilchik MW and Reed MJ, Paracine control of oestrogen production in breast cancer. *Endocrine-Related Cancer*, 1997. 4: p. 323-330.
[139] Kelly, R.W., A.E. King, and H.O. Critchley, Inflammatory mediators and endometrial function--focus on the perivascular cell. *J. Reprod. Immunol.*, 2002. 57(1-2): p. 81-93.
[140] Cheng, Y.H., A. Imir, V. Fenkci, M.B. Yilmaz, and S.E. Bulun, Stromal cells of endometriosis fail to produce paracrine factors that induce epithelial 17beta-hydroxysteroid dehydrogenase type 2 gene and its transcriptional regulator Sp1: a mechanism for defective estradiol metabolism. *Am. J. Obstet. Gynecol.*, 2007. 196(4): p. 391 e1-7; discussion 391 e7-8.
[141] Buckley C.Hilary, F.H., Bopsy Pathology of the Endometrium. 2002. Edition Number 2(I): p. 56-79.
[142] Zhu, L. and J.W. Pollard, Estradiol-17beta regulates mouse uterine epithelial cell proliferation through insulin-like growth factor 1 signaling. *Proc. Natl. Acad. Sci. USA,* 2007. 104(40): p. 15847-51.
[143] Kaaks, R., A. Lukanova, and M.S. Kurzer, Obesity, endogenous hormones, and endometrial cancer risk: a synthetic review. *Cancer Epidemiol. Biomarkers Prev.*, 2002. 11(12): p. 1531-43.
[144] Foon, K.A., Muss, H.B., *Biological and Hormonal therapies of Cancer*. 1998: p. 195-276.
[145] Serdar Serin, I., B. Ozcelik, M. Basbug, et al., Effects of hypertension and obesity on endometrial thickness. *Eur. J. Obstet. Gynecol. Reprod. Biol.*, 2003. 109(1): p. 72-5.
[146] CDC, Http://www.cdc.gov/nchs/pressroom/07newsreleases/obesity.htm.
[147] Selby, C., Sex hormone binding globulin: origin, function and clinical significance. *Ann. Clin. Biochem.*, 1990. 27 (Pt 6): p. 532-41.
[148] Brinton LA , B.M., Mortel R , Twiggs L, Barrett R, Wilbanks G Reproductive *Am. J. Obstet. Gynecol.*, 1992. 167: p. 1317-25.
[149] Hamet, P., Cancer and hypertension. An unresolved issue. *Hypertension,* 1996. 28(3): p. 321-4.
[150] Mantzoros, C.S., A. Tzonou, L.B. Signorello, et al., Insulin-like growth factor 1 in relation to prostate cancer and benign prostatic hyperplasia. *Br. J. Cancer*, 1997. 76(9): p. 1115-8.

In: Field Cancerization: Basic Science and Clinical Applications ISBN 978-1-61761-006-6
Editor: Gabriel D. Dakubo

Chapter 20

Field Cancerization in Vulvar, Vaginal and Cervical Epithelia

Ann H. Klopp and Anuja Jhingran

20.1. Introduction

Gynecologic cancers, as well as other epithelial malignancies, have significant evidence for a field effect in clinical presentation. Pre-invasive vulvar cancers in particular are recognized as frequently diffuse lesions.

Invasive vulvar and cervical cancers arise in the context of a spectrum of premalignant changes, which are often multifocal and diffuse. Furthermore, patients are at a high risk for developing a regional recurrence or a second primary cancer of pre-invasive or invasive nature. Human papilloma virus (HPV) is an important factor in creating a regional field effect in cervical and some vulvar cancers, although evidence exists for a field effect in the absence of HPV as well.

The existence of a cancerized field in vulvar and cervical cancer is also supported by molecular evidence. Molecular studies characterizing genomic changes, such as X-chromosome inactivation and loss of heterozygosity (LOH), have demonstrated that pre-malignant cervical and vulvar lesions are frequently polyclonal, suggesting that, these cancers arise independently within a region of field cancerization. Invasive cancers are more likely to be monoclonal, presumably due to regional spread of an invasive clone.

Furthermore, molecular changes characteristic of cancer have been identified in morphologically normal epithelia, demonstrating that field changes extend beyond areas of dysplasia. The effects of field cancerization have important implications for diagnosis, surgery and radiation treatment of gynecologic cancers.

20.2. Clinical Evidence for Field Effect in Gynecologic Cancer

20.2.1. Presentation of Pre-Invasive and Invasive Vulvar Cancer

A wealth of clinical data suggests that field cancerization plays an important role in oncogenesis of vulvar and cervical cancer. Vulvar intraepithelial neoplasia (VIN) is commonly multifocal with changes over a large region of the vulva. The risk of non-contiguous VIN lesions has been reported in two separate studies to occur in 82% and 93% of patients (1, 2), suggesting that this is the rule and not the exception. Identifying sites of invasive cancer in VIN can be a challenge, necessitating multiple biopsies with careful colposcopic guidance. Extensive VIN requires treatment of the regional epithelia with ablative therapy, such as CO_2 laser or drug therapy such as topical 5-FU(3), or extensive surgical approaches such as skinning vulvectomy (4). Furthermore, multifocality is an important risk factor for recurrence, even in the presence of negative margins (5). These features suggest that a field of pre-malignant changes exists for vulvar cancer and that effective treatment requires treating the entire field.

Invasive squamous cell cancer of the vulva frequently occurs contiguously with VIN. As a result, wide margins of 1 cm are recommended on excision of invasive vulvar cancer (6). This may be due to the presence of field changes in adjacent tissues, which may or may not be recognized pathologically as VIN.

In addition, pre-invasive and invasive cervical cancers and vulvar cancers are frequently found to be synchronous (7). This is particularly true of HPV positive cancers, perhaps due to a multifocal infection. In one study, 41% of patients treated with HPV associated VIN later developed a past, synchronous or future squamous malignancy of the anogenital tract (8).

20.2.2. Presentation of Pre-Invasive and Invasive Vaginal Cancer

Vaginal intraepithelial neoplasia is a less common presentation. However, it also frequently presents with multifocal lesions, and is found in the upper vagina in 80% of cases (5).

20.3. Multicentric Cancers of the Gynecologic Tract

Multicentricity is defined by the presence of intraepithelial lesions of two or three sites (cervix, vagina or vulva). Multicentricity is not an infrequent presentation. Approximately 5% of patients with cervical intraepithelial neoplasia (CIN) or vaginal intraepithelial neoplasia (VAIN) have a second lesion in other gynecologic tract (9, 10). Multicentricity has been reported to be more common in women with VIN3, with 35% of women having a second lesion in the gynecologic tract (9). Spitzer et al. reported that 85% of patients with a vulvar lesion had cervical dysplasia (11). This marked difference in multicentricity seen with vulvar as compared to cervical or vaginal lesions suggests an interesting biological difference in pre-invasive vulvar cancers. The development of vulvar cancer may be more vulnerable to field, or microenvironmental effects, or field changes may have a propensity to spread in a cranial-caudal direction in the gynecologic tract, so that a vulvar cancer is more likely to be associated with field change in adjacent cervical and vaginal mucosa.

Interestingly, multicentric lesions are not more likely to be HPV associated (9), suggesting that the field effect is not accounted for by diffuse HPV infection. Patients with multicentric lesions have a higher risk of recurrence than patients with unicentric disease. This suggests that the field changes accounting for the development of multicentric cancers also contributes to the risk of developing a future malignancy (9).

The rates of multicentricity may be underestimated for cancers involving the vagina due to staging convention. A vaginal cancer, which involves the cervix is considered to be a cervical cancer and is staged as such. However, it is possible that some of these cases may by synchronous primary cancers. Similarly, a cancer involving the vagina and vulva is staged as a vulvar cancer but may have originally represented two independent cancers. In some cases, this distinction may have treatment implications. Molecular analysis makes it possible to determine if two cancers are clonal or if they have arisen independently. The next section will discuss these molecular techniques and how they have been used to determine if gynecologic cancers are clonal and to detect molecular changes in non-malignant tumor adjacent epithelia.

20.4. Molecular Evidence for Field Cancerization in Gynecologic Cancer

20.4.1. Molecular Evidence for Field Changes in Cervical Cancer

Studies in cervical cancer have found that histologically normal appearing tissue have molecular changes such as loss of heterozygosity and genetic instability that are characteristic of malignancy. Monoclonality, measured by the pattern of X-chromosome inactivation, was found to occur in a large field of normal appearing cervical basal epithelium, spanning a distance of 500 cells. It is possible that this observation is due to a large size of "tiles" or regions of X-chromosome inactivation, which can occur developmentally. Alternatively, this may represent morphologically normal but proliferative pre-malignant areas of the cervical epithelium that represent field changes (12).

Cervical metaplasia, or replacement of the normal cuboidal epithelium with squamous epithelium, may also represent evidence of a pre-malignant change in the field of cervical cancer. Enomoto et al. investigated the clonality of cervical metaplasia with and without atypia (13). Atypical metaplasia (or atypical immature metaplasia - AIM) is squamous metaplasia with areas of nuclear atypia, which do not meet the criteria for cervical intraepithelial neoplasia. Interestingly, the authors found that histologically normal metaplasia was not likely to be clonal (10%). By contrast, metaplasia with atypia was found to be frequently clonal (89%), suggesting that it may constitute a field of proliferation, which may be a precursor of malignancy. The authors and others found that atypical immature metaplasia is likely to be associated with high-risk HPV, while typical squamous metaplasia is not (14).

Pre-cancerous cervical lesions frequently exhibit the same monoclonal pattern of X-chromosome inactivation as adjacent invasive cancers. Interestingly, pre-invasive cancers were more likely to be monoclonal when they were accompanied by an invasive component, suggesting that these monoclonal pre-invasive lesions are higher risk lesions or that fluidity exists with invasive and adjacent non-invasive cancers (15).

20.4.2. Role of HPV in Field Cancerization

Approximately 95% of cervical and 50% of vulvar cancers are HPV positive. Human papilloma virus is known to be critical etiologic factor in the development of cervical cancer, by disrupting the functions of the p53 and retinoblastoma tumor suppressor genes (16). Human papilloma virus also likely plays an important role in the formation of a field effect in gynecologic cancer. Infection with HPV may occur multifocally and infection may spread through adjacent epithelium. In addition, the inflammatory response to viral infection may alter the microenvironment, predisposing to regional transformation. The status of HPV genome changes during epithelial progression to cervical cancer. The HPV genome is generally absent in benign proliferative lesions, and is most commonly present in the episomal state in pre-invasive cancer and is clonally integrated into the genome of invasive cancers. Intraepithelial lesions, which are positive for high-grade HPV subtypes are more likely to be monoclonal while low-risk subtypes are more commonly polyclonal (17, 18). Furthermore, telomerase expression, a hallmark of immortalization, is found more commonly in monoclonal than polyclonal low-grade lesions (18). These findings are consistent with a model in which polyclonal proliferations are associated with infection with low-risk subtypes of HPV. These lesions are likely to be multi-focal. Infection with a high-risk HPV subtype leads to selection of a dominant proliferative clone. If viral integration occurs, monoclonal expansion follows and these lesions are most likely to develop into an invasive cancer. Studies of clonality of pre-malignant abnormalities may help to determine which lesions are in need of excision or ablation and which can be observed.

Human papilloma virus integration sites can also serve as a marker to determine the clonality of HPV associated lesions. Vinokurova et al. compared the integration site of HPV in patients with secondary metachronous cancers of vagina and vulva up to several years after treatment of a primary cervical cancer (19). They found that six of seven patients with a prior invasive high-grade dysplastic lesion of the cervix had identical integration in the same locus in the subsequent vaginal or vulvar lesion. This study demonstrated that intraepithelial spread occurs in the gynecology tract, creating a field of cancerization.

20.4.3. Molecular Evidence for Field Changes in Vulvar Cancer

Rosenthal et al. studied the evidence for clonality of VIN and vulvar squamous cell carcinoma (VSCC) (20). They characterized the pattern of X-chromosome inactivation in VIN and VSCC from patients who had contiguous VIN and VSCC and who had non-contiguous lesions. The pattern of X-chromosome inactivation was used to determine if malignancies were derived from a single clone. They found that 7/7 cases of VSCC with contiguous VIN had monoclonal cancers, as did 6 of 9 cases of non-contiguous VIN/VSCC. This high frequency of monoclonality suggests that VIN is the predecessor to VSCC and that pre-invasive vulvar cancers may spread throughout the epithelium.

A subset of vulvar cancers arises in areas of benign lesions, such as squamous metaplasia and lichen sclerosis. Squamous carcinomas of the vulva arise in a background of lichen sclerosis in 3-5% of cases and 20% of squamous cell hyperplasia are associated with vulvar intraepithelial neoplasia (21). A subset of squamous metaplasia and lichens sclerosis have been shown to be monoclonal but not associated with HPV infection, suggesting that they may represent an abnormal proliferative tissue that could progress following infection with HPV.

Recent studies demonstrated that some cases of lichen sclerosis adjacent to invasive vulvar cancer showed increased expression of p53 and allelic imbalance (22). These benign proliferative lesions are generally not HPV positive but may constitute a pre-malignant abnormal field, which is at risk for transformation.

20.5. Clinical utility of molecular analysis of Field Changes in Gynecologic Cancers

Molecular analysis of field changes could be used to tailor treatment. In head and neck cancer, 61% of recurrences were found to have a genetically related precursor lesion in the histologically normal tissue taken from adjacent to the primary tissue (23), suggesting that molecular analysis could be used to identify adjacent tissue at risk that should be used to define surgical margins or to design radiation treatment fields. In head and neck cancer, the risk of second primary cancers was found to decrease in the 5 years after diagnosis as compared to patients treated without radiotherapy (20, 24). This suggests that it may be possible to treat subclinical premalignant foci with radiation to prevent local recurrences or secondary primary cancers.

Identifying the clonality of pre-invasive lesions may also be useful to identify which lesions are at risk for malignant transformation. For example, multifocal, monoclonal lesions may characterize higher risk pre-invasive lesions, which have developed the capacity to spread within the epithelium and may warrant close follow-up. The studies presented here suggest that a monoclonal multifocal pre-invasive lesion is higher risk than a similar polyclonal lesion. However, a prospective analysis should be performed to determine if this is the case.

Genomic changes in histologically normal tissue may also have important prognostic value. Recently, molecular chances in pathologically normal appearing non-cancerous liver have been shown to predict late recurrence (25). A similar approach may prove to be useful in gynecologic cancers given the likely role of field changes in carcinogenesis.

Conclusion

Vulvar, vaginal and cervical cancers often present with multifocal lesions. Molecular analysis of patterns of X-chromosome inactivation, LOH and HPV integrations sites have demonstrated that these lesions can be monoclonal or polyclonal, which implies different mechanisms of field cancerization. The presence of polyclonal lesions implies that the microenvironment of the mucosa has been altered to favor the development of neoplasia. The presence of multicentric monoclonal intraepithelial lesions demonstrates that intraepithelial spread is possible. Identical HPV integration sites in metachronous vaginal and vulvar cancer provide very strong evidence for intraepithelial spread. In addition, molecular changes characteristic of cancer have been detected in adjacent normal mucosa, providing further evidence of field changes in the mucosal epithelium.

Molecular analysis to define the region at risk has a number of clinical implications. Defining the region with field changes could guide surgical management and radiation field design and may have prognostic value. These studies open the door to strategies aimed at reversing environmental effects that influence carcinogenesis or intraepithelial spread to prevent the development and progression of these cancers.

References

[1] Chafe W, Richards A, Morgan L, Wilkinson E. Unrecognized invasive carcinoma in vulvar intraepithelial neoplasia (VIN). *Gynecol. Oncol.* 1988; 31: 154-65.

[2] van Beurden M, van Der Vange N, ten Kate FJ, de Craen AJ, Schilthuis MS, Lammes FB. Restricted surgical management of vulvar intraepithelial neoplasia 3: Focus on exclusion of invasion and on relief of symptoms. *Int. J. Gynecol. Cancer* 1998; 8: 73-7.

[3] Hillemanns P, Wang X, Staehle S, Michels W, Dannecker C. Evaluation of different treatment modalities for vulvar intraepithelial neoplasia (VIN): CO(2) laser vaporization, photodynamic therapy, excision and vulvectomy. *Gynecol. Oncol.* 2006; 100: 271-5.

[4] Ayhan A, Tuncer ZS, Dogan L, Yuce K, Kucukali T. Skinning vulvectomy for the treatment of vulvar intraepithelial neoplasia 2-3: a study of 21 cases. *Eur. J. Gynaecol. Oncol.* 1998; 19: 508-10.

[5] Diakomanolis E, Stefanidis K, Rodolakis A, et al. Vaginal intraepithelial neoplasia: report of 102 cases. *Eur. J. Gynaecol. Oncol.* 2002; 23: 457-9.

[6] Heaps JM, Fu YS, Montz FJ, Hacker NF, Berek JS. Surgical-pathologic variables predictive of local recurrence in squamous cell carcinoma of the vulva. *Gynecol. Oncol.* 1990; 38: 309-14.

[7] Ayhan A, Yalcin OT, Tuncer ZS, Gurgan T, Kucukali T. Synchronous primary malignancies of the female genital tract. *Eur. J. Obstet. Gynecol. Reprod. Biol.* 1992; 45: 63-6.

[8] van de Nieuwenhof HP, van Kempen LC, de Hullu JA, et al. The etiologic role of HPV in vulvar squamous cell carcinoma fine tuned. *Cancer Epidemiol. Biomarkers Prev.* 2009; 18: 2061-7.

[9] Bornstein J, Kaufman RH, Adam E, Adler-Storthz K. Multicentric intraepithelial neoplasia involving the vulva. Clinical features and association with human papillomavirus and herpes simplex virus. *Cancer* 1988; 62: 1601-4.

[10] Audet-Lapointe P, Body G, Vauclair R, Drouin P, Ayoub J. Vaginal intraepithelial neoplasia. *Gynecol. Oncol.* 1990; 36: 232-9.

[11] Spitzer M, Krumholz BA, Seltzer VL. The multicentric nature of disease related to human papillomavirus infection of the female lower genital tract. *Obstet. Gynecol.* 1989; 73: 303-7.

[12] Ponten J, Guo Z. Precancer of the human cervix. *Cancer Surv.* 1998; 32: 201-29.
[13] Enomoto T, Haba T, Fujita M, et al. Clonal analysis of high-grade squamous intra-epithelial lesions of the uterine cervix. *Int. J. Cancer* 1997; 73: 339-44.
[14] Geng L, Connolly DC, Isacson C, Ronnett BM, Cho KR. Atypical immature metaplasia (AIM) of the cervix: is it related to high-grade squamous intraepithelial lesion (HSIL)? *Hum. Pathol.* 1999; 30: 345-51.
[15] Guo Z, Ponten F, Wilander E, Ponten J. Clonality of precursors of cervical cancer and their genetical links to invasive cancer. *Mod. Pathol.* 2000; 13: 606-13.
[16] Yugawa T, Kiyono T. Molecular mechanisms of cervical carcinogenesis by high-risk human papillomaviruses: novel functions of E6 and E7 oncoproteins. *Rev. Med. Virol.* 2009; 19: 97-113.
[17] Park TW, Richart RM, Sun XW, Wright TC, Jr. Association between human papillomavirus type and clonal status of cervical squamous intraepithelial lesions. *J. Natl. Cancer Inst.* 1996; 88: 355-8.
[18] Park TW, Riethdorf S, Schulz G, Riethdorf L, Wright T, Loning T. Clonal expansion and HPV-induced immortalization are early molecular alterations in cervical carcinogenesis. *Anticancer Res.* 2003; 23: 155-60.
[19] Vinokurova S, Wentzensen N, Einenkel J, et al. Clonal history of papillomavirus-induced dysplasia in the female lower genital tract. *J. Natl. Cancer Inst.* 2005; 97: 1816-21.
[20] Rosenthal AN, Ryan A, Hopster D, Jacobs IJ. Molecular evidence of a common clonal origin and subsequent divergent clonal evolution in vulval intraepithelial neoplasia, vulval squamous cell carcinoma and lymph node metastases. *Int. J. Cancer* 2002; 99: 549-54.
[21] Hantschmann P, Sterzer S, Jeschke U, Friese K. P53 expression in vulvar carcinoma, vulvar intraepithelial neoplasia, squamous cell hyperplasia and lichen sclerosus. *Anticancer Res* 2005; 25: 1739-45.
[22] Vanin K, Scurry J, Thorne H, Yuen K, Ramsay RG. Overexpression of wild-type p53 in lichen sclerosus adjacent to human papillomavirus-negative vulvar cancer. *J. Invest. Dermatol.* 2002; 119: 1027-33.
[23] Tabor MP, Brakenhoff RH, Ruijter-Schippers HJ, Kummer JA, Leemans CR, Braakhuis BJ. Genetically altered fields as origin of locally recurrent head and neck cancer: a retrospective study. *Clin. Cancer Res.* 2004; 10: 3607-13.
[24] Rennemo E, Zatterstrom U, Evensen J, Boysen M. Reduced risk of head and neck second primary tumors after radiotherapy. *Radiother. Oncol.* 2009; 93: 559-62.
[25] Okamoto M, Utsunomiya T, Wakiyama S, et al. Specific Gene-Expression Profiles of Noncancerous Liver Tissue Predict the Risk for Multicentric Occurrence of Hepatocellular Carcinoma in Hepatitis C Virus-Positive Patients. *Ann. Surg. Oncol.* 2006.

In: Field Cancerization: Basic Science and Clinical Applications ISBN 978-1-61761-006-6
Editor: Gabriel D. Dakubo

Chapter 21

Molecular Signatures in Ovarian Cancer

Celestine S. Tung and Kwong-Kwok Wong

Abstract

Molecular signatures are a key element in the development of new screening tools and treatment targets in ovarian cancer. The identification of molecular signatures may lead to new screening methods for early stage disease and to a more personalized approach to patient care in the future. In ovarian cancer, which has high recurrence rates and poor overall survival, the incorporation of specific chemotherapeutic and biologic agents into a treatment plan on the basis of the molecular pattern of an individual patient's disease may prolong progression-free and overall survival. These molecular patterns may also assist physicians in counseling patients regarding their overall prognosis. With advances in technology related to genomic, proteomic, and metabolomic approaches, hundreds of potential biomarkers and therapeutic targets have been identified. Much work remains to validate the clinical applicability of these molecular signatures, but the identification of novel biologic agents that target these molecules shows a promising future for individualized medicine. This chapter aims to review the various techniques used to identify molecular signatures in ovarian cancer, to discuss some of the biomarkers that have been found thus far, and to demonstrate the clinical applicability of these ovarian cancer biomarkers.

21.1. Introduction

Ovarian cancer is a leading cause of cancer death among women and is the deadliest gynecologic malignancy. In 2009, an estimated 21,550 new cases of ovarian cancer are expected in the United States, with approximately 14,600 deaths due to the disease [1]. Unfortunately, most patients present with advanced stage disease, for which the survival rate ranges from 25% to 37% [2]. When diagnosed early, the cure rate approaches 90%, but fewer than 25% of women are diagnosed with stage I ovarian cancer [2,3]. One of the challenges to early diagnosis is the paucity of effective screening tools. Currently, no standard of care exists regarding ovarian cancer screening. Both transvaginal ultrasound and the serum biomarker

CA-125 have been used to screen for ovarian cancer, as individual tools or in combination [4,5,6,7,8,9,10,11]. However, no screening modalities have had an impact on overall mortality from ovarian cancer.

In addition to poor screening tools, most ovarian cancers relapse despite initial response to chemotherapy. This is usually due to many factors, including an acquired resistance to traditional chemotherapy. It is not unusual after disease recurrence for patients to receive several chemotherapeutic regimens, but response rates to second-line agents range from only 12% to 27% [12]. The difficulty lies in determining to which drug a patient will respond and which agent will improve progression-free and overall survival.

The use of molecular signatures and identification of ovarian cancer biomarkers are crucial to tackling these issues. Many people consider ovarian cancer to be caused by a conglomeration of genetic changes, which further results in disease recurrence, progression, and resistance to treatment. The identification of these genetic alterations may provide insight into new potential screening mechanisms. Additionally, the determination of how these changes occur may identify patients who would benefit from specific chemotherapy combinations or who would be ideal candidates for novel agents targeted towards certain gene mutations. Unlike in breast cancer, where trastuzumab treatment is effective in patients with HER2/neu mutations, no such therapies have been identified and proven beneficial in ovarian cancer. However, many studies are ongoing to identify potential therapeutic targets and screening biomarkers, and the prognostic and predictive values of various molecular markers are being evaluated [13]. Further research establishing the reliability and validity of various molecular targets and predictor gene sets is still required before their clinical application.

This chapter describes the molecular and genetic heterogeneity in ovarian cancer tumorigenesis. Additionally, the various approaches to identifying and validating molecular patterns and signatures in ovarian cancer will be explored. Description of all techniques utilized to identify molecular signatures is beyond the scope of this chapter, but a summary of tools most commonly employed will be outlined. Furthermore, the potential clinical utility of biomarkers and the current limitations to their widespread integration into ovarian cancer screening and treatment will be examined. We also will discuss the future direction of biomarker discovery and the use of molecular signatures in ovarian cancer.

21.2. Definition of "Field" in Ovarian Cancer

21.2.1. Clinical and Pathologic Characteristics of Ovarian Cancer

Ovarian cancer encompasses a wide variety of histologic types. Epithelial ovarian cancer represents the most common histologic type of ovarian neoplasm, with non-epithelial malignancies comprising only 10% of all ovarian cancers [2,14]. Serous ovarian adenocarcinoma encompasses approximately 75-80% of epithelial ovarian carcinoma, and other epithelial histologies include mucinous, endometrioid, clear cell, Brenner, and undifferentiated carcinoma [2]. Each histologic subtype exhibits characteristics similar to those found in other tissues of the female genital tract such as the similarity between serous ovarian carcinoma and fallopian tube epithelia and between endometrioid and clear cell ovarian carcinomas with endometrial tissue. Overall, these malignant tumors have distinct stromal invasion, as well as nuclear pleomorphism and cytologic atypia. On the other hand, tumors of low-malignant potential (LMP) or borderline epithelial ovarian tumors usually have atypical epithelia consisting of cellular proliferation and pleomorphism, but they do not invade the basement membrane into the stroma. Non-epithelial malignancies include germ cell tumors, sex cord-stromal tumors, metastatic carcinoma to the ovaries, and other rare ovarian cancers, such as sarcomas and lipoid cell tumors. Most subtypes have similar clinical symptoms, evaluation, and treatment, but each one also has unique characteristics that require special consideration during patient assessment and treatment planning.

The mainstay of ovarian cancer treatment is aggressive debulking surgery to achieve optimal tumor reduction, followed by adjuvant chemotherapy. Patients presenting with early stage, low-risk (stage IA/IB, FIGO grade 1 or 2) ovarian cancer do not require adjuvant treatment after initial surgery [15,16]. However, stage IA/IB patients who present with high-risk characteristics, including high-grade tumor, clear cell histology, or malignant cells in ascites or peritoneal washings, will proceed with postoperative chemotherapy. Presentation at such an early disease stage is rare, with most ovarian cancer patients presenting with advanced-stage disease and requiring adjuvant therapy. The current standard of care for first-line chemotherapy consists of carboplatin and paclitaxel, and approximately 70% of patients achieve a complete clinical response [17]. Patients who recur within 6 months of completing a platinum-based chemotherapy regimen are considered to have platinum-resistant disease, and those with a greater than 6-month disease-free interval are classified as platinum sensitive. Second-line chemotherapy regimens vary depending on this platinum sensitivity classification. At this time, no tools exist to predict which patients are likely to be platinum resistant or platinum sensitive. Further study is required to develop new therapeutic regimens and to discover new tools to identify those patients who are likely to develop recurrent disease.

21.2.2. Developmental Aspects of Ovarian Cancer

Epithelial ovarian cancer is thought to originate from cells on the coelomic epithelial surface of the ovary or from the same cells trapped within the ovarian stroma during ovulation to create inclusion cysts. Nulliparity and incessant ovulation are considered risk factors for ovarian cancer due to repetitive trauma to the surface epithelial cells [18]. This results in repeated destruction of the surface epithelium, which requires increased cell proliferation and increased risk of DNA errors during DNA synthesis. This hypothesis has been substantiated by the increased number of ovulatory cycles present in women with p53-overexpressed tumors and the identification of MUC1 overexpression in ovarian cancer [19,20]. Additionally, the use of oral contraceptives to suppress ovulation has been associated with a reduced risk of ovarian cancer [21].

New hypotheses are being generated to speculate on alternative origins of ovarian cancer development. For example, a long-standing hypothesis is that ovarian epithelial tumors may be derived from Müllerian cells, such as in the fallopian tubes, endometrium, or endocervix. Embryologically, the ovary does not develop from the same tissues as the Müllerian structures, yet tumors derived from all these structures are remarkably similar. The fimbriae of the fallopian tubes have been suspected as a potential source of ovarian cancer origin, given the close proximity of the anatomic structures and the similar morphologies of malignant tumors arising from the fallopian tubes and the ovaries. Figure 21-1 depicts the coelomic epithelia versus Müllerian hypothesis for the origin of ovarian cancer. Increasing morphologic and molecular evidence has emerged to support ovarian cancer tumorigenesis from Müllerian tissue. Cheng *et al.* found the same members of the *HOX* gene family expressed in serous, endometrioid, and mucinous ovarian carcinomas as in normal fallopian tube, endometrium, and endocervix, respectively [22]. Techniques used to identify genomic expression patterns have also identified several genes, including *PAX2*, to be commonly overexpressed in ovarian tumors of low malignant potential, low-grade ovarian cancers, and Müllerian structures [23,24]. Additionally, several studies have suggested an association of the fallopian tube with ovarian tumorigenesis in patients with a genetic predisposition towards ovarian cancer, such as patients with *BRCA1/2* mutations [25,26]. In patients with *BRCA1/2* aberrations, *p53* signatures were present in early ovarian serous carcinoma and were found to be common in the distal fallopian tube [26].

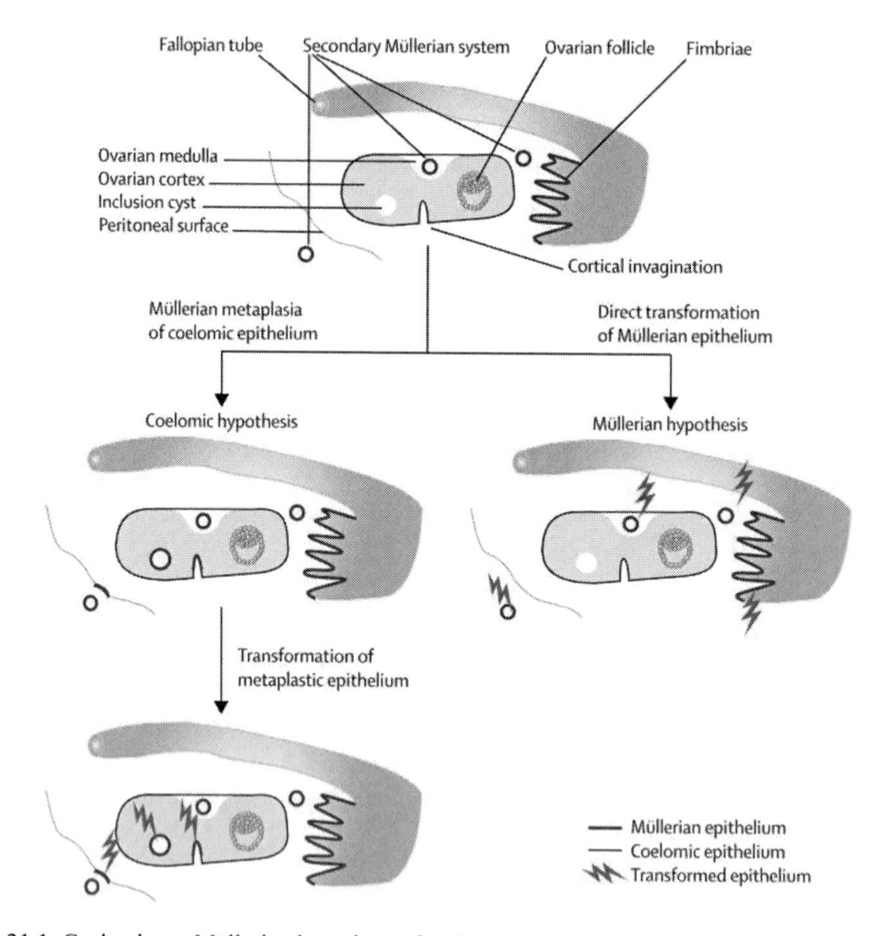

Figure 21.1. Coelomic vs. Müllerian hypotheses for the origin of ovarian, tubal, and primary peritoneal carcinomas. The coelomic hypothesis requires the ovarian epithelium (gray lines) to undergo metaplasia and change to Müllerian-like epithelium (blue lines) prior to mutation and tumorigenesis (lightning bolts). The Müllerian hypothesis does not require an intermediary step and states that Müllerian-like tumors originate directly from already existing Müllerian tumors in the fimbriae or the secondary Müllerian system [27]. (Reprinted from Dubeau, L. The cell of origin of ovarian epithelial tumours. Lancet Oncol, 2008: 9, 1191-1197 with permission from Elsevier).

Another hypothesis is that epithelial ovarian cancer develops from different cells of origin depending on tumor grade. Low-grade ovarian cancer has been commonly found in association with tumors of low malignant potential but has rare associations with high-grade ovarian carcinoma [28,29]. It has been proposed that low-grade cancers and tumors of low malignant potential develop along different pathways than high-grade ovarian carcinoma. These tumor grades differ in clinical behavior and molecular patterns. Low-grade carcinomas are typically characterized by a younger patient population, with longer overall survival, and increased platinum chemoresistance compared to high-grade carcinomas [30]. Sixty percent of ovarian low-grade cancers are found in the background of low malignant potential tumors, compared to only 2% of high-grade carcinomas [28]. Approximately 70-80% of low malignant potential tumors that recur will do so as low-grade ovarian carcinoma [31,32,33]. Furthermore, the finding that *PAX2* expression is upregulated in low-grade cancers and low malignant potential tumors, but not in high-grade cancers, further supports this hypothesis [23]. High-grade carcinomas demonstrate p53 mutations and higher expression of bcl-2 and c-kit than low-grade carcinomas, which have BRAF and KRAS mutations [34,35]. One study also reported significantly higher levels of estrogen receptor, progesterone receptor, and E-cadherin in low-grade carcinomas compared to high-grade cancer [35]. The identification of specific molecular signatures expressed by various ovarian cancer tumor specimens could help further identify the precise origins of epithelial ovarian cancer. This would enhance future research on cancer prevention and targeted cancer therapies.

21.3. Definition and Types of Molecular Signatures in Ovarian Cancer

21.3.1. Definition of Molecular Signature

Molecular signatures characterize tumors based on their genetic, protein, or translational patterns. Through the identification of these patterns, potential biomarkers may be recognized that can help identify early disease or be used to measure disease progression and treatment response. Genomic technology uncovers the DNA pattern unique to the tumor specimen. Protein signatures are usually evaluated through proteomic studies, and metabolomic signatures examining cellular metabolites are now being explored as another potential avenue for identifying unique biomarkers. Molecular signatures in the tumor, serum, or urine are being explored.

21.3.2. Genomic Expression Signatures

Genomic analysis uses various technologies to identify chromosomal abnormalities and measure the expression levels of thousands of genes. Methods such as flow cytometry and fluorescence in situ hybridization (FISH) are well-established tools for cytogenetic analysis. The measurement of DNA content in tumor cells can be evaluated with flow cytometry. Tumor ploidy is considered an independent prognostic marker in ovarian cancer [36]. Overall, early stage ovarian cancers tend to be diploid, while more advanced stage cancers are found to be aneuploid. Fluorescence in situ hybridization helps identify specific chromosomal rearrangements and can be used to detect specific loci of interest. For example, low-grade ovarian cancers frequently have increased copy numbers at 3q25-26 and 20q13, with increased copy number of 8q24 in high-grade cancers [37]. Fluorescence in situ hybridization utilizes biotin- or digioxigenin-labeled DNA probes, which are hybridized to metaphase or interphase chromosomes affixed to a microscope slide. Results are visualized by microscopy using fluorochrome reagents. Use of FISH is limited, however, owing to the high quality of cytological specimens required for the process. Additionally, chromosomal aberrations may be too complex to be identified by FISH, which may only identify crude areas of abnormality that require further investigation with more refined techniques. More recently developed applications of genomic analysis in ovarian cancer include loss of heterozygosity (LOH) analysis, comparative genomic hybridization (CGH), and transcription profiling by oligo and cDNA microarrays.

21.3.2.1. Loss of Heterozygosity

Loss of heterozygosity (LOH) analysis can identify possible locations of tumor-suppressor genes but may also provide information regarding the conglomeration of molecular and genetic alterations that has resulted in the stepwise progression of cancer development [38].

Several studies have recognized various regions deleted on LOH analysis in ovarian tumors of low malignant potential and invasive epithelial ovarian carcinoma [39]. Losses at 6q15.1-26 and 11p15 are found at higher frequency in high-grade ovarian cancers compared to all others. On the other hand, tumors of low malignant potential demonstrate a significantly lower LOH rate at most loci, with LOH occurring at 3p13-14.3 and Xq11.2-q12 in these tumors [39]. Table 21-1 lists regions frequently found to have LOH in invasive epithelial ovarian cancer.

Table 21.1. Summary of Regions Frequently Displaying LOH in Epithelial Ovarian Tumors

Chromosome	Location	Loci/Flanking loci	Physical/ Genetic distance	LOH (%)	Histopathology[a]
1p	1p36	MTHFR		43	SC
3p	3p25-pter	D3S1620		38	SC
	3p24	THRβ		33	SC
	3p13–14.3	D3S30		25–33	SC, SBOT, SBN
5q	5q13.1-21	D5S424-D5S644	22 cm	47	SC
6q	6q25.1-26	D6S473-D6S448	4 cm	44	HGSC
	6q27	D6S149	300 kb	50	SC
	6q27	D6S264-D6S297	3 cm	35–50	SC, EC, CC
7q	7q31.3	D7S655-D7S480	1300 kb	50	SC
	7q31.2	D7S486–7G14	150 kb	37	SC
	7q31.1	D7S522		73	SC
8p	8p21	D8S136		50	SC
9p	9p21	D9S171-IFNA		39	SC
	9p22-23	D9S162-D9S144		38	SC
	9q32-34	D9S16-ASS1		50	SC
10q	10q23.3	PTEN		27–42	EBN, EC, CC

Chromosome	Location	Loci/Flanking loci	Physical/ Genetic distance	LOH (%)	Histopathology[a]
11p	11p15.1	D11S1310	4 cm	47	HGSC
	11p15.3-15.5	D11S2071-D11S988	11 cm	50	HGSC
11q	11q22-23.2	D11S35-D11S925		42	SC, EC
	11q23.3-24.3	D11S934-D11S1320	8.5 mb	58–69	SC, EC
	11q23.3-qter	D11S925-D11S1336	2 mb	75	SC
		D11S912-D11S439	8 mb	67	LGSC, HGSC
12p	12p12.3-13.1	D12S89-D12S364	7 cm	26	SC
12q	12q23-qter	D12S278		30	SC
14q	14q12-13	D14S80-D14S75		45	
	14q32	D14S65-D14S267		63	
17p	17p13.3	D17S28-D17S30	15 kb	80	SC
	17q13.1	p53		35–70	SC, EC, CC, MC
17q	17q21	D17S1320-D17S1328	400 kb	65	SC
	17q25	D17S801	2 cm	60–70	SC, EC, CC, MC
18q	18q23	D18S5-D18S11		60	SC
	18q21	D18S474		36	SC
22q	22q12-q13	D22S284-CYP2D	0.5 cm	45–65	SC, EC
Xp	Xp21.1-p11.4	DXS7-DXS84		60	SC
Xq	Xq11.2-q12	DXS1161-PGK1P1	1 cm	25–60	SBOT, HGSC

[a] SC, serous carcinoma; SBOT, serous borderline ovarian tumor; SBN, serous benign tumor; HGSC, high-grade serous carcinoma; EC, endometrioid carcinoma; CC, clear cell carcinoma; EBN, endometrioid benign tumor; LGSC, low-grade serous carcinoma; MC, mucinous carcinoma. [39] (Reprinted from Mok, S. C., Elias, K. M., Wong, K. K., et al. Biomarker discovery in epithelial ovarian cancer by genomic approaches. Adv Cancer Res, 2007: 96, 1-22. with permission of Elsevier).

21.3.2.2. Comparative Genomic Hybridization

Comparative Genomic Hybridization (CGH) identifies gains and losses in DNA copy sequence through detection of gene copy number in the DNA of cells. Overexpression of tumor-promoting genes usually correlates with DNA copy gain, whereas DNA copy loss signifies underexpression of tumor-suppressing genes. The method involves differential labeling of tumor and normal DNA with distinct fluorescent molecules, followed by hybridization to normal metaphase chromosomes. The fluorescence intensities are compared using epifluorescence microscopy or quantitative image analysis, and the ratio of hybridization detected signifies the relative DNA copy number gain or loss.

Through CGH, many studies have found several areas of chromosomal gain or loss in ovarian cancer [37,40,41]. High-grade ovarian cancers typically have more copy number abnormalities than low-grade carcinomas. Gains at 1q, 2p, and 3q and losses at 4, 6q, and 8p have been found to be different in low-grade and high-grade ovarian carcinoma [42]. Poorly differentiated ovarian carcinomas have significant losses at 11p and 13q and gains at 8q and 7p compared with moderately and well differentiated ovarian cancers, which have a significant loss at 12p and gain at 18p [43]. Other regions of interest in invasive ovarian cancer identified by CGH analysis include gains at 3q26-qter, 7q32-7qter, 8q24-qter, 17q32-qter, and 20q13.2-qter and losses at 4, 13q, 16qter, 18qter, and Xq12 [40,42].

The localization of genomic aberrations can have direct clinical correlation in ovarian cancer and may signify target areas of disease progression. Several studies have examined the potential association between genome copy number and tumor grade, stage, and survival. Specifically, loss at 16q24 and the presence of more than 7 independent genome copy number abnormalities have been associated with decreased survival in ovarian cancer [40]. Other genomic aberrations found to be associated with survival include alterations present in over 20% of tumors as well as losses of chromosomes 4, 9, 16, 18, and X and gains of chromosomes 1, 3, 7, 8, and 20 [40]. Figure 21-2 shows the association between reduced survival and genomic abnormalities in ovarian cancer. Birrer *et al.* identified 4p16.3 and 5q31-5q35.3 to be strongly correlated with overall survival [44]. They found that amplification of fibroblast growth factor 1 (FGF-1) at 5q31 may lead to decreased survival in ovarian cancer patients due to increased angiogenesis. Additionally, the association between genomic alterations and recurrence of ovarian cancer has been examined. Gain of 5p, 1q41-44, 2p22-25, and 3q-26-29 and a loss of 5q14-22 are associated with higher disease recurrence rates [45,46]. Hu *et al.* found that survival time was inversely correlated with the number of genomic abnormalities in patients with recurrent ovarian cancer [46].

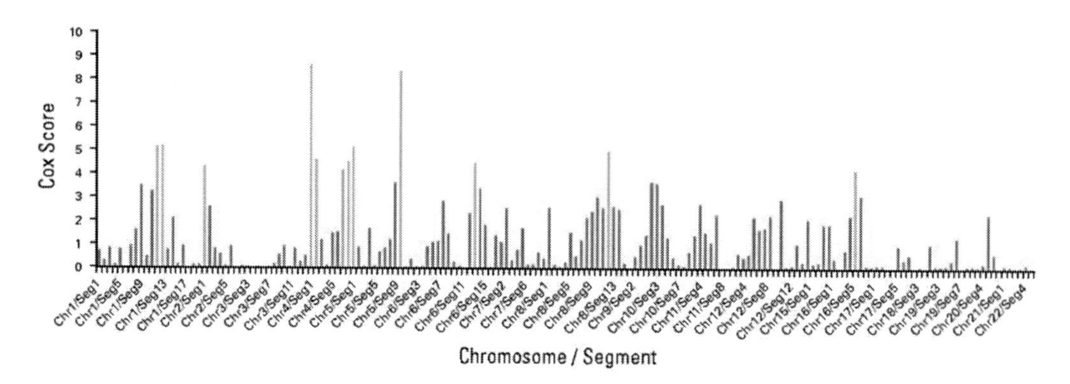

Figure 21.2. Scores for normalized chromosome segments. Bar graph showing Cox regression scores of individual chromosomal segments against overall patient survival, adjusted for debulking status. Yellow bars denote statistically significant correlation ($P < .05$) [44]. (Reprinted from Birrer, M. J., Johnson, M. E., Hao, K., et al. Whole genome oligonucleotide-based array comparative genomic hybridization analysis identified fibroblast growth factor 1 as a prognostic marker for advanced-stage serous ovarian adenocarcinomas. J. Clin. Oncol., 2007: 25, 2281-2287 with permission from the American Society of Clinical Oncology).

Associations with chemotherapy response have also been evaluated utilizing CGH. Studies have identified specific chromosomal abnormalities that occur during the development of chemotherapy resistance [47,48,49]. Kim *et al.* analyzed cancer specimens from 10 chemoresistant and 7 chemosensitive patients using high-resolution array CGH and found that the combination of losses at 13q32.1 and 8p21.1 was the most reliable marker of chemoresistant disease [48]. Additionally, Takano *et al.* identified gains of 1q21-22, including *MUC1*, in patients with platinum resistance where significantly more copy number abnormalities and higher expression levels of MUC1 were present in platinum-resistant ovarian cancer compared to platinum-sensitive disease [49].

The resolution of conventional CGH is approximately 5 Mb, and as a result, CGH is gradually being replaced by whole genome microarrays, such as the single-nucleotide polymorphism, or SNP, arrays that interrogate more than 1 million SNPs in a genome [50]. Such high-resolution SNP arrays have revealed numerous microdeletions and amplifications in ovarian cancer [50,51,52]. Etemadmoghadam *et al.* utilized SNP arrays to evaluate the association between genetic DNA copy number and primary chemoresistance in ovarian cancer [51]. They found that chemoresistant tumors had amplification of 19q12 and increased expression in cyclin E (CCNE1). Kuo *et al.* analyzed tissue from low-malignant potential tumors, low-grade, and high-grade ovarian cancers through SNP analysis. A large percentage of high-grade cancers were found to have significant amplifications and homozygous deletions compared to low-grade ovarian cancers which may identify potential tumor suppressor genes in high-grade serous ovarian carcinoma [52].

21.3.2.3. Transcription Profiling

Since the development in the mid-1990s of microarray technologies to measure the expression of slightly more than a thousand genes simultaneously [53,54], transcription profiling has changed our way of studying ovarian cancer and is becoming a standard procedure for the identification of deregulated genes/pathways in any cancer. Thousands of ovarian tumor samples and cell lines have been profiled, and the raw data are available in two public databases for further investigation [55,56]. Now, we can interrogate more than 40 thousand genes simultaneously, and even the alternative splicing variants of each gene, on a whole-genome scale.

Over the past decade, expression profiling of ovarian cancer has identified numerous potential molecular markers for early detection, prognosis, and therapeutics. Using different algorithms, such as optimized support vector machine classifiers, the use of two markers (osteopontin or kallikrein 10/matrix metalloproteinase-7) in combination with CA-125 has yielded sensitivity and specificity values for detecting early-stage disease ranging from 96% to 98.7% and 99.7% to 100%, respectively [57]. Gene signatures for chemoresistance[51] and pathways for survival have also been identified by transcription profiling [58,59]. Similarly, a 300-gene ovarian prognostic index (OPI) has been generated and validated in an independent cohort using a leave-one-out approach [60]. Transcription profiling has also identified cell-cycle- and STAT-associated targets and other pathways as potential points of therapeutic intervention for those patients with aggressive disease [61,62,63].

21.3.2.4. Mutation Signatures

Cancer is basically a genetic disease, and over the past several years, many genetic mutations have been identified in ovarian cancer. Table 21-2 lists the most common mutations that have been identified in different histological subtypes of ovarian cancer based on data retrieved from the database "The Catalogue of Somatic Mutation" [64]. Each histologic subtype has a specific gene mutation spectrum. For example, PIK3CA mutations are more commonly found in clear cell ovarian cancer, while PTEN mutations are more often found in endometrioid and mucinous ovarian cancers. CTNNB1 mutations are primarily identified in endometrioid ovarian cancer. Drugs targeting these mutations are currently being developed.

Table 21.2. Frequency of most common mutations in different histological subtypes of ovarian cancers

	BRAF	BRCA1	BRCA2	CDKN2A	CTNNB1	KRAS	PIK3CA	PTEN
Clear cell	1% (1/53)	0% (0/41)	40% (2/5)	21% (5/23)	0% (0/69)	8% (10/119)	22% (6/27)	3% (1/37)
Endometrioid	9% (8/94)	2% (1/44)	0% (0/6)	16% (10/61)	25% (70/272)	8% (21/243)	12% (19/153)	19% (31/163)
Mucinous	5% (5/86)	0% (0/40)	0% (0/2)	20% (12/60)	2% (1/41)	39% (65/163)	6% (2/30)	16% (6/36)
Serous	2% (8/327)	4% (11/246)	9% (3/34)	6% (16/239)	0% (0/190)	7% (40/518)	1% (5/360)	3% (3/118)

The number of positive samples and the total number of samples analyzed are shown in parentheses.

21.3.3. MicroRNA Signatures

MicroRNAs (miRNAs) are noncoding RNAs consisting of 19-24 nucleotides. They interact with the 3' end of targeted mRNAs, causing mRNA disruption and inhibition of translation. As a result, miRNAs have recently been shown to play a significant role in gene expression regulation [65,66]. Dysregulation of miRNA expression is increasingly recognized as a key component in human cancer development, as studies have elucidated miRNAs as either oncogenes or tumor suppressor genes [67]. MicroRNAs are found to control cell differentiation, apoptosis, and proliferation. Alterations in miRNA function may contribute to the initiation and progression of cancer [68].

Distinct miRNA signatures have been identified that can accurately distinguish tumor from normal tissue specimens and may serve as potential ovarian cancer tumor markers [69,70,71]. Iorio *et al.* identified 4 highly overexpressed miRNAs, miR-200a, miR-141, miR-200c, and miR200b, and 4 significantly underexpressed miRNAs, miR199a, miR-140, miR-145, and miR-125b1, which differentiated normal and malignant ovarian tissues [69]. They found that the expression of certain miRNA signatures correlated with specific tumor characteristics, including histology, lymphovascular invasion, and tumor involvement of the ovarian surface. Furthermore, differential levels of these miRNAs were found in circulating exosomes of ovarian cancer patients but could not be detected in normal controls, indicating the potential use of miRNA signature profiling as a diagnostic marker [72].

In addition to their diagnostic capabilities, miRNA signatures may also serve as potential prognostic indicators. Drosha and Dicer are RNAase III enzymes that function as key regulatory proteins in miRNA biogenesis and have been hypothesized to play key roles in miRNA dysfunction. Merritt *et al.* found that low Dicer expression was correlated with poor clinical outcomes in patients with epithelial ovarian cancer [73]. They observed that low Dicer expression was an independent predictor of reduced survival in ovarian cancer after examining the specimens of 111 epithelial ovarian cancer patients. Advanced tumor stage was also found to be associated with low Dicer expression levels, while low Drosha expression was associated with suboptimal surgical cytoreduction.

The *let-7* family is the best understood miRNAs. *Let*-7 miRNAs function as tumor suppressors in cancer by negatively regulating RAS, [74] HMGA2, [75,76] and c-Myc [77]. These miRNAs have been identified as potential prognostic indicators and markers of chemotherapy response. Decreased *let-7i* expression is significantly associated with reduced progression-free survival in patients with advanced ovarian cancer [68]. HMGA2 has been found to be overexpressed in advanced stage ovarian cancer and is associated with poorer prognosis [76]. Shell *et al.* identified *let-7d* as a regulator of HMGA2 expression and noted that higher *let-7d* expression was associated with lower HMGA2 expression levels [76]. In their study, the HMGA2/*let*-7 ratio was a potential prognostic indicator, since the 5-year progression-free survival rate of patients with lower ratios was 39.7%, compared to 9.6% in those with higher ratios.

Several studies have also evaluated the potential use of miRNA signatures to determine possible therapeutic regimens in the treatment of ovarian cancer. Patients with ovarian cancer resistant to cisplatin are found to have significantly reduced *let-7i* expression [68]. Various expression levels of *let-7e, miR-30c, miR-125b, miR-130a,* and *miR-335* may also play roles in the drug resistance of ovarian cancer cells to cisplatin and paclitaxel [78]. Furthermore, Boren *et al.* found 27 miRNAs and their downstream mRNA targets associated with tumor response in cell lines sensitive to cisplatin, doxorubicin, topotecan, paclitaxel, docetaxel, and gemcitabine [79]. The identification of certain miRNA signature patterns may help guide clinicians in developing patient-specific treatment plans.

21.3.4. Other Molecular Signatures

The development of advanced molecular technology has provided us with the ability to examine and search for molecular signatures specific for ovarian cancer through proteomic and metabolomic analyses. Proteomic technology evaluates the protein expression pattern of a genome, cell, tissue, or organism. Identification of novel biomarkers within the proteome can be challenging because of the many post-translational alterations that may occur based on genomic and environmental interactions as well as the differences in proteomes between cells. Recent technologic advances have graduated proteomic analysis from the basic two-dimensional polyacrylamide gel electrophoresis (PAGE) to mass spectroscopy techniques such as SELDI-TOF or MALDI-TOF, nuclear magnetic resonance (NMR) spectroscopy, and x-ray diffraction. Metabolomics evaluates signature patterns of the metabolome, which is a complex network of lipids, peptides, vitamins, protein cofactors, and other metabolic structures and products. The end product found within the metabolome ultimately depends on the interactions and alterations that occur within the genome and the proteome.

Mass spectrometry (MS) allows for determination of the mass and charge of proteins and produces large amounts of data within a very short time period. Elevated serum levels of haptoglobin-α chain and inter-α-trypsin inhibitor heavy-chain H4 (ITIH4) have been found in ovarian cancer as potential markers using MS [80,81]. Zhang *et al.* conducted a case-control study comparing serum proteomic expression patterns in 153 women with epithelial ovarian cancer, 166 women with benign pelvic masses, 142 healthy controls, and 66 women with non-epithelial ovarian cancer [81]. Downregulation of apolipoprotein A1 and transthyretin was significant in patients diagnosed with cancer, and a combination screening method assessing apolipoprotein A1, transthyretin, ITIH4, and CA-125 had higher sensitivity and specificity than CA-125 alone in an independent validation model [81]. The use of the SELDI-TOF technique with a support vector machine (SVM) has been demonstrated as a potential method to identify unique proteomic patterns that may distinguish early-stage ovarian cancer from benign conditions [82]. A seven-peak proteomic pattern was shown to distinguish between 33 advanced ovarian cancer patients and 31 control patients and was able to accurately diagnose 82% of early-stage ovarian cancers when applied to an independent validation model [82].

The use of metabolomics in ovarian cancer has been limited thus far because of the lack of an analytical platform to measure the metabolites and the large number of metabolites, which compose infinite combinations. Woo *et al.* conducted qualitative and quantitative analyses to search for potential metabolomic biomarkers in breast, ovarian, and cervical cancers [83]. They identified 3 potential ovarian biomarkers, 1-methyladenosine, 3-methyluridine, and 4-androstene-3, 17-dione, which were significantly elevated in urine specimens of patients with ovarian cancer. The clinical applicability of this technique still requires validation, however. Further investigation into the role of metabolomics as novel tumor markers in ovarian cancer is ongoing, but the approach may be promising as more advanced and mature technologic tools are developed.

21.4. Clinical Utility of Molecular Signatures in Ovarian Cancer

21.4.1. CA-125

CA-125 has been the most studied ovarian cancer biologic marker. The positive predictive value for ovarian cancer diagnosis in postmenopausal patients with an adnexal mass and CA-125 > 95 U/mL is estimated at 96% [2]. CA-125 was first identified in 1981 and is elevated in various malignant and benign diseases, including ovarian cancer, endometriosis, pregnancy, and benign conditions of the ovary. The sensitivity and specificity of CA-125 alone as a screening tool for ovarian cancer is lacking. Approximately 80% of patients with epithelial ovarian cancer have CA-125 levels >35 U/mL [84]. As a result, multiple studies have attempted to evaluate the use of CA-125 in conjunction with other tumor markers or with radiologic imaging, such as transvaginal ultrasonography, in order to improve test specificity and sensitivity.

The results of two large studies examining the effectiveness of multimodal screening have been published recently. The UK Collaborative Trial of Ovarian Cancer Screening (UKCTOCS) randomly assigned over 200,000 women between 50 and 74 years old to 3 different screening treatment arms: 1) no treatment, 2) annual CA-125 screening with follow-up transvaginal ultrasonography, or 3) annual screening with transvaginal ultrasonography alone [6]. The study found improved specificity for primary invasive ovarian and fallopian tube carcinomas of 99.8% with the combination of CA-125 and ultrasonography, but the positive predictive value was still poor at 35.1%. Similar results were found in the Prostate, Lung, Colorectal, and Ovarian (PLCO) cancer screening trial, which enrolled over 34,000 women to examine the efficacy of screening with CA-125 and transvaginal ultrasonography [11]. These trials found the approach of using CA-125 in conjunction with ultrasonography to be feasible for identifying ovarian cancer. However, the overall impact of these screening tests on mortality is still under analysis for both trials.

21.4.2. Molecular Signatures for Diagnosis of Ovarian Cancer

Detection of ovarian cancer in its early stages poses a large challenge. The identification of specific molecular signatures for the various histologic subtypes would help with biomarker identification. Oftentimes, newly identified ovarian cancer biomarkers have increased sensitivity in certain histologic types but are very poorly expressed in other types. As a result, there is no specific screening model that achieves the sensitivity and specificity necessary for accurate diagnosis. Due to the heterogeneity of the disease, early diagnosis of ovarian cancer will require a panel of tumor markers.

Several studies have examined other biomarkers to assess their sensitivity, specificity, and predictive value for detecting ovarian cancer independently or in combination. Simon *et al.* identified, through genomic analysis, B7-H4, Spondin 2, and DcR3 as differentially overexpressed genes in ovarian cancer [85]. They tested these markers in samples of healthy women and ovarian cancer patients to establish differential expression and compared their diagnostic abilities with that of CA-125. Their results demonstrated that the detection of these tumor markers may assist with early ovarian cancer diagnosis. Highly elevated expression levels of HE4 have been found in serous and endometrioid ovarian tumors, with relative specificity for ovarian cancer [86,87]. One study also analyzed the gene expression profiling of 42 epithelial ovarian cancers of different stages, grades, and subtypes and found that all tumors were detected with a combination of CLDN3, CA-125, MUC1, and VEGF [86]. They concluded that the combination of a limited number of biomarkers could identify the majority of ovarian cancer cases despite the heterogeneity of the disease. Meinhold-Heerlein *et al.* found 275 genes that encode proteins with increased or decreased expression in ovarian cancer [57]. Using a series of 67 ovarian cancer patients compared to 67 healthy controls, they recognized that various combinations of osteopontin, kallikrein 10, and metalloproteinase-7, as well as CA-125, were able to discern disease with a sensitivity of approximately 98% and specificity of 100%. Additionally, a recent study of a blood-based assay using 11 biomarkers (CA-125, CA-19-9, EGFR, C-reactive protein, myoglobin, apolipoprotein A1, apolipoprotein CIII, MIP-1alpha, IL-6, IL-18, and tenascin C) had 91.3% sensitivity and 88.5% specificity when tested on 187 controls and 176 cases of ovarian cancer [88]. Further blinded clinical validation studies are necessary to determine the appropriate combination of tumor markers for screening, but thus far, these results appear promising.

21.4.3. Molecular Signatures for Treatment Planning

Tumor markers are often also used to monitor a patient's response to surgery, chemotherapy, or radiation therapy. Gynecologic oncologists aim to reduce the disease burden to less than 1 centimeter at the time of tumor debulking surgery, but often, despite optimal cytoreduction, residual disease remains that cannot be detected on physical examination or radiologic imaging. As a result, biomarkers are often used as a surrogate indicator of disease burden and can be extremely helpful in determining if patients are responding appropriately to their prescribed treatment regimen. Rising CA-125 levels correlate with disease progression or recurrence in 90% of cases, and persistently elevated CA125 levels often indicate increasing disease burden [89].

Novel biologic therapies are emerging to target tumors that express specific proteins, growth factors, and signaling pathways. Approximately 20-30% of ovarian cancer patients overexpress ErbB2 (HER2), a growth factor noted for its role in the carcinogenesis of breast cancer [90]. Trastuzumab, a monoclonal antibody to HER2, is currently approved by the US Food and Drug Administration for use in breast cancer patients expressing HER2. The Gynecologic Oncology Group (GOG) evaluated the use of trastuzumab in a phase II trial in ovarian cancer [91]. After screening 837 patients for HER2 overexpression, 95 patients were found to be eligible for study enrollment, and only 45 of the 95 patients participated in the study. The GOG found a 7.3% response rate with trastuzumab and noted that serum HER2 levels were not associated with clinical outcome. Based on these results, they concluded that the utility of single-agent trastuzumab was limited in ovarian cancer owing to the low incidence of HER2 overexpression and poor response rate.

Several new biologic agents have been designed to target the PI3K/Akt pathway, such as the MTOR inhibitor RAD001. Amplifications and mutations of PI3K are found in 30% of ovarian cancer cases, and 12% of ovarian cancer patients overexpress AKT2, a downstream target of PI3K [92,93]. Phase I trials of drugs inhibiting these pathways are currently being conducted. One phase I trial evaluating everolimus, an MTOR inhibitor, in combination with paclitaxel has been conducted in patients with solid tumors, including 3 ovarian cancer patients, and was found to have an acceptable safety profile, warranting further clinical evaluation of the drug combination [94]. To date, no phase II trials have been conducted with these agents in ovarian cancer. The discovery of these agents is promising, however. Twenty-two percent of clear cell ovarian carcinomas have PIK3CA mutations (Table 21-2), which may be a future biologic treatment target in a disease that is traditionally extremely chemoresistant with poor prognosis.

Great strides have been made to target vascular endothelial growth factor (VEGF) in the treatment of ovarian cancer. VEGF is an angiogenic promoter and ligand that binds VEGF receptor 2 and triggers the angiogenic signaling pathway. Studies have shown that angiogenesis and neovascularization are crucial steps in tumor growth, invasion, and metastases [95,96]. Development of neutralizing anti-VEGF monoclonal antibodies has allowed for disruption of tumor angiogenesis. Bevacizumab is a monoclonal antibody that binds VEGF-A to inhibit angiogenesis. Many studies have evaluated the use of bevacizumab as a single agent or in combination with chemotherapy in ovarian cancer and have found strong response rates as well as prolonged progression-free and overall survival [97,98,99,100]. Currently, the GOG is conducting a phase III trial examining the efficacy of bevacizumab with carboplatin and paclitaxel as first-line treatment in patients with ovarian cancer. In addition to anti-VEGF monoclonal antibodies, VEGF Trap is another drug that targets VEGF to inhibit angiogenesis. It is a soluble decoy receptor with high affinity to VEGF, which prevents VEGF from binding to its physiologic receptors [101]. Phase I and II trials are being conducted to determine the potential use of VEGF Trap in ovarian cancer.

21.4.4. Molecular Signatures for Prognosis

Prognostic factors are often used to develop individualized treatment approaches in patients diagnosed with ovarian cancer. Various pathologic and clinical factors have been identified as strong prognostic markers in ovarian cancer. These include FIGO stage of disease at the time of presentation, histology, tumor grade, age, performance status, platinum sensitivity, presence of ascites, and presence of residual disease after cytoreductive surgery. The addition of molecular signatures to identify prognostic biomarkers can contribute to a clinician's ability to appropriately counsel patients regarding survival as well as to create specific treatment plans.

The prognostic value of *BRCA1* and *BRCA2* in ovarian cancer is unknown at this time. Most studies have found a favorable outcome in patients with *BRCA* mutations [102,103,104,105]. A recent case-control study compared survival in 22 *BRCA1*- and *BRCA2*-positive patients and 44 patients with sporadic ovarian cancer [102]. All patients were matched based on disease stage, histologic subtype, age, and year of diagnosis, and all had received primary platinum-based chemotherapy. *BRCA*-positive patients had higher response rates to chemotherapy and longer treatment-free intervals and overall survival compared to the control patients. Median overall survival was 8.4 years in *BRCA* patients compared to 2.9 years in the control group. The exact mechanism for this protective factor is still speculative. Some hypothesize that *BRCA*-associated tumors are more chemosensitive owing to increased cell proliferation rates [106] or the inability to repair DNA damage after chemotherapy exposure [107].

Another gene well studied in ovarian cancer for its prognostic and potential therapeutic value is *TP53*, a tumor suppressor gene found on the short arm of chromosome 17. *TP53* functions through DNA surveillance and repair during G1 of the cell cycle, and as a result, *TP53* mutations are found in over 50% of all human cancers. Overall, p53 mutations have been associated with poor patient outcome in ovarian cancer, but no consistent evidence supports the independent use of p53 as a marker of adverse prognosis. Dogan *et al.* analyzed tumor specimens from 82 patients and found that p53 expression correlated with higher-grade disease, positive cytology results, presence of residual tumor, and disease stage [108]. They noted that patients with p53 positivity had an overall survival of 36 months compared to 53 months for patients with tumor specimens that were negative for p53 ($p<0.05$). However, after multivariate analysis, p53 was not found to be a significant prognostic covariate. Bali *et al.* also demonstrated that p53 was a potential predictor of poor outcome in ovarian cancer when evaluated in combination with p21(Waf1/Cip1) [109]. Additionally, meta-analysis of the prognostic value of *TP53*, EGFR, and HER2 found a pooled hazard ratio of 1.47 (CI 1.33-1.61) for p53, 1.65 (CI 1.25-2.19) for EGFR, and 1.67 (CI 1.34-2.08) for HER2 [110]. However, the study noted significant publication bias and potential confounding factors, which influenced the published results. As a result, the utilization of p53 as a prognostic indicator is still controversial.

Many other potential molecular biomarkers are being evaluated as possible prognostic markers. Varying levels of E-cadherin and epithelial cell adhesion molecule may be associated with prognostic significance [111]. Increased claudin-3 and claudin-7 levels have also been found to indicate poorer prognosis, with decreased overall survival, in patients with ovarian carcinoma [112]'[62,63].

21.4.5. Molecular Signatures of Germ Cell and Stromal Ovarian Tumors

Germ cell tumors arise from germ cells in normal ovarian tissue and can be classified into 3 classes: benign teratomas, malignant tumors arising from teratomas, and malignant germ cell tumors. Overall, malignant germ cell tumors account for 5% of all ovarian malignancies with 30-40% of these occurring as dysgerminomas and the remaining germ cell tumors comprising of endodermal sinus tumors, embryonal carcinomas, choriocarcinomas, polyembryomas, and mixed germ cell tumors [14]. The majority of germ cell tumors occur in adolescents and young adults, with a median age at diagnosis of 16 years [113]. Stromal tumors are also rare malignancies and only account for 5-8% of all malignant ovarian neoplasm's [14]. These tumors are derived from the sex cords and ovarian stroma and are either granulosa/theca cell tumors or Sertoli/Leydig cell tumors.

Few studies have been performed to examine the molecular signatures of germ cell and stromal tumors. Diagnosis of these tumors is often based on certain tumor marker levels. Elevated alpha-fetoprotein (AFP) levels usually indicate the presence of endodermal sinus tumors, but serum levels of AFP do not appear to correlate with prognosis [114,115]. β-HCG levels are usually elevated in patients diagnosed with choriocarcinoma. Like AFP, preoperative β-HCG appears to have no prognostic value individually [115]. However, increased β-HCG in conjunction with elevated AFP levels portends a poor prognosis and may indicated poor treatment response [115]. Due to the rarity of these diseases, the identification of other molecular signatures and biomarkers specific to germ cell and stromal ovarian malignancies has not advanced greatly. However, further research is being conducted to examine the potential application of targeted chemotherapeutic and the impact on survival and progression for these tumors, similar to epithelial ovarian cancer.

21.5. Future Directions

Although over a dozen studies have reported promising molecular signatures for diagnosis, prognosis, or treatment response in ovarian cancer, these molecular signatures still need further validation. In addition to having small sample sizes, most previous studies included ovarian cancers of different histological subtypes, grades, and stages. As a result, the molecular signatures for chemoresponse or survival may be confounded by the heterogeneity of the tumor samples or other uncontrolled confounding factors such as the physiological conditions of the patients. In a recent evaluation of 21 survival biomarkers separately in each histological subtype, only 3 still correlated with survival in high-grade serous cancer [116]. Thus, a collaborative effort to archive a large collection of well-annotated tumor samples for future validation is needed. Currently, a large-scale collaborative effort, The Cancer Genome Atlas (TCGA) project, is under way to generate massive data on gene methylation patterns, exon expression, miRNA expression, somatic mutations, and copy number variations on a set of well-annotated ovarian tumor samples of advanced stage serous histological subtype. The phase I portion of the TCGA project is completed, and the molecular characterization data for ovarian cancer are available via the TCGA Data Portal [117]. This ongoing data generation and analysis study of hundreds of samples will certainly provide the next generation of integrated molecular signatures for clinical utility studies. We hope that a highly specific and sensitive test for integrated molecular signatures will be available in the near future for the early detection, therapeutic intervention, and prevention of ovarian cancer.

As the cost of whole genome sequencing has decreased substantially over the past few years, we anticipate that the sequencing of whole genomes for mutations, copy number variation (CNV), and gene expression will provide a new spectrum of mutations and integrated genomic data for cancer prevention, therapeutics, and prognosis. It is conceivable that one day whole genome sequencing analysis will be a standard test during the initial evaluation of and treatment planning for cancer patients.

Conclusion

The large-scale measurement of SNP, CNV, noncoding RNA, miRNA, mutations, mRNA, proteins, and other biomolecules in cancer cells has become feasible and will revolutionize future patient care. Over the past decade, we have gained a better understanding of the complexity and heterogeneity of ovarian cancer. By stratifying these ovarian cancers into biologically relevant subgroups using an integrated genomic approach, we should be able to develop more sensitive and specific molecular signatures for diagnosis, prognosis, and therapeutic decision-making on an individual basis in the near future.

References

[1] (2009) Overview: Ovarian Cancer; How many women get ovarian cancer? : American Cancer Society.

[2] Berek J (2005) Epithelial Ovarian Cancer. In: Berek JS, Hacker NF, editors. Practical Gynecologic Oncology. Fourth ed. Philadelphia: Lippincott Williams and Wilkins. pp. 443-510.

[3] Hoskins WJ (1995) Prospective on ovarian cancer: why prevent? *J. Cell Biochem. Suppl.* 23: 189-199.

[4] Mol BW, Boll D, De Kanter M, Heintz AP, Sijmons EA, et al. (2001) Distinguishing the benign and malignant adnexal mass: an external validation of prognostic models. *Gynecol. Oncol.* 80: 162-167.

[5] Menon U, Skates SJ, Lewis S, Rosenthal AN, Rufford B, et al. (2005) Prospective study using the risk of ovarian cancer algorithm to screen for ovarian cancer. *J. Clin. Oncol.* 23: 7919-7926.

[6] Menon U, Gentry-Maharaj A, Hallett R, Ryan A, Burnell M, et al. (2009) Sensitivity and specificity of multimodal and ultrasound screening for ovarian cancer, and stage distribution of detected cancers: results of the prevalence screen of the UK Collaborative Trial of Ovarian Cancer Screening (UKCTOCS). *Lancet Oncol.* 10: 327-340.

[7] Partridge E, Kreimer AR, Greenlee RT, Williams C, Xu JL, et al. (2009) Results from four rounds of ovarian cancer screening in a randomized trial. *Obstet. Gynecol.* 113: 775-782.

[8] van Nagell JR, Jr., DePriest PD, Ueland FR, DeSimone CP, Cooper AL, et al. (2007) Ovarian cancer screening with annual transvaginal sonography: findings of 25,000 women screened. *Cancer* 109: 1887-1896.

[9] Einhorn N, Sjovall K, Knapp RC, Hall P, Scully RE, et al. (1992) Prospective evaluation of serum CA 125 levels for early detection of ovarian cancer. *Obstet. Gynecol.* 80: 14-18.

[10] Jacobs IJ, Skates S, Davies AP, Woolas RP, Jeyerajah A, et al. (1996) Risk of diagnosis of ovarian cancer after raised serum CA 125 concentration: a prospective cohort study. *Bmj* 313: 1355-1358.

[11] Buys SS, Partridge E, Greene MH, Prorok PC, Reding D, et al. (2005) Ovarian cancer screening in the Prostate, Lung, Colorectal and Ovarian (PLCO) cancer screening trial: findings from the initial screen of a randomized trial. *Am. J. Obstet. Gynecol.* 193: 1630-1639.

[12] Armstrong DK, Armstrong DK (2002) Relapsed ovarian cancer: challenges and management strategies for a chronic disease. *Oncologist* 7 Suppl 5: 20-28.

[13] Tung CS, Wong KK, Mok SC (2008) Biomarker discovery in ovarian cancer. *Womens Health* (Lond Engl) 4: 27-40.

[14] Berek JS, Hacker NF (2005) Nonepithelial Ovarian and Fallopian Tube Cancers. In: Berek JS, Hacker NF, editors. Practical Gynecologic Oncology. 4th ed. Philadelphia, PA: Lippincott Williams and Wilkins. pp. 511-543.

[15] Guthrie D, Davy ML, Philips PR (1984) A study of 656 patients with "early" ovarian cancer. *Gynecol. Oncol.* 17: 363-369.

[16] Young RC, Walton LA, Ellenberg SS, Homesley HD, Wilbanks GD, et al. (1990) Adjuvant therapy in stage I and stage II epithelial ovarian cancer. Results of two prospective randomized trials. *N. Engl. J. Med.* 322: 1021-1027.

[17] Auersperg N, Edelson MI, Mok SC, Johnson SW, Hamilton TC (1998) The biology of ovarian cancer. *Semin Oncol* 25: 281-304.

[18] Fathalla MF (1971) Incessant ovulation--a factor in ovarian neoplasia? *Lancet* 2: 163.

[19] Schildkraut JM, Bastos E, Berchuck A (1997) Relationship between lifetime ovulatory cycles and overexpression of mutant p53 in epithelial ovarian cancer. *J. Natl. Cancer Inst.* 89: 932-938.

[20] Terry KL, Titus-Ernstoff L, McKolanis JR, Welch WR, Finn OJ, et al. (2007) Incessant ovulation, mucin 1 immunity, and risk for ovarian cancer. *Cancer Epidemiol. Biomarkers Prev.* 16: 30-35.

[21] Tworoger SS, Fairfield KM, Colditz GA, Rosner BA, Hankinson SE (2007) Association of oral contraceptive use, other contraceptive methods, and infertility with ovarian cancer risk. *Am. J. Epidemiol.* 166: 894-901.

[22] Cheng W, Liu J, Yoshida H, Rosen D, Naora H (2005) Lineage infidelity of epithelial ovarian cancers is controlled by HOX genes that specify regional identity in the reproductive tract. *Nat. Med.* 11: 531-537.

[23] Tung CS, Mok SC, Tsang YT, Zu Z, Song H, et al. (2009) PAX2 expression in low malignant potential ovarian tumors and low-grade ovarian serous carcinomas. *Mod. Pathol.*

[24] Tong GX, Chiriboga L, Hamele-Bena D, Borczuk AC (2007) Expression of PAX2 in papillary serous carcinoma of the ovary: immunohistochemical evidence of fallopian tube or secondary Mullerian system origin? *Mod. Pathol.* 20: 856-863.

[25] Colgan TJ, Murphy J, Cole DE, Narod S, Rosen B (2001) Occult carcinoma in prophylactic oophorectomy specimens: prevalence and association with BRCA germline mutation status. *Am. J. Surg. Pathol.* 25: 1283-1289.

[26] Folkins AK, Jarboe EA, Saleemuddin A, Lee Y, Callahan MJ, et al. (2008) A candidate precursor to pelvic serous cancer (p53 signature) and its prevalence in ovaries and fallopian tubes from women with BRCA mutations. *Gynecol. Oncol.* 109: 168-173.

[27] Dubeau L (2008) The cell of origin of ovarian epithelial tumours. *Lancet Oncol.* 9: 1191-1197.

[28] Malpica A, Deavers MT, Lu K, Bodurka DC, Atkinson EN, et al. (2004) Grading ovarian serous carcinoma using a two-tier system. *Am. J. Surg. Pathol.* 28: 496-504.

[29] Dehari R, Kurman RJ, Logani S, Shih Ie M (2007) The development of high-grade serous carcinoma from atypical proliferative (borderline) serous tumors and low-grade micropapillary serous carcinoma: a morphologic and molecular genetic analysis. *Am. J. Surg. Pathol.* 31: 1007-1012.

[30] Gershenson DM, Sun CC, Lu KH, Coleman RL, Sood AK, et al. (2006) Clinical behavior of stage II-IV low-grade serous carcinoma of the ovary. *Obstet. Gynecol.* 108: 361-368.

[31] Longacre TA, McKenney JK, Tazelaar HD, Kempson RL, Hendrickson MR (2005) Ovarian serous tumors of low malignant potential (borderline tumors): outcome-based study of 276 patients with long-term (> or =5-year) follow-up. *Am. J. Surg. Pathol.* 29: 707-723.

[32] Crispens MA, Bodurka D, Deavers M, Lu K, Silva EG, et al. (2002) Response and survival in patients with progressive or recurrent serous ovarian tumors of low malignant potential. *Obstet. Gynecol.* 99: 3-10.

[33] Silva EG, Gershenson DM, Malpica A, Deavers M (2006) The recurrence and the overall survival rates of ovarian serous borderline neoplasms with noninvasive implants is time dependent. *Am. J. Surg. Pathol.* 30: 1367-1371.

[34] O'Neill CJ, Deavers MT, Malpica A, Foster H, McCluggage WG (2005) An immunohistochemical comparison between low-grade and high-grade ovarian serous carcinomas: significantly higher expression of p53, MIB1, BCL2, HER-2/neu, and C-KIT in high-grade neoplasms. *Am. J. Surg. Pathol.* 29: 1034-1041.

[35] Wong KK, Lu KH, Malpica A, Bodurka DC, Shvartsman HS, et al. (2007) Significantly greater expression of ER, PR, and ECAD in advanced-stage low-grade ovarian serous carcinoma as revealed by immunohistochemical analysis. *Int. J. Gynecol. Pathol.* 26: 404-409.

[36] Foulkes W, Shelling AN (2000) Molecular Genetics of Ovarian Cancer. In: Bartlett JMS, editor. Ovarian Cancer: Methods and Protocols. Totowa, NJ: Humana Press. pp. 273-290.

[37] Iwabuchi H, Sakamoto M, Sakunaga H, Ma YY, Carcangiu ML, et al. (1995) Genetic analysis of benign, low-grade, and high-grade ovarian tumors. *Cancer Res.* 55: 6172-6180.

[38] Thiagalingam S, Laken S, Willson JK, Markowitz SD, Kinzler KW, et al. (2001) Mechanisms underlying losses of heterozygosity in human colorectal cancers. *Proc. Natl. Acad. Sci. USA* 98: 2698-2702.

[39] Mok SC, Elias KM, Wong KK, Ho K, Bonome T, et al. (2007) Biomarker discovery in epithelial ovarian cancer by genomic approaches. *Adv. Cancer Res.* 96: 1-22.

[40] Suzuki S, Moore DH, 2nd, Ginzinger DG, Godfrey TE, Barclay J, et al. (2000) An approach to analysis of large-scale correlations between genome changes and clinical endpoints in ovarian cancer. *Cancer Res.* 60: 5382-5385.

[41] Sonoda G, Palazzo J, du Manoir S, Godwin AK, Feder M, et al. (1997) Comparative genomic hybridization detects frequent overrepresentation of chromosomal material from 3q26, 8q24, and 20q13 in human ovarian carcinomas. Gen*es Chromosomes Cancer* 20: 320-328.

[42] Gray JW, Suzuki S, Kuo WL, Polikoff D, Deavers M, et al. (2003) Specific keynote: genome copy number abnormalities in ovarian cancer. *Gynecol. Oncol.* 88: S16-21; discussion S22-14.

[43] Kiechle M, Jacobsen A, Schwarz-Boeger U, Hedderich J, Pfisterer J, et al. (2001) Comparative genomic hybridization detects genetic imbalances in primary ovarian carcinomas as correlated with grade of differentiation. *Cancer* 91: 534-540.

[44] Birrer MJ, Johnson ME, Hao K, Wong KK, Park DC, et al. (2007) Whole genome oligonucleotide-based array comparative genomic hybridization analysis identified fibroblast growth factor 1 as a prognostic marker for advanced-stage serous ovarian adenocarcinomas. *J. Clin. Oncol.* 25: 2281-2287.

[45] Bruchim I, Israeli O, Mahmud SM, Aviram-Goldring A, Rienstein S, et al. (2009) Genetic alterations detected by comparative genomic hybridization and recurrence rate in epithelial ovarian carcinoma. *Cancer Genet. Cytogenet.* 190: 66-70.

[46] Hu J, Khanna V, Jones MW, Surti U (2003) Comparative study of primary and recurrent ovarian serous carcinomas: comparative genomic hybridization analysis with a potential application for prognosis. *Gynecol. Oncol.* 89: 369-375.

[47] Eckstein N, Servan K, Hildebrandt B, Politz A, von Jonquieres G, et al. (2009) Hyperactivation of the insulin-like growth factor receptor I signaling pathway is an essential event for cisplatin resistance of ovarian cancer cells. *Cancer Res.* 69: 2996-3003.

[48] Kim SW, Kim JW, Kim YT, Kim JH, Kim S, et al. (2007) Analysis of chromosomal changes in serous ovarian carcinoma using high-resolution array comparative genomic hybridization: Potential predictive markers of chemoresistant disease. *Genes. Chromosomes Cancer* 46: 1-9.

[49] Takano M, Fujii K, Kita T, Kikuchi Y, Uchida K (2004) Amplicon profiling reveals cytoplasmic overexpression of MUC1 protein as an indicator of resistance to platinum-based chemotherapy in patients with ovarian cancer. *Oncol. Rep.* 12: 1177-1182.

[50] Gorringe KL, Jacobs S, Thompson ER, Sridhar A, Qiu W, et al. (2007) High-resolution single nucleotide polymorphism array analysis of epithelial ovarian cancer reveals numerous microdeletions and amplifications. *Clin. Cancer Res.* 13: 4731-4739.

[51] Etemadmoghadam D, deFazio A, Beroukhim R, Mermel C, George J, et al. (2009) Integrated genome-wide DNA copy number and expression analysis identifies distinct mechanisms of primary chemoresistance in ovarian carcinomas. *Clin. Cancer Res.* 15: 1417-1427.

[52] Kuo KT, Guan B, Feng Y, Mao TL, Chen X, et al. (2009) Analysis of DNA copy number alterations in ovarian serous tumors identifies new molecular genetic changes in low-grade and high-grade carcinomas. *Cancer Res.* 69: 4036-4042.

[53] Schena M, Shalon D, Heller R, Chai A, Brown PO, et al. (1996) Parallel human genome analysis: microarray-based expression monitoring of 1000 genes. *Proc. Natl. Acad. Sci. USA* 93: 10614-10619.
[54] Schena M, Shalon D, Davis RW, Brown PO (1995) Quantitative monitoring of gene expression patterns with a complementary DNA microarray. *Science* 270: 467-470.
[55] GEO: http://www.ncbi.nlm.nih.gov/geo/.
[56] ArrayExpress: http://www.ebi.ac.uk/microarray-as/ae/.
[57] Meinhold-Heerlein I, Bauerschlag D, Zhou Y, Sapinoso LM, Ching K, et al. (2007) An integrated clinical-genomics approach identifies a candidate multi-analyte blood test for serous ovarian carcinoma. *Clin. Cancer Res.* 13: 458-466.
[58] Murph MM, Liu W, Yu S, Lu Y, Hall H, et al. (2009) Lysophosphatidic acid-induced transcriptional profile represents serous epithelial ovarian carcinoma and worsened prognosis. *PLoS One* 4: e5583.
[59] Crijns AP, Fehrmann RS, de Jong S, Gerbens F, Meersma GJ, et al. (2009) Survival-related profile, pathways, and transcription factors in ovarian cancer. *PLoS Med.* 6: e24.
[60] Denkert C, Budczies J, Darb-Esfahani S, Gyorffy B, Sehouli J, et al. (2009) A prognostic gene expression index in ovarian cancer - validation across different independent data sets. *J. Pathol.* 218: 273-280.
[61] Meinhold-Heerlein I, Bauerschlag D, Hilpert F, Dimitrov P, Sapinoso LM, et al. (2005) Molecular and prognostic distinction between serous ovarian carcinomas of varying grade and malignant potential. *Oncogene* 24: 1053-1065.
[62] Yap TA, Carden CP, Kaye SB (2009) Beyond chemotherapy: targeted therapies in ovarian cancer. *Nat. Rev. Cancer* 9: 167-181.
[63] Bast RC, Jr., Hennessy B, Mills GB (2009) The biology of ovarian cancer: new opportunities for translation. *Nat. Rev. Cancer* 9: 415-428.
[64] Bartel DP (2004) MicroRNAs: genomics, biogenesis, mechanism, and function. *Cell* 116: 281-297.
[65] Coticchia CM, Yang J, Moses MA (2008) Ovarian cancer biomarkers: current options and future promise. *J. Natl. Compr. Canc. Netw.* 6: 795-802.
[66] Zhang L, Volinia S, Bonome T, Calin GA, Greshock J, et al. (2008) Genomic and epigenetic alterations deregulate microRNA expression in human epithelial ovarian cancer. *Proc. Natl. Acad. Sci. USA* 105: 7004-7009.
[67] Yang N, Kaur S, Volinia S, Greshock J, Lassus H, et al. (2008) MicroRNA microarray identifies Let-7i as a novel biomarker and therapeutic target in human epithelial ovarian cancer. *Cancer Res.* 68: 10307-10314.
[68] Iorio MV, Visone R, Di Leva G, Donati V, Petrocca F, et al. (2007) MicroRNA signatures in human ovarian cancer. *Cancer Res.* 67: 8699-8707.
[69] Resnick KE, Alder H, Hagan JP, Richardson DL, Croce CM, et al. (2009) The detection of differentially expressed microRNAs from the serum of ovarian cancer patients using a novel real-time PCR platform. *Gynecol. Oncol.* 112: 55-59.
[70] Bearfoot JL, Choong DY, Gorringe KL, Campbell IG (2008) Genetic analysis of cancer-implicated MicroRNA in ovarian cancer. *Clin. Cancer Res.* 14: 7246-7250.
[71] Taylor DD, Gercel-Taylor C (2008) MicroRNA signatures of tumor-derived exosomes as diagnostic biomarkers of ovarian cancer. *Gynecol. Oncol.* 110: 13-21.
[72] Merritt WM, Lin YG, Han LY, Kamat AA, Spannuth WA, et al. (2008) Dicer, Drosha, and outcomes in patients with ovarian cancer. *N. Engl. J. Med.* 359: 2641-2650.

[73] Johnson SM, Grosshans H, Shingara J, Byrom M, Jarvis R, et al. (2005) RAS is regulated by the let-7 microRNA family. *Cell* 120: 635-647.

[74] Lee YS, Dutta A (2007) The tumor suppressor microRNA let-7 represses the HMGA2 oncogene. *Genes Dev.* 21: 1025-1030.

[75] Shell S, Park SM, Radjabi AR, Schickel R, Kistner EO, et al. (2007) Let-7 expression defines two differentiation stages of cancer. *Proc. Natl. Acad. Sci. USA* 104: 11400-11405.

[76] Sampson VB, Rong NH, Han J, Yang Q, Aris V, et al. (2007) MicroRNA let-7a down-regulates MYC and reverts MYC-induced growth in Burkitt lymphoma cells. *Cancer Res.* 67: 9762-9770.

[77] Sorrentino A, Liu CG, Addario A, Peschle C, Scambia G, et al. (2008) Role of microRNAs in drug-resistant ovarian cancer cells. *Gynecol. Oncol.* 111: 478-486.

[78] Boren T, Xiong Y, Hakam A, Wenham R, Apte S, et al. (2009) MicroRNAs and their target messenger RNAs associated with ovarian cancer response to chemotherapy. *Gynecol. Oncol.* 113: 249-255.

[79] Ye B, Cramer DW, Skates SJ, Gygi SP, Pratomo V, et al. (2003) Haptoglobin-alpha subunit as potential serum biomarker in ovarian cancer: identification and characterization using proteomic profiling and mass spectrometry. *Clin. Cancer Res.* 9: 2904-2911.

[80] Zhang Z, Bast RC, Jr., Yu Y, Li J, Sokoll LJ, et al. (2004) Three biomarkers identified from serum proteomic analysis for the detection of early stage ovarian cancer. *Cancer Res.* 64: 5882-5890.

[81] Wang J, Zhang X, Ge X, Guo H, Xiong G, et al. (2008) Proteomic studies of early-stage and advanced ovarian cancer patients. *Gynecol. Oncol.* 111: 111-119.

[82] Woo HM, Kim KM, Choi MH, Jung BH, Lee J, et al. (2009) Mass spectrometry based metabolomic approaches in urinary biomarker study of women's cancers. *Clin. Chim. Acta.* 400: 63-69.

[83] Canney PA, Moore M, Wilkinson PM, James RD (1984) Ovarian cancer antigen CA125: a prospective clinical assessment of its role as a tumour marker. *Br. J. Cancer* 50: 765-769.

[84] Simon I, Liu Y, Krall KL, Urban N, Wolfert RL, et al. (2007) Evaluation of the novel serum markers B7-H4, Spondin 2, and DcR3 for diagnosis and early detection of ovarian cancer. *Gynecol. Oncol.* 106: 112-118.

[85] Lu KH, Patterson AP, Wang L, Marquez RT, Atkinson EN, et al. (2004) Selection of potential markers for epithelial ovarian cancer with gene expression arrays and recursive descent partition analysis. *Clin. Cancer Res.* 10: 3291-3300.

[86] Huhtinen K, Suvitie P, Hiissa J, Junnila J, Huvila J, et al. (2009) Serum HE4 concentration differentiates malignant ovarian tumours from ovarian endometriotic cysts. *Br. J. Cancer* 100: 1315-1319.

[87] Amonkar SD, Bertenshaw GP, Chen TH, Bergstrom KJ, Zhao J, et al. (2009) Development and preliminary evaluation of a multivariate index assay for ovarian cancer. *PLoS ONE* 4: e4599.

[88] Bast RC, Jr., Badgwell D, Lu Z, Marquez R, Rosen D, et al. (2005) New tumor markers: CA125 and beyond. *Int. J. Gynecol. Cancer* 15 Suppl 3: 274-281.

[89] Hellstrom I, Goodman G, Pullman J, Yang Y, Hellstrom KE (2001) Overexpression of HER-2 in ovarian carcinomas. *Cancer Res.* 61: 2420-2423.

[90] Bookman MA, Darcy KM, Clarke-Pearson D, Boothby RA, Horowitz IR (2003) Evaluation of monoclonal humanized anti-HER2 antibody, trastuzumab, in patients with recurrent or refractory ovarian or primary peritoneal carcinoma with overexpression of HER2: a phase II trial of the Gynecologic Oncology Group. *J. Clin. Oncol.* 21: 283-290.

[91] Campbell IG, Russell SE, Choong DY, Montgomery KG, Ciavarella ML, et al. (2004) Mutation of the PIK3CA gene in ovarian and breast cancer. *Cancer Res.* 64: 7678-7681.

[92] Bellacosa A, de Feo D, Godwin AK, Bell DW, Cheng JQ, et al. (1995) Molecular alterations of the AKT2 oncogene in ovarian and breast carcinomas. *Int. J. Cancer* 64: 280-285.

[93] Campone M, Levy V, Bourbouloux E, Berton Rigaud D, Bootle D, et al. (2009) Safety and pharmacokinetics of paclitaxel and the oral mTOR inhibitor everolimus in advanced solid tumours. *Br. J. Cancer* 100: 315-321.

[94] Folkman J (1995) Angiogenesis in cancer, vascular, rheumatoid and other disease. *Nat Med* 1: 27-31.

[95] Fidler IJ, Ellis LM (1994) The implications of angiogenesis for the biology and therapy of cancer metastasis. *Cell* 79: 185-188.

[96] Burger RA, Sill MW, Monk BJ, Greer BE, Sorosky JI (2007) Phase II trial of bevacizumab in persistent or recurrent epithelial ovarian cancer or primary peritoneal cancer: a Gynecologic Oncology Group Study. *J. Clin. Oncol.* 25: 5165-5171.

[97] Cannistra SA, Matulonis UA, Penson RT, Hambleton J, Dupont J, et al. (2007) Phase II study of bevacizumab in patients with platinum-resistant ovarian cancer or peritoneal serous cancer. *J. Clin. Oncol.* 25: 5180-5186.

[98] Chura JC, Van Iseghem K, Downs LS, Jr., Carson LF, Judson PL (2007) Bevacizumab plus cyclophosphamide in heavily pretreated patients with recurrent ovarian cancer. *Gynecol. Oncol.* 107: 326-330.

[99] Cohn DE, Valmadre S, Resnick KE, Eaton LA, Copeland LJ, et al. (2006) Bevacizumab and weekly taxane chemotherapy demonstrates activity in refractory ovarian cancer. *Gynecol. Oncol.* 102: 134-139.

[100] Holash J, Davis S, Papadopoulos N, Croll SD, Ho L, et al. (2002) VEGF-Trap: a VEGF blocker with potent antitumor effects. *Proc. Natl. Acad. Sci. USA* 99: 11393-11398.

[101] Tan DS, Rothermundt C, Thomas K, Bancroft E, Eeles R, et al. (2008) "BRCAness" syndrome in ovarian cancer: a case-control study describing the clinical features and outcome of patients with epithelial ovarian cancer associated with BRCA1 and BRCA2 mutations. *J. Clin. Oncol.* 26: 5530-5536.

[102] Majdak EJ, Debniak J, Milczek T, Cornelisse CJ, Devilee P, et al. (2005) Prognostic impact of BRCA1 pathogenic and BRCA1/BRCA2 unclassified variant mutations in patients with ovarian carcinoma. *Cancer* 104: 1004-1012.

[103] Cass I, Baldwin RL, Varkey T, Moslehi R, Narod SA, et al. (2003) Improved survival in women with BRCA-associated ovarian carcinoma. *Cancer* 97: 2187-2195.

[104] Ben David Y, Chetrit A, Hirsh-Yechezkel G, Friedman E, Beck BD, et al. (2002) Effect of BRCA mutations on the length of survival in epithelial ovarian tumors. *J. Clin. Oncol.* 20: 463-466.

[105] Levine DA, Federici MG, Reuter VE, Boyd J (2002) Cell proliferation and apoptosis in BRCA-associated hereditary ovarian cancer. *Gynecol. Oncol.* 85: 431-434.

[106] Edwards SL, Brough R, Lord CJ, Natrajan R, Vatcheva R, et al. (2008) Resistance to therapy caused by intragenic deletion in BRCA2. *Nature* 451: 1111-1115.

[107] Dogan E, Saygili U, Tuna B, Gol M, Gurel D, et al. (2005) p53 and mdm2 as prognostic indicators in patients with epithelial ovarian cancer: a multivariate analysis. *Gynecol. Oncol.* 97: 46-52.

[108] Bali A, O'Brien PM, Edwards LS, Sutherland RL, Hacker NF, et al. (2004) Cyclin D1, p53, and p21Waf1/Cip1 expression is predictive of poor clinical outcome in serous epithelial ovarian cancer. *Clin. Cancer Res.* 10: 5168-5177.

[109] de Graeff P, Crijns AP, de Jong S, Boezen M, Post WJ, et al. (2009) Modest effect of p53, EGFR and HER-2/neu on prognosis in epithelial ovarian cancer: a meta-analysis. *Br. J. Cancer*.

[110] Shim HS, Yoon BS, Cho NH (2009) Prognostic significance of paired epithelial cell adhesion molecule and E-cadherin in ovarian serous carcinoma. *Hum. Pathol.* 40: 693-698.

[111] Kleinberg L, Holth A, Trope CG, Reich R, Davidson B (2008) Claudin upregulation in ovarian carcinoma effusions is associated with poor survival. *Hum. Pathol.* 39: 747-757.

[112] Gershenson DM, Del Junco G, Copeland LJ, Rutledge FN (1984) Mixed germ cell tumors of the ovary. *Obstet. Gynecol.* 64: 200-206.

[113] Umezu T, Kajiyama H, Terauchi M, Shibata K, Ino K, et al. (2008) Long-term outcome and prognostic factors for yolk sac tumor of the ovary. *Nagoya J. Med. Sci.* 70: 29-34.

[114] Murugaesu N, Schmid P, Dancey G, Agarwal R, Holden L, et al. (2006) Malignant ovarian germ cell tumors: identification of novel prognostic markers and long-term outcome after multimodality treatment. *J. Clin. Oncol.* 24: 4862-4866.

[115] Kobel M, Kalloger SE, Boyd N, McKinney S, Mehl E, et al. (2008) Ovarian carcinoma subtypes are different diseases: implications for biomarker studies. *PLoS Med* 5: e232.

[116] Hede K (2008) Superhighway or blind alley? The cancer genome atlas releases first results. *J. Natl. Cancer Inst.* 100: 1566-1569.

In: Field Cancerization: Basic Science and Clinical Applications ISBN 978-1-61761-006-6
Editor: Gabriel D. Dakubo

Chapter 22

Epigenetic Changes in Prostatic Tissues: Evidence of Field Cancerization

Devendar Katkoori, Rakesh Singal and Murugesan Manoharan

Abstract

Prostate cancer (PC) alone accounts for 25% of incident cases of cancer in men and is the most frequently diagnosed cancer in American men. Early diagnosis is essential for successful management of PC. Current diagnostic methods have significant drawbacks leading to a significant dilemma in selecting the appropriate management strategy. The need for improving both the diagnostic accuracy and prognostic prediction is evident. There is overwhelming evidence to support the view that epigenetic markers in PC can have diagnostic, therapeutic and prognostic implications. Two of the well-studied epigenetic mechanisms are aberrant DNA methylation and histone modifications. The identification of specific genetic alterations can help in both establishing a diagnosis and also provide useful prognostic information. It is also exciting to know that epigenetic changes are heritable and potentially reversible. Hence, it is reasonable to expect that these can be used as potential therapeutic targets. Currently there are several drugs that are at different stages of development. More recent evidence has focused on a field cancer effect in PC. Epigenetic changes as evidence to this field cancerization have important clinical implications in chemoprevention, early diagnosis, prognostic prediction and active surveillance.

22.1. Introduction

In the United States for the year 2009 it is estimated that 192,280 new cases of prostate cancer will be diagnosed [1]. Prostate cancer (PC) alone accounts for 25% of incident cases of cancer in men and is the most frequently diagnosed cancer in American men. With an estimated 27,360 deaths in 2009, prostate cancer is the second leading cause of death in men

[1]. More than 90% of newly diagnosed prostate cancer is localized and the 5-yr survival for patients diagnosed at this stage approaches 100% [1]. Hence, diagnosis at an early stage is imperative for successful management of prostate cancer. However, diagnosing prostate cancer early is a challenging task considering the fact that early prostate cancer is asymptomatic. The introduction of PSA screening for early detection has lead to a dramatic increase in prostate cancer diagnosis [2]. The American cancer society (ACS) recommends annual screening for men above the age of 50 with PSA and digital rectal examination [3]. However these diagnostic methods have significant limitations and hence ACS emphasizes that before any decision about testing, a discussion should take place about the potential benefits, limitations, and harms associated with testing. Although PSA is arguably one of the best tumor markers, its poor specificity means that nearly two-thirds of men with an elevated PSA (more than 4ng/ml) have normal histology on biopsy [4]. Subjecting all men with elevated PSA to a transrectal ultrasound (TRUS) guided biopsy has significant drawbacks, mainly because of the detection of "clinically insignificant tumors" and procedure related anxiety. On the other hand, 25% of patients with a normal PSA may have prostate cancer [5]. All these limitations lead to significant clinical dilemmas in patient management. Clearly, with these methods it is not possible to differentiate a latent clinically insignificant tumor from an aggressive tumor. The field of epigenetics has the potential to resolve these issues. There is considerable data that suggests that DNA methylation may be useful in early diagnosis of prostate cancer. There is also increasing evidence of an association between specific gene methylation and clinicopathologic indicators of poor prognosis in prostate cancer.

Epigenetics is one of the most rapidly growing fields in cancer research. Epigenetic changes, particularly DNA methylation is found to be involved in a variety of cancers including colon, lung, breast and ovarian cancers apart from prostate cancer [6]. Environmental and dietary factors may influence the risk of developing a cancer through epigenetic mechanisms. For example, monozygotic twins are epigenetically identical at birth and early in life; however with ageing, differences in DNA methylation, histone modification and gene expression develop, the difference being more if they live apart and have different environmental and dietary influences. Epigenetic changes are an early event in cancer development and hence can be used to assess the risk of developing cancer. The potential reversibility of epigenetic changes makes it an attractive target for therapeutic intervention. The role of epigenetics in prostate cancer is still being evaluated. The potential role for epigenetic markers is considerable [7]. In this chapter, we will first discuss the epigenetic changes seen in prostate cancer, then discuss the concept of field cancerization in prostate cancer and finally discuss the clinical implications.

22.2. Epigenetic Changes

Considerable evidence is now available supporting the role of epigenetic changes in prostate cancer development. The term "epigenetic" refers to a change in gene expression without a change in DNA sequence or copy number. Conventionally, this includes CpG island methylation, histone modification and gene imprinting; more recent evidence also suggests a role for small RNA in directing epigenetic silencing. The epigenetic changes can control gene expression and in doing so can contribute to tumor angiogenesis, invasiveness, mobility and proliferation [8]. The identification of specific genetic alterations can help in both establishing a diagnosis and also provide useful prognostic information. Two of the well-studied epigenetic mechanisms are aberrant DNA methylation and histone modifications such as acetylation. Both these factors can act independently and/or together affecting gene expression and in turn oncogenesis.

22.2.1. Aberrant DNA Methylation

DNA methylation is a covalent chemical modification, in the form of addition of a methyl (CH3) group at the C-5 position of the Cytosine ring in the DNA. The human genome is not uniformly methylated. The "CpG islands" are small areas within the genome, rich in Cytosine and Guanine bases and are mostly unmethylated [9]. Epigenetic alterations target this region thereby affecting gene expression. Both hyper- and hypo-methylation can affect gene expression.

22.2.2. DNA Hypermethylation

DNA hypermethylation is a well-established epigenetic abnormality seen in several malignancies, more importantly in prostate cancer [10]. Carcinogenesis is a multistep process and hypermethylation is hypothesized as an early event in the development and progression of prostate cancer [11]. Hypermethylation of a gene is facilitated by a group of enzymes known as DNA methyltransferases (DNMT), which includes DNMT1, DNMT1b, DNMT1o, DNMT1p, DNMT2, DNMT3a, DNMT3b and DNMT3L [12]. The hypermethylation involves CpG islands in the promoter regions of genes and that results in the silencing of genes that are involved in tumor suppressor activity, DNA repair and other critical cellular mechanisms. Some of the important genes that are frequently hypermethylated in prostate cancer are listed in table 22-1. Glutathione S-transferase P1 (GSTP1) is a protector gene and silencing this gene by hypermethylation leads to DNA damage and may contribute to cancer initiation [13,14].

Table 22.1. Hypermethylated genes in prostate cancer and their role

Role	Genes
DNA repair	GSTP1, MGMT
Tumor invasion and architecture	APC, CD44, *E-cadherin, H-cadherin,* CAV1, LAMA3, LAMB3, LAMC2
Hormone response	AR, RARB, ERα, ERβ
Signal transduction	RASSF1, DAB21P,DAPK1, EDNRB
Cell cycle control	CDKN2A, CCND2, CDKN1A, SFN

Methyl Guanine DNA methyl transferase (MGMT) is another DNA repair gene, which is silenced by hypermethylation [15]. Putative tumor suppressor genes such as Ras association domain family 1 gene (RASSF1A) [16,17], KAI 1 [18], Inhibin-alpha [19] and DAB21P [20] are inactivated by hypermethylation. Hypermethylation promotes carcinogenesis in prostate cancer by affecting cell cycle control, hormonal response, cell adhesions and architecture [11]. A recent study identified that hypermethylation of HOXD3 and BMP7 genes may play a role in development of high- grade tumors [21]. In this study the methylation pattern correlated with tumor grade according to Gleason pattern.

22.2.3. DNA Hypomethylation

DNA hypomethylation is a second type of methylation related epigenetic aberration seen in a variety of malignancies including prostate cancer [22]. Hypomethylation is facilitated by the demethylase enzyme group, which includes 5-methylcytosine glycosylase and MBD2b [23]. Methylation of normal genomes act as defensive mechanism against cancer, for example, oncogenes can be transcriptionally silenced and prevented from activation by being methylated. The hypomethylation of such genes causes breakdown of this defense mechanism and is implicated in oncogenesis. The hypomethylation can be "global" or "localized". Global hypomethylation refers to overall decrease in methylation content in the genome. Bedford et al. reported that global hypomethylation is significantly lower in patients with metastatic prostate cancer compared to non metastatic prostate cancer [22]. Localized or gene specific hypomethylation refers to a decrease in cytosine methylation relative to normal levels. This affects the specific regions within the genome such as promoter regions of oncogenes that are highly methylated [10].

22.2.4. Histone Code

Histones have emerged as important regulators of chromatin, thereby controlling gene expression. In each nucleosome, two super helical turns of DNA containing around 146 base pairs wrap an octomer of histone core made of four histone partners (an H3-H4 tetramer and two H2A-H2B diamers [24]. Histones consist of a globular domain and a more flexible and charged NH2 terminal known as histone "tail". These tails, which are placed peripherally, are susceptible to a variety of covalent modifications, such as acetylation, methylation, phosphorylation and ubiquitination (called 'marks'). These modifications are referred to as "the histone code" and are effective epigenetic mechanisms regulating gene expression [25]. Histone acetylation and deacetylations are mediated by histone acetyl transferases (HAT) and histone deacetylases (HDAC) respectively. Huang et al. and Tsubaki et al. reported that treatment of prostate cancer cells with HDAC inhibitors results in increased expression of specific genes such as CPA3 [26] and Insulin like growth factor binding protein 3 [27]. Coxsackie and adenovirus receptor (CAR) gene and Vitamin D receptor gene have been shown to be affected by histone acetylation in prostate cancer. Decreased CAR expression is associated with an increased Gleason score [28].

Histone methylation affects the chromatin function depending on the specific amino acid being modified and the extent of methylation [29]. Methylation of H3 at lysine 4 is associated with inactive transcription of the PSA gene in prostate cancer cell line LNCaP and decreased di and trimethylated H3 at lysine 4 is associated with androgen receptor-mediated transcription of the PSA gene [10].

22.2.5. Loss of Imprinting

Imprinting is a normal cellular genetic phenomenon that allows specific expression of either the paternal or maternal allele. Nearly forty genes are known to demonstrate imprinting. IGF2 is a gene that is normally imprinted and its altered expression is known to affect prostate and other cancers [8]. Biallelic expression of IGF2 due to reactivation of maternal allele has been described in both tumor and adjacent tissue from radical prostatectomy specimens. In contrast BPH specimens did not show such an altered expression [30]. Loss of IGF2 imprinting is known to occur with ageing and may explain the higher risk of prostate cancer with ageing. P57, a tumor suppressor gene is also modulated by imprinting and this gene is altered in nearly 56% of all prostate cancer cases [31]. DNA methylation controls p57 imprinting.

22.2.6. RNA-Mediated Transcriptional Gene Silencing

Recent evidence also suggests a role for small RNA in directing epigenetic silencing. Small interfering RNA (si RNA) may have a role in controlling the epigenetic state. The role is still being evaluated [32,33].

22.2.7. DNA Methylation - Histone Code Interplay

DNA promoter methylation and histone deacetylation can act synergistically resulting in inactive chromatin state resulting in suppression of gene expression (figure 22-1).

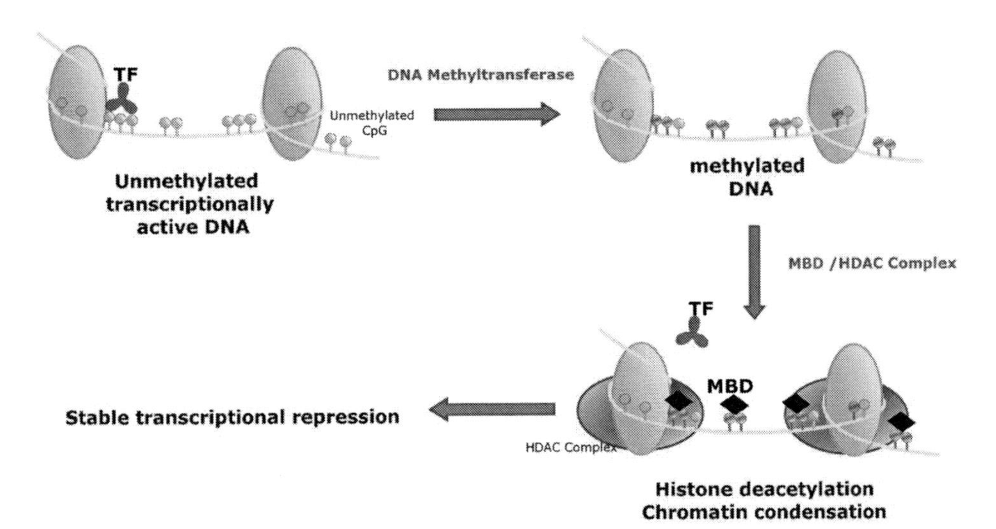

Figure 22.1. Epigenetic silencing of gene expression. DNA methyl-transferases carry out the methylation of CpG dinucleotides, which triggers the process of gene silencing by recruitment of methyl binding domain (MBD) and Histone deacetylases (HDAC) to bind to the methylated DNA. This results in histone deacetylation and chromatin condensation leading to loss of transcription factor binding and subsequent repression of transcription.

Methylated DNA binding proteins such as MeCP2 may play an important role. Retinoic acid receptor beta gene (RARB) that is silenced in prostate cancer tissues and cell lines is regulated by both methylation and histone acetylation. This indicates that combined treatment targeting methylation and histone acetylation may result in reversal of epigenetic silencing of tumor suppressor genes [10,34]. Similarly, DNA methylation and histone methylation may interact to facilitate chromatin silencing. However, it is unclear which event takes place first [10].

22.3. Field Cancerization

The term field cancerization is used to describe the process whereby cells in a particular tissue or organ are transformed, such that genetically altered but histologically normal appearing cells predate the development of neoplasia or coexist with malignant cells, irrespective of clonality. The concept of field Cancerization was first proposed by Slaughter et al. while studying oral cancer, to explain the occurrence of multiple primary tumors and local recurrences [35]. They observed that the normal appearing cells adjacent to the malignant cells were histologically abnormal and therefore were part of the transformed cells in a particular tumor field and hence were responsible for the local tumor recurrence. The lateral spread of a tumor could be explained as a progressive transformation of the cells adjacent to the tumor and not due to spread and destruction of adjacent epithelium by pre-existing cancer cells [35]. They proposed that "cancer does not arise as an isolated cellular phenomenon, but rather as an anaplastic tendency involving many cells at once" [36]. Modern molecular techniques have provided unequivocal evidence to support the proposals of Slaughter et al. Organ systems in which field cancerization has been described since then are: head and neck (oral cavity, oropharynx, and larynx), lung, vulva, esophagus, cervix, breast, skin, colon, bladder and recently prostate.

It is not surprising to note that field cancerization has been documented for these epithelial tumors. The epithelial cells have important physiologic functions and their protective role exposes them to a variety of environmental influences including carcinogens. The turnover of epithelial cells is high and the risk of abnormal proliferation is significant. This can result in a large genetically altered cancer field. Relatively little research has been conducted on field cancerization in prostate cancer. Multifocality is a hallmark of prostate cancer [37], suggesting the possibility that the organ itself is genetically altered. It is likely that multiple tumors arising in the prostate are a result of the organ being genetically altered by a particular carcinogen.

Genomic instability, gene expression studies and analysis of mitochondrial genome alterations have recently been reported to show field cancerization in prostate cancer. Hanson et al reported that methylation of GSTP1 and RARbeta2 was seen in prostate tumor epithelium, stromal tissue adjacent to the tumor cells and also normal glands adjacent to the tumor showing a field effect, while normal epithelia and stromal tissue from a benign prostatic hyperplasia specimen did not show methylation of GSTP1 and RARbeta2 [38]. Finding gene methylation in normal appearing epithelial and normal stromal cells adjacent to tumor suggests a field cancer effect. Yu et al performed a comprehensive gene expression analysis of prostate cancer tissues, prostate tissues adjacent to tumor, and organ donor prostate tissues, obtained from men of various ages. They reported that gene expression pattern in normal tissue adjacent to the tumor closely resembled that of the tumor and was different from the normal donor prostate samples supporting a cancer field effect [39]. Several other studies also support a field cancer effect in prostate. Fordyce et al evaluated the telomere DNA content (TC) in prostate tumor tissue and its relation to prostate cancer recurrence. A subblot analysis was done to measure TC in tumor tissue and histologically normal nearby prostate tissue from radical prostatectomy specimens. They reported that decreased TC in prostate tissues obtained from radical prostatectomy specimen is an independent predictor of prostate cancer recurrence. The interesting finding however was that, TC in tumor tissue is associated with the TC in histologically normal prostate tissue. Thus they concluded that the genomic instability was operative in the entire field well beyond the tumor margins [40]. In another interesting study, injection of prostate cancer cell lines into athymic nude mice caused cytogenetic abnormalities in stromal cells, suggesting that at least in prostate cancer, tumor cells might have the potential of transforming adjacent normal glands [41]. Field cancerization in prostate cancer is expected to have some important clinical implications in both diagnosis and management.

22.4. Clinical Implications of Epigenetic Changes

There are several areas of prostate cancer management, which can benefit from the use of epigenetic markers.

22.4.1. Prostate Cancer Diagnosis

Prostate cancer rarely causes symptoms early in the course of the disease. Prostate cancer arises in the peripheral zone and hence a mass effect and consequential voiding symptoms are seen only in advanced disease. Presently the diagnosis is primarily by biochemical testing along with a digital rectal examination and a prostate biopsy in suspected prostate cancer. The biochemical marker presently used, prostate specific antigen (PSA), is a less than optimal tumor marker. Epigenetic markers, particularly aberrant DNA methylation, have the potential as a useful diagnostic tumor marker. These markers can be detected in cancer tissues, serum and body fluids. The methylation markers have several advantages over the mutation-based genetic markers. The detection of these markers is technically simple and can be sensitively detected both quantitatively and qualitatively by polymerase chain reaction (PCR). Furthermore, the incidence of aberrant DNA methylation is higher than that of mutations and can be discovered by genome wide screening procedures [42].

In recent years, the role of GSTP1 as a prostate cancer marker is being widely studied. GSTP1 hypermethylation is seen in more than 90% of patients with of prostate cancer [8]. GSTP1 methylation is specific to prostate cancer and it can be detected easily in body fluids containing prostate cell such as blood, urine and semen. Goessl et al. examined the urine after prostatic massage and methylation was detected in 68% patients with early prostate cancer and 78% of patients with locally advanced cancer [43]. Table 22-2 shows methylation of GSTP1 in different tissues and body fluids. Harden et al. reported 73% GSTP1 methylation in prostate cancer tissue samples. They also reported that methylation assay with histological analysis improves the diagnostic specificity [44]. Methylation of several other genes have been studied in the diagnosis of prostate cancer including, RARB, CD44, E-cadherin (ECAD), RASSF1A, APC and tazarotene induced gene 1 (T1G1) [13,45]. Recent studies by Yegnasubramanian et al [46] and others have reported that use of a panel of methylation markers including GSTP1 improves the diagnosis of prostate cancer in both body fluids and tissues. Further studies are needed before these markers can be used as diagnostic markers in the routine clinical practice.

Table 22.2. GSTP1 methylation in prostate cancer

Specimen	Methylation (%)
Tissue	90
Serum	72
Ejaculate	50
Urine after prostate massage	76

22.4.2. Prostate Cancer Prognosis

Kollerman et al. demonstrated that GSTP1 hypermethylation is seen in 40% of pre-operative bone marrow aspirate in patients with advanced PC [47]. They also found evidence of GSTP1 hypermethylation in 90% of PC patients with lymph node involvement where as in only 11% of lymph nodes in non-cancer group. Genes such as CAV1, CDH1, CD 44 and T1G1 may exhibit specific methylation in high risk and metastatic tumors that can be used in the molecular staging and predictors of disease progression [11]. Prostate cancers with high Gleason score are correlated with a higher degree of methylation of many genes, such as RARβ, RASSF1A, GSTP1 and CDH13 [9]. Further studies also indicate that use of a panel of multiple methylation makers can be better predictors than individual genes [48]. Hypermethylation of GSTP1 gene in combination with APC and cyclinD2 were shown to be significant predictors of time to relapse in prostate cancer [49].

Seligson et al. reported that histone modification patterns could predict prostate cancer outcome independent of tumor stage, preoperative PSA and capsular invasion [50]. This finding could help in further stratifying patients with low-risk prostate cancer, and help in predicting the biological behavior of tumors.

22.4.3. Therapeutic Targets

Epigenetic changes are not heritable and potentially reversible. Hence, it is reasonable to expect that these can be used as potential therapeutic targets. Currently there are several drugs, which are at different stages of development. They can be broadly classified in two groups: (i) DNMT inhibitors and (ii) Histone Deacetylase (HDAC) inhibitors. Some of the drugs in both groups, which are being tested and used currently, are shown in table 22-3.

Table 22.3. Drugs used for epigenetic modifications

DNMT inhibitors	HDAC inhibitors
5-aza-2'-Deoxycytidine	Trichostatin A (TSA)
Zebularine	Sodium butyrate
Procainamide	Suberoylanilide hydroxamic acid (SAHA)
Procaine	Valproic acid
Epigallocatechin-3-gallate (EGCG)	Pyroxamide
MG98	Phenyl butyrate
5-azacytidine	

22.4.3.1. DNMT Inhibitors

5-aza-2' - Deoxycytidine (5-aza-dC) is one of the early drugs identified as DNMT inhibitor after being used as cytotoxic drug in the1990s. This drug forms irreversible covalent bonds with DNMT1 after its incorporation in to DNA, thereby inducing degradation of DNMT1 [51] Issa et al. [52] demonstrated that low dose continuous administration of 5-aza-dC is more effective than higher doses. Myelosuppression is a known side effect of this drug, which is otherwise well tolerated. 5-aza-dC has been recently approved by the FDA for clinical use in certain hematological conditions. Another drug in the same group, Zebularine can be administered orally or intraperitoneally. It has to be given in high doses, however, it is chemically stable and has low toxicity [53]. Other drugs in this group, which are being studied, include Epigallocatechin-3-Gallate (EGCG), Procainamide, Procaine and MG 98 [42]. The significant problem with this group of drugs is the nonselective nature of the inhibition and requirement that the cell is actively dividing [8].

22.4.3.2. Histone Deacetylases Inhibitors

A variety of natural products exhibit HDAC inhibitory activity. Commonly used HDAC inhibitors, which are being tested, include trichostatin A (TSA), Suberoylanilide hydroxamic acid (SAHA) and valproic acid [10]. Many of these drugs have exhibited antitumor activity. SAHA and sodium butyrate have shown prostate cancer inhibition in animal models [54,55]. Overall, low toxicity rates of these drugs are encouraging for them to be considered in conducting further studies. The combination of HDAC and DNMT inhibitors has synergistic effects in the reactivation of silenced genes [10]. Another interesting possibility is the combination of epigenetic drugs and conventional anti androgens and chemotherapeutic agents. It should be cautioned that the epigenetic drugs currently lack gene specificity and some of them are associated with significant toxicity. Hence, efforts are being made to develop gene-specific epigenetic drugs [42].

22.5. Clinical implications for a "Field Cancer Effect" in Prostate Cancer

22.5.1. Chemoprevention

Prostate cancer is an appropriate candidate for chemoprevention. Prostate cancer is a multistep molecular process induced by genetic and epigenetic changes. Genetic changes in normal appearing cells can be identified, allowing recruitment of individuals at risk of developing PC in to primary chemoprevention regimes. Knowledge of methylation patterns and their role in malignant transformation will enable controlled use of methylation reversal agents in primary chemoprevention. Similarly secondary chemoprevention can be adopted for preventing the progression of precancerous lesions into invasive cancers.

22.5.2. Early Detection and Improving the Accuracy of Biopsy

An important clinical utility of field cancerization will be in interpretation of needle biopsy specimen. Conventional histological methods rely on abnormal cell morphology and hence absence of abnormal cells precludes the diagnosis of cancer. However, if cells with aberrant DNA methylation surround tumor regions, then either a tumor was missed by the biopsy or some cells in the tissue are progressing towards malignancy and require further evaluation or surveillance. This can bring down the false negative rate of a prostate needle biopsy considerably.

22.5.3. Role in Active Surveillance

Active surveillance is being used increasingly in the management of "select" low risk prostate cancer patients. However one of the important concerns with this approach is the lack of tools to predict the likelihood of progression in these patients. In light of previous evidence, a prostate biopsy showing epigenetic field change can significantly alter the risk of progression and this finding can guide the selection of patients for active surveillance.

22.5.4. Interpretation of Margins and Risk of Recurrence

Not all surgical margin-positive patients develop biochemical recurrence following radical prostatectomy [56]. The presence or absence of genetically altered field at the site of positive surgical margin can help in evaluating the risk of recurrence and also if any additional therapy is required.

22.6. Summary and Future Directions

Epigenetic changes in prostate cancer are being studied extensively at present and genome wide screening will lead to development of novel epigenetic markers. Epigenetic changes are an early event in cancer development and hence can be used to assess the risk of developing cancer. Li et al. suggest that genes such as CAV1, CDH1, CD44 and T1G1 should be explored further as "risk markers", particularly to differentiate the indolent tumors from others with bad prognostic potential [11]. The recognition of a field cancer effect in PC has significant clinical implications. Epigenetic molecular classification will help to identify patients at high risk of recurrence following definitive treatments such as radical prostatectomy. Therapeutic drugs, which reverse these epigenetic changes, have the potential to be an effective adjunct treatment for prostate cancer. However, they need to be studied both for efficacy and safety profile. Gene specific epigenetic drugs need to be developed for better targeting the disease. As the epigenetic changes are early events in prostate cancer development, these drugs have a potential to play a role in disease prevention. Two main features of epigenetic changes, "reversibility" and being an "early event" in oncogenesis, makes epigenetic targeting an important future research area for cancer diagnosis, risk stratification, treatment and prevention resulting in effective cancer control.

References

[1] Kamp DW (2009) Asbestos-induced lung diseases: an update. *Transl Res.* 153: 143-152.

[2] Crawford ED (2003) Epidemiology of prostate cancer. *Urology* 62: 3-12.

[3] Smith RA, Cokkinides V, Brawley OW (2008) Cancer screening in the United States, 2008: a review of current American Cancer Society guidelines and cancer screening issues. *CA Cancer J. Clin.* 58: 161-179.

[4] Frankel S, Smith GD, Donovan J, Neal D (2003) Screening for prostate cancer. *Lancet* 361: 1122-1128.

[5] Hernandez J, Thompson IM (2004) Prostate-specific antigen: a review of the validation of the most commonly used cancer biomarker. *Cancer* 101: 894-904.

[6] Manoharan M, Ramachandran K, Soloway MS, Singal R (2007) Epigenetic targets in the diagnosis and treatment of prostate cancer. *Int. Braz. J. Urol.* 33: 11-18.

[7] Ramachandran K, Soloway MS, Singal R, Manoharan M (2007) The emerging role of epigenetics in urological cancers. *Can. J. Urol.* 14: 3535-3541.

[8] Dobosy JR, Roberts JL, Fu VX, Jarrard DF (2007) The expanding role of epigenetics in the development, diagnosis and treatment of prostate cancer and benign prostatic hyperplasia. *J. Urol.* 177: 822-831.

[9] Das PM, Singal R (2004) DNA methylation and cancer. *J. Clin. Oncol.* 22: 4632-4642.

[10] Li LC, Carroll PR, Dahiya R (2005) Epigenetic changes in prostate cancer: implication for diagnosis and treatment. *J. Natl. Cancer Inst.* 97: 103-115.

[11] Li LC, Okino ST, Dahiya R (2004) DNA methylation in prostate cancer. *Biochim. Biophys. Acta.* 1704: 87-102.

[12] Robertson KD (2002) DNA methylation and chromatin - unraveling the tangled web. *Oncogene* 21: 5361-5379.

[13] Singal R, Ferdinand L, Reis IM, Schlesselman JJ (2004) Methylation of multiple genes in prostate cancer and the relationship with clinicopathological features of disease. *Oncol. Rep.* 12: 631-637.

[14] Nelson CP, Kidd LC, Sauvageot J, Isaacs WB, De Marzo AM, et al. (2001) Protection against 2-hydroxyamino-1-methyl-6-phenylimidazo[4,5-b]pyridine cytotoxicity and DNA adduct formation in human prostate by glutathione S-transferase P1. *Cancer Res.* 61: 103-109.

[15] Konishi N, Nakamura M, Kishi M, Nishimine M, Ishida E, et al. (2002) DNA hypermethylation status of multiple genes in prostate adenocarcinomas. *Jpn J. Cancer Res.* 93: 767-773.

[16] Song MS, Song SJ, Ayad NG, Chang JS, Lee JH, et al. (2004) The tumour suppressor RASSF1A regulates mitosis by inhibiting the APC-Cdc20 complex. *Nat. Cell Biol.* 6: 129-137.

[17] Oh HJ, Lee KK, Song SJ, Jin MS, Song MS, et al. (2006) Role of the tumor suppressor RASSF1A in Mst1-mediated apoptosis. *Cancer Res.* 66: 2562-2569.

[18] Sekita N, Suzuki H, Ichikawa T, Kito H, Akakura K, et al. (2001) Epigenetic regulation of the KAI1 metastasis suppressor gene in human prostate cancer cell lines. *Jpn J. Cancer Res.* 92: 947-951.

[19] Schmitt JF, Millar DS, Pedersen JS, Clark SL, Venter DJ, et al. (2002) Hypermethylation of the inhibin alpha-subunit gene in prostate carcinoma. *Mol. Endocrinol.* 16: 213-220.

[20] Chen H, Toyooka S, Gazdar AF, Hsieh JT (2003) Epigenetic regulation of a novel tumor suppressor gene (hDAB2IP) in prostate cancer cell lines. *J. Biol. Chem.* 278: 3121-3130.

[21] Kron K, Pethe V, Briollais L, Sadikovic B, Ozcelik H, et al. (2009) Discovery of novel hypermethylated genes in prostate cancer using genomic CpG island microarrays. *PLoS ONE* 4: e4830.

[22] Bedford MT, van Helden PD (1987) Hypomethylation of DNA in pathological conditions of the human prostate. *Cancer Res.* 47: 5274-5276.

[23] Bhattacharya SK, Ramchandani S, Cervoni N, Szyf M (1999) A mammalian protein with specific demethylase activity for mCpG DNA. *Nature* 397: 579-583.

[24] Luger K, Mader AW, Richmond RK, Sargent DF, Richmond TJ (1997) Crystal structure of the nucleosome core particle at 2.8 A resolution. *Nature* 389: 251-260.

[25] Jenuwein T, Allis CD (2001) Translating the histone code. *Science* 293: 1074-1080.

[26] Huang H, Reed CP, Zhang JS, Shridhar V, Wang L, et al. (1999) Carboxypeptidase A3 (CPA3): a novel gene highly induced by histone deacetylase inhibitors during differentiation of prostate epithelial cancer cells. *Cancer Res.* 59: 2981-2988.

[27] Tsubaki J, Hwa V, Twigg SM, Rosenfeld RG (2002) Differential activation of the IGF binding protein-3 promoter by butyrate in prostate cancer cells. *Endocrinology* 143: 1778-1788.

[28] Rauen KA, Sudilovsky D, Le JL, Chew KL, Hann B, et al. (2002) Expression of the coxsackie adenovirus receptor in normal prostate and in primary and metastatic prostate carcinoma: potential relevance to gene therapy. *Cancer Res.* 62: 3812-3818.

[29] Moggs JG, Goodman JI, Trosko JE, Roberts RA (2004) Epigenetics and cancer: implications for drug discovery and safety assessment. *Toxicol. Appl. Pharmacol.* 196: 422-430.

[30] Jarrard DF, Bussemakers MJ, Bova GS, Isaacs WB (1995) Regional loss of imprinting of the insulin-like growth factor II gene occurs in human prostate tissues. *Clin. Cancer Res.* 1: 1471-1478.

[31] Lodygin D, Epanchintsev A, Menssen A, Diebold J, Hermeking H (2005) Functional epigenomics identifies genes frequently silenced in prostate cancer. *Cancer Res.* 65: 4218-4227.

[32] Morris KV (2008) RNA-mediated transcriptional gene silencing in human cells. *Curr. Top. Microbiol. Immunol.* 320: 211-224.

[33] Han J, Kim D, Morris KV (2007) Promoter-associated RNA is required for RNA-directed transcriptional gene silencing in human cells. *Proc. Natl. Acad. Sci. USA* 104: 12422-12427.

[34] Nakayama T, Watanabe M, Yamanaka M, Hirokawa Y, Suzuki H, et al. (2001) The role of epigenetic modifications in retinoic acid receptor beta2 gene expression in human prostate cancers. *Lab. Invest.* 81: 1049-1057.

[35] Slaughter DP, Southwick HW, Smejkal W (1953) Field cancerization in oral stratified squamous epithelium; clinical implications of multicentric origin. *Cancer* 6: 963-968.

[36] Slaughter DP (1944) The multiplicity of origin of malignant tumors: collective review. *Internat. Abstr. Surg.* 79: 89-98.

[37] Epstein JI, Oesterling JE, Walsh PC (1988) The volume and anatomical location of residual tumor in radical prostatectomy specimens removed for stage A1 prostate cancer. *J. Urol.* 139: 975-979.

[38] Hanson JA, Gillespie JW, Grover A, Tangrea MA, Chuaqui RF, et al. (2006) Gene promoter methylation in prostate tumor-associated stromal cells. *J. Natl. Cancer Inst.* 98: 255-261.

[39] Yu YP, Landsittel D, Jing L, Nelson J, Ren B, et al. (2004) Gene expression alterations in prostate cancer predicting tumor aggression and preceding development of malignancy. *J. Clin. Oncol.* 22: 2790-2799.

[40] Fordyce CA, Heaphy CM, Joste NE, Smith AY, Hunt WC, et al. (2005) Association between cancer-free survival and telomere DNA content in prostate tumors. *J. Urol.* 173: 610-614.

[41] Pathak S, Nemeth MA, Multani AS, Thalmann GN, von Eschenbach AC, et al. (1997) Can cancer cells transform normal host cells into malignant cells? *Br. J. Cancer* 76: 1134-1138.

[42] Miyamoto K, Ushijima T (2005) Diagnostic and therapeutic applications of epigenetics. *Jpn J. Clin. Oncol.* 35: 293-301.

[43] Goessl C, Krause H, Muller M, Heicappell R, Schrader M, et al. (2000) Fluorescent methylation-specific polymerase chain reaction for DNA-based detection of prostate cancer in bodily fluids. *Cancer Res.* 60: 5941-5945.

[44] Harden SV, Guo Z, Epstein JI, Sidransky D (2003) Quantitative GSTP1 methylation clearly distinguishes benign prostatic tissue and limited prostate adenocarcinoma. *J. Urol.* 169: 1138-1142.

[45] Tokumaru Y, Harden SV, Sun DI, Yamashita K, Epstein JI, et al. (2004) Optimal use of a panel of methylation markers with GSTP1 hypermethylation in the diagnosis of prostate adenocarcinoma. *Clin. Cancer Res.* 10: 5518-5522.

[46] Yegnasubramanian S, Kowalski J, Gonzalgo ML, Zahurak M, Piantadosi S, et al. (2004) Hypermethylation of CpG islands in primary and metastatic human prostate cancer. *Cancer Res.* 64: 1975-1986.

[47] Kollermann J, Muller M, Goessl C, Krause H, Helpap B, et al. (2003) Methylation-specific PCR for DNA-based detection of occult tumor cells in lymph nodes of prostate cancer patients. *Eur. Urol.* 44: 533-538.

[48] Rhodes DR, Sanda MG, Otte AP, Chinnaiyan AM, Rubin MA (2003) Multiplex biomarker approach for determining risk of prostate-specific antigen-defined recurrence of prostate cancer. *J. Natl. Cancer Inst.* 95: 661-668.

[49] Rosenbaum E, Hoque MO, Cohen Y, Zahurak M, Eisenberger MA, et al. (2005) Promoter hypermethylation as an independent prognostic factor for relapse in patients with prostate cancer following radical prostatectomy. *Clin Cancer Res* 11: 8321-8325.

[50] Seligson DB, Horvath S, Shi T, Yu H, Tze S, et al. (2005) Global histone modification patterns predict risk of prostate cancer recurrence. *Nature* 435: 1262-1266.

[51] Christman JK (2002) 5-Azacytidine and 5-aza-2'-deoxycytidine as inhibitors of DNA methylation: mechanistic studies and their implications for cancer therapy. *Oncogene* 21: 5483-5495.

[52] Issa JP, Garcia-Manero G, Giles FJ, Mannari R, Thomas D, et al. (2004) Phase 1 study of low-dose prolonged exposure schedules of the hypomethylating agent 5-aza-2'-deoxycytidine (decitabine) in hematopoietic malignancies. *Blood* 103: 1635-1640.

[53] Cheng JC, Weisenberger DJ, Gonzales FA, Liang G, Xu GL, et al. (2004) Continuous zebularine treatment effectively sustains demethylation in human bladder cancer cells. *Mol. Cell Biol.* 24: 1270-1278.

[54] Butler LM, Agus DB, Scher HI, Higgins B, Rose A, et al. (2000) Suberoylanilide hydroxamic acid, an inhibitor of histone deacetylase, suppresses the growth of prostate cancer cells in vitro and in vivo. *Cancer Res.* 60: 5165-5170.

[55] Kuefer R, Hofer MD, Altug V, Zorn C, Genze F, et al. (2004) Sodium butyrate and tributyrin induce in vivo growth inhibition and apoptosis in human prostate cancer. *Br. J. Cancer* 90: 535-541.

[56] Simon MA, Kim S, Soloway MS (2006) Prostate specific antigen recurrence rates are low after radical retropubic prostatectomy and positive margins. *J. Urol.* 175: 140-144; discussion 144-145.

In: Field Cancerization: Basic Science and Clinical Applications ISBN 978-1-61761-006-6
Editor: Gabriel D. Dakubo

Chapter 23

Epigenetic Mechanisms in Solid Tumours of Infancy and Childhood

Kornelius Kerl and Michael C. Frühwald

23.1. Introduction

Malignant tumors in childhood represent a rather heterogenous group of neoplasms. Among solid tumours the largest group is the one arising in the central nervous system, followed by neuroblastomas and Wilms tumors. In the last 20 years, the treatment and prognosis of many of these entities has improved dramatically. However some prove resistant to chemotherapy, even with high dose chemotherapy and radiotherapy. More aggresive therapeutic approaches only seem to add toxicity but do not increase cure rates. Thus alternatives are desperately sought.

In the last several years our knowledge of the biological behaviour of the tumors and potential ways to influence tumor-pathways has grown. One appealing approach is to perturb the *epigenetic code* of high-risk tumors. Conrad Waddington initially used the term "epigenetic" in the 1940s to describe the interaction of genes with their environment to create a phenotype. Today, the term epigenetic is used to describe heritable informations on gene expression mediated by dynamic mechanisms other than nucleotide sequence [1].

In the nuclei of all eukaryotes, genomic DNA is folded, constrained, packaged and associated with proteins in a complex known as chromatin. Chromatin consists of regularly repeating units, known as nucleosomes. Each nucleosome is made up of 146bp of DNA tightly wrapped around the core of eight histone proteins, two units of each histone H2A, H2B, H3 and H4. Two states of chromatin may be found in the human genome: transcriptionally active *euchromatin* accessible to components of the transcriptional machinery and silent *heterochromatin*. The balance between euchromatin and heterochromatin guarantees the maintenance of gene expression patterns of a certain cell type in its daughter cells as heritable traits[2]. The epigenetic regulation of gene expression is mediated by mechanisms such as DNA methylation and histone modification [3].

23.2. The Histone Complex and Its Modifications

There are eight distinct types and over 60 different known modifications on histones, which are dynamic and rapidly changing. Enzymes have been identified for acetylation [4], methylation [5], phosphorylation [6], ubiquitination [7], sumoylation [8], ADP-ribosylation [9], deamination[10] and proline isomerization[11]. In general acetylation, methylation, phosphorylation and ubiquitination result in "activation", whereas methylation, ubiquitination, sumoylation, deamination, and proline isomerization induce repression. Most enzymes, which transduce histone tail modifications, are highly specific for particular amino acid positions [12]. Histone modifications have two major functions: disruption of contacts between nucleosomes to ''unravel'' chromatin and the recruitment of nonhistone proteins (figure 23.1; *Epigenetic regulation of gene transcription*).

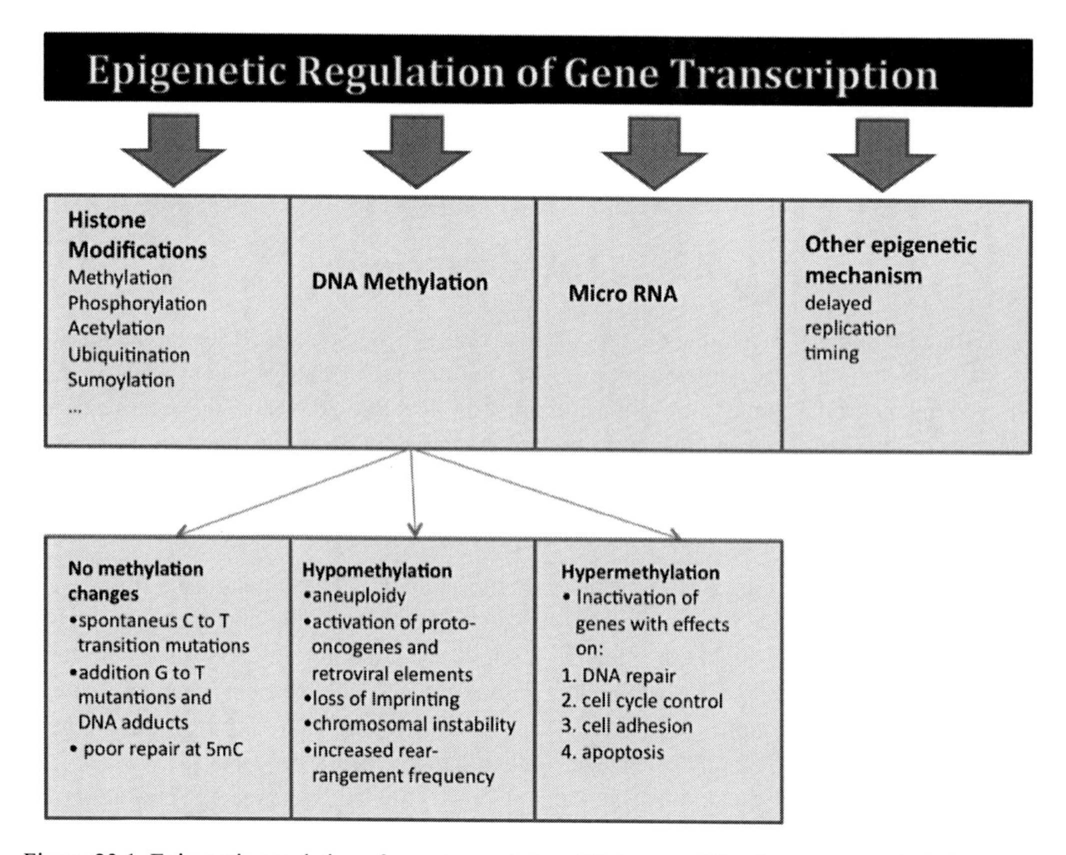

Figure 23.1. Epigenetic regulation of gene transcription. Histone modifications (e.g., methylation, acetylation, phosphorylation and many others), DNA methylation and other mechanisms (e.g., delayed replication timing) result in the modulation of transcription.

The *histone code hypothesis* predicts that modification marks on histone tails provide binding sites for effector proteins:

- Methylation is recognized by chromo-like domains of the royal family (chromo, tudor, MBT) and nonrelated PHD domains. Several chromodomains have been characterized: The chromodomain of HP1 is highly selective for methylated H3K9 and less for H3K4 and is associated with deacetylase and methyltransferase activities [13,14,15]. Methylation of H3K27 (H3K27me) recruits the chromodomain of polycomb protein PC2, which is associated with ubiquitin ligase activity specific for H2A [16]. Furthermore Su (var) 3-9 HMTase family members and several repressive chromatin remodelling complexes such as MI-2/CHD ATPase subunit of the NURD complex contain chromodomains [17,18]. Other important chromodomains are for example: BPTF, a component of the NURF chromatin-remodeling complex [19], the PHD-finger protein ING2 [20] and JMJD2A, a histone lysine demethylase that binds via a tudor domain [21,22].

- Acetylation is recognized by bromodomains. The bromodomain (found in *SNF2*, *TAFII 250*, mammalian trithorax (*HRX/MII*) and other transcriptional regulators possessing intrinsic histone acetyltransferase activity (e.g. GCN5, PCAF, TAF I 250)) interact with an acetylated lysine in the histone NH2-terminal tail (reviewed by Mujtaba et al. 2007) [23].
- Phosphorylation is recognized by a domain within 14-3-3 proteins (for review see Mohammad *et al.*[24]).

23.3. Epigenetic Changes Can Lead to the Formation of Cancer

An array of epigenetic mechanisms may contribute to the origin of neoplastic diseases. As two predominant examples, acetylation of histones and methylation of promoter DNA will be described in more detail in this chapter.

Acetylation of histones is controlled by histone acetyltransferases (HAT) and their removal by histone deacetylases (HDACs). Acetylation is generally associated with transcriptional activation. *Acetyltransferases* can be divided into three main groups: GNAT, MYST, and CBP/p300 [4]. Most acetyltransferases modify more than one lysine residue and most of the acetylation sites are in the N-terminal tail of the histones. In the presence of DNA damage the deacetylases for H3K56, Hst3, and Hst4 (two paralogs of Sir2) are downregulated, whereas acetylation of H3K56, by Rtt109, is deposited on newly synthesized histones during S phase [25].

The 18 currently characterized different histone deacetylases (*HDACs)* can be classified into four main groups. The “classical 11 HDACs” of group I, II and IV are involved in controlling hallmarks of cancer such as proliferation, apoptosis, differentiation, angiogenesis, migration and drug resistance. Class III consists of the NAD-dependent group of the SIR-family. In several tumors, for example colorectal cancer, pancreatic carcinoma and gastric cancer, but also pediatric malignancies, such as neuroblastoma, one or more HDACs are overexpressed [26,27,28]. The knockdown of HDAC I, II and III results in cell cycle arrest, increased sensitivity to chemotherapy and apoptosis [29,30]. A novel tool in cancer therapy is the inhibition of HDACs by small molecular compounds (see below). For more information on cancer relevant changes of histones by phosphorylation, methylation, sumoylation, ADP ribosylation, proline isomerization and ubiquitynation consult the excellent review by Kouzarides *et al.*, 2007 [31].

23.4. Epigenetic Regulation through DNA-Methylation

DNA is generally hypermethylated in intergenic regions and hypomethylated at gene promoters. Genes are actively transcribed if these regions are unmethylated [32], while methylation of promoter CpG islands (regions of the genome, occurring on average every 100 kb at least 200 kb in length displaying a CpG density of more than 50%)[33], results in a compact arrangement of nucleosomes and correlates with transcriptional inactivation[34]. DNA-methylation may posttranscriptionally affect cytosine residues in CpG dinucleotides [35] at CpG islands. But there is also a strong correlation between gene expression and methylation of non-CpG islands [36]. DNA-methylation may repress transcription in different ways:

- The direct binding of transcription factors to the promoter can be sterically inhibited [37].
- The binding of methyl-CpG-binding proteins (MBP) to methylated DNA sites, which recruits histone deacetylases and other factors, can be inhibited.

In contrast to normal cells, the DNA in cancer cells is globally hypomethylated (especially in solid tumors), and the degree of hypomethylation increases with the grading of the tumor [38]. Cancer cells also exhibit aberrant methylation in the regulatory regions of genes [39]. DNA hypomethylation seems to play an independent role in tumorigenesis by causing chromosomal instability, the reaction of transposable elements with viruses and by loss of imprinting (LOI). The methylation of cytosines in coding regions may increase mutation rates, by elevating spontaneous hydrolytic deamination of methylated cytosines leading to increased C-T transitions [40].

23.5. The Epigenetics of Solid Malignancies in Children and Young Adults

23.5.1. Tumors of the Central Nervous System

Tumors of the Central Nervous System (CNS) are the most common solid tumors in childhood. Foremost, gliomas comprise approximately 60% of pediatric CNS tumors, whereas the remaining 40% are heterogeneous and consist of medulloblastomas and other embryonal tumors (24%), craniopharyngiomas (4%), pineal tumors (1%), meningiomas (1%), and others (10%) [41].

The molecular mechanisms inducing pediatric brain tumors are largely unknown. Environmental factors do not appear to play a major role in the predisposition to develop brain tumors [42]. There are a number of hereditary gene defects known in brain tumors: e.g., mutations of the *p53* gene in Li-Fraumeni-Syndrome or *APC* in Turcot I Syndrome (for review see Bont et al. [43]). Survival rates for pediatric brain tumor patients have significantly improved over the years due to developments in diagnostic techniques, neurosurgery, chemotherapy, and supportive care, but prognosis is still highly dependent on clinical characteristics, such as age of the patient, tumor type, stage and anatomical localization.

It has become clear that the (epigenetic) deregulation of signalling pathways, essential for brain development, for example, sonic hedgehog (SHH), Wnt and Notch pathways, play important roles in pathogenesis and biological behaviour of brain tumors [43]. It is important to learn more about the biological characteristics of these tumors to facilitate diagnosis, contribute to better risk-group stratification and foremost to detect novel therapeutic targets.

23.5.1.1. Medulloblastoma and cerebral Primitive Neuroectodermal Tumors (cPNET)

Medulloblastoma (MB) is the most common embryonal CNS tumor of infants and comprises several biologically different entities arising from stem and progenitor cells of the cerebellum [43]. The most commonly reported cytogenetic change in medulloblastoma is a loss of 17p in up to 50% of tumors most commonly of the classic histologic subtype. Apart from gene mutations several epigenetic dysregulated pathways are found in medulloblastoma: Distinct methylation patterns have been detected in MB and cPNET alike. In these tumors up to 1% of all CpG islands seem to be methylated [39,44,45]. Aberrant methylation in the major chromosomal breakpoint cluster region in 17p11.2, affected by genomic disruption in these tumors, might be linked to chromosomal instability and formation of an isochromosome 17q, which is detected in up to 50% of MB [44]. Genes hypermethylated in medulloblastomas encode proteins that play a role in diverse functions, including cell cycle control (*TP53, TP74, RB1*, $p14^{ARF}$ and p 16^{INK4A}), microtubule stabilization and the regulation of mitosis (*RASSF1A*), transcription (*HIC1*), apoptosis (*CASP8, DAPK*) cell adhesion (*CDH1*), extracellular matrix (*TIMP3*), DNA repair (*MGMT*), and response to chemotherapeutic agents (*MCJ*) [46].

Epigentically dysregulated pathways in medulloblastoma and cPNET: The Sonic Hedgehog Signaling Pathway (SHH) is involved in apoptosis and angiogenesis. In Drosophila in the absence of Hedgehog (Hh), a cell-surface transmembrane protein called Patched (PTCH) prevents high expression and activity of a 7-membrane spanning receptor called Smoothened (SMO) [47]. When Patched is inhibited by Hh, Smoothened accumulates and inhibits the proteolytic cleavage of Cubitus interruptus (Ci), which accumulates in the cell cytoplasm. Consequently levels of CiR (a fragment of Ci) decrease [48] and CiR diffuses into the nucleus, where it acts as a co-repressor for Hh target genes [49]. Cubitus interruptus forms a complex with kinesin-like protein Costal leading to Ci protein proteolysis. In vertebrates the SHH pathway acts in a similar fashion: SHH binds to the Patched-1 (PTCH1) receptor. In the absence of ligand, PTCH1 inhibits Smoothened (SMO) [50]. The binding of SHH relieves SMO inhibition, leading to activation of the GLI transcription factors (activators: Gli1 and Gli2; repressor: Gli3). GLI controls the transcription of hedgehog target genes (Rb and the p53 pathway) [51]. Activation of the Hedgehog pathway leads to an increase in angiogenic factors (angiopoietin-1 and angiopoietin-2), cyclins (cyclin D1 and B1) [52], anti-apoptotic genes and a decrease in apoptotic genes (for review Jenkins et al. 2009) [53].

The sonic hedgehog-patched signalling pathway controls normal development of the external granular layer of the cerebellum [54], eyes, limbs and foregut. SHH disruption during critical periods of embryogenesis leads to developmental disorders (e.g., holoprosencephaly, the VATER-association) [55]. The tumor suppressor gene Patched 1 (PTCH1) on chromosome 9p22.3, is mutated in Gorlin Syndrome, an autosomal dominant disorder that is characterized by multiple developmental defects and a predisposition for basal cell carcinoma, rhabdomyosarcoma and medulloblastoma [56]. In 30% of medulloblastomas, mutations in different components of the SHH pathway such as *PTCH1* and *SMO* are detected, but cancer-specific methylation changes in primary medulloblastomas are also found including Sonic hedgehog (Shh) [57]. Diede *et al* demonstrated that the PTCH1-1C promoter, a negative regulator of the SHH pathway is methylated in both primary patient samples and human medulloblastoma cell lines. Treatment with the DNA methyltransferase inhibitor 5-aza-2`deoxycytidine (5-aza-dC) increases the expression of PTCH1[57].

Medulloblastoma is derived from cells important for cerebellar development, which is in mouse composed of a thin layer of cerebellar granule neuronal precursors (CGNPs). The proliferation of CGNPs is driven by Shh. The INK4c promoter was found methylated in human medulloblastomas. In mice disruption of Ink4c collaborates independently with loss of p53 or with inactivation of Ptch1 [58,59].

The *Wnt/Wingless pathway* is critical for normal development, determining cell fate, proliferation, migration and polarity. The canonical *β*-catenin/Tcf-mediated pathway, which is associated with the Wnt pathway plays an important role in regulating the balance between cell proliferation and differentiation [60]. *β-catenin* mutations and *APC* gene mutations are present in many cancers of adults, but also in childhood (e.g. medulloblastoma, cPNET, hepatoblastoma, Wilms tumors...). The activation of the Wnt/Wg pathway is an independent marker of favourable outcome in medulloblastoma [61]. The genetic defects identified to date only describe limited number of medulloblastomas. Axin2, a negative regulator of the WNT-pathway was found methylated in denaturation analyses of methylation differences (DAMD) by Diede *et al*, in primary medulloblastomas [57]. Hypermethylation of promoter-associated CpG islands leading to transcriptional silencing of the WNT-pathway is seen in many other tumors (ALL and many carcinomas in adults) [62,63,64].

Dickkopf (DKK1) is silenced in some medulloblastoma samples by histone acetylation in the promoter region. *DKK1* is an important antagonist of WNT and therefore an important suppressor of cell growth and inducer of apoptosis [65].

Deleted in liver cancer 1 (DLC1) located in chromosome 8p21.3-22, was identified in hepatocellular carcinomas (HCC) and encodes a protein with high homology to rat p122 RhoGAP[66]. RhoGAPs, is one major class of regulators of Rho GTPase. It stimulates the intrinsic GTPase activity of Rho to convert the active GTP-bound Rho protein into the inactive GDP-bound form. Rho GTPase are involved in various cellular functions: cytoskeletal organization and migration, growth, differentiation, apoptosis, neuronal development and synaptic function [67]. DLC1 induces apoptosis by activating caspase 3 and inhibits migration *in vitro* [68]. Reduction and loss of *DLC1* gene expression in several human tumors is associated with promoter hypermethylation, e.g. in supratentorial primitive neuroectodermal tumors (cPNET), but the reduced expression of *DLC1* found in medulloblastoma is not due to hypermethylation of the promoter region.

The *hypermethylated in cancer (HIC1)* gene is located on 17p13.3 and is a candidate tumor suppressor gene, which may play a role in several human tumors including brain tumors (e.g., medulloblastoma) [57], but also breast tumors, hepatocellular carcinomas, lung cancer, ALL and colorectal tumors [69,70,71,72,73]. HIC1 methylation is independently predictive of poor overall survival in medulloblastoma and promoter hypermethylation was found in 72% of medulloblastoma [74,75]. *HIC1* encodes a zinc finger transcription factor that functions as a transcription repressor containing five Krüppel-like C_2H_2 zinc finger motifs and a N-terminal autonomous transcriptional repression domain [76,77]. HIC-1 contains a TP53 binding site in the 5′flanking region and its expression is activated by wild-type TP53 [78]. HIC-1 mediates transcriptional repression by both HDAC-independent and HDAC-dependent mechanisms [76] and negatively regulates the Shh pathway [79]. *HIC-1* deficient mice die perinatally, show reduction in overall size, developmental defects and mice that lack one copy of *HIC-1* develop many different spontaneous malignant tumors [80].

O^6 –methylguanine-DNA methyltransferase (MGMT), a DNA repair protein, is involved in cancer development through alkylation of DNA at the O^6-position of guanine. O^6-methylguanine tends to pair with thymine during replication resulting in a conversion of G:C to A:T pairs in DNA. O^6-methylguanine also cross-links with opposite cytosine residues and blocks replication [81]. The O^6-methylguanine-DNA methyltransferase removes cytotoxic chlorethyl and methyl adducts from the O^6 position of guanine to its own cysteine residues leading to inactivation of one MGMT molecule for each repaired lesion [82]. Thus MGMT does not only protect cells from accumulating mutations, but also exerts a protective effect to tumor cells and contributes to the resistance of tumors to alkylating chemotherapeutics like temozolomide and carmustin [83,84]. MGMT activity is generally higher in malignant tumors, including pediatric brain tumors (94% MGMT activity) [85], indicating that tumorigenesis of pediatric brain tumors is accompanied by increased MGMT activity. Hypermethylation of the *MGMT* gene promoter has been demonstrated in medulloblastomas, malignant astrocytomas, oligodendrogliomas, ependymomas and choroid plexus tumors [86,87,88,89,90,91]. Some researchers do not see any relation between promoter hypermethylation and gene silencing [87]. In glioblastoma and oligodendroglial tumors, patients in which the MGMT promoter is methylated have a favourable outcome following treatment with alkylating agents [92]. This indicates that MGMT *inhibitors* such as the pseudosubstrate O^6-benzylguanine (BG) may have potential in the therapy of patients with an unmethylated *MGMT* promoter [84]. Lack of MGMT activity has two consequences for cancer cells: it may lead to accumulation of mutations in cancer related genes such as *TP53* [81], but it makes tumors also more susceptible to chemotherapy with alkylating drugs [83].

The *S100 protein family* is a large family of EF hand calcium-binding proteins of approximately 20 members [93,94] involved in the regulation of a variety of cellular processes including cell growth and cell cycle regulation. Members of the S100 gene family have been demonstrated to be aberrantly methylated in up to 20% of medulloblastomas. S100A6 is found hypermethylated, S100A4, hypomethylated, leading to prometastatic signals by direct targeting of ErbB2 [95,96].

The role of the *HGF/MET signal pathway* in the formation and progression of brain tumors is well established. The hepatocyte growth factor (HGF or "scatter factor") and its tyrosine kinase receptor c-Met play an important role in medulloblastoma [97]. HGF induces c-Myc levels via transcriptional and posttranscriptional modification involving MAPK and PI3K, inhibition of GSK-3b and translocation of β-catenin to the nucleus. Induction of Cdk2 kinase activity mediates cell cycle progression [98]. SPINT2, an inhibitor of the HGF/MET pathway, is found silenced by methylation of its promoter region potentially inducing medulloblastoma pathogenesis [99].

MCJ (DNAJC15, DnaJ (HSP49) homolog, subfamily C, member 15) is methylated and epigenetically silenced in malignant brain tumors in children such as medulloblastoma, cPNET and ependymoma, while no methylation has been detected in normal brain tissue

[100]. *MCJ* belongs to the DNAJ-protein family, which contains a 70-amino-acid functional J-domain and acts as co-chaperones, recruits Hsp70 chaperone partners and accelerates the ATP-hydrolysis step of the chaperone cycle [101]. In ovarian cancer, loss of *MCJ* due to methylation is associated with chemotherapeutic drug resistance [102].

RASSF1A regulates cyclin D1 expression, which is important in controling the cell cycle. In contrast to other malignancies, hypermethylation of *RASSF1A* in medulloblastoma is not accompanied by allelic loss of 3p21.3 or mutation, but by biallelic hypermethylation [103]. For more information about *RASSF1*, see the section on "neuroblastoma".

Promoter hypermethylation of *CASP8,* a cysteine-aspartyl-protease involved in death-receptor-mediated apoptosis, leads to loss of CASP8 mRNA expression. Loss of *CASP8* leads to apoptotic resistance by inducing tumor necrosis factor-related apoptosis-inducing ligand (TRAIL) [104,105]. Low expression of CASP8 protein has been reported as an independent indicator of poor survival in medulloblastoma patients [46]. Figure 23.2 depicts five of the most commonly dysregulated tumor pathways in medulloblastoma and other brain tumors.

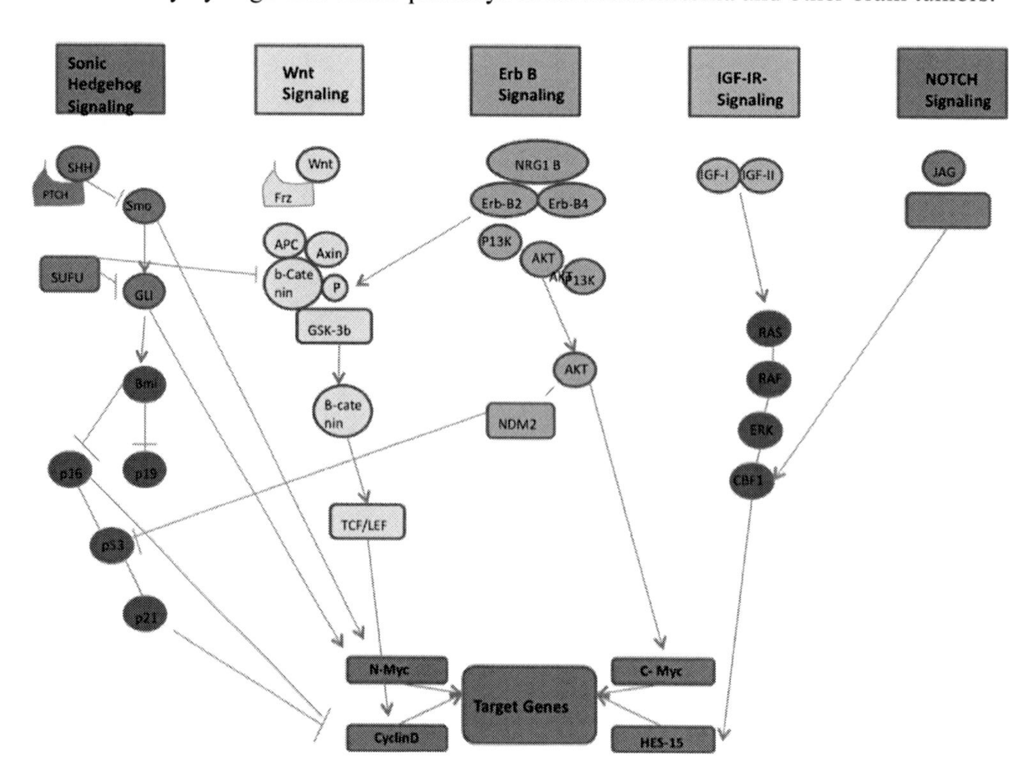

Figure 23.2. Five important signaling pathways often deregulated by epigenetic mechanisms in pediatric tumors.

23.5.1.2. The Epigenetics of Glioma in Childhood

Gliomas comprise about 60% of all pediatric brain tumors [106], and may arise from any glial cell of the central nervous system, e.g., astrocytes giving rise to astrocytomas of various WHO grades or glioblastoma multiforme. Oligodendrocytes may develop into oligodendrogliomas and ependymal cells may develop into ependymomas. Adult gliomas may represent a different biological entity. The epigenome of glioma in adults has been extensively much more studied than gliomas in children. In infants embryonal tumors such as medulloblastoma, supratentorial primitive neuroectodermal tumors predominate, whereas in children older than three years pilocytic astrocytomas prevail (for review see Pfister and Witt [41]).

In gliomas, as in many other pediatric tumors, genes that participate in various cellular processes such as apoptosis, cell cycle control, angiogenesis and DNA repair are epigenetically changed. The *p14*^{ARF} and *p16*^{INK4A} tumor suppressor genes belong to the cyclin-dependent kinase inhibitors 2A (CDKN2A) and are frequently lost in brain tumors [107]. P14 stabilizes TP53 by binding and promoting the degradation of MDM, leading to cell cycle arrest [108,109]. P14 also prevents the nuclear export of TP53. In astrocytomas, hypermethylation of *p14*^{ARF} has been detected and seems to be an early event in the progression to secondary glioblastoma [107]. Methylation of *p14*^{ARF} is independent from the *p16*^{INK4A} methylation status, even though those two genes share an overlapping reading frame on chromosome 9p21 [110]. Promoter hypermethylation of *p14*^{ARF} has also been found in many brain tumors of adults such as ependymoma and oligodendroglioma [110].

P15^{INK4b} and *p16*^{INK4A} inhibit the exit from G1 to the S-phase of the cell cycle via inhibiting phosphorylation of the retinoblastoma protein (RB) through inactivating CDK4 and CDK6 [111,112,113,114]. Methylation of *p15*^{INK4b} and *p16*^{INK4A} are uncommon in childhood brain tumors, but promoter hypermethylation associated with loss of *p16*^{INK4A} expression and inactivation of *p15*^{INK4b} through CpG island methylation has been reported in glioma [115]. The retinoblastoma protein 1 (Rb1) and *TP73*, a gene related to *TP53*, both involved in cell cycle control, have been found methylated in several brain tumors: e.g., medulloblastomas, astrocytomas and glioblastomas [116,117], but also in oligodendrogliomas and ependymomas [118].

Tissue inhibitor of metalloproteinase-3 (TIMP3) on chromosome 22q12.1.13.2 is silenced by promoter methylation in astrocytic tumors such as glioblastomas, but also in some ependymomas, oligodendrogliomas and medulloblastomas [119,120,121]. TIMP proteins inhibit the proteolytic activity of matrix metalloproteinases (MMPs) [122]. There is an MMP-dependent, but also an MMP-independent role of TIMP3 in the development of cancer. The balance between TIMP and MMPs plays a crucial role in remodelling the extracellular matrix during normal development, but also in cancer [123]. TIMP3 blocks MMP-independent VEGF (vascular endothelial growth factor) binding to the VEGF-receptor-2 and inhibits angiogenesis in this way [124]. Loss of TIMP3 allows tumor cell expansion due to MMP loss and angiogenesis [123]. In pediatric anaplastic astrocytomas and glioblastomas the tumor suppressor Phosphatase and *TEN*sin homologue (PTEN), which is located on chromosome 11q23 has been found mutated (astrocytomas - 6%, glioblastoma - 8%) and is associated with a dismal prognosis [125].

PTEN induces growth suppression by blocking cell cycle progression through negatively regulating the p13-kinase/Akt signaling pathway [126]. Epigenetic silencing of *PTEN* has been observed in oligodendroglial tumors (42.9%) [127], astrocytomas [128] and in adult patients with glioblastoma [129].

23.5.1.3. Epigenetic Lesions in AT/RT (Atypical Teratoid/Rhabdoid Tumors)

Rhabdoid tumors are rare but highly aggressive neoplasms with an incidence that peaks between birth and 3 years of age [130]. Rhabdoid tumors of the kidney are termed RTK (rhabdoid tumors of the kidney), their central nervous system counterparts are atypical teratoid/rhabdoid tumors and those of soft tissues are termed MRT (malignant rhabdoid tumors). The cell of origin for these tumors is unknown and because of the presence of mixed cell types, varied anatomic locations, and early onset it is hypothesized, that these tumors may arise from pluripotent stem cells. Prognosis for patients with rhabdoid tumors is poor despite the use of potent chemotherapeutic, radiotherapeutic, and surgical interventions [131] (2-year survival rate is between 15% to 55% for children with atypical teratoid rhabdoid tumors) [132, 133]. Cytogenetic and molecular genetic studies of rhabdoid tumors have indicated that the majority of rhabdoid tumors harbour recurrent biallelic alterations in the *SMARCB1INI1/hSNF5* gene, located on chromosome 22q11.2.4. Mutations in *SMARCB1INI1/hSNF5* predispose individuals to various types of cancers including AT/RT and other tumors of central nervous system [134]. Targeted disruption of *SMARCB1/INI1/hSNF5* in mice demonstrated that heterozygous mice develop tumours at a high frequency, while homozygous deletions are embryonic lethal [135]. *SMARCB1/INI1/hSNF5* also known as *BAF47* is a component of the human chromatin remodelling SWI/SNF complex [136]. There are two broad classes of chromatin remodelling machines: those that remodel chromatin mediated by covalent modification such as acetylation, deacetylation and methylation (as described above), and those that modify chromatin by disrupting and/or repositioning the nucleosomes in an ATP-dependent manner. The most important three-chromatin remodelling complexes are: The first, the *Swi/Snf complex* removes histones from DNA or mediates the transfer of histones from one DNA strand to another [137]. The second, the *NuRD complex* is associated with repressed gene expression [138]. The third important group of chromatin remodelers include the *polycomb proteins* (see below), which influence many cell cycle genes and genes of early development and are conserved through vertebrates [139].

The *SWI/SNF* complex, which was initially identified in screens for genes that regulate mating-type switching (SWI) and sucrose non-fermenting (SNF) phenotypes in yeast [140] consists of nine subunits that are conserved among eukaryotes. Among these are four core subunits that are required for chromatin remodelling, including SWI2/SNF2, the key ATPase subunit, and INI1/hSNF5, another critical component of the SWI/SNF complex. The Drosophila orthologue of ATPase subunit SWI2/SNF2 is termed Brahma, from which the two human paralogues derive their name, the *hBRM* and *BRG1* (brahma-related gene). In drosophila *brm* or *brahma* was identified as a trithorax group gene that suppresses the Polycomp [141], activate *hox* genes [142] and being involved in chromatin remodelling [143,144]. Mammalian cells express BRM as well as a closely related protein Brahma-related gene-1 (BRG1), and in addition 8-10 subunits, which are referred to as BRM or BRG1-associated factors or BAF [145].

The SWI/SNF complexes act as ATP-dependent chromatin-remodelers. Alternative models show how SWI/SNF complexes act, including ATP-dependent movement (from catalytic subunit BRM and BRG) of histone octamers in cis along the DNA, transfer of histone octamers from one nucleosomal array to another or replacement of nucleosomal histones [146]. The yeast SWI/SNF moves bidirectionally along the DNA, resulting in a continuous positional re-distribution around a characteristic distance of motion of approximately 28bp [147]. The result is an altered structure that is hypersensitive to nuclease digestion and exhibits increased affinity for transcription factors [148] and the transcriptional machinery [149]. For a brilliant review on SWI/SNF complex and its relation to cancer see Reisman *et al.* [150].

BRM is epigenetically silenced in several tumor cell lines [151,152,153,154] and histone deacetylase inhibitors (HDACs) can restore BRM mRNA and protein expression in a variety of BRM null cell lines [151,154]. A large number of tumor cells have lost both *BRM* and *BRG1* expression and re-expression of either *BRG1* or *BRM* inhibits growth of such cells in culture [155]. In *BRM* null mice, the expression levels of *BRG1* is threefold higher than in wild-type BRM mice [156] and embryonic fibroblasts from BRM knockout mice demonstrate striking abnormalities in cell cycle control and *BRM* null mice are larger than wild-type mice [156,157,158]. BRM functions in;

- cell cycle control by interacting with RB family members (RB1, p107 and p 130) [159]. Thus SWI/SNF is required for E2F-dependent transcription [160]. Re-expression of *BRG1* induces p21, which inhibits RB phosphorylation by cyclin dependent kinases (CDKs) [161].
- DNA repair by controlling p53, BRCA1 and Fanconi anemia proteins [162,163].
- controlling the expression of genes that are involved in cellular adhesion (CD44, E-cadherin; MMP1, MMP2, transgelin, GALS3BP P8, PODXL, Integrin A5, LGALS1, Integrin A3, TIMP3, PLAU) [164,165,166,167].
- regulating the activity of some nuclear receptors (glucocorticoid receptor, androgen / estrogen receptor, retinoic acid receptor) [154,168,169,170], which could be responsible for resistance of tumors to treatment with steroids and other hormones [171,172].

As described for BRM and BRG1 there is evidence that several other subunits of the SWI/SNF complex play a central role in the development of cancer [173,174], but BAF47 (INI1) has the most tumorigenic defect that has been engineered to date [175,176]. INI1 was initially discovered as a protein that binds HIV integrase[177] and is identical to BAF47 (SNF5, SMARCB1) (located on chromosome 22q11). A conditional knockdown of BAF47 results in CML, Hodgkin´s lymphomas and rhabdoid tumors with a penetrance of 100% [175,178]. In adult tumors loss of BAF47 is very rare. The dominant deletion of the SWI/SNF complex in adults is the loss of *BRG1* and *BRM* (e.g., 30% of lung cancer cell lines) [179,180]. In rhabdoid tumours, one allele of BAF47 is consistently deleted and the other is either mutated or silenced by methylation [181,182]. About 5% of all genes are regulated by SWI/SNF5. *SMARCB1/INI1/hSNF5* is present in any of the SWI/SNF complexes, implicating a multiple and varied function for this protein in mammalian cells. The SWI/SNF activity is maintained at some level even in the absence of BAF47, which seems to act more as an enhancer of remodelling activity, rather than an obligatory component of the chromatin-remodelling complex [183].

Reintroduction of *SMARCB1/INI1/hSNF5* into rhabdoid cells alone is sufficient to block S-Phase entry and to cause G0/G1 arrest and senescence. *SMARCB1/INI1/hSNF5* directly represses cyclin D1 (not Cyclin D2 and D3) by recruiting HDAC1 complex to its promoter [184,185,186]. Cyclin D1 serves as a key sensor and integrator of extracellular stimuli in early to mid-G1 phase of the cell cycle [187]. Cyclin D1 activates cyclin dependent kinases 4 and 6, which in turn phosphorylate the retinoblastoma protein (RB). Overexpressed cyclin D1 also sequesters p21cip1 (cdks inhibitor), activating cyclin E-cdk2 holoenzyme, resulting in

G1-S transition. Targeting cyclinD1 by cyclinD-inhibitors like Fenretinide, leads to G0-arrest and apoptosis [188].

Another valid option to influence this pathway is to use HDIs (histone deacetylase inhibitors). The exact mechanism of how HDIs act in this pathway is not completely understood, but *in vitro* data demonstrate a strong inhibitory effect on tumor cell growth and induction of apoptosis in rhabdoid tumor cell lines [189]. Figure 23.3 shows the SWI/SNF complex and the dependent tumor pathway.

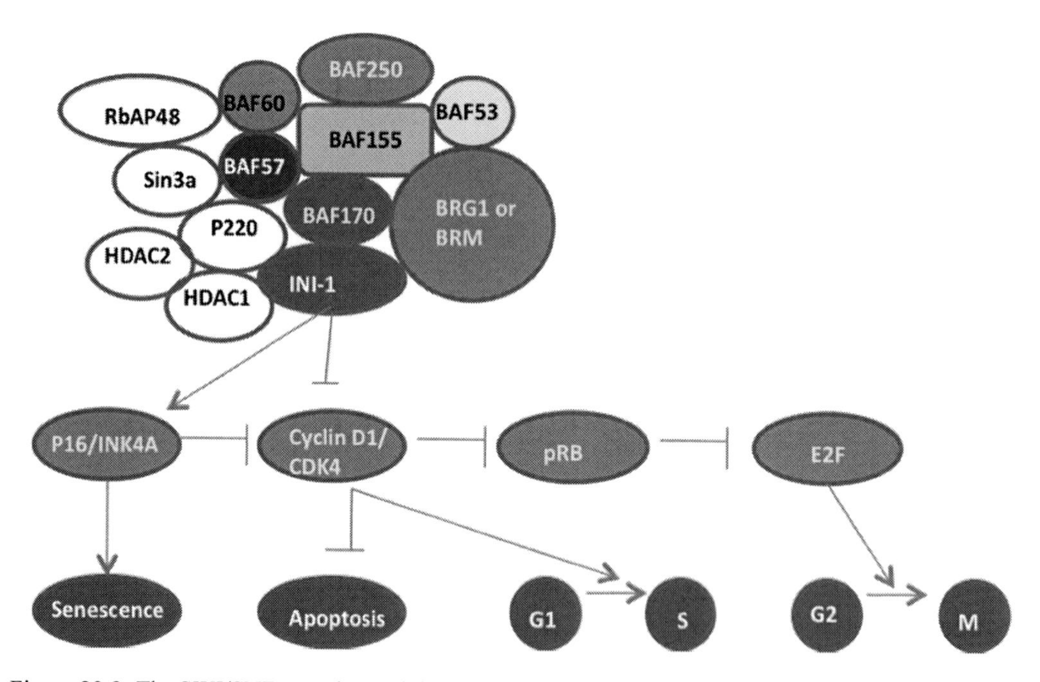

Figure 23.3. The SWI/SNF complex and the regulation of the CyclinD-CDK-Rb-Pathway by INI1/SNF5. INI1 is regularly mutated in rhabdoid tumors. This results in deregulation of CyclinD, phosphorylation of Rb and activation of E2F target genes.

23.5.2. The Epigenome of Wilms' Tumor

Wilms tumor, derived from embryonic rests of the kidney has uncovered important principles in cancer genetics i.e., the recognition of the Wilms' tumor-aniridia (WAGR) syndrome, its mapping to chromosome 11p13 [190] and the discovery of the *WT1* tumor suppressor gene [191,192]. *WT1* is mutated in 10% of Wilms' tumors overall, predominantly in the setting of WAGR and Denys-Drash syndromes but also in a small subset of sporadic Wilms' tumors [193]. Sporadic Wilms' tumors show LOH of several regions, most frequently 11p15 but also 1p, 4q, 7p, 11q, 14q, 16q, and 17p.

23.5.2.1. Aberrant Methylation in Wilms' Tumor

The *IGF pathway* plays an important role in neuronal development. Three ligands are involved in insulin-like growth factor (IGF) signaling: IGF-I, IGF-II, and insulin. IGF-I and IGF-II build a complex, bound to one of six IGF binding proteins (IGFBP-1 to IGFBP-6) [194]. Three receptors form six distinct receptor combinations: IGF receptors type 1 and type

2 (IGF-1R and IGF-2R), insulin receptors A and B (IR-A and IR-B), and hybrid receptors (IGF-1R/IR-A and IGF-1R/IR-B) [195]. IGF-1R consists of two α-subunits (extracellular, binding IGF) and two β-subunits (transmembrane, linked by disulfide bonds and contain an intracellular tyrosine kinase domain) [196]. Binding of IGF-I or IGF-II ligand to IGF-1R leads to phosphorylation of three key tyrosine residues in the kinase domain and the phosphorylation of downstream substrates [197]. Phosphorylation of additional tyrosine residues in other areas of the β-subunit allows the recruitment of adaptor proteins [196], inducing signal transduction along several specific pathways (increases proliferation (mitogen-activated protein kinase), decreased apoptosis (phosphatidylinositol 3' kinase), translational adaption (mammalian target of rapamycin (mTOR) [198]. There are many other adaptor proteins that are known to play an important role in IGF-1R signaling, beside the insulin receptor substrate family [198].

Epigenetic dysregulation of the IGF-pathway is found in Wiedemann-Beckwith-Syndrome (see below), which is associated with embryonal tumors such as Wilms' tumors, rhabdomyosarcomas, neuroblastomas, adrenal cortical carcinomas and gonadoblastomas [199,200,201,202,203,204,205].

About 40% of Wilms' tumors exhibit loss of heterozygosity (LOH) of chromosome 11p comprising tumors with LOH restricted to the *WT1* locus on 11p13. Thirty to fifty percent of Wilms' tumors exhibit loss of imprinting (LOI) of the *WT2* locus on 11p15, which corresponds to the closely linked and oppositely imprinted genes, *IGF2* and *H19* on this chromosomal band. In 45% of sporadic Wilms' tumors that have 11p15.5 LOH, there is a selective loss of maternal alleles and duplication of paternal alleles (reviewed by Feinberg et al. 2004) [206]. *IGF2* has four promoter regions. The allelic expression of *IGF2* is regulated by the methylation status of the sixth CTCF (CCCTC-binding factor) site in the H19 differentially methylated region (DMR) that represents the parental origin of the IGF2 allele. Whereas the paternal CTCF6 allele is methylated, the maternal allele is unmethylated in normal tissues [207,208]. IGF2 and *H19* promoters compete on the same chromosome for a shared enhancer, and access of the maternal IGF2 allele to this enhancer is blocked by H19 DMR when unmethylated because of the insulator activity of CTCF binding to unmethylated H19 DMR [207,208]. In Wilms' tumors aberrant methylation of the maternal CTCF6 prevents insulator binding and leads to loss of imprinting (LOI) (32–38% of WTs), resulting in the overexpression of IGF2 [209] and loss of heterozygosity (LOH), leading to uniparental disomy (UPD) of the paternal IGF2, which occurs in 36–50% of WTs [210].

Other solid tumors in children exhibit changes in the epigenetic patterns of IGF genes as well. In a study of germ-line genetics in osteosarcoma, another common solid tumor in children, variation in growth pathway genes of the insulin-like growth factor 2 receptor (IGF2R) Ex16+88G>A and IVS16+15C>T single nucleotide polymorphisms (SNPs) have been identified. Both SNPs results in loss of methylation at a CpG island and are associated with increased risk of osteosarcoma [211].

Most medulloblastomas overexpress the IGF-1 receptor (IGF-1R) and the activated phosphorylated form of IGF-1R that causes the activation of downstream targets of IGF-1 such as IRS-1 (insulin receptor substrate-1), AKT/PKB, PI3K, Erk-1 and Erk-2. Inhibition of IGF-1R signaling reduce medulloblastoma tumor growth, augmented by constitutive GSK3-β phosphorylation [212]. Epigenetic changes in the IGF pathway in medulloblastoma have not been explored in enough detail as of now.

Other regions of LOH in Wilms' tumors have been described in the *CXCR 4* gene on chromosome 4q24-q25, a repressor gene of the WNT pathway[210] and *nephronectin* on chromosome 4q24-q25, which is an extracellular matrix component that is a ligand for α_8/β_1 integrin, which is in turn a molecule that is essential for metanephric kidney maturation [213].

23.5.2.2. Loss of Imprinting (LOI)

In somatic cells of diploid organisms autosomal genes are represented by two copies, or alleles, with one copy from the mother and one copy from the father. Both alleles are simultaneously expressed in most autosomal genes, but in mammals a small proportion (<1%, meaning~80 genes in humans) of genes are imprinted. Imprinted means that gene expression occurs from only one allele [214]. The expressed allele is dependent upon its parental origin (Insulin-like growth factor 2 (IGF2/Igf2) is only expressed from the allele inherited from the father) [215]. Many of the imprinted genes are involved in embryonic and placental growth and development [216]. In germline cells the imprint is erased, and then re-established according to the sex of the individual, which is epigenetically controlled by DNA methylation and histone modifications. Regulatory elements, such as non-coding RNAs and differentially methylated regions (DMRs), control the imprinting of one or more genes (imprinting control regions (ICR)) [217].

23.5.3. Neuroblastoma as a Paradigm for Epigenetic Lesions

Apart from brain tumors neuroblastomas are the most frequently occurring solid tumors in children below 5 years of age. Neuroblastomas are neuro-ectodermal tumors of embryonic neural crest-derived cells and the spectrum of these tumors ranges from undifferentiated, malignant neuroblastomas, via ganglioneuroblastomas to well-differentiated mostly benign ganglioneuromas. One of the most prominent regions of loss of heterozygosity in neuroblastoma is 1p36. Epigenetic mechanisms do not seem to play an important role in gene silencing of this region [218].

23.5.3.1. Apoptotic Pathways in Neuroblastoma

Apoptosis or programmed cell death is a major form of cell death that influences the growth of tumor cell populations. Chromosome 2q33, the location of *caspase 8*, is associated with LOH. In neuroblastomas but also medulloblastomas, rhabdomyosarcomas, retinoblastomas and neuroendocrine lung cancer, alterations of *caspase 8* can be found [219,220]. Caspase 8 is a cysteine protease and a member of the caspase family of proteolytic enzymes, which are active in programmed cell death. Caspase 8 can be activated by most members of the TNF-receptor super family (TNFRSF members, e.g., Fas, Death Receptor 3, DR4, DR5, TNFR2, p75TNR) through an intermediate FADD (FAS-associating protein with death domain). Activated caspase 8 leads to activation of pro-caspase 3 and initiation of the final pathway to apoptosis. Tumor cells with loss of *CASP8* do not respond to TNF-receptor mediated triggers like TNF receptor apoptosis inducing ligand (TRAIL) or Fas ligand (FasL) [221,222,223]. The *caspase 8* promoter region is found hypermethylated in 35% of neuroblastomas [224] and *caspase 8* is re-expressed in neuroblastoma cell lines after 5-AZA treatment [225]. An important regulator of caspase 8 is the flice inhibitory protein (FLIP), a caspase 8-related protein, which is also often found hypermethylated in neuroblastoma [221].

Furthermore, genes of the intrinsic apoptosis pathway can be found to be dysregulated: increased levels of *BCL2* and *BCLXL* have been observed, and correlate with decreased apoptosis [226]. Overexpression of *BCL2* blocks TRAIL-induced apoptosis in neuroblastoma cell lines [227] and correlates with poor prognosis [228].

Expression of lysosomal associated protein multispanning transmembrane 5 (*LAPTM5*) is usually down-regulated through DNA methylation in favourable and unfavourable NB tumor samples, and is found upregulated in degenerating NB cells. Overexpression of *LAPTM5* induces caspase-independent lysosomal cell death due to lysosomal destabilization with lysosomal-membrane permeabilization, with the accumulation of immature autophagic vacuoles and ubiquitinated proteins [229].

23.5.3.2. Hypermethylation of RASSF1A

RASSF1 is silenced and frequently inactivated by promoter region hypermethylation in many adult and childhood cancers, including lung-, breast-, kidney-, gastric-, bladder-cancer, neuroblastoma, medulloblastoma and glioma [220,230]. In addition it plays an important role in cell cycle regulation, apoptosis and microtubule stability (reviewed by Agathanggelou [231]).

Allelic loss of the short arm of chromosome 3 (location of *RASSF1A*) is common in neuroblastomas (chromosomal band 3p21.3) [232]. Hypermethylation of *RASSF1A* in neuroblastomas is common with a frequency of 40–55% of tumors and 86% of cell lines. There is a relationship to concomitant hypermethylation of *CASP8*: methylation of *CASP8* was detected in 56% of tumors with *RASSF1A* methylation and only in 17% in tumors without *RASSF1A* methylation [231]. Two CpG islands are associated with the promoter region of *RASSF1* (the first spans the promoter region of *RASSF1A* (and *RASSF1D*, *RASSF1E*, *RASSF1F*, and *RASSF1G*) and the second for *RASSF1B* and *RASSF1C*). A Ras association or RalGDS/AF-6 domain is located at the COOH terminus of RASSF1 isoforms A-E, which mediates interactions with Ras and other small GTPases. Ras is a small inner membrane GTPase that relays proliferative signals from cell surface receptors such as receptor tyrosine kinases. Ras becomes activated by binding to GTP causing a shift in conformation revealing cytoplasmic epitopes that mediate interactions with effector proteins such as Raf kinases [231]. Ras is an important modulator of the apoptotic response and is thought to mediate cell survival in response to hyperproliferative signals in transformed cells through PI3-K– and Tiam-1–pathways and to induce apoptosis in untransformed cells through pathways mediated by RASSF1 and NORE1 [233]. NORE1A and two RASSF1 homologues (AD037and RASSF2) are downregulated by hypermethylation of the CpG islands in the promoter region of adult tumors such as non-small lung-cancer [234,235,236,237].

23.5.3.3. Epigenetic Aspects of MYCN in Neuroblastoma

MYCN is associated with a number of tumors including neuroblastoma, but also plays a central role in the function of normal neural stem and precursor cells (NSC). *MYCN* is associated with a wide variety of cellular functions including proliferation, apoptosis, cellular metabolism and DNA synthesis (reviewed by Eilers et al.) [238]. Myc genes encode transcription factors of the basic helix-loop-helix-zipper (bHLHZ) superfamily and regulate both specific gene transcription through discrete chromatin events usually at target gene promoters and maintain very large euchromatic domains [239]. At specific promoters and much larger chromatin domains, Myc is strongly linked to euchromatic marks including acetylation of lysine 9 (AcK9) and methylation of lysine 4 of histone H3 (triMeK4). MYCN regulates the expression of a number of genes encoding stem-related factors in neuroblastoma and in neuronal stem cells, including lif, klf2, klf4, and lin28b suggesting enforced expression of aspects of a pluripotency program [240]. MYCN regulates trimethylation of lysine 4 of histone H3 in the promoter of lif and possibly in the promoters of several other stem-related genes, indicating that MYCN regulates overlapping stem-related gene expression programs in neuroblastoma and NSC [240].

23.5.3.4. CpG Island Methylator Phenotype in Neuroblastoma

The CpG island (CGI) methylator phenotype (CIMP), which is characterized by methylation of multiple CGIs, has been detected in various tumors [241]. In neuroblastomas CIMP was found to be associated with poor survival [242]. Neuroblastoma cases with CIMP included almost all cases with *MYCN* amplification, but even among cases without *MYCN* amplification CIMP is a significant and strong prognostic marker [242]. In NBL CIMP is most sensitively detected by methylation of nonpromoter CGIs (PCDH-α gene family, P CDH-β gene family, HLP and its pseudogene and CYP26C1) [242]. Their methylation does not appear to repress transcription [243], but methylation of nonpromoter CGI is associated with methylation of promoter CGIs of tumor suppressor genes, such as *RASSF1A* and *BLU* [242] or genes involved in neuronal development like *FERD3L* and *PCDHGC4* [244]. CIMP invariably induces methylation of susceptible CGIs (specific nonpromoter CGIs) and occasionally induces methylation of resistant CGIs (promoter CGIs), causing gene silencing [244].

23.5.3.5. The Histone Code of Neuroblastomas

The upregulation of HDAC8 is a prognostic factor in neuroblastoma just as the loss of 1p and 11q and older age. It thus indicates poor long-term overall and event-free survival [26]. Targeting of HDAC8 in neuroblastoma cell lines and tumor cells induces differentiation, cell cycle arrest and reduced clonogenic growth. In chemotherapy resistant neuroblastoma cell lines, HDAC1 was found up-regulated and knockdown of HDAC1 resulted in re-sensitization of cells to chemotherapy [30]. It was furthermore involved in mediating the repressing effects of the *MYCN* oncogene in neuroblastoma cells.

23.5.4. Epigenome Changes in Ewing Sarcoma and Osteosarcoma

Osteosarcoma is the most frequent primary bone sarcoma, comprising approximately 20% of all bone tumors and about 5% of pediatric tumors overall. The most common locations in young adults are regions with rapid bone growth, including the distal femur, proximal tibia, and proximal humerus. Although osteosarcoma development is associated with several genetic predisposition conditions, most osteosarcomas are sporadic without familial patterns [245,246,247].

Amplifications are rather common and have been detected in the following chromosomal regions 6p12–p21 (28%), 17p11.2 (32%), and 12q13–q14 (8%), but also other chromosomal losses (2q, 3p, 9, 10p, 13q, 14q, 15q, 16, 17p, 18q) and chromosomal gains (Xp, Xq, 5q, 6p, 8q, 17p, and 20q) have been identified [248].

Terminal differentiation of osteoblasts, which are derived from multipotent mesenchymal stem cells, is a well orchestrated process and controlled by a cascade of regulatory signalling [249]. Bone development is relatively well understood at a cellular and molecular level (reviewed by Aubin [250]) including two key steps in cellular differentiation that appear critical to tumorigenesis. The first key transition point is the step between a mesenchymal stem cell and a lineage-restricted progenitor cell; the second one initiates terminal differentiation and permanent cell cycle withdrawal. Epigenetic mechanisms are critical in both steps. The crossover from a stem cell to a transit amplifying compartment is regulated by the polycomb (PcG) family [251]. PcG proteins are one of three groups of chromatin remodelling proteins and play critical roles in the assignment of epigenetic states, through histone modification. Due to the huge importance in chromatin remodelling and the importance in the development of osteosarcoma, the role of the three PcG complexes that have been characterized to date are briefly described.

- The first, polycomb repressive complex 2 (PRC2) initiates silencing through methylation of lysine residues on histones H3 and H1.
- The second, PRC1, is involved in the maintenance of stable states of gene repression by recognizing methylated lysines on histone H3.
- The third complex, PRC3, targets specific lysine residues (K27 on H3 and K26 on H1) via Eed proteins [252].

Polycomb genes affect epigenetic processes important to maintenance of the stem cell phenotype. *Bmi-1* is a main subunit of the PRC1-complex and *Bmi-1*-deficient mice manifest defects in hemopoietic and neuronal development [253]. *Bmi-1* is overexpressed in a variety of human cancers and stimulates proliferation by repression of the Ink4a/Arf locus [254,255].

Bmi-1 is regulated by hedgehog, which is a key morphogen in skeletal development. Ectopic expression of Bmi-1 in mesenchymal stem cells resulted in immortalization without loss of differentiation [256]. BMI-1 is highly expressed in Ewing Sarcoma cells and actively promotes growth *in vitro* and tumorigenicity *in vivo* [257].

Histone methyltransferase Enhancer of Zeste (*EZH2*), the enzymatic subunit of the polycomb PRC2 complex methylates histone H3K27 to mediate gene silencing. *EZH2* is required for blastocyst development and the generation of embryonic stem cell lines, implying a role in early embryonic stem cell function. The expression levels of *Ezh2* mRNA in bone and bone marrow are very high in the adult mouse [258].

Ewing tumors are defined by *ews/ets* translocations, which generate the expression of the *EWS-FLI*-fusion gene. The human Ewing Sarcoma (EWS) protein belongs to the TET family of RNA-binding proteins and consists of an N-terminal transcriptional activation domain (EAD) and a C-terminal RNA-binding domain (RBD), which is extensively methylated at arginine residues. This multifunctional protein acts in transcriptional co-activation, DNA-recombination, -pairing and -repair, in splicing, and mRNA transport. The role of the EWS protein arginine methylation, which occurs immediately after translation remains unclear [259]. The EWS protein interacts via its RBD with RNase-sensitive protein complexes consisting of mainly heterogeneous nuclear ribonucleoproteins (hnRNPs) and RNA helicases [259]. *EWS-FLI1* binds to the *EZH2* promoter *in vivo*. *EZH2* suppression results in a generalized loss of H3K27me3 as well as an increase in H3 acetylation and suppresses tumor development and metastasis [260,261].

Other PcG members such as polyhomeotic-like 3 (PHC3) also seem to play a role in development of primary pediatrics bone tumors [262].

At the transition between the transamplifying compartment and terminal differentiation, *Rb* has a key role in the establishment of chromatin structures in senescence, in a manner reminiscent of polycomb functions. Dysregulation of the Rb-pathway is found in osteosarcomas through different mechanism [263,264,265]. *PRb* controls histone methyltransferase activity by direct interactions with SUV4-20H1 and SUV4- 20H2, which methylate lysine 20 on histone H4 [266]. The trimethylation of histone H4 is associated with pericentric and telomeric heterochromatin. In cells lacking pRb there is a decrease in global cytosine methylation, an increase in histone H1 and 3 acetylation, and a decrease in histone H4 methylation. pRb is involved in maintaining overall chromatin structure and in particular constitutive heterochromatin, which leads to genomic instability and aneuploidy [266]. Osteosarcomas are characteristically aneuploid tumors. PRb also interacts with the polycomb pathway, either directly [267], or by regulation of polycomb proteins such as EZH2 [268].

Apart from these epigenetic modifications of the polycomb complexes and the pRB pathways in the development of osteosarcoma and Ewing Sarcoma, an array of other tumor pathways are suggested to be epigenetically modified. Several major signaling pathways, such WNT-, BMP-, FGF-, and hedgehog signaling, play an important role in regulating osteogenic differentiation [269,270]. The WNT-pathway (see above) is epigenetically silenced in some osteosarcomas by expressing high levels of the *WNT-inhibitory factor 1(WIF1)*[271]. Kansara *et al.* analyzed five osteosarcoma cell lines using high-throughput mass spectrometry. *Wif1* is highly expressed in the developing and mature mouse skeleton. In primary human osteosarcomas, silencing of *WIF*1 by promoter hypermethylation was associated with differentiation, increased *β-catenin* levels and increased proliferation [271].

Several transcription factors have been identified as important regulators of osteogenic lineage commitment and terminal differentiation: *Runx2, Osterix, ATF4*, and *TAZ* [272,273,274,275]. *RUNX2* (CBFA1/Osf2/PEBP2a) is a key transcriptional regulator of osteoblast differentiation. RUNX2 belongs to the runt family of transcription factors[276]. *RUNX2* postnatally regulates expression of bone-specific genes such as *osteopontin* and *osteocalcin*, and controls bone matrix deposition [277]. Changes in promoter methylation of the *osteocalcin* gene have been suggested to play a role in osteoblast differentiation and carcinogenesis [278,279]. Osteocalcin (OC), a bone-specific protein and marker of the mature osteoblast, is expressed only in nonproliferating osteoblasts in a mineralizing extracellular matrix, and is down-regulated upon treatment with transforming growth factor (TGF)-beta 1. TGFb family members play important roles in regulating cell growth and development [280].

Aberrant DNA methylation of the imprinted *IGF2* and *H19* loci has also been observed and suggested to play a role in osteosarcoma tumorigenesis [281]. *RASSF1* was frequently hypermethylated in pediatric tumours including osteosarcoma and Ewing Sarcoma (68% in Ewing Sarcoma and 75% in ES cell lines) [282,283] and is associated with poor prognosis in Ewing Sarcoma [283].

HIC1 encodes a zinc finger transcriptional factor that represses transcription dependent and independent of class I histone deacetylases [76,284] (see above). In double-transgenic mice for *HIC1* and *TP53,* lymphomas and osteosarcomas are found, with a high degree of metastasis. Somatic *TP53* mutations in human osteosarcomas range from 19% to 38%

[285,286]. The presence of *TP53* mutations correlates with high levels of genomic instability in osteosarcomas [286]. Hypermethylation of *HIC1* has been found in 17% of pediatric osteosarcomas [287]. *HIC1* is likely involved in a feedback regulation of p53 in tumor suppression, so that loss of *HIC1* by hypermethylation may complement *p53* mutations in the development of a subset of human osteosarcomas [288].

LSAMP, also known as LAMP, is a neuronal surface glycoprotein [289] and is one of four IgLONs constituting a subfamily of glycoproteins that belong to the immunoglobulin superfamily. The IgLONs are cell adhesion molecules that are involved in modification of neurite outgrowth and cell-cell recognition [290]. *LSAMP* has previously been identified as a translocation breakpoint-spanning gene in familial clear cell renal carcinoma [291]. Loss of heterozygosity (LOH) of *LSAMP* was observed in several tumors, both with and without promoter methylation. Hypermethylation was also detected in osteosarcoma cell lines and primary tumors and was associated with reduced gene expression compared to normal bone [292].

In two osteosarcoma cell lines, U2OS and MG63, eight genes (in both cell lines) were hypermethylated and repressed (*SLIT3, DLC1, GLT25D2, LMO3. GDNF, PCSK1, FLJ 37440, LHX9*) and several genes were significantly hypomethylated and overexpressed (76 genes in U2OS and 92 genes in MG63 cells) [293]. These data suggest that, in addition to the hypermethylation and possible loss of gene expression, increases in gene expression driven by hypomethylation may play a role in osteosarcoma [293]. The majority of these genes are located in the regions that are amplified in the tumors, including chromosomes 6p, 8q, 9p, and17p in tumors and cell lines [294,295], consistent with the emerging evidence in other cancers linking DNA hypomethylation and regions of genomic imbalance and genomic instability [296,297].

23.5.5. The Epigenetics of Hepatoblastoma

Hepatoblastoma (HB) represents the most common malignant liver tumor in children with a median age at presentation of 6 to 36 months [298]. The incidence in Western countries amounts to about one HB case per million children [299], with an increasing trend corresponding to an improved survival of very-low-birth-weight babies [300].

The molecular mechanisms suggested to be involved in the development and progression of HB include among others downregulation of *RASSF1A* by promoter hypermethylation [282,301,302] in 30-45% of hepatoblastomas. This correlates with poor outcome [302]; hypermethylation of *SOCS1* (33%) and *CASP8* (15%)[302]. Furthermore alterations of genes in the Wnt signalling pathway and most notably, a high incidence of *CTNNB1* (catenin, b1) mutations [303] have been observed.

Hedgehog (Hh) signaling (see above) is implicated in embryonic development of the liver and its regeneration in the adult [304,305,306]. The Hh target genes *glioma-associated oncogene homologue 1* (*GLI1*) and *Patched* (*PTCH1*) showed increased transcript levels in 65% and 30% of HB samples compared with normal liver tissues [307]. The gene encoding the hedgehog interacting protein (HHIP) is transcriptionally silenced by CpG island promoter hypermethylation in 26% of HB cases [307]. The Hh-interacting protein functions as a negative regulator of the Hh pathway [308]. *HHIP* hypermethylation is found in other tumors such as pancreatic [309], gastrointestinal [310] and hepatocellular cancer [311].

IGF2 is a maternally imprinted gene and encodes a fetal peptide hormone that regulates cellular proliferation and differentiation (see above) [312]. IGF2 P3 is the most active promoter in the fetal liver [313]. IGF2 is downregulated in normal tissues after birth, except for liver tissue, and is overexpressed in a wide variety of childhood and adult cancers [314]. Epigenetic alterations in the IGF2-H19 region with elevated expression of IGF2 mRNA identified in Wilms' tumors were also found in the great majority of hepatoblastomas[315]. In hepatoblastoma, LOH of IGF2 is found 20–30% [315].

23.5.6. The Methylation Status of Multidrug Resistance Genes and Other Mechanisms of Chemotherapy Resistance in Childhood Tumors

Alterations in cell cycle checkpoints, failure of apoptotic mechanisms, altered DNA repair pathways and increased drug efflux are responsible for the onset of acquired resistance to chemotherapy in childhood cancer [316]. The multidrug resistance (*MDR1*) gene encodes P-glycoprotein (P-gp), which is a phosphoglycoprotein that functions as a drug efflux pump to decrease intracellular drug concentrations [317]. The *MDR1* promoter is usually methylated and down-regulated to a non-functional silent state [318]. It is assembled into chromatin with methyl binding protein-2 (MeCP2) and deacetylated histones. DNA demethylation causes the release of MeCP2, leading to histone acetylation and transcription of *MDR1* in several human cancers [319].

Table 23.1. Examples of aberrant methylated gene promoters in different pediatric tumors

Gene	Tumor Type	Methylation Frequency	Ref.
RASSF1A	Glioma	36/63 (57%)	[236]
(3p21.3)	Ependymoma	17/20 (85%)	[322]
		27/14 (56%)	[323]
	Medulloblastoma	41/44 (93%)	[46]
		14/16 (88%)	[282]
		5/5 (100%)	[324]
		19/21 (91%)	[325]
	sPNET	19/24 (79%)	[326]
		5/6 (83%)	[325]
	AT/RT	4/6 (66%)	[91]
	Willms Tumours	13/31 (42%)	[282]
		21/39 (51%)	[327]
	Neuroblastoma	42/45 (93%)	[224]
		41/49 (83%)	[328]
	Ewing Sarcoma	21/31 (68%)	[283]
	Osteosarcoma	4/10 (40%)	[329]
	Hepatoblastoma	5/27 (19%)	[282]
		15/39 (39%)	[301]
HIC1	Ependymoma	43/52 (83%)	[330]

Gene	Tumor Type	Methylation Frequency	Ref.
(17p13.3)	Medulloblastoma	17/44 (39%)	[46]
		33/39 (85%)	[331]
		12/15 (80%)	[287]
		26/36 (72%)	[75]
	Neuroblastoma	12/28 (43%)	[287]
MGMT	Glioblastoma	4/10 (40%)	[332]
(10q26)	Oligodendroglial tumors	25/49 (51%)	[127]
	Choroid plexus tumors	17/31 (58%)	[91]
	Medulloblastoma	28/37 (76%)	[333]
	Willms Tumors	12/40 (30%)	[334]
CASP8	Ependymoma	1/27 (4%)	[120]
(2q33-34)		4/20 (20%)	[322]
	Medulloblastoma	36/40 (90%)	[121]
		14/39 (36%)	[46]
		13/16 (81%)	[220]
		6/11 (55%)	[335]
	sPNET	8/24 (33%)	[91]
	AT/RT	4/6 (67%)	[91]
	Willms Tumors	6/31 (19%)	[220]
		17/40 (43%)	[334]
	Neuroblastoma	17/45 (38%)	[224]
		25/41 (60%)	[328]
		17/27 (42%)	[220]
	Hepatoblastoma	15/97 (16%)	[302]
p14ARF/	Ependymoma	23/108 (21%)	[336]
CDKN2A	Medulloblastoma	2/44 (5%)	[46]
(9p21)		11/42 (25%)	[337]
	Neuroblastoma	12/41 (29%)	[338]
	Osteosarcoma	15/32 (47%)	[339]
p16INK4a/	Glioma	10/42 (24%)	[115]
CDKN2A	Glioblastoma	14/23 (61%)	[340]
	Ependymoma	25%	[118]
		5/27 (19%)	[120]
	Medulloblastoma	4/ 23 (17%)	[45]
		3/44 (6%)	[46]
		17/43 (40%)	[337]
	Neuroblastoma	23/23 (100%)	[341]
	Osteosarcoma	5/32 (16%)	[339]
	Hepatoblastoma	12/24 (50%)	[342]
p15INK4b/	Osteosarcoma	3/21 (14%)	[343]

Table 23.1 (Continued)

Gene	Tumor Type	Methylation Frequency	Ref.
CDKN2B	Ewing Sarcoma	4/24 (17%)	[343]
(1p36.3)	Astrocytoma	25/53 (47%)	[128]
	Ependymoma	9/27 (33%)	[120]
		1/7 (14%)	[118]
		1/20 (5%)	[322]
CD 44	Neuroblastoma	29/42 (69%)	[344]
CDH1/ECAD	Medulloblastoma	3/36 (8%)	[121]
(16q22.1)		3/23 (14%)	[45]
		31/41 (75%)	[337]
	Neuroblastoma	3/42 (8%)	[344]
		2/6 (33%)	[282]
	Osteosarcoma	2/18 (11%)	[282]
TIMP3	Ewing Sarcoma	4/24 (17%)	[343]
(22q12.1-13.2)	Oligodendroglioma	10/41 (24%)	[118]
	Medulloblastoma	3/36 (8%)	[121]
		3/23 (14%)	[45]
		31/41 (75%)	[337]
	Neuroblastoma	23/45 (51%)	[224]
DcR1 (9q32-33)	Neuroblastoma	11/45 (25%)	[224]
DcR2	Neuroblastoma	5/45 (11%)	[224]
NORE 1	Neuroblastoma	1/41 (3%)	[328]
MCJ/DNAJC15	Ependymoma	2/20 (10%)	[345]
(13q14.1)	Medulloblastoma	2/28 (7%)	[345]
	sPNET	3/10 (30%)	[345]
BLU/ZMYND10 (3p21.3)	Glioma	35/44 (80%)	[236]
	Neuroblastoma	15/45 (34%)	[224]
		3/41 (8%)	[224]
PTEN (10q23.3)	Neuroblastoma	10/43 (25%)	[344]

Chemotherapeutic resistance of tumors may also be the result of disrupted apoptosis programs. In several tumors (e.g., Ewing sarcomas, neuroblastomas, malignant brain tumors and melanoma) *caspase-8* expression acts as a key determinant of sensitivity to apoptosis induced by death-inducing ligands or cytotoxic drugs. In tumor cell lines resistant to TRAIL, anti-CD95 or TNFa, caspase-8 protein and mRNA expression is decreased by promoter hypermethylation [320].

Decreased folate carrier expression is a common mechanism of methotrexate resistance in osteogenic sarcomas. The folate carrier promoter has been found hypermethylated in 84.3% of osteosarcomas with a subsequent reduction of expression [321].

23.6. Approaches towards Epigenetic Therapy in Children with Cancer

Epigenetic alterations in tumor formation are catalysed by enzymes, which can be pharmacologically influenced. Strategies for targeting the epigenome might also be the basis for cancer prevention, as epigenetic changes may occur early in malignant progression and have the potential to be detected even in precancerous tissues [346]. Moreover the combinatorial use of conventional chemotherapeutic agents and epigenetics-based therapies may provide the opportunity to sensitize drug resistant tumors to established therapeutic approaches such as conventional chemotherapy or radiotherapeutic approaches [347]. Current targets for epigenetic cancer therapy are DNA methyltransferases (DNMT) and histone deacetylases.

23.6.1. Demethylating Agents

5-Azacitidine has been the first epigentically active drug to be approved by the US Food and Drug Administration for the treatment of myelodysplastic syndromes in May 2004 [348]. 5-Azacytidine and 5-aza 2′-deoxycyctidine (decitabine) act through incorporation into DNA and covalent binding of DNMT leading to its inactivation by replacing cytosines during DNA-replication [349]. Azacitidine binds to RNA and interrupts protein translation, whereas decitabine binds to DNA only. Through the incorporation into DNA these compounds have typical side effects like myelosuppression, gastrointestinal disturbances, fever, rigors, ecchymoses, petechiae, arthralgia and dizziness. Azacitidine and 5-aza-2′deoxycitidine are degraded rapidly in serum. More hydrolytically stable cytidine analogs such as zebularine are amenable for oral adminstration. Zebularine can be given continuously at lower doses to maintain demethylation for a prolonged period, which is only possible because of its low toxicity [350]. This molecule is an effective inhibitor of DNMT and cytidine deaminase and targets tumor cells preferentially.

Non-nucleoside DNMT inhibitors such as procainamide and procaine target DNA-methylation without incorporating into DNA (originally approved for cardiac dysrhythmias and as local anaesthetics) [351]. There are also novel DNMT-inhibitors in development (which also do not incorporate into DNA): RG108 suits the catalytic DNMT1-domain and seems to act via blocking the active site of this enzyme [352]. Other approaches use analogues of the methyl donor SAM (S-adenosylmethionine) to inhibit cellular methyltransferase, target DNA-methylation through antisense constructs against the DNA methyltransferases or other component of the DNA methylation machinery [353].

Clinical experience with demethylating agents in childhood is rare: 5-aza-2′deoxycytidine has been used in a study in 21 children with ALL and AML [354]. These authors describe a dose dependent reduction in blast counts. There are few clinical trials in children with DNMTs in combination with other chemotherapeutic agents: 5-aza-2′deoxycytidine plus valproic acid is used in children with MDS [355]. No patient achieved a complete remission, but one of 3 patients achieved a complete marrow response and toxicity was low. In another clinical trial the combination of 5-aza-2′deoxycytidine, valproic acid and all-trans retinoic acid was used. No toxicity was observed and one child achieved a bone marrow response.

While data for children are rare, in adult patients 5-azacytidine and 5-aza-2´deoxycytidine have been employed for the treatment of myelodysplatic syndrome (MDS) [356]. In a randomized controlled trial involving 191 poor-risk myelodysplastic syndrome patients, where 5-azacytidine was tested, the overall response rate (complete or part normalization of blood cell counts and bone marrow morphology) was 23% in the azacitidine arm versus none in the best supportive care arm (control) [357]. Decitabine was tested in a study with 170 patients with poor-risk myelodysplastic syndrome[358]. The patients who received the study drug had a significantly higher overall response rate (17% complete response plus partial response) than those receiving best supportive care (0%). Even if first clinical tests did not show severe side effects, long term effects are not clear until today [358]. DNMT inibitors are illustrated in table 23.2.

Table 23.2. DNA methyltransferase inhititors in development

DNMT Inhibitor	Stage of development	References
5-Azacytidine (Vidaza)	- phase III approved for myelodysplastic syndromes (MDS with response rates: 30-60%) - low dose: DNA hypomethylation - high dose: Inhibition of DNA synthesis (side effects) - combined use with phenylbutyrate, valpoic acid (leukemias, MDS)	[357]
5-Aza-2´-deoxycytidine (Decitabine)	- phase II trials, active against leukemia and MDS - limited activity against solid tumors - Combined use with valproic acid (leukemias), IL2 (melanoma, renal tumors), carboplatin (relapsed solid tumors)	[354,359,360, 361,362],[35 8,363]
1,2-di-hydro-pyrimidin-2-Zebularine	- stable in aqueous solution - increased electrophilic character making oral application possible	[350]
Procainamide/ Procaine	- 4-aminobenzoic acid derivative - agent to treat cardiac arrhythmias (procainamide); anesthetic (procaine)	[351,364,365]
MG98	- 20-mer antisense oligonucleotide with phosphorothioate backbone - binds to DNMT1 and causes mRNA degradation - phase I and II trial	[366,367]
RG108	- novel class of DNMT inhibitor, which blocks DNA-methylation in human cancer cell lines	[368]

23.6.2. Histone Deacetylase Inhibitors

The second group of anti-cancer drugs targeting the epigenome comprises histone deacetylase inhibitors (HDIs) (Table 23.3). Histone deacetylase inhibitors induce cell cycle arrest, apoptosis and cell differentiation through acetylation of histones by inhibiting transcription factors and other proteins such as p53, α-tubulin, HSP90 or β-catenin [369] and reactivate tumor suppressor genes such as *p21WAF* [370].

Table 23.3. HDAC inhibitors in development

HDAC Inhibitor	Comment	References
Hydroxamic acids		
Vorinostat (SAHA)	- approved by the FDA for adult cutaneous T-cell lymphoma - broad range of anti-tumor activities against solid and hematologic malignancies in phase I/II trials in adults - interesting compound for brain tumors (penetrates blood brain barrier) - active against several pediatric tumor models in vitro and in vivo - side effects: gastrointestinal, thrombozytopenia, fatigue	[401,402]
LBH589 and PXD101	- targets HDAC class I and II - Stage of development: phase I and II trial in adult patients	[403]
Benzamides		
MS-275	- phase I/II trials in adults - active against several pediatric tumor models in vitro and in vivo (inhibitis HDAC1+9 > HDAC2+3)	[178,404]
N-acetyldinaline (CI-994) and MGCD0103	- ongoing Phase I/II clinical trials in adults with AML and MDS - N-acetyldinaline: penetrates blood-brain barrier - MGCD0103: selective class I HDAC-inhibitor	[405,406, 407]
Cyclic tetrapeptides		
Depsipeptide (FK228)	- phase II trials in adults - completed phase I dose finding study in pediatric oncology - moderate activity in pre-clinical pediatric tumor models, but in neuroblastoma cells: re-sensitizes resistant cells - HDAC activity HDAC1>HDAC2+4 - long half-time	[408,409, 410]
Short chain fatty acids		
Valproic acid (VPA)	- low potency inhibitor acting in the millimolar range - approved anti-epileptic drug in pediatrics - applied in the HIT GBM C study	[381,411,412,413, 414]
Phenylbutyrate	- preclinical effects in several pediatric and adult tumors - Phase II trials	[415,416]

HDIs comprise a group of small molecule compounds with different chemical structures that demonstrate anti-tumor activities *in vitro* and *in vivo*. HDIs act through binding to the active site pocket and chelation of the catalytic zinc-ion located at its base [371]. Due to the highly conserved nature of the enzymatic pocket, most HDAC-inhibitors do not selectively inhibit individual HDAC isoenzymes, and either inhibit all HDACs or at least several members simultaneously. HDIs such as trichostatin A are also currently investigated in clinical trials [372].

Vorinostat (SAHA) was the first HDAC inhibitor to be approved by the US Food and Drug Administration for cutaneous T-cell lymphoma in 2006 [373]. The broad-spectrum HDAC inhibitors such as vorinostat and trichostatin A are unselective in inhibiting HDACs and affect the expression of 2–10% of all genes investigated, corresponding to several hundreds to thousands of genes in the human genome. Currently, over 100 phase I and II clinical trials are underway to evaluate the safety and efficacy of HDAC inhibitors [374] and show promising results in adult patients with leukemias and solid tumors.

In pediatric cancer, HDIs of different chemical classes have shown anti-tumoral effects (ALL, Ewing sarcoma, osteosarcoma, neuroblastoma, medulloblastoma, cPNET, retinoblastoma, AT/RT, glioblastoma) [189,375,376,377,378,379,380,381]. HDIs also cause numerous side effects (bone marrow depression, diarrhoea, weight loss, taste disturbances, electrolyte changes, disordered clotting, fatigue, and cardiac arrhythmias) [382]. VPA plus radiotherapy has been evaluated in a retrospective analysis of 66 pediatric patients with glioblastoma multiforme and anaplastic astrocytomas, and the response rates are encouraging [383]. VPA was employed in the German pediatric high-grade glioma trial HIT GBM-C as maintenance therapy after surgery, radiation and chemotherapy. In these heavily pretreated 44 patients, VPA showed a median overall survival of 1.33 years, with large differences between first-line (5-year overall survival, 44%) and relapse therapy (5-year overall survival, 14%) [384]. Vorinostat crosses the blood-brain barrier in mouse models, which makes it suitable for the treatment of brain tumors. Because of the severe side effects of unselective HDIs, one major goal is to develop more specific drugs. Over the last several years the role of each HDAC has become clearer and more *selective HDAC inhibitors* targeting classical HDAC family members of classes I, II, and IV have been developed. Experiences with selective HDAC inhibitors in clinical trials are mainly derived from adults.

Class I selective HDAC inhibitors induce cell cycle block and inhibition of proliferation. Class I selective inhibitors targeting HDAC1 or HDAC2 such as MS275 [385], apicidin and depsipeptide are like pan HDAC inhibitors with potent induction of p21Waf1/Cip1 *in vitro* and *in vivo* suggesting that targeting of HDACs 1 and 2 is sufficient to activate expression of this critical tumor suppressor gene. Induction of p21Waf1/Cip1 through HDAC inhibition is associated with acetylation of lysines 5, 8, 12 of histone H4, acetylation of lysines 9 and 14 of histone H3, and methylation of lysine 4 of histone 3 in the p21Waf1/Cip1 promoter region [386]. The protein complex associated with the proximal region of the p21Waf1/Cip1 promoter includes HDAC1, HDAC2, myc, BAF155, Brg-1, GCN5, p300, and SP1 [386]. Induction of p21Waf1/Cip1 by HDAC inhibition is critical for mediating the anti-proliferative effects of these compounds [387].

MS-275 is relatively selective for HDAC1 compared with the other class I HDACs 2 and 3, but also inhibits HDAC9 [388]. At low concentrations, MS-275 induces p21Waf1/Cip1 expression, cell cycle block and differentiation, while at higher concentrations, the compound causes marked induction of reactive oxygen species (ROS), mitochondrial damage, caspase activation and apoptosis [385]. The compound induces histone but not tubulin-acetylation and is currently evaluated in phase I/II clinical trials. MGCD0103, structurally related to MS-275, is very potent against HDAC1 and 2, acting in the nanomolar range, but less effective against other class I and II family members [389]. The compound exerts growth inhibitory activity against various cancer cells and is being tested in phase II clinical trials.

The cyclic tetrapeptide, depsipeptide (FK228, romidepsine) is particularly active against HDAC1, to a lesser extent against HDAC2 and at higher concentrations against HDAC4. Depsipeptide is active in several cancer cell models and has been tested in a phase I dose finding and pharmacokinetic trial in pediatric patients. Depsipeptide causes p53 acetylation at lysines 373/382 thereby protecting it from proteasomal degradation and recruits histone acetyl transferases to the p21Waf1/Cip1 promoter with subsequent transcriptional (indirect) activation of p21.

Depsipeptide (but not the pan-HDAC trichostatin) also exhibits significant demethylating activities on the promoters of several genes, including *p16*^{INK4A}, *SALL3*, and *GATA4*. The expression of DNMT1 was not affected, but Depsipeptide decreased the binding of DNMT1 to the promoter of these genes [390]. Depsipeptide also suppressed expression of histone methyltransferases G9A and SUV39H1, which in turn resulted in a decrease of di- and trimethylated H3K9 around these gene promoters. Depsipeptide reduced loading of heterochromatin-associated protein 1 to methylated H3K9 and binding of DNMT1 to these genes [390].

In the first clinical trial of MS 275, MGCD0103 and FK228 pharmacodynamic investigations document induction of histone acetylation as a surrogate parameter for *in vivo* HDAC inhibition.

Toxicity profiles of the class I selective HDAC inhibitors are similar to the ones observed with unselective pan-HDAC inhibitors and includes fatigue, nausea, vomiting, diarrhoea, thrombocytopenia, and neutropenia. Clinical development of MGCD0103 has been suspended due to reports of pericarditis [391]. MGCD0103 was used in a phase I trial in patients with AML (76%) and MDS (24%). Three of the 29 pretreated patients showed a complete bone marrow response [392].

There are selective HDAC8 inhibitors: SB-379278A inhibits HDAC8, but not HDAC1 and 3. PCI-34051, which induces apoptosis in T-cell lymphoma or leukemia cell lines, was found to selectively target HDAC8, but not HDACs1, 2, 3, 6, and 10. In neuroblastoma cells, the HDAC8 selective compound Cpd2 induced neuronal differentiation, inhibition of proliferation, and decreases in clonogenic growth [26,393].

These HDAC8 selective compounds do not alter histone acetylation in contrast to class I HDAC selective inhibitors, but induce apoptosis, cell cycle block, and differentiation by changing the acetylation level of non-histone target proteins.

Tubacin is a HDAC6-selective compound that causes tubulin acetylation in mammalian cells [394]. Cell motility and invasion is inhibited by tubacin through inhibition of epithelial-mesenchymal transition of tumor cells by interference with the TGFb-SMAD3 signalling pathway [395].

The thiolate analogues, NCT-10a and NCT-14a are HDAC6 selective inhibitors, which significantly increase the effect of paclitaxel on cancer cell growth [396]. In contrast to pan-HDAC inhibitors, HDAC6 selective inhibition did not significantly change gene expression signatures in microarray analysis suggesting that HDAC6 inhibition in clinical settings may not cause major side effects [397]. Other class II selective inhibitors include APHA derivatives (selectivity for HDAC4) and trifluoroacetylthiophenes showing HDAC4 and HDAC6 selectivity [398,399].

The combinatorial use of DNMT-inhibitors and HDI is appealing in some cases. Ongoing studies have explored the combination of standard dose 5-azacytidine with MGCD0103, 5-azacitidine with vorinostat and others.

These studies have shown that such combinations are tolerable at doses near single agent application, but outcome remains to be evaluated [357]. Hypermethylated genes such as *TIMP3*, *p15*^{INK4b}, *p14*^{ARF} and *p16*^{INK4a} are reactivated by TSA after combinatorial use with 5-aza-2′-deoxycytidine [400]. Figure 23.4 depicts different HDACs in controlling tumor cell development.

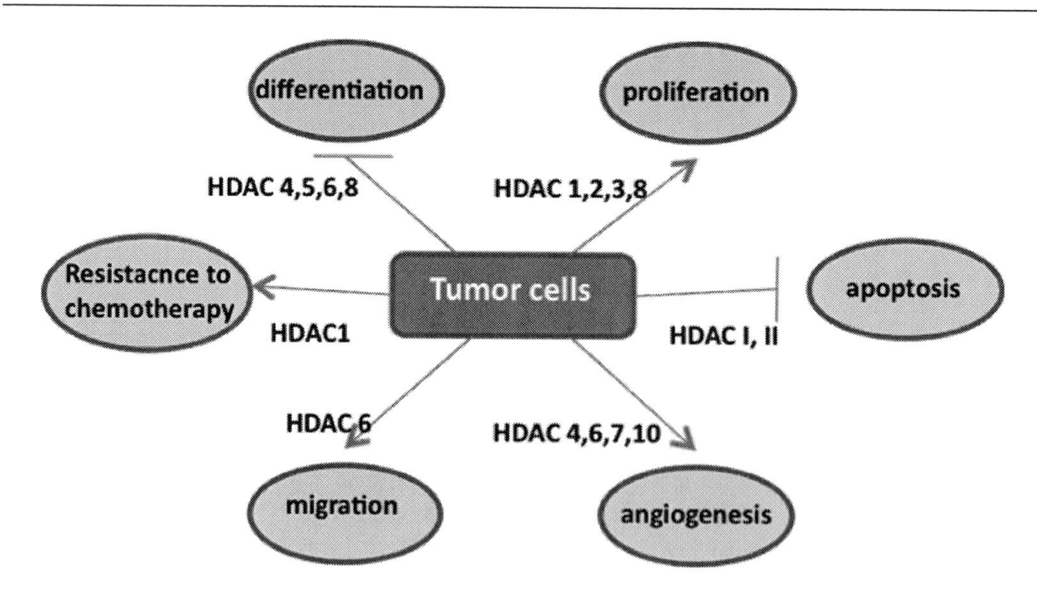

Figure 23.4. The role of HDAC in tumor cell growth. HDACs influence differentiation, proliferation, apoptosis, angiogenesis, migration and resistance to chemotherapy.

23.7. Lessons Learned from the Study of Epigenetics in Solid Tumors of Childhood and Adolescence

Over the last years, knowledge of epigenetic changes, which may induce solid tumors in childhood, has grown expeditiously and it is now evident that aberrant epigenetic regulation is a fundamental process in cancer development and progression. Even if many mechanisms are incompletely understood (e.g., the exact mechanism of mutated SNF5 leading to formation of AR/TR and other tumors) the relevance of epigenetics in these circumstances is undoubted.

Processes such as cell cycle control, apoptosis and many others, which lead to cancer formation when deregulated, are controlled by epigenetic mechanisms. These processes include reversible enzymatic reactions by DNMT and HDAC activity, which can be targeted by small molecule inhibitors. These compounds show promising anti-cancer activity at least *in vitro* and in animal models. Many phase I/II clinical trials are currently running.

Major clinical approaches towards epigenetic-based therapy in different pediatric tumors are currently missing. Over the next years, epigenetic mechanisms in pediatric oncology have to be further evaluated and these results have to be implemented into clinical research. There is evidence of potential synergy of HDAC inhibitors in combination with many other chemotherapeutic drugs, which will be an important focus in the future.

On the other hand biomarkers such as HDAC expression have to be correlated with response to epigenetic therapy, to make a prediction possible for the individual patient. Phase I/II trials with unselective HDAC inhibitors and inhibitors of DNMT have shown side effects like myelotoxicity and gastrointestinal disturbances. Selective inhibitors have to be tested in pediatric patients. Although no severe long-term side effects have been recognized in the few patients treated with epigenetic drugs, it has to be evaluated whether long-term effects for example on bone marrow or endocrine function appear.

References

[1] Esteller M (2008) Epigenetics in cancer. *N. Engl. J. Med.* 358: 1148-1159.

[2] Bird A (2002) DNA methylation patterns and epigenetic memory. *Genes. Dev.* 16: 6-21.

[3] Lujambio A, Ropero S, Ballestar E, Fraga MF, Cerrato C, et al. (2007) Genetic unmasking of an epigenetically silenced microRNA in human cancer cells. *Cancer Res.* 67: 1424-1429.

[4] Sterner DE, Berger SL (2000) Acetylation of histones and transcription-related factors. *Microbiol. Mol. Biol. Rev.* 64: 435-459.

[5] Zhang Y, Reinberg D (2001) Transcription regulation by histone methylation: interplay between different covalent modifications of the core histone tails. *Genes. Dev.* 15: 2343-2360.

[6] Nowak SJ, Corces VG (2004) Phosphorylation of histone H3: a balancing act between chromosome condensation and transcriptional activation. *Trends Genet.* 20: 214-220.

[7] Shilatifard A (2006) Chromatin modifications by methylation and ubiquitination: implications in the regulation of gene expression. *Annu. Rev. Biochem.* 75: 243-269.

[8] Nathan D, Ingvarsdottir K, Sterner DE, Bylebyl GR, Dokmanovic M, et al. (2006) Histone sumoylation is a negative regulator in Saccharomyces cerevisiae and shows dynamic interplay with positive-acting histone modifications. *Genes. Dev.* 20: 966-976.

[9] Hassa PO, Haenni SS, Elser M, Hottiger MO (2006) Nuclear ADP-ribosylation reactions in mammalian cells: where are we today and where are we going? *Microbiol. Mol. Biol. Rev.* 70: 789-829.

[10] Wang Y, Wysocka J, Sayegh J, Lee YH, Perlin JR, et al. (2004) Human PAD4 regulates histone arginine methylation levels via demethylimination. *Science* 306: 279-283.

[11] Nelson CJ, Santos-Rosa H, Kouzarides T (2006) Proline isomerization of histone H3 regulates lysine methylation and gene expression. *Cell* 126: 905-916.

[12] Strahl BD, Allis CD (2000) The language of covalent histone modifications. *Nature* 403: 41-45.

[13] Paro R, Hogness DS (1991) The Polycomb protein shares a homologous domain with a heterochromatin-associated protein of Drosophila. *Proc. Natl. Acad. Sci. USA* 88: 263-267.

[14] Jones PA, Baylin SB (2002) The fundamental role of epigenetic events in cancer. *Nat. Rev. Genet.* 3: 415-428.

[15] Bannister AJ, Zegerman P, Partridge JF, Miska EA, Thomas JO, et al. (2001) Selective recognition of methylated lysine 9 on histone H3 by the HP1 chromo domain. *Nature* 410: 120-124.

[16] Valk-Lingbeek ME, Bruggeman SW, van Lohuizen M (2004) Stem cells and cancer; the polycomb connection. *Cell* 118: 409-418.

[17] Ivanova AV, Bonaduce MJ, Ivanov SV, Klar AJ (1998) The chromo and SET domains of the Clr4 protein are essential for silencing in fission yeast. *Nat. Genet.* 19: 192-195.

[18] Ahringer J (2000) NuRD and SIN3 histone deacetylase complexes in development. *Trends Genet.* 16: 351-356.

[19] Wysocka J, Allis CD, Coonrod S (2006) Histone arginine methylation and its dynamic regulation. *Front Biosci.* 11: 344-355.

[20] Pena PV, Davrazou F, Shi X, Walter KL, Verkhusha VV, et al. (2006) Molecular mechanism of histone H3K4me3 recognition by plant homeodomain of ING2. *Nature* 442: 100-103.

[21] Pray-Grant MG, Daniel JA, Schieltz D, Yates JR, 3rd, Grant PA (2005) Chd1 chromodomain links histone H3 methylation with SAGA- and SLIK-dependent acetylation. *Nature* 433: 434-438.

[22] Sims RJ, 3rd, Chen CF, Santos-Rosa H, Kouzarides T, Patel SS, et al. (2005) Human but not yeast CHD1 binds directly and selectively to histone H3 methylated at lysine 4 via its tandem chromodomains. *J. Biol. Chem.* 280: 41789-41792.

[23] Mujtaba S, Zeng L, Zhou MM (2007) Structure and acetyl-lysine recognition of the bromodomain. *Oncogene* 26: 5521-5527.

[24] Mohammad DH, Yaffe MB (2009) 14-3-3 proteins, FHA domains and BRCT domains in the DNA damage response. *DNA Repair* (Amst) 8: 1009-1017.

[25] Celic I, Masumoto H, Griffith WP, Meluh P, Cotter RJ, et al. (2006) The sirtuins hst3 and Hst4p preserve genome integrity by controlling histone h3 lysine 56 deacetylation. *Curr. Biol.* 16: 1280-1289.

[26] Oehme I, Deubzer HE, Wegener D, Pickert D, Linke JP, et al. (2009) Histone deacetylase 8 in neuroblastoma tumorigenesis. *Clin. Cancer Res.* 15: 91-99.

[27] Weichert W (2009) HDAC expression and clinical prognosis in human malignancies. *Cancer Lett.* 280: 168-176.

[28] Witt O, Deubzer HE, Lodrini M, Milde T, Oehme I (2009) Targeting histone deacetylases in neuroblastoma. *Curr. Pharm. Des.* 15: 436-447.

[29] Glaser KB, Li J, Staver MJ, Wei RQ, Albert DH, et al. (2003) Role of class I and class II histone deacetylases in carcinoma cells using siRNA. *Biochem. Biophys. Res. Commun.* 310: 529-536.

[30] Keshelava N, Davicioni E, Wan Z, Ji L, Sposto R, et al. (2007) Histone deacetylase 1 gene expression and sensitization of multidrug-resistant neuroblastoma cell lines to cytotoxic agents by depsipeptide. *J. Natl. Cancer Inst.* 99: 1107-1119.

[31] Kouzarides T (2007) Chromatin modifications and their function. Cell 128: 693-705.

[32] Jones PA, Baylin SB (2007) The epigenomics of cancer. *Cell* 128: 683-692.

[33] Gardiner-Garden M, Frommer M (1987) CpG islands in vertebrate genomes. *J. Mol. Biol.* 196: 261-282.

[34] Fouladi M, Furman WL, Chin T, Freeman BB, 3rd, Dudkin L, et al. (2006) Phase I study of depsipeptide in pediatric patients with refractory solid tumors: a Children's Oncology Group report. *J. Clin. Oncol.* 24: 3678-3685.

[35] Ting AH, McGarvey KM, Baylin SB (2006) The cancer epigenome--components and functional correlates. *Genes. Dev.* 20: 3215-3231.

[36] Futscher BW, Oshiro MM, Wozniak RJ, Holtan N, Hanigan CL, et al. (2002) Role for DNA methylation in the control of cell type specific maspin expression. *Nat. Genet* 31: 175-179.

[37] Singal R, Ginder GD (1999) DNA methylation. *Blood* 93: 4059-4070.

[38] Ehrlich M (2002) DNA methylation in cancer: too much, but also too little. *Oncogene* 21: 5400-5413.

[39] Fruhwald MC, Plass C (2002) Global and gene-specific methylation patterns in cancer: aspects of tumor biology and clinical potential. *Mol. Genet. Metab.* 75: 1-16.

[40] Cooper DN, Krawczak M (1989) Cytosine methylation and the fate of CpG dinucleotides in vertebrate genomes. *Hum. Genet.* 83: 181-188.

[41] Pfister S, Witt O (2009) Pediatric gliomas. *Recent Results Cancer Res.* 171: 67-81.

[42] Wrensch M, Minn Y, Chew T, Bondy M, Berger MS (2002) Epidemiology of primary brain tumors: current concepts and review of the literature. *Neuro. Oncol.* 4: 278-299.

[43] de Bont JM, Packer RJ, Michiels EM, den Boer ML, Pieters R (2008) Biological background of pediatric medulloblastoma and ependymoma: a review from a translational research perspective. *Neuro Oncol.* 10: 1040-1060.

[44] Fruhwald MC, O'Dorisio MS, Dai Z, Rush LJ, Krahe R, et al. (2001) Aberrant hypermethylation of the major breakpoint cluster region in 17p11.2 in medulloblastomas but not supratentorial PNETs. *Genes. Chromosomes Cancer* 30: 38-47.

[45] Fruhwald MC, O'Dorisio MS, Dai Z, Tanner SM, Balster DA, et al. (2001) Aberrant promoter methylation of previously unidentified target genes is a common abnormality in medulloblastomas--implications for tumor biology and potential clinical utility. *Oncogene* 20: 5033-5042.

[46] Lindsey JC, Lusher ME, Anderton JA, Bailey S, Gilbertson RJ, et al. (2004) Identification of tumour-specific epigenetic events in medulloblastoma development by hypermethylation profiling. *Carcinogenesis* 25: 661-668.

[47] Chen W, Ren XR, Nelson CD, Barak LS, Chen JK, et al. (2004) Activity-dependent internalization of smoothened mediated by beta-arrestin 2 and GRK2. *Science* 306: 2257-2260.

[48] Apionishev S, Katanayeva NM, Marks SA, Kalderon D, Tomlinson A (2005) Drosophila Smoothened phosphorylation sites essential for Hedgehog signal transduction. *Nat. Cell Biol.* 7: 86-92.

[49] Collins RT, Cohen SM (2005) A genetic screen in Drosophila for identifying novel components of the hedgehog signaling pathway. *Genetics* 170: 173-184.

[50] Strutt H, Thomas C, Nakano Y, Stark D, Neave B, et al. (2001) Mutations in the sterol-sensing domain of Patched suggest a role for vesicular trafficking in Smoothened regulation. *Curr. Biol.* 11: 608-613.

[51] Leung C, Lingbeek M, Shakhova O, Liu J, Tanger E, et al. (2004) Bmi1 is essential for cerebellar development and is overexpressed in human medulloblastomas. *Nature* 428: 337-341.

[52] Lee SW, Moskowitz MA, Sims JR (2007) Sonic hedgehog inversely regulates the expression of angiopoietin-1 and angiopoietin-2 in fibroblasts. *Int. J. Mol. Med.* 19: 445-451.

[53] Jenkins D (2009) Hedgehog signalling: Emerging evidence for non-canonical pathways. Cell Signal.

[54] Wechsler-Reya RJ, Scott MP (1999) Control of neuronal precursor proliferation in the cerebellum by Sonic Hedgehog. *Neuron* 22: 103-114.

[55] Arsic D, Qi BQ, Beasley SW (2002) Hedgehog in the human: a possible explanation for the VATER association. *J. Paediatr Child Health* 38: 117-121.

[56] Cowan R, Hoban P, Kelsey A, Birch JM, Gattamaneni R, et al. (1997) The gene for the naevoid basal cell carcinoma syndrome acts as a tumour-suppressor gene in medulloblastoma. *Br. J. Cancer* 76: 141-145.

[57] Diede SJ, Guenthoer J, Geng LN, Mahoney SE, Marotta M, et al. (2009) DNA methylation of developmental genes in pediatric medulloblastomas identified by denaturation analysis of methylation differences. *Proc. Natl. Acad. Sci. USA*.

[58] Uziel T, Zindy F, Sherr CJ, Roussel MF (2006) The CDK inhibitor p18Ink4c is a tumor suppressor in medulloblastoma. *Cell Cycle* 5: 363-365.

[59] Uziel T, Zindy F, Xie S, Lee Y, Forget A, et al. (2005) The tumor suppressors Ink4c and p53 collaborate independently with Patched to suppress medulloblastoma formation. *Genes. Dev.* 19: 2656-2667.

[60] Giles RH, van Es JH, Clevers H (2003) Caught up in a Wnt storm: Wnt signaling in cancer. *Biochim Biophys Acta* 1653: 1-24.

[61] Clifford SC, Lusher ME, Lindsey JC, Langdon JA, Gilbertson RJ, et al. (2006) Wnt/Wingless pathway activation and chromosome 6 loss characterize a distinct molecular sub-group of medulloblastomas associated with a favorable prognosis. *Cell Cycle* 5: 2666-2670.

[62] Roman-Gomez J, Jimenez-Velasco A, Cordeu L, Vilas-Zornoza A, San Jose-Eneriz E, et al. (2007) WNT5A, a putative tumour suppressor of lymphoid malignancies, is inactivated by aberrant methylation in acute lymphoblastic leukaemia. *Eur. J. Cancer* 43: 2736-2746.

[63] Su HY, Lai HC, Lin YW, Liu CY, Chen CK, et al. (2009) Epigenetic silencing of SFRP5 is related to malignant phenotype and chemoresistance of ovarian cancer through Wnt signaling pathway. *Int. J. Cancer*.

[64] Gotze S, Wolter M, Reifenberger G, Muller O, Sievers S (2009) Frequent promoter hypermethylation of Wnt pathway inhibitor genes in malignant astrocytic gliomas. *Int. J. Cancer*.

[65] Vibhakar R, Foltz G, Yoon JG, Field L, Lee H, et al. (2007) Dickkopf-1 is an epigenetically silenced candidate tumor suppressor gene in medulloblastoma. *Neuro. Oncol.* 9: 135-144.

[66] Yuan BZ, Miller MJ, Keck CL, Zimonjic DB, Thorgeirsson SS, et al. (1998) Cloning, characterization, and chromosomal localization of a gene frequently deleted in human liver cancer (DLC-1) homologous to rat RhoGAP. *Cancer Res.* 58: 2196-2199.

[67] Moon SY, Zheng Y (2003) Rho GTPase-activating proteins in cell regulation. *Trends Cell Biol* 13: 13-22.

[68] Zhou X, Thorgeirsson SS, Popescu NC (2004) Restoration of DLC-1 gene expression induces apoptosis and inhibits both cell growth and tumorigenicity in human hepatocellular carcinoma cells. *Oncogene* 23: 1308-1313.

[69] Ahuja N, Mohan AL, Li Q, Stolker JM, Herman JG, et al. (1997) Association between CpG island methylation and microsatellite instability in colorectal cancer. *Cancer Res.* 57: 3370-3374.

[70] Fujii H, Biel MA, Zhou W, Weitzman SA, Baylin SB, et al. (1998) Methylation of the HIC-1 candidate tumor suppressor gene in human breast cancer. *Oncogene* 16: 2159-2164.

[71] Eguchi K, Kanai Y, Kobayashi K, Hirohashi S (1997) DNA hypermethylation at the D17S5 locus in non-small cell lung cancers: its association with smoking history. *Cancer Res*. 57: 4913-4915.

[72] Kanai Y, Hui AM, Sun L, Ushijima S, Sakamoto M, et al. (1999) DNA hypermethylation at the D17S5 locus and reduced HIC-1 mRNA expression are associated with hepatocarcinogenesis. *Hepatology* 29: 703-709.

[73] Melki JR, Vincent PC, Clark SJ (1999) Cancer-specific region of hypermethylation identified within the HIC1 putative tumour suppressor gene in acute myeloid leukaemia. *Leukemia* 13: 877-883.

[74] Salvesen GS (2002) Caspases and apoptosis. *Essays Biochem.* 38: 9-19.

[75] Rood BR, Zhang H, Weitman DM, Cogen PH (2002) Hypermethylation of HIC-1 and 17p allelic loss in medulloblastoma. *Cancer Res*. 62: 3794-3797.

[76] Deltour S, Pinte S, Guerardel C, Wasylyk B, Leprince D (2002) The human candidate tumor suppressor gene HIC1 recruits CtBP through a degenerate GLDLSKK motif. *Mol. Cell Biol.* 22: 4890-4901.

[77] Guerardel C, Deltour S, Pinte S, Monte D, Begue A, et al. (2001) Identification in the human candidate tumor suppressor gene HIC-1 of a new major alternative TATA-less promoter positively regulated by p53. *J. Biol. Chem.* 276: 3078-3089.

[78] Wales MM, Biel MA, el Deiry W, Nelkin BD, Issa JP, et al. (1995) p53 activates expression of HIC-1, a new candidate tumour suppressor gene on 17p13.3. *Nat. Med.* 1: 570-577.

[79] Briggs KJ, Corcoran-Schwartz IM, Zhang W, Harcke T, Devereux WL, et al. (2008) Cooperation between the Hic1 and Ptch1 tumor suppressors in medulloblastoma. *Genes. Dev*. 22: 770-785.

[80] Chen WY, Zeng X, Carter MG, Morrell CN, Chiu Yen RW, et al. (2003) Heterozygous disruption of Hic1 predisposes mice to a gender-dependent spectrum of malignant tumors. *Nat. Genet.* 33: 197-202.

[81] Esteller M, Hamilton SR, Burger PC, Baylin SB, Herman JG (1999) Inactivation of the DNA repair gene O6-methylguanine-DNA methyltransferase by promoter hypermethylation is a common event in primary human neoplasia. *Cancer Res*. 59: 793-797.

[82] Xu-Welliver M, Pegg AE (2002) Degradation of the alkylated form of the DNA repair protein, O(6)-alkylguanine-DNA alkyltransferase. *Carcinogenesis* 23: 823-830.

[83] Silber JR, Blank A, Bobola MS, Ghatan S, Kolstoe DD, et al. (1999) O6-methylguanine-DNA methyltransferase-deficient phenotype in human gliomas: frequency and time to tumor progression after alkylating agent-based chemotherapy. *Clin. Cancer Res.* 5: 807-814.

[84] Bobola MS, Silber JR, Ellenbogen RG, Geyer JR, Blank A, et al. (2005) O6-methylguanine-DNA methyltransferase, O6-benzylguanine, and resistance to clinical alkylators in pediatric primary brain tumor cell lines. *Clin. Cancer Res.* 11: 2747-2755.

[85] Bobola MS, Berger MS, Ellenbogen RG, Roberts TS, Geyer JR, et al. (2001) O6-Methylguanine-DNA methyltransferase in pediatric primary brain tumors: relation to patient and tumor characteristics. *Clin. Cancer Res.* 7: 613-619.

[86] Watanabe T, Katayama Y, Komine C, Yoshino A, Ogino A, et al. (2005) O6-methylguanine-DNA methyltransferase methylation and TP53 mutation in malignant astrocytomas and their relationships with clinical course. *Int. J. Cancer* 113: 581-587.

[87] Rood BR, Zhang H, Cogen PH (2004) Intercellular heterogeneity of expression of the MGMT DNA repair gene in pediatric medulloblastoma. *Neuro. Oncol.* 6: 200-207.

[88] Gonzalez-Gomez P, Bello MJ, Arjona D, Lomas J, Alonso ME, et al. (2003) Promoter hypermethylation of multiple genes in astrocytic gliomas. *Int. J. Oncol.* 22: 601-608.

[89] Balana C, Ramirez JL, Taron M, Roussos Y, Ariza A, et al. (2003) O6-methyl-guanine-DNA methyltransferase methylation in serum and tumor DNA predicts response to 1,3-bis(2-chloroethyl)-1-nitrosourea but not to temozolamide plus cisplatin in glioblastoma multiforme. *Clin. Cancer Res.* 9: 1461-1468.

[90] Gonzalez-Gomez P, Bello MJ, Lomas J, Arjona D, Alonso ME, et al. (2003) Aberrant methylation of multiple genes in neuroblastic tumours. relationship with MYCN amplification and allelic status at 1p. *Eur. J. Cancer* 39: 1478-1485.

[91] Hasselblatt M, Muhlisch J, Wrede B, Kallinger B, Jeibmann A, et al. (2009) Aberrant MGMT (O6-methylguanine-DNA methyltransferase) promoter methylation in choroid plexus tumors. *J. Neurooncol.* 91: 151-155.

[92] Mollemann M, Wolter M, Felsberg J, Collins VP, Reifenberger G (2005) Frequent promoter hypermethylation and low expression of the MGMT gene in oligodendroglial tumors. *Int. J. Cancer* 113: 379-385.

[93] Donato R (2003) Intracellular and extracellular roles of S100 proteins. *Microsc Res Tech* 60: 540-551.

[94] Marenholz I, Heizmann CW, Fritz G (2004) S100 proteins in mouse and man: from evolution to function and pathology (including an update of the nomenclature). *Biochem. Biophys. Res. Commun.* 322: 1111-1122.

[95] Hernan R, Fasheh R, Calabrese C, Frank AJ, Maclean KH, et al. (2003) ERBB2 up-regulates S100A4 and several other prometastatic genes in medulloblastoma. *Cancer Res.* 63: 140-148.

[96] Garrett SC, Varney KM, Weber DJ, Bresnick AR (2006) S100A4, a mediator of metastasis. *J. Biol. Chem.* 281: 677-680.

[97] Abounader R, Laterra J (2005) Scatter factor/hepatocyte growth factor in brain tumor growth and angiogenesis. *Neuro. Oncol.* 7: 436-451.

[98] Li Y, Guessous F, Johnson EB, Eberhart CG, Li XN, et al. (2008) Functional and molecular interactions between the HGF/c-Met pathway and c-Myc in large-cell medulloblastoma. *Lab. Invest.* 88: 98-111.

[99] Kongkham PN, Northcott PA, Ra YS, Nakahara Y, Mainprize TG, et al. (2008) An epigenetic genome-wide screen identifies SPINT2 as a novel tumor suppressor gene in pediatric medulloblastoma. *Cancer Res.* 68: 9945-9953.

[100] Lindsey T, Watts-Tate N, Southwood E, Routhieaux J, Beatty J, et al. (2005) Chronic blood transfusion therapy practices to treat strokes in children with sickle cell disease. *J. Am. Acad. Nurse Pract.* 17: 277-282.

[101] Kelley WL (1998) The J-domain family and the recruitment of chaperone power. *Trends Biochem. Sci.* 23: 222-227.

[102] Strathdee G, Davies BR, Vass JK, Siddiqui N, Brown R (2004) Cell type-specific methylation of an intronic CpG island controls expression of the MCJ gene. *Carcinogenesis* 25: 693-701.

[103] Lusher ME, Lindsey JC, Latif F, Pearson AD, Ellison DW, et al. (2002) Biallelic epigenetic inactivation of the RASSF1A tumor suppressor gene in medulloblastoma development. *Cancer Res.* 62: 5906-5911.

[104] Debatin KM, Krammer PH (2004) Death receptors in chemotherapy and cancer. *Oncogene* 23: 2950-2966.

[105] Grotzer MA, Eggert A, Zuzak TJ, Janss AJ, Marwaha S, et al. (2000) Resistance to TRAIL-induced apoptosis in primitive neuroectodermal brain tumor cells correlates with a loss of caspase-8 expression. *Oncogene* 19: 4604-4610.

[106] Kaatsch P, Rickert CH, Kuhl J, Schuz J, Michaelis J (2001) Population-based epidemiologic data on brain tumors in German children. *Cancer* 92: 3155-3164.

[107] Nakamura M, Watanabe T, Klangby U, Asker C, Wiman K, et al. (2001) p14ARF deletion and methylation in genetic pathways to glioblastomas. *Brain Pathol.* 11: 159-168.

[108] Zhang Y, Xiong Y, Yarbrough WG (1998) ARF promotes MDM2 degradation and stabilizes p53: ARF-INK4a locus deletion impairs both the Rb and p53 tumor suppression pathways. *Cell* 92: 725-734.

[109] Weber JD, Taylor LJ, Roussel MF, Sherr CJ, Bar-Sagi D (1999) Nucleolar Arf sequesters Mdm2 and activates p53. *Nat. Cell Biol.* 1: 20-26.

[110] Yin D, Xie D, Hofmann WK, Miller CW, Black KL, et al. (2002) Methylation, expression, and mutation analysis of the cell cycle control genes in human brain tumors. *Oncogene* 21: 8372-8378.

[111] Serrano M, Hannon GJ, Beach D (1993) A new regulatory motif in cell-cycle control causing specific inhibition of cyclin D/CDK4. *Nature* 366: 704-707.

[112] Lukas J, Parry D, Aagaard L, Mann DJ, Bartkova J, et al. (1995) Retinoblastoma-protein-dependent cell-cycle inhibition by the tumour suppressor p16. *Nature* 375: 503-506.

[113] Koh J, Enders GH, Dynlacht BD, Harlow E (1995) Tumour-derived p16 alleles encoding proteins defective in cell-cycle inhibition. *Nature* 375: 506-510.

[114] Hannon GJ, Beach D (1994) p15INK4B is a potential effector of TGF-beta-induced cell cycle arrest. *Nature* 371: 257-261.

[115] Costello JF, Berger MS, Huang HS, Cavenee WK (1996) Silencing of p16/CDKN2 expression in human gliomas by methylation and chromatin condensation. *Cancer Res.* 56: 2405-2410.

[116] Gonzalez-Gomez P, Bello MJ, Arjona D, Alonso ME, Lomas J, et al. (2003) CpG island methylation of tumor-related genes in three primary central nervous system lymphomas in immunocompetent patients. *Cancer Genet. Cytogenet.* 142: 21-24.

[117] Watanabe T, Huang H, Nakamura M, Wischhusen J, Weller M, et al. (2002) Methylation of the p73 gene in gliomas. *Acta. Neuropathol.* 104: 357-362.

[118] Alonso ME, Bello MJ, Gonzalez-Gomez P, Arjona D, Lomas J, et al. (2003) Aberrant promoter methylation of multiple genes in oligodendrogliomas and ependymomas. *Cancer Genet. Cytogenet.* 144: 134-142.

[119] Nakamura M, Ishida E, Shimada K, Kishi M, Nakase H, et al. (2005) Frequent LOH on 22q12.3 and TIMP-3 inactivation occur in the progression to secondary glioblastomas. *Lab Invest* 85: 165-175.

[120] Alonso ME, Bello MJ, Gonzalez-Gomez P, Arjona D, de Campos JM, et al. (2004) Aberrant CpG island methylation of multiple genes in ependymal tumors. *J. Neurooncol.* 67: 159-165.

[121] Ebinger M, Senf L, Wachowski O, Scheurlen W (2004) Promoter methylation pattern of caspase-8, P16INK4A, MGMT, TIMP-3, and E-cadherin in medulloblastoma. *Pathol. Oncol. Res.* 10: 17-21.

[122] Gomez DE, Alonso DF, Yoshiji H, Thorgeirsson UP (1997) Tissue inhibitors of metalloproteinases: structure, regulation and biological functions. *Eur. J. Cell Biol* 74: 111-122.

[123] Anand-Apte B, Bao L, Smith R, Iwata K, Olsen BR, et al. (1996) A review of tissue inhibitor of metalloproteinases-3 (TIMP-3) and experimental analysis of its effect on primary tumor growth. *Biochem Cell Biol* 74: 853-862.

[124] Qi JH, Ebrahem Q, Moore N, Murphy G, Claesson-Welsh L, et al. (2003) A novel function for tissue inhibitor of metalloproteinases-3 (TIMP3): inhibition of angiogenesis by blockage of VEGF binding to VEGF receptor-2. *Nat. Med.* 9: 407-415.

[125] Raffel C, Frederick L, O'Fallon JR, Atherton-Skaff P, Perry A, et al. (1999) Analysis of oncogene and tumor suppressor gene alterations in pediatric malignant astrocytomas reveals reduced survival for patients with PTEN mutations. *Clin. Cancer Res.* 5: 4085-4090.

[126] Li DM, Sun H (1998) PTEN/MMAC1/TEP1 suppresses the tumorigenicity and induces G1 cell cycle arrest in human glioblastoma cells. *Proc. Natl. Acad. Sci. USA* 95: 15406-15411.

[127] Kuo LT, Kuo KT, Lee MJ, Wei CC, Scaravilli F, et al. (2009) Correlation among pathology, genetic and epigenetic profiles, and clinical outcome in oligodendroglial tumors. *Int. J. Cancer* 124: 2872-2879.

[128] Yu J, Zhang H, Gu J, Lin S, Li J, et al. (2004) Methylation profiles of thirty four promoter-CpG islands and concordant methylation behaviours of sixteen genes that may contribute to carcinogenesis of astrocytoma. *BMC Cancer* 4: 65.

[129] Baeza N, Weller M, Yonekawa Y, Kleihues P, Ohgaki H (2003) PTEN methylation and expression in glioblastomas. *Acta. Neuropathol.* 106: 479-485.

[130] Biegel JA (2006) Molecular genetics of atypical teratoid/rhabdoid tumor. *Neurosurg Focus* 20: E11.

[131] Packer RJ, Biegel JA, Blaney S, Finlay J, Geyer JR, et al. (2002) Atypical teratoid/rhabdoid tumor of the central nervous system: report on workshop. *J. Pediatr. Hematol. Oncol.* 24: 337-342.

[132] Versteege I, Sevenet N, Lange J, Rousseau-Merck MF, Ambros P, et al. (1998) Truncating mutations of hSNF5/INI1 in aggressive paediatric cancer. *Nature* 394: 203-206.

[133] Chi SN, Zimmerman MA, Yao X, Cohen KJ, Burger P, et al. (2009) Intensive multimodality treatment for children with newly diagnosed CNS atypical teratoid rhabdoid tumor. *J. Clin. Oncol.* 27: 385-389.

[134] Sevenet N, Sheridan E, Amram D, Schneider P, Handgretinger R, et al. (1999) Constitutional mutations of the hSNF5/INI1 gene predispose to a variety of cancers. *Am. J. Hum. Genet.* 65: 1342-1348.

[135] Guidi CJ, Sands AT, Zambrowicz BP, Turner TK, Demers DA, et al. (2001) Disruption of Ini1 leads to peri-implantation lethality and tumorigenesis in mice. *Mol. Cell Biol.* 21: 3598-3603.

[136] Biegel JA, Kalpana G, Knudsen ES, Packer RJ, Roberts CW, et al. (2002) The role of INI1 and the SWI/SNF complex in the development of rhabdoid tumors: meeting

summary from the workshop on childhood atypical teratoid/rhabdoid tumors. Cancer Res. 62: 323-328.
[137] Fan HY, He X, Kingston RE, Narlikar GJ (2003) Distinct strategies to make nucleosomal DNA accessible. Mol Cell 11: 1311-1322.
[138] Zhang Y, Ng HH, Erdjument-Bromage H, Tempst P, Bird A, et al. (1999) Analysis of the NuRD subunits reveals a histone deacetylase core complex and a connection with DNA methylation. Genes. Dev. 13: 1924-1935.
[139] Lund AH, van Lohuizen M (2004) Polycomb complexes and silencing mechanisms. Curr Opin Cell Biol 16: 239-246.
[140] Carlson M, Osmond BC, Botstein D (1981) Mutants of yeast defective in sucrose utilization. Genetics 98: 25-40.
[141] Tamkun JW, Deuring R, Scott MP, Kissinger M, Pattatucci AM, et al. (1992) brahma: a regulator of Drosophila homeotic genes structurally related to the yeast transcriptional activator SNF2/SWI2. Cell 68: 561-572.
[142] Armstrong JA, Papoulas O, Daubresse G, Sperling AS, Lis JT, et al. (2002) The Drosophila BRM complex facilitates global transcription by RNA polymerase II. Embo J 21: 5245-5254.
[143] Tamkun JW (1995) The role of brahma and related proteins in transcription and development. Curr Opin Genet Dev 5: 473-477.
[144] Kal AJ, Mahmoudi T, Zak NB, Verrijzer CP (2000) The Drosophila brahma complex is an essential coactivator for the trithorax group protein zeste. Genes. Dev. 14: 1058-1071.
[145] Wang W, Xue Y, Zhou S, Kuo A, Cairns BR, et al. (1996) Diversity and specialization of mammalian SWI/SNF complexes. Genes. Dev. 10: 2117-2130.
[146] Saha A, Wittmeyer J, Cairns BR (2006) Mechanisms for nucleosome movement by ATP-dependent chromatin remodeling complexes. Results Probl Cell Differ 41: 127-148.
[147] Shundrovsky A, Smith CL, Lis JT, Peterson CL, Wang MD (2006) Probing SWI/SNF remodeling of the nucleosome by unzipping single DNA molecules. Nat Struct Mol Biol 13: 549-554.
[148] Schnitzler G, Sif S, Kingston RE (1998) Human SWI/SNF interconverts a nucleosome between its base state and a stable remodeled state. Cell 94: 17-27.
[149] Imbalzano AN, Kwon H, Green MR, Kingston RE (1994) Facilitated binding of TATA-binding protein to nucleosomal DNA. Nature 370: 481-485.
[150] Reisman D, Glaros S, Thompson EA (2009) The SWI/SNF complex and cancer. Oncogene 28: 1653-1668.
[151] Mizutani T, Ito T, Nishina M, Yamamichi N, Watanabe A, et al. (2002) Maintenance of integrated proviral gene expression requires Brm, a catalytic subunit of SWI/SNF complex. J. Biol. Chem. 277: 15859-15864.
[152] Bourachot B, Yaniv M, Muchardt C (2003) Growth inhibition by the mammalian SWI-SNF subunit Brm is regulated by acetylation. Embo J 22: 6505-6515.
[153] Yamamichi N, Yamamichi-Nishina M, Mizutani T, Watanabe H, Minoguchi S, et al. (2005) The Brm gene suppressed at the post-transcriptional level in various human cell lines is inducible by transient HDAC inhibitor treatment, which exhibits antioncogenic potential. Oncogene 24: 5471-5481.

[154] Glaros S, Cirrincione GM, Muchardt C, Kleer CG, Michael CW, et al. (2007) The reversible epigenetic silencing of BRM: implications for clinical targeted therapy. Oncogene 26: 7058-7066.

[155] Khavari PA, Peterson CL, Tamkun JW, Mendel DB, Crabtree GR (1993) BRG1 contains a conserved domain of the SWI2/SNF2 family necessary for normal mitotic growth and transcription. Nature 366: 170-174.

[156] Reyes JC, Barra J, Muchardt C, Camus A, Babinet C, et al. (1998) Altered control of cellular proliferation in the absence of mammalian brahma (SNF2alpha). Embo J 17: 6979-6991.

[157] Muchardt C, Yaniv M (1999) ATP-dependent chromatin remodelling: SWI/SNF and Co. are on the job. J Mol Biol 293: 187-198.

[158] Coisy-Quivy M, Disson O, Roure V, Muchardt C, Blanchard JM, et al. (2006) Role for Brm in cell growth control. Cancer Res. 66: 5069-5076.

[159] Strober BE, Dunaief JL, Guha, Goff SP (1996) Functional interactions between the hBRM/hBRG1 transcriptional activators and the pRB family of proteins. *Mol. Cell Biol.* 16: 1576-1583.

[160] Liu K, Luo Y, Lin FT, Lin WC (2004) TopBP1 recruits Brg1/Brm to repress E2F1-induced apoptosis, a novel pRb-independent and E2F1-specific control for cell survival. *Genes. Dev.* 18: 673-686.

[161] Kang H, Cui K, Zhao K (2004) BRG1 controls the activity of the retinoblastoma protein via regulation of p21CIP1/WAF1/SDI. *Mol. Cell Biol.* 24: 1188-1199.

[162] Bochar DA, Wang L, Beniya H, Kinev A, Xue Y, et al. (2000) BRCA1 is associated with a human SWI/SNF-related complex: linking chromatin remodeling to breast cancer. *Cell* 102: 257-265.

[163] Wang W (2007) Emergence of a DNA-damage response network consisting of Fanconi anaemia and BRCA proteins. *Nat. Rev. Genet.* 8: 735-748.

[164] Banine F, Bartlett C, Gunawardena R, Muchardt C, Yaniv M, et al. (2005) SWI/SNF chromatin-remodeling factors induce changes in DNA methylation to promote transcriptional activation. *Cancer Res.* 65: 3542-3547.

[165] Liu R, Liu H, Chen X, Kirby M, Brown PO, et al. (2001) Regulation of CSF1 promoter by the SWI/SNF-like BAF complex. *Cell* 106: 309-318.

[166] Hendricks KB, Shanahan F, Lees E (2004) Role for BRG1 in cell cycle control and tumor suppression. *Mol. Cell Biol.* 24: 362-376.

[167] Wang L, Baiocchi RA, Pal S, Mosialos G, Caligiuri M, et al. (2005) The BRG1- and hBRM-associated factor BAF57 induces apoptosis by stimulating expression of the cylindromatosis tumor suppressor gene. *Mol. Cell Biol.* 25: 7953-7965.

[168] Sumi-Ichinose C, Ichinose H, Metzger D, Chambon P (1997) SNF2beta-BRG1 is essential for the viability of F9 murine embryonal carcinoma cells. *Mol. Cell Biol.* 17: 5976-5986.

[169] Ichinose H, Garnier JM, Chambon P, Losson R (1997) Ligand-dependent interaction between the estrogen receptor and the human homologues of SWI2/SNF2. *Gene* 188: 95-100.

[170] Flajollet S, Lefebvre B, Cudejko C, Staels B, Lefebvre P (2007) The core component of the mammalian SWI/SNF complex SMARCD3/BAF60c is a coactivator for the nuclear retinoic acid receptor. *Mol. Cell Endocrinol.* 270: 23-32.

[171] Agalioti T, Lomvardas S, Parekh B, Yie J, Maniatis T, et al. (2000) Ordered recruitment of chromatin modifying and general transcription factors to the IFN-beta promoter. *Cell* 103: 667-678.

[172] Morshead KB, Ciccone DN, Taverna SD, Allis CD, Oettinger MA (2003) Antigen receptor loci poised for V(D)J rearrangement are broadly associated with BRG1 and flanked by peaks of histone H3 dimethylated at lysine 4. *Proc. Natl. Acad. Sci. USA* 100: 11577-11582.

[173] Sekine I, Sato M, Sunaga N, Toyooka S, Peyton M, et al. (2005) The 3p21 candidate tumor suppressor gene BAF180 is normally expressed in human lung cancer. *Oncogene* 24: 2735-2738.

[174] Link KA, Burd CJ, Williams E, Marshall T, Rosson G, et al. (2005) BAF57 governs androgen receptor action and androgen-dependent proliferation through SWI/SNF. *Mol. Cell Biol.* 25: 2200-2215.

[175] Roberts CW, Leroux MM, Fleming MD, Orkin SH (2002) Highly penetrant, rapid tumorigenesis through conditional inversion of the tumor suppressor gene Snf5. Cancer *Cell* 2: 415-425.

[176] Decristofaro MF, Betz BL, Rorie CJ, Reisman DN, Wang W, et al. (2001) Characterization of SWI/SNF protein expression in human breast cancer cell lines and other malignancies. *J. Cell Physiol.* 186: 136-145.

[177] Kalpana GV, Marmon S, Wang W, Crabtree GR, Goff SP (1994) Binding and stimulation of HIV-1 integrase by a human homolog of yeast transcription factor SNF5. *Science* 266: 2002-2006.

[178] Yuge M, Nagai H, Uchida T, Murate T, Hayashi Y, et al. (2000) HSNF5/INI1 gene mutations in lymphoid malignancy. *Cancer Genet. Cytogenet.* 122: 37-42.

[179] Muchardt C, Yaniv M (2001) When the SWI/SNF complex remodels...the cell cycle. *Oncogene* 20: 3067-3075.

[180] Reisman DN, Sciarrotta J, Bouldin TW, Weissman BE, Funkhouser WK (2005) The expression of the SWI/SNF ATPase subunits BRG1 and BRM in normal human tissues. *Appl. Immunohistochem. Mol. Morphol.* 13: 66-74.

[181] Biegel JA, Fogelgren B, Zhou JY, James CD, Janss AJ, et al. (2000) Mutations of the INI1 rhabdoid tumor suppressor gene in medulloblastomas and primitive neuroectodermal tumors of the central nervous system. *Clin. Cancer Res.* 6: 2759-2763.

[182] Biegel JA, Fogelgren B, Wainwright LM, Zhou JY, Bevan H, et al. (2000) Germline INI1 mutation in a patient with a central nervous system atypical teratoid tumor and renal rhabdoid tumor. *Genes Chromosomes Cancer* 28: 31-37.

[183] Phelan ML, Sif S, Narlikar GJ, Kingston RE (1999) Reconstitution of a core chromatin remodeling complex from SWI/SNF subunits. *Mol. Cell* 3: 247-253.

[184] Versteege I, Medjkane S, Rouillard D, Delattre O (2002) A key role of the hSNF5/INI1 tumour suppressor in the control of the G1-S transition of the cell cycle. *Oncogene* 21: 6403-6412.

[185] Tsikitis M, Zhang Z, Edelman W, Zagzag D, Kalpana GV (2005) Genetic ablation of Cyclin D1 abrogates genesis of rhabdoid tumors resulting from Ini1 loss. *Proc. Natl. Acad. Sci. USA* 102: 12129-12134.

[186] Zhang ZK, Davies KP, Allen J, Zhu L, Pestell RG, et al. (2002) Cell cycle arrest and repression of cyclin D1 transcription by INI1/hSNF5. *Mol. Cell Biol.* 22: 5975-5988.

[187] Ewen ME, Lamb J (2004) The activities of cyclin D1 that drive tumorigenesis. *Trends Mol. Med.* 10: 158-162.

[188] Dragnev KH, Pitha-Rowe I, Ma Y, Petty WJ, Sekula D, et al. (2004) Specific chemopreventive agents trigger proteasomal degradation of G1 cyclins: implications for combination therapy. *Clin. Cancer Res.* 10: 2570-2577.

[189] Furchert SE, Lanvers-Kaminsky C, Juurgens H, Jung M, Loidl A, et al. (2007) Inhibitors of histone deacetylases as potential therapeutic tools for high-risk embryonal tumors of the nervous system of childhood. *Int. J. Cancer* 120: 1787-1794.

[190] Kaneko Y, Egues MC, Rowley JD (1981) Interstitial deletion of short arm of chromosome 11 limited to Wilms' tumor cells in a patient without aniridia. *Cancer Res.* 41: 4577-4578.

[191] Call KM, Glaser T, Ito CY, Buckler AJ, Pelletier J, et al. (1990) Isolation and characterization of a zinc finger polypeptide gene at the human chromosome 11 Wilms' tumor locus. *Cell* 60: 509-520.

[192] Gessler M, Poustka A, Cavenee W, Neve RL, Orkin SH, et al. (1990) Homozygous deletion in Wilms tumours of a zinc-finger gene identified by chromosome jumping. *Nature* 343: 774-778.

[193] Little M, Wells C (1997) A clinical overview of WT1 gene mutations. *Hum. Mutat.* 9: 209-225.

[194] Bach LA, Headey SJ, Norton RS (2005) IGF-binding proteins--the pieces are falling into place. *Trends Endocrinol. Metab.* 16: 228-234.

[195] De Meyts P, Whittaker J (2002) Structural biology of insulin and IGF1 receptors: implications for drug design. *Nat. Rev. Drug Discov.* 1: 769-783.

[196] Butler AA, Yakar S, Gewolb IH, Karas M, Okubo Y, et al. (1998) Insulin-like growth factor-I receptor signal transduction: at the interface between physiology and cell biology. *Comp. Biochem. Physiol. B Biochem. Mol. Biol.* 121: 19-26.

[197] Adams TE, Epa VC, Garrett TP, Ward CW (2000) Structure and function of the type 1 insulin-like growth factor receptor. *Cell Mol. Life Sci.* 57: 1050-1093.

[198] Dearth RK, Cui X, Kim HJ, Hadsell DL, Lee AV (2007) Oncogenic transformation by the signaling adaptor proteins insulin receptor substrate (IRS)-1 and IRS-2. *Cell Cycle* 6: 705-713.

[199] Henry I, Bonaiti-Pellie C, Chehensse V, Beldjord C, Schwartz C, et al. (1991) Uniparental paternal disomy in a genetic cancer-predisposing syndrome. *Nature* 351: 665-667.

[200] Wilkin F, Gagne N, Paquette J, Oligny LL, Deal C (2000) Pediatric adrenocortical tumors: molecular events leading to insulin-like growth factor II gene overexpression. *J. Clin. Endocrinol. Metab.* 85: 2048-2056.

[201] Schneider DT, Schuster AE, Fritsch MK, Hu J, Olson T, et al. (2001) Multipoint imprinting analysis indicates a common precursor cell for gonadal and nongonadal pediatric germ cell tumors. *Cancer Res.* 61: 7268-7276.

[202] Geryk-Hall M, Hughes DP (2009) Critical signaling pathways in bone sarcoma: candidates for therapeutic interventions. *Curr. Oncol. Rep.* 11: 446-453.

[203] Sartelet H, Oligny LL, Vassal G (2008) AKT pathway in neuroblastoma and its therapeutic implication. *Expert Rev. Anticancer. Ther.* 8: 757-769.

[204] Engstrom W, Granerus M (2009) The Expression of the Insulin-like Growth Factor II, JIP-1 and WT1 Genes in Porcine Nephroblastoma. *AntiCancer Res.* 29: 4999-5003.

[205] Cao L, Yu Y, Darko I, Currier D, Mayeenuddin LH, et al. (2008) Addiction to elevated insulin-like growth factor I receptor and initial modulation of the AKT pathway define the responsiveness of rhabdomyosarcoma to the targeting antibody. *Cancer Res*. 68: 8039-8048.

[206] Feinberg AP, Tycko B (2004) The history of cancer epigenetics. *Nat. Rev. Cancer* 4: 143-153.

[207] Bell AC, Felsenfeld G (2000) Methylation of a CTCF-dependent boundary controls imprinted expression of the Igf2 gene. *Nature* 405: 482-485.

[208] Hark AT, Schoenherr CJ, Katz DJ, Ingram RS, Levorse JM, et al. (2000) CTCF mediates methylation-sensitive enhancer-blocking activity at the H19/Igf2 locus. *Nature* 405: 486-489.

[209] Ravenel JD, Broman KW, Perlman EJ, Niemitz EL, Jayawardena TM, et al. (2001) Loss of imprinting of insulin-like growth factor-II (IGF2) gene in distinguishing specific biologic subtypes of Wilms tumor. *J. Natl. Cancer Inst.* 93: 1698-1703.

[210] Yuan E, Li CM, Yamashiro DJ, Kandel J, Thaker H, et al. (2005) Genomic profiling maps loss of heterozygosity and defines the timing and stage dependence of epigenetic and genetic events in Wilms' tumors. *Mol. Cancer Res*. 3: 493-502.

[211] Savage SA, Woodson K, Walk E, Modi W, Liao J, et al. (2007) Analysis of genes critical for growth regulation identifies Insulin-like Growth Factor 2 Receptor variations with possible functional significance as risk factors for osteosarcoma. *Cancer Epidemiol. Biomarkers Prev.* 16: 1667-1674.

[212] Urbanska K, Trojanek J, Del Valle L, Eldeen MB, Hofmann F, et al. (2007) Inhibition of IGF-I receptor in anchorage-independence attenuates GSK-3beta constitutive phosphorylation and compromises growth and survival of medulloblastoma cell lines. *Oncogene* 26: 2308-2317.

[213] Brandenberger R, Schmidt A, Linton J, Wang D, Backus C, et al. (2001) Identification and characterization of a novel extracellular matrix protein nephronectin that is associated with integrin alpha8beta1 in the embryonic kidney. *J. Cell Biol.* 154: 447-458.

[214] Wilkinson LS, Davies W, Isles AR (2007) Genomic imprinting effects on brain development and function. *Nat. Rev. Neurosci.* 8: 832-843.

[215] DeChiara TM, Robertson EJ, Efstratiadis A (1991) Parental imprinting of the mouse insulin-like growth factor II gene. *Cell* 64: 849-859.

[216] Reik W, Lewis A (2005) Co-evolution of X-chromosome inactivation and imprinting in mammals. *Nat. Rev. Genet.* 6: 403-410.

[217] Sasaki H, Ishihara K, Kato R (2000) Mechanisms of Igf2/H19 imprinting: DNA methylation, chromatin and long-distance gene regulation. *J. Biochem.* 127: 711-715.

[218] van Noesel MM, Pieters R, Voute PA, Versteeg R (2003) The N-myc paradox: N-myc overexpression in neuroblastomas is associated with sensitivity as well as resistance to apoptosis. *Cancer Lett.* 197: 165-172.

[219] Shivapurkar N, Toyooka S, Eby MT, Huang CX, Sathyanarayana UG, et al. (2002) Differential inactivation of caspase-8 in lung cancers. *Cancer Biol. Ther.* 1: 65-69.

[220] Harada K, Toyooka S, Shivapurkar N, Maitra A, Reddy JL, et al. (2002) Deregulation of caspase 8 and 10 expression in pediatric tumors and cell lines. *Cancer Res*. 62: 5897-5901.

[221] van Noesel MM, van Bezouw S, Voute PA, Herman JG, Pieters R, et al. (2003) Clustering of hypermethylated genes in neuroblastoma. *Genes. Chromosomes Cancer* 38: 226-233.

[222] Teitz T, Wei T, Valentine MB, Vanin EF, Grenet J, et al. (2000) Caspase 8 is deleted or silenced preferentially in childhood neuroblastomas with amplification of MYCN. *Nat. Med.* 6: 529-535.

[223] Fulda S, Lutz W, Schwab M, Debatin KM (2000) MycN sensitizes neuroblastoma cells for drug-triggered apoptosis. *Med. Pediatr. Oncol.* 35: 582-584.

[224] Michalowski MB, de Fraipont F, Plantaz D, Michelland S, Combaret V, et al. (2008) Methylation of tumor-suppressor genes in neuroblastoma: The RASSF1A gene is almost always methylated in primary tumors. *Pediatr Blood Cancer* 50: 29-32.

[225] Kamimatsuse A, Matsuura K, Moriya S, Fukuba I, Yamaoka H, et al. (2009) Detection of CpG island hypermethylation of caspase-8 in neuroblastoma using an oligonucleotide array. *Pediatr Blood Cancer* 52: 777-783.

[226] Ikeda H, Hirato J, Akami M, Matsuyama S, Suzuki N, et al. (1995) Bcl-2 oncoprotein expression and apoptosis in neuroblastoma. *J. Pediatr Surg.* 30: 805-808.

[227] Fulda S, Meyer E, Debatin KM (2002) Inhibition of TRAIL-induced apoptosis by Bcl-2 overexpression. *Oncogene* 21: 2283-2294.

[228] Castle VP, Heidelberger KP, Bromberg J, Ou X, Dole M, et al. (1993) Expression of the apoptosis-suppressing protein bcl-2, in neuroblastoma is associated with unfavorable histology and N-myc amplification. *Am. J. Pathol.* 143: 1543-1550.

[229] Inoue J, Misawa A, Tanaka Y, Ichinose S, Sugino Y, et al. (2009) Lysosomal-associated protein multispanning transmembrane 5 gene (LAPTM5) is associated with spontaneous regression of neuroblastomas. *PLoS One* 4: e7099.

[230] Dammann R, Schagdarsurengin U, Strunnikova M, Rastetter M, Seidel C, et al. (2003) Epigenetic inactivation of the Ras-association domain family 1 (RASSF1A) gene and its function in human carcinogenesis. *Histol. Histopathol.* 18: 665-677.

[231] Agathanggelou A, Cooper WN, Latif F (2005) Role of the Ras-association domain family 1 tumor suppressor gene in human cancers. *Cancer Res.* 65: 3497-3508.

[232] Ejeskar K, Aburatani H, Abrahamsson J, Kogner P, Martinsson T (1998) Loss of heterozygosity of 3p markers in neuroblastoma tumours implicate a tumour-suppressor locus distal to the FHIT gene. *Br. J. Cancer* 77: 1787-1791.

[233] Agathanggelou A, Bieche I, Ahmed-Choudhury J, Nicke B, Dammann R, et al. (2003) Identification of novel gene expression targets for the Ras association domain family 1 (RASSF1A) tumor suppressor gene in non-small cell lung cancer and neuroblastoma. *Cancer Res.* 63: 5344-5351.

[234] Hesson L, Dallol A, Minna JD, Maher ER, Latif F (2003) NORE1A, a homologue of RASSF1A tumour suppressor gene is inactivated in human cancers. *Oncogene* 22: 947-954.

[235] Lerman MI, Minna JD (2000) The 630-kb lung cancer homozygous deletion region on human chromosome 3p21.3: identification and evaluation of the resident candidate tumor suppressor genes. The International Lung Cancer Chromosome 3p21.3 Tumor Suppressor Gene Consortium. *Cancer Res.* 60: 6116-6133.

[236] Hesson L, Bieche I, Krex D, Criniere E, Hoang-Xuan K, et al. (2004) Frequent epigenetic inactivation of RASSF1A and BLU genes located within the critical 3p21.3 region in gliomas. *Oncogene* 23: 2408-2419.

[237] Eckfeld K, Hesson L, Vos MD, Bieche I, Latif F, et al. (2004) RASSF4/AD037 is a potential ras effector/tumor suppressor of the RASSF family. *Cancer Res.* 64: 8688-8693.

[238] Eilers M, Eisenman RN (2008) Myc's broad reach. *Genes. Dev.* 22: 2755-2766.

[239] Guccione E, Martinato F, Finocchiaro G, Luzi L, Tizzoni L, et al. (2006) Myc-binding-site recognition in the human genome is determined by chromatin context. *Nat. Cell Biol.* 8: 764-770.

[240] Cotterman R, Knoepfler PS (2009) N-Myc regulates expression of pluripotency genes in neuroblastoma including lif, klf2, klf4, and lin28b. *PLoS One* 4: e5799.

[241] Issa JP, Shen L, Toyota M (2005) CIMP, at last. *Gastroenterology* 129: 1121-1124.

[242] Abe M, Ohira M, Kaneda A, Yagi Y, Yamamoto S, et al. (2005) CpG island methylator phenotype is a strong determinant of poor prognosis in neuroblastomas. *Cancer Res.* 65: 828-834.

[243] Nguyen C, Liang G, Nguyen TT, Tsao-Wei D, Groshen S, et al. (2001) Susceptibility of nonpromoter CpG islands to de novo methylation in normal and neoplastic cells. *J. Natl. Cancer Inst.* 93: 1465-1472.

[244] Abe M, Watanabe N, McDonell N, Takato T, Ohira M, et al. (2008) Identification of genes targeted by CpG island methylator phenotype in neuroblastomas, and their possible integrative involvement in poor prognosis. *Oncology* 74: 50-60.

[245] Hansen MF (2002) Genetic and molecular aspects of osteosarcoma. *J. Musculoskelet. Neuronal. Interact.* 2: 554-560.

[246] Helman LJ, Meltzer P (2003) Mechanisms of sarcoma development. *Nat. Rev. Cancer* 3: 685-694.

[247] Wang LL (2005) Biology of osteogenic sarcoma. *Cancer J.* 11: 294-305.

[248] Sandberg AA, Bridge JA (2003) Updates on the cytogenetics and molecular genetics of bone and soft tissue tumors: osteosarcoma and related tumors. *Cancer Genet. Cytogenet.* 145: 1-30.

[249] Luu HH, Song WX, Luo X, Manning D, Luo J, et al. (2007) Distinct roles of bone morphogenetic proteins in osteogenic differentiation of mesenchymal stem cells. *J. Orthop. Res.* 25: 665-677.

[250] Aubin JE (1998) Bone stem cells. *J. Cell Biochem. Suppl.* 30-31: 73-82.

[251] Feinberg AP, Ohlsson R, Henikoff S (2006) The epigenetic progenitor origin of human cancer. *Nat. Rev. Genet.* 7: 21-33.

[252] Kuzmichev A, Margueron R, Vaquero A, Preissner TS, Scher M, et al. (2005) Composition and histone substrates of polycomb repressive group complexes change during cellular differentiation. *Proc. Natl. Acad. Sci. USA* 102: 1859-1864.

[253] van der Lugt NM, Domen J, Linders K, van Roon M, Robanus-Maandag E, et al. (1994) Posterior transformation, neurological abnormalities, and severe hematopoietic defects in mice with a targeted deletion of the bmi-1 proto-oncogene. *Genes. Dev.* 8: 757-769.

[254] Vonlanthen S, Heighway J, Altermatt HJ, Gugger M, Kappeler A, et al. (2001) The bmi-1 oncoprotein is differentially expressed in non-small cell lung cancer and correlates with INK4A-ARF locus expression. *Br. J. Cancer* 84: 1372-1376.

[255] Jacobs JJ, Kieboom K, Marino S, DePinho RA, van Lohuizen M (1999) The oncogene and Polycomb-group gene bmi-1 regulates cell proliferation and senescence through the ink4a locus. *Nature* 397: 164-168.

[256] Takeda Y, Mori T, Imabayashi H, Kiyono T, Gojo S, et al. (2004) Can the life span of human marrow stromal cells be prolonged by bmi-1, E6, E7, and/or telomerase without affecting cardiomyogenic differentiation? *J. Gene. Med.* 6: 833-845.

[257] Douglas D, Hsu JH, Hung L, Cooper A, Abdueva D, et al. (2008) BMI-1 promotes ewing sarcoma tumorigenicity independent of CDKN2A repression. *Cancer Res.* 68: 6507-6515.

[258] Su AI, Wiltshire T, Batalov S, Lapp H, Ching KA, et al. (2004) A gene atlas of the mouse and human protein-encoding transcriptomes. *Proc. Natl. Acad. Sci. USA* 101: 6062-6067.

[259] Pahlich S, Quero L, Roschitzki B, Leemann-Zakaryan RP, Gehring H (2009) Analysis of Ewing sarcoma (EWS)-binding proteins: interaction with hnRNP M, U, and RNA-helicases p68/72 within protein-RNA complexes. *J. Proteome Res.* 8: 4455-4465.

[260] Burdach S, Plehm S, Unland R, Dirksen U, Borkhardt A, et al. (2009) Epigenetic maintenance of stemness and malignancy in peripheral neuroectodermal tumors by EZH2. *Cell Cycle* 8: 1991-1996.

[261] Riggi N, Suva ML, Suva D, Cironi L, Provero P, et al. (2008) EWS-FLI-1 expression triggers a Ewing's sarcoma initiation program in primary human mesenchymal stem cells. *Cancer Res.* 68: 2176-2185.

[262] Deshpande AM, Akunowicz JD, Reveles XT, Patel BB, Saria EA, et al. (2007) PHC3, a component of the hPRC-H complex, associates with E2F6 during G0 and is lost in osteosarcoma tumors. *Oncogene* 26: 1714-1722.

[263] Quelle DE, Zindy F, Ashmun RA, Sherr CJ (1995) Alternative reading frames of the INK4a tumor suppressor gene encode two unrelated proteins capable of inducing cell cycle arrest. *Cell* 83: 993-1000.

[264] Pomerantz J, Schreiber-Agus N, Liegeois NJ, Silverman A, Alland L, et al. (1998) The Ink4a tumor suppressor gene product, p19Arf, interacts with MDM2 and neutralizes MDM2's inhibition of p53. *Cell* 92: 713-723.

[265] Nielsen GP, Burns KL, Rosenberg AE, Louis DN (1998) CDKN2A gene deletions and loss of p16 expression occur in osteosarcomas that lack RB alterations. *Am. J. Pathol.* 153: 159-163.

[266] Gonzalo S, Garcia-Cao M, Fraga MF, Schotta G, Peters AH, et al. (2005) Role of the RB1 family in stabilizing histone methylation at constitutive heterochromatin. *Nat. Cell Biol.* 7: 420-428.

[267] Dahiya A, Wong S, Gonzalo S, Gavin M, Dean DC (2001) Linking the Rb and polycomb pathways. *Mol. Cell* 8: 557-569.

[268] Bracken AP, Pasini D, Capra M, Prosperini E, Colli E, et al. (2003) EZH2 is downstream of the pRB-E2F pathway, essential for proliferation and amplified in cancer. *Embo J.* 22: 5323-5335.

[269] Reya T, Clevers H (2005) Wnt signalling in stem cells and cancer. *Nature* 434: 843-850.

[270] Reya T, Morrison SJ, Clarke MF, Weissman IL (2001) Stem cells, cancer, and cancer stem cells. *Nature* 414: 105-111.

[271] Kansara M, Tsang M, Kodjabachian L, Sims NA, Trivett MK, et al. (2009) Wnt inhibitory factor 1 is epigenetically silenced in human osteosarcoma, and targeted disruption accelerates osteosarcomagenesis in mice. *J. Clin. Invest.* 119: 837-851.

[272] Chien KR, Karsenty G (2005) Longevity and lineages: toward the integrative biology of degenerative diseases in heart, muscle, and bone. *Cell* 120: 533-544.

[273] Karsenty G (2003) The complexities of skeletal biology. *Nature* 423: 316-318.

[274] Winslow MM, Pan M, Starbuck M, Gallo EM, Deng L, et al. (2006) Calcineurin/NFAT signaling in osteoblasts regulates bone mass. *Dev. Cell* 10: 771-782.

[275] Yang X, Karsenty G (2004) ATF4, the osteoblast accumulation of which is determined post-translationally, can induce osteoblast-specific gene expression in non-osteoblastic cells. *J. Biol. Chem.* 279: 47109-47114.

[276] Ogawa E, Inuzuka M, Maruyama M, Satake M, Naito-Fujimoto M, et al. (1993) Molecular cloning and characterization of PEBP2 beta, the heterodimeric partner of a novel Drosophila runt-related DNA binding protein PEBP2 alpha. *Virology* 194: 314-331.

[277] Ducy P, Starbuck M, Priemel M, Shen J, Pinero G, et al. (1999) A Cbfa1-dependent genetic pathway controls bone formation beyond embryonic development. *Genes. Dev.* 13: 1025-1036.

[278] Locklin RM, Oreffo RO, Triffitt JT (1998) Modulation of osteogenic differentiation in human skeletal cells in Vitro by 5-azacytidine. *Cell Biol. Int.* 22: 207-215.

[279] Ryhanen S, Pirskanen A, Jaaskelainen T, Maenpaa PH (1997) State of methylation of the human osteocalcin gene in bone-derived and other types of cells. *J. Cell Biochem.* 66: 404-412.

[280] Massague J, Chen YG (2000) Controlling TGF-beta signaling. *Genes. Dev.* 14: 627-644.

[281] Ulaner GA, Vu TH, Li T, Hu JF, Yao XM, et al. (2003) Loss of imprinting of IGF2 and H19 in osteosarcoma is accompanied by reciprocal methylation changes of a CTCF-binding site. *Hum. Mol. Genet.* 12: 535-549.

[282] Harada K, Toyooka S, Maitra A, Maruyama R, Toyooka KO, et al. (2002) Aberrant promoter methylation and silencing of the RASSF1A gene in pediatric tumors and cell lines. *Oncogene* 21: 4345-4349.

[283] Avigad S, Shukla S, Naumov I, Cohen IJ, Ash S, et al. (2009) Aberrant methylation and reduced expression of RASSF1A in Ewing sarcoma. *Pediatr Blood Cancer* 53: 1023-1028.

[284] Deltour S, Guerardel C, Leprince D (1999) Recruitment of SMRT/N-CoR-mSin3A-HDAC-repressing complexes is not a general mechanism for BTB/POZ transcriptional repressors: the case of HIC-1 and gammaFBP-B. *Proc. Natl. Acad. Sci. USA* 96: 14831-14836.

[285] Gokgoz N, Wunder JS, Mousses S, Eskandarian S, Bell RS, et al. (2001) Comparison of p53 mutations in patients with localized osteosarcoma and metastatic osteosarcoma. *Cancer* 92: 2181-2189.

[286] Overholtzer M, Rao PH, Favis R, Lu XY, Elowitz MB, et al. (2003) The presence of p53 mutations in human osteosarcomas correlates with high levels of genomic instability. *Proc. Natl. Acad. Sci. USA* 100: 11547-11552.

[287] Rathi A, Virmani AK, Harada K, Timmons CF, Miyajima K, et al. (2003) Aberrant methylation of the HIC1 promoter is a frequent event in specific pediatric neoplasms. *Clin. Cancer Res.* 9: 3674-3678.

[288] Chen W, Cooper TK, Zahnow CA, Overholtzer M, Zhao Z, et al. (2004) Epigenetic and genetic loss of Hic1 function accentuates the role of p53 in tumorigenesis. *Cancer Cell* 6: 387-398.

[289] Pimenta AF, Zhukareva V, Barbe MF, Reinoso BS, Grimley C, et al. (1995) The limbic system-associated membrane protein is an Ig superfamily member that mediates selective neuronal growth and axon targeting. *Neuron* 15: 287-297.

[290] Eagleson KL, Pimenta AF, Burns MM, Fairfull LD, Cornuet PK, et al. (2003) Distinct domains of the limbic system-associated membrane protein (LAMP) mediate discrete effects on neurite outgrowth. *Mol. Cell Neurosci.* 24: 725-740.

[291] Chen J, Lui WO, Vos MD, Clark GJ, Takahashi M, et al. (2003) The t(1;3) breakpoint-spanning genes LSAMP and NORE1 are involved in clear cell renal cell carcinomas. *Cancer Cell* 4: 405-413.

[292] Kresse SH, Ohnstad HO, Paulsen EB, Bjerkehagen B, Szuhai K, et al. (2009) LSAMP, a novel candidate tumor suppressor gene in human osteosarcomas, identified by array comparative genomic hybridization. *Genes. Chromosomes. Cancer* 48: 679-693.

[293] Sadikovic B, Yoshimoto M, Al-Romaih K, Maire G, Zielenska M, et al. (2008) In vitro analysis of integrated global high-resolution DNA methylation profiling with genomic imbalance and gene expression in osteosarcoma. *PLoS One* 3: e2834.

[294] Lim G, Karaskova J, Vukovic B, Bayani J, Beheshti B, et al. (2004) Combined spectral karyotyping, multicolor banding, and microarray comparative genomic hybridization analysis provides a detailed characterization of complex structural chromosomal rearrangements associated with gene amplification in the osteosarcoma cell line MG-63. *Cancer Genet. Cytogenet.* 153: 158-164.

[295] Squire JA, Pei J, Marrano P, Beheshti B, Bayani J, et al. (2003) High-resolution mapping of amplifications and deletions in pediatric osteosarcoma by use of CGH analysis of cDNA microarrays. *Genes. Chromosomes. Cancer* 38: 215-225.

[296] Roman-Gomez J, Jimenez-Velasco A, Agirre X, Castillejo JA, Navarro G, et al. (2008) Repetitive DNA hypomethylation in the advanced phase of chronic myeloid leukemia. *Leuk Res.* 32: 487-490.

[297] Schulz WA, Elo JP, Florl AR, Pennanen S, Santourlidis S, et al. (2002) Genomewide DNA hypomethylation is associated with alterations on chromosome 8 in prostate carcinoma. *Genes. Chromosomes. Cancer* 35: 58-65.

[298] Weinberg AG, Finegold MJ (1983) Primary hepatic tumors of childhood. *Hum. Pathol.* 14: 512-537.

[299] Mann JR, Kasthuri N, Raafat F, Pincott JR, Parkes SE, et al. (1990) Malignant hepatic tumours in children: incidence, clinical features and aetiology. *Paediatr Perinat. Epidemiol.* 4: 276-289.

[300] Ross JA, Gurney JG (1998) Hepatoblastoma incidence in the United States from 1973 to 1992. *Med. Pediatr Oncol.* 30: 141-142.

[301] Sugawara W, Haruta M, Sasaki F, Watanabe N, Tsunematsu Y, et al. (2007) Promoter hypermethylation of the RASSF1A gene predicts the poor outcome of patients with hepatoblastoma. *Pediatr Blood Cancer* 49: 240-249.

[302] Honda S, Haruta M, Sugawara W, Sasaki F, Ohira M, et al. (2008) The methylation status of RASSF1A promoter predicts responsiveness to chemotherapy and eventual cure in hepatoblastoma patients. *Int. J. Cancer* 123: 1117-1125.

[303] Taniguchi K, Roberts LR, Aderca IN, Dong X, Qian C, et al. (2002) Mutational spectrum of beta-catenin, AXIN1, and AXIN2 in hepatocellular carcinomas and hepatoblastomas. *Oncogene* 21: 4863-4871.

[304] Deutsch G, Jung J, Zheng M, Lora J, Zaret KS (2001) A bipotential precursor population for pancreas and liver within the embryonic endoderm. *Development* 128: 871-881.

[305] Sicklick JK, Li YX, Choi SS, Qi Y, Chen W, et al. (2005) Role for hedgehog signaling in hepatic stellate cell activation and viability. *Lab. Invest.* 85: 1368-1380.

[306] Sicklick JK, Li YX, Melhem A, Schmelzer E, Zdanowicz M, et al. (2006) Hedgehog signaling maintains resident hepatic progenitors throughout life. *Am. J. Physiol. Gastrointest Liver Physiol.* 290: G859-870.

[307] Eichenmuller M, Gruner I, Hagl B, Haberle B, Muller-Hocker J, et al. (2009) Blocking the hedgehog pathway inhibits hepatoblastoma growth. *Hepatology* 49: 482-490.

[308] Chuang PT, Kawcak T, McMahon AP (2003) Feedback control of mammalian Hedgehog signaling by the Hedgehog-binding protein, Hip1, modulates Fgf signaling during branching morphogenesis of the lung. *Genes. Dev.* 17: 342-347.

[309] Martin ST, Sato N, Dhara S, Chang R, Hustinx SR, et al. (2005) Aberrant methylation of the Human Hedgehog interacting protein (HHIP) gene in pancreatic neoplasms. *Cancer Biol. Ther.* 4: 728-733.

[310] Taniguchi H, Yamamoto H, Akutsu N, Nosho K, Adachi Y, et al. (2007) Transcriptional silencing of hedgehog-interacting protein by CpG hypermethylation and chromatic structure in human gastrointestinal cancer. *J. Pathol.* 213: 131-139.

[311] Tada M, Kanai F, Tanaka Y, Tateishi K, Ohta M, et al. (2008) Down-regulation of hedgehog-interacting protein through genetic and epigenetic alterations in human hepatocellular carcinoma. *Clin. Cancer Res.* 14: 3768-3776.

[312] Foulstone E, Prince S, Zaccheo O, Burns JL, Harper J, et al. (2005) Insulin-like growth factor ligands, receptors, and binding proteins in cancer. *J. Pathol.* 205: 145-153.

[313] Li X, Gray SG, Flam F, Pietsch T, Ekstrom TJ (1998) Developmental-dependent DNA methylation of the IGF2 and H19 promoters is correlated to the promoter activities in human liver development. *Int. J. Dev Biol* 42: 687-693.

[314] Toretsky JA, Helman LJ (1996) Involvement of IGF-II in human cancer. *J. Endocrinol.* 149: 367-372.

[315] Honda S, Arai Y, Haruta M, Sasaki F, Ohira M, et al. (2008) Loss of imprinting of IGF2 correlates with hypermethylation of the H19 differentially methylated region in hepatoblastoma. *Br. J. Cancer* 99: 1891-1899.

[316] Scotto KW (2003) Transcriptional regulation of ABC drug transporters. *Oncogene* 22: 7496-7511.

[317] Ling V (1995) P-glycoprotein: its role in drug resistance. *Am. J. Med.* 99: 31S-34S.

[318] Tada Y, Wada M, Kuroiwa K, Kinugawa N, Harada T, et al. (2000) MDR1 gene overexpression and altered degree of methylation at the promoter region in bladder cancer during chemotherapeutic treatment. *Clin. Cancer Res.* 6: 4618-4627.

[319] El-Osta A, Kantharidis P, Zalcberg JR, Wolffe AP (2002) Precipitous release of methyl-CpG binding protein 2 and histone deacetylase 1 from the methylated human multidrug resistance gene (MDR1) on activation. *Mol. Cell Biol.* 22: 1844-1857.

[320] Fulda S, Kufer MU, Meyer E, van Valen F, Dockhorn-Dworniczak B, et al. (2001) Sensitization for death receptor- or drug-induced apoptosis by re-expression of caspase-8 through demethylation or gene transfer. *Oncogene* 20: 5865-5877.

[321] Yang R, Qin J, Hoang BH, Healey JH, Gorlick R (2008) Polymorphisms and methylation of the reduced folate carrier in osteosarcoma. *Clin. Orthop. Relat. Res.* 466: 2046-2051.

[322] Hamilton DW, Lusher ME, Lindsey JC, Ellison DW, Clifford SC (2005) Epigenetic inactivation of the RASSF1A tumour suppressor gene in ependymoma. *Cancer Lett.* 227: 75-81.

[323] Michalowski MB, de Fraipont F, Michelland S, Entz-Werle N, Grill J, et al. (2006) Methylation of RASSF1A and TRAIL pathway-related genes is frequent in childhood intracranial ependymomas and benign choroid plexus papilloma. *Cancer Genet. Cytogenet.* 166: 74-81.

[324] Horiguchi K, Tomizawa Y, Tosaka M, Ishiuchi S, Kurihara H, et al. (2003) Epigenetic inactivation of RASSF1A candidate tumor suppressor gene at 3p21.3 in brain tumors. *Oncogene* 22: 7862-7865.

[325] Inda MM, Castresana JS (2007) RASSF1A promoter is highly methylated in primitive neuroectodermal tumors of the central nervous system. *Neuropathology* 27: 341-346.

[326] Muhlisch J, Schwering A, Grotzer M, Vince GH, Roggendorf W, et al. (2006) Epigenetic repression of RASSF1A but not CASP8 in supratentorial PNET (sPNET) and atypical teratoid/rhabdoid tumors (AT/RT) of childhood. *Oncogene* 25: 1111-1117.

[327] Wagner KJ, Cooper WN, Grundy RG, Caldwell G, Jones C, et al. (2002) Frequent RASSF1A tumour suppressor gene promoter methylation in Wilms' tumour and colorectal cancer. *Oncogene* 21: 7277-7282.

[328] Lazcoz P, Munoz J, Nistal M, Pestana A, Encio I, et al. (2006) Frequent promoter hypermethylation of RASSF1A and CASP8 in neuroblastoma. *BMC Cancer* 6: 254.

[329] Lim S, Yang MH, Park JH, Nojima T, Hashimoto H, et al. (2003) Inactivation of the RASSF1A in osteosarcoma. *Oncol Rep.* 10: 897-901.

[330] Waha A, Koch A, Hartmann W, Mack H, Schramm J, et al. (2004) Analysis of HIC-1 methylation and transcription in human ependymomas. *Int. J. Cancer* 110: 542-549.

[331] Waha A, Koch A, Meyer-Puttlitz B, Weggen S, Sorensen N, et al. (2003) Epigenetic silencing of the HIC-1 gene in human medulloblastomas. *J. Neuropathol. Exp. Neurol.* 62: 1192-1201.

[332] Donson AM, Addo-Yobo SO, Handler MH, Gore L, Foreman NK (2007) MGMT promoter methylation correlates with survival benefit and sensitivity to temozolomide in pediatric glioblastoma. *Pediatr Blood Cancer* 48: 403-407.

[333] Rood BR, Zhang H, Cogen PH (2004) Intercellular heterogeneity of expression of the MGMT DNA repair gene in pediatric medulloblastoma. *Neuro-oncol.* 6: 200-207.

[334] Morris MR, Hesson LB, Wagner KJ, Morgan NV, Astuti D, et al. (2003) Multigene methylation analysis of Wilms' tumour and adult renal cell carcinoma. *Oncogene* 22: 6794-6801.

[335] Zuzak TJ, Steinhoff DF, Sutton LN, Phillips PC, Eggert A, et al. (2002) Loss of caspase-8 mRNA expression is common in childhood primitive neuroectodermal brain tumour/medulloblastoma. *Eur. J. Cancer* 38: 83-91.

[336] Rousseau E, Ruchoux MM, Scaravilli F, Chapon F, Vinchon M, et al. (2003) CDKN2A, CDKN2B and p14ARF are frequently and differentially methylated in ependymal tumours. *Neuropathol. Appl. Neurobiol.* 29: 574-583.
[337] Muhlisch J, Bajanowski T, Rickert CH, Roggendorf W, Wurthwein G, et al. (2007) Frequent but borderline methylation of p16 (INK4a) and TIMP3 in medulloblastoma and sPNET revealed by quantitative analyses. *J. Neurooncol.* 83: 17-29.
[338] Carr-Wilkinson J, O'Toole K, Wood KM, Challen CC, Baker AG, et al. High Frequency of p53/MDM2/p14ARF Pathway Abnormalities in Relapsed Neuroblastoma. *Clin. Cancer Res.* 16: 1108-1118.
[339] Oh JH, Kim HS, Kim HH, Kim WH, Lee SH (2006) Aberrant methylation of p14ARF gene correlates with poor survival in osteosarcoma. *Clin. Orthop. Relat. Res.* 442: 216-222.
[340] Park SH, Jung KC, Ro JY, Kang GH, Khang SK (2000) 5' CpG island methylation of p16 is associated with absence of p16 expression in glioblastomas. *J. Korean Med. Sci.* 15: 555-559.
[341] Aktas S, Celebiler AC, Zadeoglulari Z, Diniz G, Kargi A, et al. (2009) Expression and Methylation Pattern of p16 in Neuroblastoma Tumorigenesis. *Pathol. Oncol. Res.*
[342] Shim YH, Park HJ, Choi MS, Kim JS, Kim H, et al. (2003) Hypermethylation of the p16 gene and lack of p16 expression in hepatoblastoma. *Mod. Pathol.* 16: 430-436.
[343] Tsuchiya T, Sekine K, Hinohara S, Namiki T, Nobori T, et al. (2000) Analysis of the p16INK4, p14ARF, p15, TP53, and MDM2 genes and their prognostic implications in osteosarcoma and Ewing sarcoma. *Cancer Genet. Cytogenet.* 120: 91-98.
[344] Hoebeeck J, Michels E, Pattyn F, Combaret V, Vermeulen J, et al. (2009) Aberrant methylation of candidate tumor suppressor genes in neuroblastoma. *Cancer Lett.* 273: 336-346.
[345] Lindsey JC, Lusher ME, Strathdee G, Brown R, Gilbertson RJ, et al. (2005) Epigenetic inactivation of MCJ (DNAJD1) in malignant paediatric brain tumours. *Int. J. Cancer.*
[346] Kopelovich L, Crowell JA, Fay JR (2003) The epigenome as a target for cancer chemoprevention. *J. Natl. Cancer Inst.* 95: 1747-1757.
[347] Balch C, Montgomery JS, Paik HI, Kim S, Kim S, et al. (2005) New anti-cancer strategies: epigenetic therapies and biomarkers. *Front Biosci.* 10: 1897-1931.
[348] Issa JP, Kantarjian H (2005) Azacitidine. *Nat. Rev. Drug Discov. Suppl*: S6-7.
[349] Lyko F, Brown R (2005) DNA methyltransferase inhibitors and the development of epigenetic cancer therapies. *J. Natl. Cancer Inst.* 97: 1498-1506.
[350] Weisenberger DJ, Velicescu M, Cheng JC, Gonzales FA, Liang G, et al. (2004) Role of the DNA methyltransferase variant DNMT3b3 in DNA methylation. *Mol.. Cancer Res.* 2: 62-72.
[351] Villar-Garea A, Fraga MF, Espada J, Esteller M (2003) Procaine is a DNA-demethylating agent with growth-inhibitory effects in human cancer cells. *Cancer Res.* 63: 4984-4989.
[352] Brueckner B, Garcia Boy R, Siedlecki P, Musch T, Kliem HC, et al. (2005) Epigenetic reactivation of tumor suppressor genes by a novel small-molecule inhibitor of human DNA methyltransferases. *Cancer Res.* 65: 6305-6311.
[353] Esteller M (2005) DNA methylation and cancer therapy: new developments and expectations. *Curr. Opin. Oncol.* 17: 55-60.

[354] Momparler RL, Bouchard J, Samson J (1985) Induction of differentiation and inhibition of DNA methylation in HL-60 myeloid leukemic cells by 5-AZA-2'-deoxycytidine. *Leuk Res.* 9: 1361-1366.

[355] Garcia-Manero G, Kantarjian HM, Sanchez-Gonzalez B, Yang H, Rosner G, et al. (2006) Phase 1/2 study of the combination of 5-aza-2'-deoxycytidine with valproic acid in patients with leukemia. *Blood* 108: 3271-3279.

[356] Kantarjian H, Oki Y, Garcia-Manero G, Huang X, O'Brien S, et al. (2007) Results of a randomized study of 3 schedules of low-dose decitabine in higher-risk myelodysplastic syndrome and chronic myelomonocytic leukemia. *Blood* 109: 52-57.

[357] Silverman LR, Demakos EP, Peterson BL, Kornblith AB, Holland JC, et al. (2002) Randomized controlled trial of azacitidine in patients with the myelodysplastic syndrome: a study of the cancer and leukemia group B. *J. Clin. Oncol.* 20: 2429-2440.

[358] Kantarjian H, Issa JP, Rosenfeld CS, Bennett JM, Albitar M, et al. (2006) Decitabine improves patient outcomes in myelodysplastic syndromes: results of a phase III randomized study. *Cancer* 106: 1794-1803.

[359] Kantarjian HM, O'Brien S, Cortes J, Giles FJ, Faderl S, et al. (2003) Results of decitabine (5-aza-2'deoxycytidine) therapy in 130 patients with chronic myelogenous leukemia. *Cancer* 98: 522-528.

[360] Issa JP, Garcia-Manero G, Giles FJ, Mannari R, Thomas D, et al. (2004) Phase 1 study of low-dose prolonged exposure schedules of the hypomethylating agent 5-aza-2'-deoxycytidine (decitabine) in hematopoietic malignancies. *Blood* 103: 1635-1640.

[361] Aparicio A, Eads CA, Leong LA, Laird PW, Newman EM, et al. (2003) Phase I trial of continuous infusion 5-aza-2'-deoxycytidine. *Cancer Chemother. Pharmacol.* 51: 231-239.

[362] Pohlmann P, DiLeone LP, Cancella AI, Caldas AP, Dal Lago L, et al. (2002) Phase II trial of cisplatin plus decitabine, a new DNA hypomethylating agent, in patients with advanced squamous cell carcinoma of the cervix. *Am. J. Clin. Oncol.* 25: 496-501.

[363] Wijermans P, Lubbert M, Verhoef G, Bosly A, Ravoet C, et al. (2000) Low-dose 5-aza-2'-deoxycytidine, a DNA hypomethylating agent, for the treatment of high-risk myelodysplastic syndrome: a multicenter phase II study in elderly patients. *J. Clin. Oncol.* 18: 956-962.

[364] Segura-Pacheco B, Trejo-Becerril C, Perez-Cardenas E, Taja-Chayeb L, Mariscal I, et al. (2003) Reactivation of tumor suppressor genes by the cardiovascular drugs hydralazine and procainamide and their potential use in cancer therapy. *Clin. Cancer Res.* 9: 1596-1603.

[365] Lin X, Asgari K, Putzi MJ, Gage WR, Yu X, et al. (2001) Reversal of GSTP1 CpG island hypermethylation and reactivation of pi-class glutathione S-transferase (GSTP1) expression in human prostate cancer cells by treatment with procainamide. *Cancer Res.* 61: 8611-8616.

[366] Dreyer ZE, Kadota RP, Stewart CF, Friedman HS, Mahoney DH, et al. (2003) Phase 2 study of idarubicin in pediatric brain tumors: Pediatric Oncology Group study POG 9237. *Neuro-oncol.* 5: 261-267.

[367] Plummer R, Vidal L, Griffin M, Lesley M, de Bono J, et al. (2009) Phase I study of MG98, an oligonucleotide antisense inhibitor of human DNA methyltransferase 1, given as a 7-day infusion in patients with advanced solid tumors. *Clin. Cancer Res.* 15: 3177-3183.

[368] Brueckner B, Boy RG, Siedlecki P, Musch T, Kliem HC, et al. (2005) Epigenetic reactivation of tumor suppressor genes by a novel small-molecule inhibitor of human DNA methyltransferases. *Cancer Res*. 65: 6305-6311.

[369] Bhalla KN (2005) Epigenetic and chromatin modifiers as targeted therapy of hematologic malignancies. *J. Clin. Oncol.* 23: 3971-3993.

[370] Bolden JE, Peart MJ, Johnstone RW (2006) Anticancer activities of histone deacetylase inhibitors. *Nat. Rev. Drug Discov.* 5: 769-784.

[371] Finnin MS, Donigian JR, Cohen A, Richon VM, Rifkind RA, et al. (1999) Structures of a histone deacetylase homologue bound to the TSA and SAHA inhibitors. *Nature* 401: 188-193.

[372] Vigushin DM, Coombes RC (2004) Targeted histone deacetylase inhibition for cancer therapy. *Curr. Cancer Drug Targets* 4: 205-218.

[373] Marks PA (2007) Discovery and development of SAHA as an anticancer agent. *Oncogene* 26: 1351-1356.

[374] Dokmanovic M, Clarke C, Marks PA (2007) Histone deacetylase inhibitors: overview and perspectives. *Mol. Cancer Res*. 5: 981-989.

[375] Einsiedel HG, Kawan L, Eckert C, Witt O, Fichtner I, et al. (2006) Histone deacetylase inhibitors have antitumor activity in two NOD/SCID mouse models of B-cell precursor childhood acute lymphoblastic leukemia. *Leukemia* 20: 1435-1436.

[376] Deubzer HE, Ehemann V, Kulozik AE, Westermann F, Savelyeva L, et al. (2008) Anti-neuroblastoma activity of Helminthosporium carbonum (HC)-toxin is superior to that of other differentiating compounds in vitro. *Cancer Lett.* 264: 21-28.

[377] Deubzer HE, Ehemann V, Westermann F, Heinrich R, Mechtersheimer G, et al. (2008) Histone deacetylase inhibitor Helminthosporium carbonum (HC)-toxin suppresses the malignant phenotype of neuroblastoma cells. *Int. J. Cancer* 122: 1891-1900.

[378] Jaboin J, Wild J, Hamidi H, Khanna C, Kim CJ, et al. (2002) MS-27-275, an inhibitor of histone deacetylase, has marked in vitro and in vivo antitumor activity against pediatric solid tumors. *Cancer Res*. 62: 6108-6115.

[379] Sonnemann J, Kumar KS, Heesch S, Muller C, Hartwig C, et al. (2006) Histone deacetylase inhibitors induce cell death and enhance the susceptibility to ionizing radiation, etoposide, and TRAIL in medulloblastoma cells. *Int. J. Oncol* 28: 755-766.

[380] Witt O, Monkemeyer S, Ronndahl G, Erdlenbruch B, Reinhardt D, et al. (2003) Induction of fetal hemoglobin expression by the histone deacetylase inhibitor apicidin. *Blood* 101: 2001-2007.

[381] Witt O, Schweigerer L, Driever PH, Wolff J, Pekrun A (2004) Valproic acid treatment of glioblastoma multiforme in a child. *Pediatr Blood Cancer* 43: 181.

[382] Bruserud O, Stapnes C, Ersvaer E, Gjertsen BT, Ryningen A (2007) Histone deacetylase inhibitors in cancer treatment: a review of the clinical toxicity and the modulation of gene expression in cancer cell. *Curr. Pharm. Biotechnol.* 8: 388-400.

[383] Masoudi A, Elopre M, Amini E, Nagel ME, Ater JL, et al. (2008) Influence of valproic acid on outcome of high-grade gliomas in children. *AntiCancer Res*. 28: 2437-2442.

[384] Wolff JE, Kramm C, Kortmann RD, Pietsch T, Rutkowski S, et al. (2008) Valproic acid was well tolerated in heavily pretreated pediatric patients with high-grade glioma. *J. Neurooncol.* 90: 309-314.

[385] Rosato RR, Almenara JA, Grant S (2003) The histone deacetylase inhibitor MS-275 promotes differentiation or apoptosis in human leukemia cells through a process

regulated by generation of reactive oxygen species and induction of p21CIP1/WAF1 1. *Cancer Res.* 63: 3637-3645.

[386] Gui CY, Ngo L, Xu WS, Richon VM, Marks PA (2004) Histone deacetylase (HDAC) inhibitor activation of p21WAF1 involves changes in promoter-associated proteins, including HDAC1. *Proc. Natl. Acad. Sci. USA* 101: 1241-1246.

[387] Archer SY, Meng S, Shei A, Hodin RA (1998) p21(WAF1) is required for butyrate-mediated growth inhibition of human colon cancer cells. *Proc. Natl. Acad. Sci. USA* 95: 6791-6796.

[388] Khan N, Jeffers M, Kumar S, Hackett C, Boldog F, et al. (2008) Determination of the class and isoform selectivity of small-molecule histone deacetylase inhibitors. *Biochem. J.* 409: 581-589.

[389] Khandelwal A, Gediya L, Njar V (2008) MS-275 synergistically enhances the growth inhibitory effects of RAMBA VN/66-1 in hormone-insensitive PC-3 prostate cancer cells and tumours. *Br. J. Cancer* 98: 1234-1243.

[390] Wu LP, Wang X, Li L, Zhao Y, Lu S, et al. (2008) Histone deacetylase inhibitor depsipeptide activates silenced genes through decreasing both CpG and H3K9 methylation on the promoter. *Mol. Cell Biol.* 28: 3219-3235.

[391] Jones LK, Saha V (2002) Chromatin modification, leukaemia and implications for therapy. *Br. J. Haematol* 118: 714-727.

[392] Garcia-Manero G, Assouline S, Cortes J, Estrov Z, Kantarjian H, et al. (2008) Phase 1 study of the oral isotype specific histone deacetylase inhibitor MGCD0103 in leukemia. *Blood* 112: 981-989.

[393] Krennhrubec K, Marshall BL, Hedglin M, Verdin E, Ulrich SM (2007) Design and evaluation of 'Linkerless' hydroxamic acids as selective HDAC8 inhibitors. *Bioorg Med Chem Lett.* 17: 2874-2878.

[394] Haggarty SJ, Koeller KM, Wong JC, Grozinger CM, Schreiber SL (2003) Domain-selective small-molecule inhibitor of histone deacetylase 6 (HDAC6)-mediated tubulin deacetylation. *Proc. Natl. Acad. Sci. USA* 100: 4389-4394.

[395] Shan B, Yao TP, Nguyen HT, Zhuo Y, Levy DR, et al. (2008) Requirement of HDAC6 for transforming growth factor-beta1-induced epithelial-mesenchymal transition. *J. Biol. Chem.* 283: 21065-21073.

[396] Itoh Y, Suzuki T, Kouketsu A, Suzuki N, Maeda S, et al. (2007) Design, synthesis, structure--selectivity relationship, and effect on human cancer cells of a novel series of histone deacetylase 6-selective inhibitors. *J. Med. Chem.* 50: 5425-5438.

[397] Zhang Y, Kwon S, Yamaguchi T, Cubizolles F, Rousseaux S, et al. (2008) Mice lacking histone deacetylase 6 have hyperacetylated tubulin but are viable and develop normally. *Mol. Cell Biol.* 28: 1688-1701.

[398] Mai A, Massa S, Pezzi R, Simeoni S, Rotili D, et al. (2005) Class II (IIa)-selective histone deacetylase inhibitors. 1. Synthesis and biological evaluation of novel (aryloxopropenyl)pyrrolyl hydroxyamides. *J. Med. Chem.* 48: 3344-3353.

[399] Jones P, Altamura S, De Francesco R, Paz OG, Kinzel O, et al. (2008) A novel series of potent and selective ketone histone deacetylase inhibitors with antitumor activity in vivo. *J. Med. Chem.* 51: 2350-2353.

[400] Cameron EE, Bachman KE, Myohanen S, Herman JG, Baylin SB (1999) Synergy of demethylation and histone deacetylase inhibition in the re-expression of genes silenced in cancer. *Nat. Genet.* 21: 103-107.

[401] Kelly WK, Richon VM, O'Connor O, Curley T, MacGregor-Curtelli B, et al. (2003) Phase I clinical trial of histone deacetylase inhibitor: suberoylanilide hydroxamic acid administered intravenously. *Clin. Cancer Res.* 9: 3578-3588.

[402] Blumenschein G, Lu G, Kies M, Glisson B, Papadimitrakopoulou V, et al. Phase II clinical trial of suberoylanilide hydroxamic acid (SAHA) in patients with recurrent and/or metastatic head and neck cancer(SCCHN); 2004 July 15.

[403] Prince HM, Bishton MJ, Harrison SJ (2009) Clinical studies of histone deacetylase inhibitors. *Clin. Cancer Res.* 15: 3958-3969.

[404] Ryan QC, Headlee D, Acharya M, Sparreboom A, Trepel JB, et al. (2005) Phase I and pharmacokinetic study of MS-275, a histone deacetylase inhibitor, in patients with advanced and refractory solid tumors or lymphoma. *J. Clin. Oncol.* 23: 3912-3922.

[405] Kraker AJ, Mizzen CA, Hartl BG, Miin J, Allis CD, et al. (2003) Modulation of histone acetylation by [4-(acetylamino)-N-(2-amino-phenyl) benzamide] in HCT-8 colon carcinoma. *Mol. Cancer Ther.* 2: 401-408.

[406] Pauer LR, Olivares J, Cunningham C, Williams A, Grove W, et al. (2004) Phase I study of oral CI-994 in combination with carboplatin and paclitaxel in the treatment of patients with advanced solid tumors. *Cancer Invest.* 22: 886-896.

[407] Prakash S, Foster BJ, Meyer M, Wozniak A, Heilbrun LK, et al. (2001) Chronic oral administration of CI-994: a phase 1 study. *Invest New Drugs* 19: 1-11.

[408] Varambally S, Dhanasekaran SM, Zhou M, Barrette TR, Kumar-Sinha C, et al. (2002) The polycomb group protein EZH2 is involved in progression of prostate cancer. *Nature* 419: 624-629.

[409] Piekarz RL, Robey R, Sandor V, Bakke S, Wilson WH, et al. (2001) Inhibitor of histone deacetylation, depsipeptide (FR901228), in the treatment of peripheral and cutaneous T-cell lymphoma: a case report. *Blood* 98: 2865-2868.

[410] Byrd JC, Marcucci G, Parthun MR, Xiao JJ, Klisovic RB, et al. (2005) A phase 1 and pharmacodynamic study of depsipeptide (FK228) in chronic lymphocytic leukemia and acute myeloid leukemia. *Blood* 105: 959-967.

[411] Chavez-Blanco A, Segura-Pacheco B, Perez-Cardenas E, Taja-Chayeb L, Cetina L, et al. (2005) Histone acetylation and histone deacetylase activity of magnesium valproate in tumor and peripheral blood of patients with cervical cancer. A phase I study. *Mol. Cancer* 4: 22.

[412] Oberndorfer S, Piribauer M, Marosi C, Lahrmann H, Hitzenberger P, et al. (2005) P450 enzyme inducing and non-enzyme inducing antiepileptics in glioblastoma patients treated with standard chemotherapy. *J. Neurooncol.* 72: 255-260.

[413] Kramer OH, Zhu P, Ostendorff HP, Golebiewski M, Tiefenbach J, et al. (2003) The histone deacetylase inhibitor valproic acid selectively induces proteasomal degradation of HDAC2. *Embo J.* 22: 3411-3420.

[414] Gottlicher M, Minucci S, Zhu P, Kramer OH, Schimpf A, et al. (2001) Valproic acid defines a novel class of HDAC inhibitors inducing differentiation of transformed cells. *Embo J.* 20: 6969-6978.

[415] Hurtubise A, Bernstein ML, Momparler RL (2008) Preclinical evaluation of the antineoplastic action of 5-aza-2'-deoxycytidine and different histone deacetylase inhibitors on human Ewing's sarcoma cells. *Cancer Cell Int.* 8: 16.
[416] Svechnikova I, Almqvist PM, Ekstrom TJ (2008) HDAC inhibitors effectively induce cell type-specific differentiation in human glioblastoma cell lines of different origin. *Int. J. Oncol.* 32: 821-827.

In: Field Cancerization: Basic Science and Clinical Applications ISBN 978-1-61761-006-6
Editor: Gabriel D. Dakubo

Chapter 24

Epigenetics in Hematological Malignancies

Ulrich Lehmann

Abstract

Epigenetic alterations are now recognized as important as genetic defects in the development and progression of hematological malignancies. Because the aberrant DNA methylation of growth-regulatory genes in lymphoid malignancies and leukemia is well described in several excellent up-to-date reviews, this contribution will focus on; i) aberrant DNA methylation in chronic myeloproliferative diseases (CMPD), ii) aberrant reduction of DNA methylation (DNA hypomethylation), and iii) altered methylation patterns in imprinted genes. The principal reversibility of epigenetic mechanisms makes them also an attractive target for pharmacological intervention.

Keywords: DNA methylation, hypomethylation, chronic myeloproliferative disease (CMPD), imprinting, myelodysplastic syndromes (MDS).

24.1. Introduction

In 2004, we were invited to review epigenetic alterations in hematological malignancies [1]. At that time, it was not possible to provide a comprehensive coverage of the primary literature about DNA methylation aberrations in lymphoid malignancies and leukemia. Since then, the field of "epigenetics" has literally exploded and expanded with such a speed in many directions that it is now difficult to keep track of all relevant reviews dealing with epigenetic alterations in human malignancies. This development is fueled to a great deal by technological innovations [2]. Therefore, this contribution does not attempt to be a comprehensive coverage of the primary literature, which is no longer possible, but tries to outline the concepts and focuses on several topics that are clearly underrepresented in the literature (see below). In addition, throughout the chapter, methodological developments and technical difficulties will be discussed, because the literature about epigenetic alterations in human malignancies is marred by not only a few methodologically flawed publications. Since the aberrant hypermethylation of tumor suppressor genes and other regulatory genes, which antagonize the development and progression of hematological malignancies is well described for lymphomas and leukemia in several excellent reviews (for example: [3,4]), this contribution will focus on the following issues, which are underrepresented in the literature; i) aberrant hypermethylation in chronic myeloproliferative diseases (CMPD), ii) DNA hypomethylation, and iii) altered methylation patterns in imprinted genes

24.2. Definition of Epigenetics

The term epigenetics was originally coined by Conrad Waddington nearly 70 years ago in describing the developmental processes of an organism (ontogeny) [5,6]. Since then this word has been used in quiet different contexts with slightly or clearly different meanings. A common theme of all usages or definitions is that epigenetic mechanisms and phenomena are not reflected in the primary genetic material (i.e., the DNA or RNA sequence of the genome of a given organism). They are somehow "beyond" or "around" genomics. In this chapter we follow the most recent definition put forward by Berger et al. in 2009 [7]: "An epigenetic trait is a stably heritable phenotype resulting from changes in a chromosome without alterations in the DNA sequence." This definition can involve the heritability of a phenotype, passed on through either mitosis or meiosis. It has to be pointed out that most of the epigenetic mechanisms and phenomena described in the literature are heritable through mitosis, whereas heritability through meiosis, that means transgenerational inheritance, has not been proven for most phenomena, especially for higher multicellular organisms. The complicated topic of transgenerational epigenetic effects have been recently reviewed elsewhere [8].

24.3. Epigenetic Systems

In a very good 2002 review by Adrian Bird, it was stated that only two molecular mechanisms are *bona fide* epigenetic mechanisms: DNA methylation and Polycomb/trithorax protein complexes [9]. Histone modifications and non-coding RNAs are the next best candidates for epigenetic mechanisms. Because the heritability of histone modifications is still not yet proven under many circumstances, "the term "epigenetics" is not always a correct term to define histone modifications" [7]. Whether the expression of non-protein coding RNAs (e.g., microRNAs, long ncRNA) define stably inherited mRNA expression patterns has to be shown in the future. A just emerging and far from comprehensively explored epigenetic mechanism is the internal compartmentalization of the nucleus into so called "chromosomal territories" [10]. It is now clear that the transcriptional activity of a genomic locus depends also on it's localization inside the nucleus. This implies that architectural rearrangements of chromosomes can modify gene expression patterns and that perturbations of these delicate mechanisms may lead to cancer development [11]. However, the analysis of chromosomal territories is technically very challenging and notoriously difficult, especially in small clinical specimens. Several components of Poylcomb complexes turned out to have histone modifying enzymatic activity (for overview: [12]). Therefore, the classification and definition of "epigenetic systems" is still an ongoing endeavor.

24.4. DNA Methylation – Some Basic Facts

DNA methylation in higher eukaryotes affects only the base cytosine, which becomes covalently modified at the carbon atom number 5. This modification takes place only when the cytosine is followed by a guanine base (CpG methylation). Methylated cytosine is a target for point mutations because deamination of 5'-methyl-cytosine leads to the formation of the naturally occurring DNA base thymidine, which cannot be recognized as mutated by the DNA repair machinery of the cell. Because deamination is constantly taking place under physiological conditions, albeit at a low frequency, there is a selective pressure to reduce the number of methylated cytosine bases throughout the genome, leading to a significant underrepresentation of the dinucleotide CpG in the human genome. Since active transcription seems to protect against DNA methylation [13], only the physiologically unmethylated CpG sites in the promoter region and first exons of transcribed genes remain unaltered. These mostly unmethylated CpG-rich stretches of DNA form the so-called "CpG islands" in the "sea" of the CpG depleted genome. These CpG islands comprise 1-2% of the genome and are characterized by an overall CG-content of more than 55% and an approximately five times more frequent occurrence of the dinucleotide CpG [14,15,16].

DNA methylation leads in concert to histone modification, namely histone deacetylation, to the formation of a dense, more compact chromatin structure, which reduces the accessibility of promoter regions for the basal transcription machinery and accessory factors, thereby inhibiting gene expression.

A few studies have reported the identification of non-CpG methylation in human cells [17,18,19,20,21]. Until very recently, these reports remained a bit isolated in the literature, not followed-up or confirmed by other groups. However, the first nearly complete DNA methylation map of a human cell with single nucleotide resolution accomplished by high throughput next-generation sequencing technology provides strong evidence for frequent non-CpG methylation in embryonic stem cells and induced pluripotent cells [22]. Because tumor cells recapitulate many features of stem cells and many human malignancies might be driven by so-called cancer stem cells [23], it is reasonable to expect the identification of frequent non-CpG methylation in tumor cells in the near future.

24.5. Methodology Matters

In 2007 Capel et al. [24] published a very interesting and important study about the relationship between *MLH1* promoter methylation and gene expression and a survey of the literature dealing with this question. In accordance with an earlier study by Deng et al. [25] they found out that only methylation of the proximal promoter correlated with reduction or absence of *MLH1* expression and that several samples with an intact mismatch repair system were found to be methylated in the distal promoter. This clearly demonstrates that many methylation events easily picked up by methylation–specific PCR might be of no functional relevance. Astonishingly, ~ 60% of all studies appearing after the publication of Deng et al. and surveyed by Capel et al. used primers amplifying the distal promoter region. An unknown percentage of samples in all these studies scored as "methylated" will have an unmethylated proximal promoter and will show uncompromised mismatch repair capability. Therefore, the true prevalence of epigenetic inactivation of *MLH1* in human malignancies by aberrant DNA methylation cannot be derived from the literature. Despite the fact that aberrant *MLH1* methylation is quite a rare event in hematological malignancies, this example serves as a general warning for the above mentioned inaccuracies of some data in the DNA methylation literature from methodologically flawed publications.

In the context of hematological malignancies, the question of which region of the SOCS-1 gene has to be analyzed is still under discussion. Several studies reporting frequent methylation of *SOCS-1* in CMPDs [26,27,28] analyzed the CpG islands spanning intron 1 and exon 2. By contrast, Fourouclas et al. found no evidence for *SOCS-1* promoter methylation in 68 samples from CMPD patients whereas 53% of their controls displayed *SOCS-1* exon 2 methylation [29]. These results are in accordance with earlier studies showing aberrant *SOCS-1* exon 2 methylation in a high proportion of control samples [30,31]. For more details, see the section below about aberrant hypermethylation in CMPD.

Another topic still under discussion is the choice of detection methodology. Liu et al., for example, reported high frequency (77%) of aberrant *PTEN* methylation in juvenile myelomonocytic leukemia (JMML) using conventional non-quantitative methylation-specific PCR [32]. Analyzing a really large cohort of this rare entity (n = 90) with semi-quantitative DHPLC, Batz et al. challenged this report by finding no methylation at all in three regions within the 1 kbp CpG islands spanning the *PTEN* promoter in their JMML cohort [33]. Most probably, the very sensitive, non-quantitative methylation-specific PCR is exaggerating spurious methylation events representing biological background.

Many DNA methylation studies rely on the use of fresh-frozen specimens. However, under many circumstances such specimens are not available. In addition, the archives of institutes of pathology around the world contain millions of formalin-fixed and paraffin-embedded (FFPE) blocks with detailed documentation of histopathological diagnosis and clinical data. This represents an invaluable treasure trove for retrospective molecular studies.[34] Also, in prospective trials, often only FFPE material is preserved, because many subtle morphological differences are only detectable in appropriately stained FFPE sections and these specimens can easily be exchanged between participating institutions. Several years ago we showed for selected loci that quantitative methylation analysis can be performed reliably with DNA extracted from tissue biopsies stored as FFPE blocks [35,36]. More recently, Killian et al. demonstrated in a very important and well-performed study the suitability of using archival lymphoid tissue for large-scale, comprehensive quantitative methylation studies [37]. The analysis of 1505 CpG sites in 20 paired fresh-frozen and FFPE specimens revealed correlation coefficients between 0.95 and 0.99.

Methodological advances in the field of high-content microarrays and massive parallel sequencing technologies brought the possibility of a genome-wide study of the human methylome in large series of patient samples much closer to reality [2,38]. However, today the costs and the efforts required, especially concerning data analysis, are still restricting these endeavors to the analysis of a few samples, and to highly specialized centers.

Nevertheless, the first large-scale studies of the methylation pattern in various cell-types revealed interesting new insights.

Using the bead-based platform from Illumina [39], which measures the methylation level of ~1500 individual CpG sites selected from about 800 cancer-associated genes, Martin-Subero et al. analyzed 83 mature aggressive B-cell non-Hodgkin lymphoma (maB-NHL) comprised of several subtypes [40]. The authors identified 56 genes methylated *de novo* in all lymphoma subtypes. This group of genes was significantly enriched for polycomb targets in embryonic stem cells. From this finding, the authors concluded that maB-NHL originates from cells with stem cell features or that stemness was acquired during lymphomagensis by epigenetic remodeling. Continuing with this project, the authors analyzed 367 hematological malignancies (comprising 16 of the most representative B-cell, T-cell, and myeloid neoplasias) using the same methodology [41]. Hypermethylation of six genes (*DBC1, DIO3, FZD9, HS3ST2, MOS*, and *MYOD1*) was found in all entities indicating an important role of methylation of these genes in the development of different hematological neoplasias. Employing the same methodology Jiang et al. analyzed DNA methylation patterns in 184 patients with MDS or AML and compared the methylation data with the karyotypes of the patients assessed by high-density single nucleotide polymorphism arrays [42]. The results indicate that aberrant DNA methylation can cooperate with deletions in the silencing of tumor suppressor genes (TSG).

The ubiquity, extent, and correlation with disease progression of DNA methylation aberrations led the authors to the conclusion that this is a dominant mechanism for TSG silencing and clonal variation in progression from MDS to AML. Utilizing a completely different, more comprehensive methodology for a genome-wide survey of DNA methylation patterns (the so called "HELP assay" [43]), Figueroa et al. analyzed bone marrow samples from 14 patients with MDS, secondary AML or CMML and from 15 patients with *de novo* AML [44].

As a control 8 CD34+ bone marrow fractions from healthy controls were analyzed. Because CD34-sorted samples are available only from quite a small subset of samples, the authors compared in a first step the DNA methylation profile of CD34+ sorted versus CD34- bone marrow cells from 3 patients and 4 healthy controls. They found a very good correlation of the methylation levels measured between the two fractions from every patient and control ($r < 0.95$) and an intraindividual variability, which is much lower than the interindividual variability.

The same group compared AML samples with a mutated CCAAT/enhancer binding protein alpha (CEBPA) locus versus samples with an epigenetically silenced CEBPA locus using the already mentioned HELP assay [45]. Silencing of the CEBPA locus by DNA methylation was associated with the presence of an aberrant DNA hypermethylation signature, which was not present in the CEBPA mutant group. This former subgroup showed a markedly worse treatment response than the CEBPA mutant group and might represent a new candidate group for epigenetic therapy (see below).

A completely different approach for the genome-wide screening for epigenetically regulated genes is the treatment of cell lines with demethylating agents and/or inhibitors of histone modifying enzymes and the subsequent search for differentially expressed genes employing microarray technology. This approach has recently been reviewed elsewhere [46].

24.6. DNA Hypomethylation

It is now firmly established that loss of DNA methylation is as widespread and important as aberrant gain of DNA methylation in the development and progression of human malignancies [47]. However, despite the fact that hypomethylation in human tumor cells was described well before single-copy gene hypermethylation was discovered [48,49], it is much less thoroughly examined. There are two main reasons for this imbalance: Firstly, reduction of a signal (i.e., loss of methylation) is methodologically under many circumstances much more difficult to assess reliably in comparison to measuring a signal that arises *de novo* (such as aberrant hypermethylation of a specific locus). Secondly, the direct primary functional consequences of hypomethylation are not as clearly defined as the primary consequence of hypermethylation, i.e., loss of expression of the affected gene. In addition, the majority of studies that analyze gene-specific or global hypomethylation are focused on solid tumors [50,51].

The list of loci affected by hypomethylation in hematological malignancies presented in Table 24-1 contains also several somewhat older studies not mentioned in the text. In these studies the methylation status of single or multiple CpG dinucleotides was analyzed by using methylation-sensitive restriction enzymes followed by Southern blotting or PCR, a method with limited sensitivity and low resolution.

In addition to the ectopic expression of hypomethylated single-copy genes, hypomethylation contributed to the development of chromosomal instability [62], which subsequently led to the development of aggressive T cell lymphomas in a mouse model [63]. Bollati et al. employed quantitative high-resolution pyrosequencing to assess for the first time the methylation status of LINE-1, Alu, and Sat-alpha sequences in multiple myeloma [54]. They found a statistically significant decrease by 5 – 10 percentage points for these repetitive elements, which correlated somewhat paradoxically with an increase in DNMT1 mRNA expression. This increase in DNMT1 expression might reflect increased proliferation rate accompanied by disturbance of the DNA methylation machinery in the myeloma cells. In chronic myeloid leukemia, Roman-Gomez et al. also found a positive correlation between mRNA expression of DNMT3b4 and hypomethylation of LINE-1 sequences [55].

Table 24.1. Hypomethylation in hematological malignancies

DNA	Disease	Reference
LINE-1	B-CLL	[52,53]
LINE-1/Alu/Sat-alpha	MM	[54]
LINE-1	CML	[55]
Bcl-2	B-CLL	[56]
MDR1	AML	[57]
TCL1	B-Lymphoma	[58]
c-Myc	sec. AML	[59]
MPO	APL	[60]
ODC	CLL	[61]

This study also showed that in CML, LINE-1 hypomethylation correlates with disease progression and poorer prognosis, a result confirmed in a follow-up study by the same group in the analysis of other repetitive sequence elements in the human genome [64]. The correlation between hypomethylation and disease progression as well as poorer prognosis in CML is in direct contrast to the situation described in acute lymphoblastic leukemia. In this lymphoid malignancy, hypomethylation is a highly significant indicator of good prognosis, and it is even able to define a very low-risk ALL subgroup among CpG island methylator phenotype ("CIMP") negative patients [65]. These findings highlight the cell-type and disease entity-specific effects of aberrant DNA methylation.

A very interesting link between chromatin remodeling, DNA hypomethylation, and development of malignancy was described by Fan et al. [66]. Observing the occurrence of erythroleukemia in Lsh(-/-) mice, the authors analyzed the DNA methylation status in leukemic cells of these animals. They found widespread hypomethylation of repetitive sequences and specific retroviral elements within the PU.1 gene, accompanied by increased expression of *PU.1*.

24.7. Global Hypermethylation

The now firmly established textbook schema describes gene-specific hypermethylation in the context of global hypomethylation for cancer cells. However, analyzing a large series of bone marrow samples from patients with myelodysplastic syndromes (MDS), Römermann et al. [67] found unexpectedly high global DNA methylation level, instead of a decrease, which is well described for solid tumors [68] and selected haematological malignancies [54,55]. This increase was confirmed by three independent methods and correlated highly significantly with the risk score according to the International Prognostic Scoring System (IPSS), the blast count and the karyotype ("good, intermediate, and poor").

24.8. Aberrant Hypermethylation in Chronic Myeloproliferative Diseases

In 2005 several publications reported more or less in parallel, a new genetic defect in CMPD. A point mutation in the tyrosine kinase JAK2 (at codon 617) turned out to be a frequent event in CMPDs and has revolutionized since then the understanding and molecular diagnosis of CMPDs [69]. The excitement about the discovery of this point mutation, which caused a real flood of publications, is in part due to the fact that the etiology of CMPDs and underlying molecular defects were largely unknown before (and are still not completely resolved). Interestingly, epigenetic aberrations are not very well investigated in CMPDs. In contrast to lymphoid malignancies or overt leukemia, which are already quite well characterized on the epigenetic level, CMPDs are still clearly underrepresented in the epigenetic literature. This is especially true for the "non-CML-CMPDs" such as polycythemia vera, primary myelofibrosis, and essential thrombocythemia. Only a few studies focusing on a handful of genes are published.

Since JAK-2 kinase belongs to the JAK/STAT signaling pathway, most interest focused on the DNA methylation analysis of other components of this pathway, namely *SOCS-1*, *SOCS-2*, and *SOCS-3* [26,27,28,29,70], with somewhat contradicting results. This might primarily be due to methodological reasons (see section on "Methodology matters" and discussion in [29]). Overall, the frequencies of aberrant gene methylation reported in the literature are quite low for most genes studied so far. Only frequent hypermethylation of the *SOCS-3* (30 – 50%) and concomitant transcriptional down-regulation seems to be confirmed by two independent groups in a sufficient number of cases (50 and 112, respectively) without a publication reporting contradicting results [27,29]. The high frequency of RARβ2 gene methylation (16 out of 18 cases analyzed) reported by Jones et al. [71] could not be confirmed by Jost et al. [26].

Table 24-2 lists the genes for which the presence or absence of aberrant DNA methylation has been reported in CMPD. The frequent listing of genes in the upper (presence of methylation) and the lower (absence of methylation) parts of the table gives a first impression of the contradictions present in the literature. The majority of studies employed conventional non-quantitative methylation-specific PCR (MSP) and scored samples as "methylated" if a band was detected employing primers assumed to be specific for methylated DNA. It is very difficult to compare results obtained by this method from different laboratories even if identical primer pairs are used, because the sensitivity of this method depends on the amount of DNA input, the precise reaction conditions, the efficiency of the enzyme used, the cycle number, the performance of the thermocycler among other factors.

Table 24.2. DNA methylation in chronic myeloproliferative disease

Presence of aberrant DNA methylation reported	
Gene	Reference
ABL1	[73]
Calcitonin	[74]
CXCR4	[75]
DAPK	[26]
E-Cadherin	[26]
MGMT	[26]
NPM1	[76]
p14	[77]
p15	[26] [77] [78]
p16	[26] [78]
p73	[26]
PRV-1	[79]
PTPN6	[27]
RARβ2	[71]
SOCS-1	[26] [27,28]
SOCS-2	[70]
SOCS-3	[27] [28]
TIMP-2	[26]

Absence of aberrant DNA methylation reported	
Gene	Reference
APC	[77]
DAPK	[77]
hMLH1	[26] [77]
hMSH2	[77]
p16	[77]
RASSF1A	[26]
RARβ2	[26]
Rb	[77]
SHP-1	[26]
SOCS-1	[29]
SOCS-2	[28]
TGFbeta1RII	[76] [80]
TIMP-3	[26]

Referring to the first description of MSP by Herman et al. in 1996 [72], it is often stated that MSP has a sensitivity of 1 in 1000 [26]. This is clearly an oversimplification. In addition, different primer pairs will contribute to an even greater variability of the detection sensitivity and, as explained above, not all regions in a gene of interest are equally informative for methylation studies. Also the sample type used for methylation analyses varies between different studies (e.g., peripheral blood versus bone marrow, whole bone marrow versus CD34+ sorted bone marrow, whole peripheral blood versus mononuclear cells or granulocytes etc.). Therefore, Table 24-2 can serve only as a first overview for those planning to study DNA methylation in CMPDs.

24.9. Imprinting and Hematological Malignancies

In humans, all autosomal (i.e., not on a sex chromosomes) genes are expressed from the maternal and the paternal alleles (bi-allelic expression). However, this does not hold true for a small group of genes (a few hundred out of ~25,000), which display parent-of-origin specific monoallelic expression. This phenomenon is termed "imprinting" (see [81] for an excellent general introduction). Genomic imprinting is for several reasons an intellectually and methodologically challenging phenomenon. It raises the question of why a silencing mechanism evolved in diploid organisms that renders a small fraction of the genome "pseudo-haploid". Intriguingly, many imprinted genes code for factors regulating embryonic and neonatal growth, implying a specific role in mammalian reproduction. In studying imprinted genes, one faces the problem that this is a very tissue- and cell-type-specific phenomenon, and that the monoallelic expression is not always maintained 100% in different cell types. For many genes healthy controls show quite a lot of variability regarding the extent of "monoallelic expression", which might be recorded adequately only if analyzing a sufficient number of control individuals (see below). A cell-type-specific analysis is mandatory, the results from one organ cannot be assigned to another organ, and quantitative measurements and threshold definitions ("how skewed is monoallelic?") have to be applied. This might explain some confusions and contradictory results presented in the literature (see below).

The physiological imprinting pattern can be lost ("loss of imprinting", LOI) in cancer by several mechanisms: microdeletion of the imprinting control region (ICR, [82]), hypomethylation of promoter or control regions [83], biallelic methylation [84], or uniparental disomy (UPD, [85]).

In the context of disease, and especially neoplasia, the most thoroughly studied imprinted region in the human genome is the *IGF2/H19* locus on chromosome 11p15.5 [86]. For several solid tumors, loss of imprinting of *IGF-2* (i.e. biallelic expression) has been described [87,88,89,90,91,92,93,94,95]. In fact, it turned out to be one of the most frequent molecular alterations in cancer [91,96]. However, the functional consequences of *IGF-2* biallelic expression in terms of quantitative mRNA levels have been addressed only in a few studies using different methodologies and reporting conflicting results [88,90,97,98,99]. In some instances biallelic *IGF-2* expression is accompanied by reduced or absent *H19* expression [97], while in others *H19* expression is completely independent of *IGF-2* dysregulation [88,90]. Concerning the expression level and the imprinting status of these two genes in normal and malignant hematopoiesis, only a few studies have been reported in the literature [98,100,101,102,103,104,105] with contradictory results. Bone marrow samples from healthy controls were analyzed by only three groups, each with a small sample size [98,102,104]. Exclusive monoallelic [104] or exclusive biallelic [102,106] expression has been reported. These contradictory results led to divergent conclusions concerning alterations of the imprinting status during normal hematopoiesis (bone marrow versus peripheral blood [98,100,102,105]) and during leukemogenesis (normal versus leukemic samples and incipient or stable disease versus progression) [98,102,103,107]. Analyzing a large series of peripheral blood samples from healthy controls (n = 98), Tessema et al. could confirm the strict monoallelic expression of *H19* in all informative samples [108]. However, *IGF-2* showed a heterogeneous pattern with mono- and bi-allelic expression in the control series. This makes any conclusion about the association of biallelic *IGF2* expression with development or progression of disease (as put forward by e.g., Randhawa et al. [107]) difficult. It also demonstrates the necessity to analyze a sufficiently large series of control samples because if only a few controls are analyzed the impression of strict monoallelic expression could be produced, leading to false conclusions about loss of imprinting in the course of disease.

More recently, the "paternally expressed gene 10" (PEG10) from the imprinted locus on chromosome 7q21 was shown to be strongly overexpressed in high-risk B-CLL. However, this overexpression is obviously not linked to loss of monoallelic expression or altered methylation patterns [109], indicating that perhaps imprinting-independent mechanisms might lead to deregulation of imprinted genes.

24.10. Therapeutic and Diagnostic Potential

The potential reversibility of epigenetic alterations makes them conceptually an attractive target for pharmacological intervention. The first FDA approved "epigenetic drugs" are Decitabine (aza-deoxycytidine) and Vidaza (aza-cytidine) for the treatment of high risk myelodysplastic syndromes and acute myelogenous leukemia [124]. Both substances are inhibitors of DNA methyltransferases, which lead to successive reduction of DNA methylation levels by inhibition of methylation of newly synthesized DNA strands during replication.

Table 24.3. Examples for hypermethylation events associated with poor prognosis

Gene	Disease	Reference
$p15^{INK4b}$	acute leukemia	[110]
$p15^{INK4b}$	APL	[111]
$p16^{INK4a}$	MM	[112]
p21	ALL	[113]
CDH1	MDS, sec. AML	[114]
DKK1	AML	[115]
HOXA4/HOXA5	CML	[116]
lamin A/C	B-DLCL	[117]
MEG3	AML	[118]
MGMT	B-DLCL	[119]
miR-124a	ALL	[120]
RIL	MDS	[121]
SOCS-1	MDS	[122]
WNT5A	ALL	[123]

ALL: acute lymphoblastic leukemia; APL: acute promylemonocytic leukemia; MM: multiple myeloma; B-DLCL: diffuse large B-cell lymphoma; MDS: myelodysplastic syndromes.

The total lack of sequence specificity, the induction of malignancy by reducing methylation levels in a mouse model [63] and cytotoxic side-effects are the major reasons for concern using these drugs. However, encouraging results have been reported, especially using low-dose therapy regiments [125,126]. These demethylating agents have also been combined with histone-deacetylase inhibitors in order to increase clinical efficacy due to molecular synergy [127]. The detailed discussion of the different clinical trials (dose, time intervals, combination therapy, selection of patients, monitoring of therapy etc.) is beyond the scope of this chapter. Therefore, the interested reader is referred to several excellent up-to-date reviews [128,129,130]. Also the adequate discussion of the diagnostic and prognostic potential of the detection of epigenetic aberrations in hematological malignancies would require an additional chapter. Table 24-3 gives several examples for hypermethylation events reported to be associated with poor prognosis as a starting point for the interested reader.

References

[1] Lehmann U, Brakensiek K, Kreipe H (2004) Role of epigenetic changes in hematological malignancies. *Ann. Hematol.* 83: 137-152.

[2] Estecio MR, Issa JP (2009) Tackling the methylome: recent methodological advances in genome-wide methylation profiling. *Genome Med.* 1: 106.

[3] Boultwood J, Wainscoat JS (2007) Gene silencing by DNA methylation in haematological malignancies. *Br. J. Haematol.* 138: 3-11.
[4] Iacobuzio-Donahue CA (2008) Epigenetic Changes in Cancer. *Annu. Rev. Pathol.*
[5] Lederberg J (2001) The meaning of Epigenetics. *The Scientist* 15: 6.
[6] Holliday R (2006) Epigenetics: a historical overview. *Epigenetics* 1: 76-80.
[7] Berger SL, Kouzarides T, Shiekhattar R, Shilatifard A (2009) An operational definition of epigenetics. Genes. Dev. 23: 781-783.
[8] Youngson NA, Whitelaw E (2008) Transgenerational epigenetic effects. *Annu. Rev. Genomics Hum Genet* 9: 233-257.
[9] Bird A (2002) DNA methylation patterns and epigenetic memory. *Genes. Dev.* 16: 6-21.
[10] Cremer T, Cremer M, Dietzel S, Muller S, Solovei I, et al. (2006) Chromosome territories--a functional nuclear landscape. *Curr. Opin. Cell Biol.* 18: 307-316.
[11] Lever E, Sheer D The role of nuclear organization in cancer. *J. Pathol.* 220: 114-125.
[12] Gieni RS, Hendzel MJ (2009) Polycomb group protein gene silencing, non-coding RNA, stem cells, and cancer. *Biochem. Cell Biol.* 87: 711-746.
[13] Clark SJ, Melki J (2002) DNA methylation and gene silencing in cancer: which is the guilty party? *Oncogene* 21: 5380-5387.
[14] Bird AP (1986) CpG-rich islands and the function of DNA methylation. *Nature* 321: 209-213.
[15] Gardiner-Garden M, Frommer M (1987) CpG islands in vertebrate genomes. *J. Mol. Biol.* 196: 261-282.
[16] Takai D, Jones PA (2002) Comprehensive analysis of CpG islands in human chromosomes 21 and 22. *Proc. Natl. Acad. Sci. USA* 99: 3740-3745.
[17] Clark SJ, Harrison J, Frommer M (1995) CpNpG methylation in mammalian cells. *Nat. Genet.* 10: 20-27.
[18] Ramsahoye BH, Biniszkiewicz D, Lyko F, Clark V, Bird AP, et al. (2000) Non-CpG methylation is prevalent in embryonic stem cells and may be mediated by DNA methyltransferase 3a. *Proc. Natl. Acad. Sci. USA* 97: 5237-5242.
[19] Malone CS, Miner MD, Doerr JR, Jackson JP, Jacobsen SE, et al. (2001) CmC(A/T)GG DNA methylation in mature B cell lymphoma gene silencing. *Proc. Natl. Acad. Sci. USA* 98: 10404-10409.
[20] White GP, Watt PM, Holt BJ, Holt PG (2002) Differential patterns of methylation of the IFN-gamma promoter at CpG and non-CpG sites underlie differences in IFN-gamma gene expression between human neonatal and adult CD45RO- T cells. *J. Immunol.* 168: 2820-2827.
[21] Agirre X, Vizmanos JL, Calasanz MJ, Garcia-Delgado M, Larrayoz MJ, et al. (2003) Methylation of CpG dinucleotides and/or CCWGG motifs at the promoter of TP53 correlates with decreased gene expression in a subset of acute lymphoblastic leukemia patients. *Oncogene* 22: 1070-1072.
[22] Lister R, Pelizzola M, Dowen RH, Hawkins RD, Hon G, et al. (2009) Human DNA methylomes at base resolution show widespread epigenomic differences. *Nature* 462: 315-322.
[23] Maenhaut C, Dumont JE, Roger P, van Staveren WC (2009) Cancer Stem Cells : A Reality, A Myth, A Fuzzy Concept or A Misnomer ? An Analysis. *Carcinogenesis.*

[24] Capel E, Flejou JF, Hamelin R (2007) Assessment of MLH1 promoter methylation in relation to gene expression requires specific analysis. *Oncogene* 26: 7596-7600.

[25] Deng G, Chen A, Hong J, Chae HS, Kim YS (1999) Methylation of CpG in a small region of the hMLH1 promoter invariably correlates with the absence of gene expression. *Cancer Res.* 59: 2029-2033.

[26] Jost E, do ON, Dahl E, Maintz CE, Jousten P, et al. (2007) Epigenetic alterations complement mutation of JAK2 tyrosine kinase in patients with BCR/ABL-negative myeloproliferative disorders. *Leukemia* 21: 505-510.

[27] Capello D, Deambrogi C, Rossi D, Lischetti T, Piranda D, et al. (2008) Epigenetic inactivation of suppressors of cytokine signalling in Philadelphia-negative chronic myeloproliferative disorders. *Br. J. Haematol.* 141: 504-511.

[28] Teofili L, Martini M, Cenci T, Guidi F, Torti L, et al. (2008) Epigenetic alteration of SOCS family members is a possible pathogenetic mechanism in JAK2 wild type myeloproliferative diseases. *Int. J. Cancer* 123: 1586-1592.

[29] Fourouclas N, Li J, Gilby DC, Campbell PJ, Beer PA, et al. (2008) Methylation of the suppressor of cytokine signaling 3 gene (SOCS3) in myeloproliferative disorders. *Haematologica* 93: 1635-1644.

[30] Chim CS, Fung TK, Cheung WC, Liang R, Kwong YL (2004) SOCS1 and SHP1 Hypermethylation in Multiple Myeloma: Implications for Epigenetic Activation of the Jak/STAT pathway. *Blood.*

[31] Johan MF, Bowen DT, Frew ME, Goodeve AC, Reilly JT (2005) Aberrant methylation of the negative regulators RASSFIA, SHP-1 and SOCS-1 in myelodysplastic syndromes and acute myeloid leukaemia. *Br. J. Haematol.* 129: 60-65.

[32] Liu YL, Castleberry RP, Emanuel PD (2009) PTEN deficiency is a common defect in juvenile myelomonocytic leukemia. *Leuk Res.* 33: 671-677.

[33] Batz C, Sandrock I, Niemeyer CM, Flotho C (2009) Methylation of the PTEN gene CpG island is infrequent in juvenile myelomonocytic leukemia: Comments on "PTEN deficiency is a common defect in juvenile myelomonocytic leukemia" [Leuk. Res. 2009;33:671-677 (Epub 2008 November 17)]. *Leuk Res.* 33: 1578-1579; author reply 1580.

[34] Lewis F, Maughan NJ, Smith V, Hillan K, Quirke P (2001) Unlocking the archive--gene expression in paraffin-embedded tissue. *J. Pathol.* 195: 66-71.

[35] Lehmann U, Hasemeier B, Lilischkis R, Kreipe H (2001) Quantitative analysis of promoter hypermethylation in laser-microdissected archival specimens. *Lab. Invest.* 81: 635-638.

[36] Lehmann U, Berg-Ribbe I, Wingen LU, Brakensiek K, Becker T, et al. (2005) Distinct methylation patterns of benign and malignant liver tumors revealed by quantitative methylation profiling. *Clin. Cancer Res.* 11: 3654-3660.

[37] Killian JK, Bilke S, Davis S, Walker RL, Killian MS, et al. (2009) Large-scale profiling of archival lymph nodes reveals pervasive remodeling of the follicular lymphoma methylome. *Cancer Res.* 69: 758-764.

[38] Beck S, Rakyan VK (2008) The methylome: approaches for global DNA methylation profiling. Trends Genet 24: 231-237.

[39] Bibikova M, Lin Z, Zhou L, Chudin E, Garcia EW, et al. (2006) High-throughput DNA methylation profiling using universal bead arrays. *Genome Res.* 16: 383-393.

[40] Martin-Subero JI, Kreuz M, Bibikova M, Bentink S, Ammerpohl O, et al. (2009) New insights into the biology and origin of mature aggressive B-cell lymphomas by combined epigenomic, genomic, and transcriptional profiling. *Blood* 113: 2488-2497.

[41] Martin-Subero JI, Ammerpohl O, Bibikova M, Wickham-Garcia E, Agirre X, et al. (2009) A comprehensive microarray-based DNA methylation study of 367 hematological neoplasms. *PLoS One* 4: e6986.

[42] Jiang Y, Dunbar A, Gondek LP, Mohan S, Rataul M, et al. (2009) Aberrant DNA methylation is a dominant mechanism in MDS progression to AML. *Blood* 113: 1315-1325.

[43] Khulan B, Thompson RF, Ye K, Fazzari MJ, Suzuki M, et al. (2006) Comparative isoschizomer profiling of cytosine methylation: the HELP assay. *Genome Res.* 16: 1046-1055.

[44] Figueroa ME, Skrabanek L, Li Y, Jiemjit A, Fandy TE, et al. (2009) MDS and secondary AML display unique patterns and abundance of aberrant DNA methylation. *Blood* 114: 3448-3458.

[45] Figueroa ME, Wouters BJ, Skrabanek L, Glass J, Li Y, et al. (2009) Genome-wide epigenetic analysis delineates a biologically distinct immature acute leukemia with myeloid/T-lymphoid features. *Blood* 113: 2795-2804.

[46] Cairns P (2009) 5'-azacytidine expression arrays. *Methods Mol. Biol.* 507: 165-174.

[47] Ehrlich M (2006) Cancer-linked DNA hypomethylation and its relationship to hypermethylation. *Curr. Top. Microbiol. Immunol.* 310: 251-274.

[48] Feinberg AP, Vogelstein B (1983) Hypomethylation distinguishes genes of some human cancers from their normal counterparts. *Nature* 301: 89-92.

[49] Gama-Sosa MA, Slagel VA, Trewyn RW, Oxenhandler R, Kuo KC, et al. (1983) The 5-methylcytosine content of DNA from human tumors. *Nucleic Acids Res* 11: 6883-6894.

[50] Ehrlich M (2002) DNA methylation in cancer: too much, but also too little. *Oncogene* 21: 5400-5413.

[51] Wilson AS, Power BE, Molloy PL (2007) DNA hypomethylation and human diseases. *Biochim. Biophys. Acta.* 1775: 138-162.

[52] Dante R, Dante-Paire J, Rigal D, Roizes G (1992) Methylation patterns of long interspersed repeated DNA and alphoid repetitive DNA from human cell lines and tumors. *AntiCancer Res.* 12: 559-563.

[53] Wahlfors J, Hiltunen H, Heinonen K, Hamalainen E, Alhonen L, et al. (1992) Genomic hypomethylation in human chronic lymphocytic leukemia. *Blood* 80: 2074-2080.

[54] Bollati V, Fabris S, Pegoraro V, Ronchetti D, Mosca L, et al. (2009) Differential repetitive DNA methylation in multiple myeloma molecular subgroups. *Carcinogenesis* 30: 1330-1335.

[55] Roman-Gomez J, Jimenez-Velasco A, Agirre X, Cervantes F, Sanchez J, et al. (2005) Promoter hypomethylation of the LINE-1 retrotransposable elements activates sense/antisense transcription and marks the progression of chronic myeloid leukemia. *Oncogene* 24: 7213-7223.

[56] Hanada M, Delia D, Aiello A, Stadtmauer E, Reed JC (1993) bcl-2 gene hypomethylation and high-level expression in B-cell chronic lymphocytic leukemia. *Blood* 82: 1820-1828.

[57] Nakayama M, Wada M, Harada T, Nagayama J, Kusaba H, et al. (1998) Hypomethylation status of CpG sites at the promoter region and overexpression of the human MDR1 gene in acute myeloid leukemias. *Blood* 92: 4296-4307.

[58] Yuille MR, Condie A, Stone EM, Wilsher J, Bradshaw PS, et al. (2001) TCL1 is activated by chromosomal rearrangement or by hypomethylation. *Genes Chromosomes Cancer* 30: 336-341.

[59] Tsukamoto N, Morita K, Karasawa M, Omine M (1992) Methylation status of c-myc oncogene in leukemic cells: hypomethylation in acute leukemia derived from myelodysplastic syndromes. *Exp. Hematol.* 20: 1061-1064.

[60] Lubbert M, Oster W, Ludwig WD, Ganser A, Mertelsmann R, et al. (1992) A switch toward demethylation is associated with the expression of myeloperoxidase in acute myeloblastic and promyelocytic leukemias. *Blood* 80: 2066-2073.

[61] Lipsanen V, Leinonen P, Alhonen L, Janne J (1988) Hypomethylation of ornithine decarboxylase gene and erb-A1 oncogene in human chronic lymphatic leukemia. *Blood* 72: 2042-2044.

[62] Lengauer C (2003) Cancer. An unstable liaison. *Science* 300: 442-443.

[63] Gaudet F, Hodgson JG, Eden A, Jackson-Grusby L, Dausman J, et al. (2003) Induction of tumors in mice by genomic hypomethylation. *Science* 300: 489-492.

[64] Roman-Gomez J, Jimenez-Velasco A, Agirre X, Castillejo JA, Navarro G, et al. (2008) Repetitive DNA hypomethylation in the advanced phase of chronic myeloid leukemia. *Leuk Res.* 32: 487-490.

[65] Roman-Gomez J, Jimenez-Velasco A, Agirre X, Castillejo JA, Navarro G, et al. (2006) Promoter hypermethylation and global hypomethylation are independent epigenetic events in lymphoid leukemogenesis with opposing effects on clinical outcome. *Leukemia* 20: 1445-1448.

[66] Fan T, Schmidtmann A, Xi S, Briones V, Zhu H, et al. (2008) DNA hypomethylation caused by Lsh deletion promotes erythroleukemia development. *Epigenetics* 3: 134-142.

[67] Romermann D, Hasemeier B, Metzig K, Gohring G, Schlegelberger B, et al. (2008) Global increase in DNA methylation in patients with myelodysplastic syndrome. *Leukemia* 22: 1954-1956.

[68] Ehrlich M (2000) DNA Hypomethylation and Cancer. In: Ehrlich M, editor. DNA Alterations in Cancer: Genetic and Epigenetic Changes. Natick: Eaton Publishing. pp. 273-292.

[69] Kilpivaara O, Levine RL (2008) JAK2 and MPL mutations in myeloproliferative neoplasms: discovery and science. *Leukemia* 22: 1813-1817.

[70] Quentmeier H, Geffers R, Jost E, Macleod RA, Nagel S, et al. (2008) SOCS2: inhibitor of JAK2V617F-mediated signal transduction. *Leukemia* 22: 2169-2175.

[71] Jones LC, Tefferi A, Idos GE, Kumagai T, Hofmann WK, et al. (2004) RARbeta2 is a candidate tumor suppressor gene in myelofibrosis with myeloid metaplasia. *Oncogene* 23: 7846-7853.

[72] Herman JG, Graff JR, Myohanen S, Nelkin BD, Baylin SB (1996) Methylation-specific PCR: a novel PCR assay for methylation status of CpG islands. *Proc. Natl. Acad. Sci. USA* 93: 9821-9826.

[73] Aviram A, Witenberg B, Shaklai M, Blickstein D (2003) Detection of methylated ABL1 promoter in philadelphia-negative myeloproliferative disorders. *Blood Cells Mol. Dis.* 30: 100-106.

[74] Ihalainen J, Juvonen E, Savolainen ER, Ruutu T, Palotie A (1994) Calcitonin gene methylation in chronic myeloproliferative disorders. *Leukemia* 8: 230-235.

[75] Bogani C, Ponziani V, Guglielmelli P, Desterke C, Rosti V, et al. (2008) Hypermethylation of CXCR4 promoter in CD34+ cells from patients with primary myelofibrosis. *Stem. Cells* 26: 1920-1930.

[76] Oki Y, Jelinek J, Beran M, Verstovsek S, Kantarjian HM, et al. (2006) Mutations and promoter methylation status of NPM1 in myeloproliferative disorders. *Haematologica* 91: 1147-1148.

[77] Kumagai T, Tefferi A, Jones L, Koeffler HP (2005) Methylation analysis of the cell cycle control genes in myelofibrosis with myeloid metaplasia. *Leuk Res.* 29: 511-515.

[78] Wang JC, Chen W, Nallusamy S, Chen C, Novetsky AD (2002) Hypermethylation of the P15INK4b and P16INK4a in agnogenic myeloid metaplasia (AMM) and AMM in leukaemic transformation. *Br. J. Haematol.* 116: 582-586.

[79] Jelinek J, Li J, Mnjoyan Z, Issa JP, Prchal JT, et al. (2007) Epigenetic control of PRV-1 expression on neutrophils. *Exp. Hematol.* 35: 1677-1683.

[80] Li J, Bench AJ, Huntly BJ, Green AR (2001) Mutation and methylation analysis of the transforming growth factor beta receptor II gene in polycythaemia vera. *Br. J. Haematol.* 115: 872-880.

[81] Prawitt D, Enklaar T, Gartner-Rupprecht B, Spangenberg C, Lausch E, et al. (2005) Microdeletion and IGF2 loss of imprinting in a cascade causing Beckwith-Wiedemann syndrome with Wilms' tumor. *Nat. Genet.* 37: 785-786; author reply 786-787.

[82] Gicquel C, Rossignol S, Cabrol S, Houang M, Steunou V, et al. (2005) Epimutation of the telomeric imprinting center region on chromosome 11p15 in Silver-Russell syndrome. *Nat. Genet.* 37: 1003-1007.

[83] Nakagawa H, Chadwick RB, Peltomaki P, Plass C, Nakamura Y, et al. (2001) Loss of imprinting of the insulin-like growth factor II gene occurs by biallelic methylation in a core region of H19-associated CTCF-binding sites in colorectal cancer. *Proc. Natl. Acad. Sci. USA* 98: 591-596.

[84] Tuna M, Knuutila S, Mills GB (2009) Uniparental disomy in cancer. *Trends Mol. Med.* 15: 120-128.

[85] Paulsen M, Ferguson-Smith AC (2001) DNA methylation in genomic imprinting, development, and disease. *J. Pathol.* 195: 97-110.

[86] Wu MS, Wang HP, Lin CC, Sheu JC, Shun CT, et al. (1997) Loss of imprinting and overexpression of IGF2 gene in gastric adenocarcinoma. *Cancer Lett.* 120: 9-14.

[87] Chen CL, Ip SM, Cheng D, Wong LC, Ngan HY (2000) Loss of imprinting of the IGF-II and H19 genes in epithelial ovarian cancer. *Clin. Cancer Res.* 6: 474-479.

[88] el-Naggar AK, Lai S, Tucker SA, Clayman GL, Goepfert H, et al. (1999) Frequent loss of imprinting at the IGF2 and H19 genes in head and neck squamous carcinoma. *Oncogene* 18: 7063-7069.

[89] Oda H, Kume H, Shimizu Y, Inoue T, Ishikawa T (1998) Loss of imprinting of igf2 in renal-cell carcinomas. *Int. J. Cancer* 75: 343-346.

[90] Cui H, Cruz-Correa M, Giardiello FM, Hutcheon DF, Kafonek DR, et al. (2003) Loss of IGF2 imprinting: a potential marker of colorectal cancer risk. *Science* 299: 1753-1755.

[91] Uyeno S, Aoki Y, Nata M, Sagisaka K, Kayama T, et al. (1996) IGF2 but not H19 shows loss of imprinting in human glioma. *Cancer Res.* 56: 5356-5359.

[92] Ulaner GA, Vu TH, Li T, Hu JF, Yao XM, et al. (2003) Loss of imprinting of IGF2 and H19 in osteosarcoma is accompanied by reciprocal methylation changes of a CTCF-binding site. *Hum. Mol. Genet.* 12: 535-549.

[93] Kim HT, Choi BH, Niikawa N, Lee TS, Chang SI (1998) Frequent loss of imprinting of the H19 and IGF-II genes in ovarian tumors. *Am. J. Med. Genet.* 80: 391-395.

[94] Nonomura N, Miki T, Nishimura K, Kanno N, Kojima Y, et al. (1997) Altered imprinting of the H19 and insulin-like growth factor II genes in testicular tumors. *J. Urol.* 157: 1977-1979.

[95] Feinberg AP, Cui H, Ohlsson R (2002) DNA methylation and genomic imprinting: insights from cancer into epigenetic mechanisms. *Semin. Cancer Biol.* 12: 389-398.

[96] Steenman MJ, Rainier S, Dobry CJ, Grundy P, Horon IL, et al. (1994) Loss of imprinting of IGF2 is linked to reduced expression and abnormal methylation of H19 in Wilms' tumour. *Nat. Genet.* 7: 433-439.

[97] Hofmann WK, de Vos S, Komor M, Hoelzer D, Wachsman W, et al. (2002) Characterization of gene expression of CD34+ cells from normal and myelodysplastic bone marrow. *Blood* 100: 3553-3560.

[98] Wang WH, Duan JX, Vu TH, Hoffman AR (1996) Increased expression of the insulin-like growth factor-II gene in Wilms' tumor is not dependent on loss of genomic imprinting or loss of heterozygosity. *J. Biol. Chem.* 271: 27863-27870.

[99] Vorwerk P, Wex H, Bessert C, Hohmann B, Schmidt U, et al. (2003) Loss of imprinting of IGF-II gene in children with acute lymphoblastic leukemia. *Leuk Res.* 27: 807-812.

[100] Nunez C, Bashein AM, Brunet CL, Hoyland JA, Freemont AJ, et al. (2000) Expression of the imprinted tumour-suppressor gene H19 is tightly regulated during normal haematopoiesis and is reduced in haematopoietic precursors of patients with the myeloproliferative disease polycythaemia vera. *J. Pathol.* 190: 61-68.

[101] Morison IM, Eccles MR, Reeve AE (2000) Imprinting of insulin-like growth factor 2 is modulated during hematopoiesis. *Blood* 96: 3023-3028.

[102] Hattori H, Matsuzaki A, Suminoe A, Ihara K, Eguchi M, et al. (2000) Genomic imprinting of insulin-like growth factor-2 in infant leukemia and childhood neuroblastoma. *Cancer* 88: 2372-2377.

[103] Wu HK, Weksberg R, Minden MD, Squire JA (1997) Loss of imprinting of human insulin-like growth factor II gene, IGF2, in acute myeloid leukemia. *Biochem. Biophys. Res. Commun.* 231: 466-472.

[104] Giannoukakis N, Deal C, Paquette J, Kukuvitis A, Polychronakos C (1996) Polymorphic functional imprinting of the human IGF2 gene among individuals, in blood cells, is associated with H19 expression. *Biochem. Biophys. Res. Commun.* 220: 1014-1019.

[105] Hofmann WK, Takeuchi S, Frantzen MA, Hoelzer D, Koeffler HP (2002) Loss of genomic imprinting of insulin-like growth factor 2 is strongly associated with cellular proliferation in normal hematopoietic cells. *Exp. Hematol.* 30: 318-323.

[106] Randhawa GS, Cui H, Barletta JA, Strichman-Almashanu LZ, Talpaz M, et al. (1998) Loss of imprinting in disease progression in chronic myelogenous leukemia. *Blood* 91: 3144-3147.

[107] Tessema M, Langer F, Bock O, Seltsam A, Metzig K, et al. (2005) Down-regulation of the IGF-2/H19 locus during normal and malignant hematopoiesis is independent of the imprinting pattern. *Int. J. Oncol* 26: 499-507.

[108] Kainz B, Shehata M, Bilban M, Kienle D, Heintel D, et al. (2007) Overexpression of the paternally expressed gene 10 (PEG10) from the imprinted locus on chromosome 7q21 in high-risk B-cell chronic lymphocytic leukemia. *Int. J. Cancer* 121: 1984-1993.

[109] Wong IH, Ng MH, Huang DP, Lee JC (2000) Aberrant p15 promoter methylation in adult and childhood acute leukemias of nearly all morphologic subtypes: potential prognostic implications. *Blood* 95: 1942-1949.

[110] Chim CS, Wong SY, Kwong YL (2003) Aberrant gene promoter methylation in acute promyelocytic leukaemia: profile and prognostic significance. *Br. J. Haematol.* 122: 571-578.

[111] Galm O, Wilop S, Reichelt J, Jost E, Gehbauer G, et al. (2004) DNA methylation changes in multiple myeloma. *Leukemia* 18: 1687-1692.

[112] Roman-Gomez J, Castillejo JA, Jimenez A, Gonzalez MG, Moreno F, et al. (2002) 5' CpG island hypermethylation is associated with transcriptional silencing of the p21(CIP1/WAF1/SDI1) gene and confers poor prognosis in acute lymphoblastic leukemia. *Blood* 99: 2291-2296.

[113] Grovdal M, Khan R, Aggerholm A, Antunovic P, Astermark J, et al. (2007) Negative effect of DNA hypermethylation on the outcome of intensive chemotherapy in older patients with high-risk myelodysplastic syndromes and acute myeloid leukemia following myelodysplastic syndrome. *Clin. Cancer Res.* 13: 7107-7112.

[114] Suzuki R, Onizuka M, Kojima M, Shimada M, Fukagawa S, et al. (2007) Preferential hypermethylation of the Dickkopf-1 promoter in core-binding factor leukaemia. *Br. J. Haematol.* 138: 624-631.

[115] Strathdee G, Holyoake TL, Sim A, Parker A, Oscier DG, et al. (2007) Inactivation of HOXA genes by hypermethylation in myeloid and lymphoid malignancy is frequent and associated with poor prognosis. *Clin. Cancer Res.* 13: 5048-5055.

[116] Agrelo R, Setien F, Espada J, Artiga MJ, Rodriguez M, et al. (2005) Inactivation of the lamin A/C gene by CpG island promoter hypermethylation in hematologic malignancies, and its association with poor survival in nodal diffuse large B-cell lymphoma. *J. Clin. Oncol.* 23: 3940-3947.

[117] Benetatos L, Hatzimichael E, Dasoula A, Dranitsaris G, Tsiara S, et al. (2009) CpG methylation analysis of the MEG3 and SNRPN imprinted genes in acute myeloid leukemia and myelodysplastic syndromes. *Leuk Res.*.

[118] Esteller M, Gaidano G, Goodman SN, Zagonel V, Capello D, et al. (2002) Hypermethylation of the DNA repair gene O(6)-methylguanine DNA methyltransferase and survival of patients with diffuse large B-cell lymphoma. *J. Natl. Cancer Inst.* 94: 26-32.

[119] Agirre X, Vilas-Zornoza A, Jimenez-Velasco A, Martin-Subero JI, Cordeu L, et al. (2009) Epigenetic silencing of the tumor suppressor microRNA Hsa-miR-124a regulates CDK6 expression and confers a poor prognosis in acute lymphoblastic leukemia. *Cancer Res.* 69: 4443-4453.

[120] Boumber YA, Kondo Y, Chen X, Shen L, Gharibyan V, et al. (2007) RIL, a LIM gene on 5q31, is silenced by methylation in cancer and sensitizes cancer cells to apoptosis. *Cancer Res.* 67: 1997-2005.

[121] Wu SJ, Yao M, Chou WC, Tang JL, Chen CY, et al. (2006) Clinical implications of SOCS1 methylation in myelodysplastic syndrome. *Br. J. Haematol.* 135: 317-323.

[122] Roman-Gomez J, Jimenez-Velasco A, Cordeu L, Vilas-Zornoza A, San Jose-Eneriz E, et al. (2007) WNT5A, a putative tumour suppressor of lymphoid malignancies, is inactivated by aberrant methylation in acute lymphoblastic leukaemia. *Eur. J. Cancer* 43: 2736-2746.

[123] Jabbour E, Issa JP, Garcia-Manero G, Kantarjian H (2008) Evolution of decitabine development: accomplishments, ongoing investigations, and future strategies. C*ancer* 112: 2341-2351.

[124] Issa JP, Gharibyan V, Cortes J, Jelinek J, Morris G, et al. (2005) Phase II study of low-dose decitabine in patients with chronic myelogenous leukemia resistant to imatinib mesylate. *J. Clin. Oncol.* 23: 3948-3956.

[125] Kantarjian H, Oki Y, Garcia-Manero G, Huang X, O'Brien S, et al. (2007) Results of a randomized study of 3 schedules of low-dose decitabine in higher-risk myelodysplastic syndrome and chronic myelomonocytic leukemia. *Blood* 109: 52-57.

[126] Griffiths EA, Gore SD (2008) DNA methyltransferase and histone deacetylase inhibitors in the treatment of myelodysplastic syndromes. *Semin Hematol* 45: 23-30.

[127] Oki Y, Aoki E, Issa JP (2007) Decitabine--bedside to bench. *Crit. Rev. Oncol. Hematol.* 61: 140-152.

[128] Oki Y, Issa JP (2007) Treatment options in advanced myelodysplastic syndrome, with emphasis on epigenetic therapy. *Int. J. Hematol* 86: 306-314.

[129] Altucci L, Minucci S (2009) Epigenetic therapies in haematological malignancies: searching for true targets. *Eur. J. Cancer* 45: 1137-1145.

Part IV – Biomarker Development and Therapy Targeting of Epigenetics

In: Field Cancerization: Basic Science and Clinical Applications ISBN 978-1-61761-006-6
Editor: Gabriel D. Dakubo

Chapter 25

Molecular Signatures as Cancer Biomarkers: Methodologic Issues in Discovery, Validation, Qualification, and Standardization

Laura B. Pritzker and Kenneth P.H. Pritzker

Abstract

Molecular signatures appear particularly well suited as biomarkers for cancer processes as this type of biomarker has promise to associate particular genomic patterns with progression. However, the discovery and development of molecular-signature cancer biomarkers is characterized by daunting methodologic challenges derived from the complexity of analyzing multiple analytes present in small concentrations, and the extensive associated bioinformatics. Molecular signatures can be discovered either by empiric association studies using high throughput genomic and proteomic analysis or by hypothesis-generated research, which selects key molecules in cellular pathways to pathogenesis. Biomarker development involves the processes of validation, qualification and standardization. Molecular-signature validation seeks to establish a reliable association of the cancer feature with the biomarker. This involves utilization of rigorous analytical techniques with appropriate clinical data sets. Biomarker qualification, the formal assessment of clinical utility, requires further assessment including assessment against current biomarkers using clinical data sets independent from the validation set. Biomarker standardization is the quantitative comparison of the biomarker in practice with other methods that measure the same biomarker. Characteristic of molecular signatures, at all stages of biomarker discovery and development, extensive bioinformatics are employed in the correlative clinical-chemical analysis. Accelerating the implementation of molecular signature biomarkers in cancer diagnosis and therapy is dependent on lower cost, more reliable analysis, more transparent bioinformatics strategies as well as minimizing the number of signature components and clinical parameters studied.

25.1. Introduction

Field cancerization, the development of cancer by progressive genomic alteration and subsequent phenotypic changes in groups of cells within a tissue, is a process common to many, if not most types of epithelial cancers [1] as well as some forms of sarcoma and hematologic malignancies. Clinically, assessment of field cancerization has diagnostic and therapeutic implications aligned along both temporal and spatial dimensions. As time progresses, the cells of the cancer field develop incremental genomic alterations, which lead to progressive phenotypic atypia. In some cancers, genomic alterations occur at specific susceptible gene and chromosomal locations. These can result in detectible phenotypic characteristics that are indicators of therapy, e.g., estrogen, progesterone, HER2 sensitivity in breast cancer or alternatively, specific diagnostic markers, such as chromosome translocation/fusion in specific sarcomas and leukemias. However, the specificity of most genomic abnormalities in tumors at this time is not known and, therefore, the observed genomic changes appear to be random. Spatially, some domains of the cancer field continue to have fewer genomic alterations and appear phenotypically less advanced or even, as at the earliest phases, phenotypically undetectable. The different domains within the cancer field are usually contiguous, indicative that as the field itself expands, domains with particular genomic characteristics also expand by clonal replication of the genomic abnormalities.

Using an epithelial cancer such as squamous cell carcinoma as an example, neoplasia is characterized first by genomic abnormality in the epithelium, the phenotype of which is unlikely to be macroscopically or histologically detectable. Over time, and with clonal proliferation, more cells are recruited that have the genomic abnormalities. Meanwhile, further episodes of genomic alteration give rise to additional groups of cells, which demonstrate cytologic abnormality, perhaps characterized by nuclear atypia, but the organization of the epithelium itself remains intact.

The first clinical manifestation of neoplasia is often dysfunction of the tissue in the cancer field. For surface epithelium, this is manifested by increased permeability, which may give rise to inflammation and to an epithelial reaction by the neoplastic cells themselves, as well as by cells in the adjacent fields. In the skin, this is seen as focal thickening or hyperkeratization; in the mucosa by "leukoplakia" that is mucosal thickening with a parakeratin layer. However, in this phase, the phenotypic pattern is not restricted to neoplasia as reactive processes may have similar appearances. Therefore, with conventional histologic examination, detection of the cancer field in tissues at this stage is a considerable challenge.

Further genomic alterations result in groups of cells with recognizable cytologic atypia, such as increased nuclear cytoplasmic ratio, enlarged nuclei, coarse nuclear chromatin, followed by loss of tissue organization amongst the cells. At this phase, if biopsied, the neoplastic cells can be recognized as dysplastic or with further progression, as carcinoma *in situ*. The natural history for these cancer fields is to develop further genomic abnormalities, resulting in cell groups migrating beyond their natural boundary to invade adjacent local tissues and with further genomic change, to metastasize to distant sites. However, the time course for these events is highly variable and requires additional biomarker indicators beyond tests currently available. Except from historical clinical pathologic information regarding similar classes of tumors, there is usually little knowledge about the capacity of a particular tumor studied to progress to invasive cancer or to metastasis. In this description of cancer progression, we have omitted general and local preconditions, which permit the cancer field to develop and retain cells with genomic changes.

Predisposition to neoplasia may be enabled by heritable genetic changes, which predispose to cancer development in specific organs, e.g., BRCA1, BRCA2 in breast and ovary [2,3]; FAP and HNPCC genes in colon [4], or by acquired changes that give rise to genomic abnormalities. The development of elastotic degeneration of dermal collagen from prolonged sun exposure is an example of acquired changes that can contribute to development of the neoplastic epithelial fields in the overlying epidermis.

Ideally, cancer fields would be identified and removed by therapy prior to tumor invasion. Failing this for established cancers, parameters of biologic aggressiveness such as the extent of invasion, the capacity for metastasis or susceptibility to therapy could be determined by biomarkers. As direct observation or imaging of the cancer field of adjacent tissues may not be sufficiently sensitive to detect early changes, biomarkers, particularly biomarkers based on molecular signatures are a widely proposed method for assessing cancer fields. Potentially, biomarker deployment could facilitate targeted therapy and decrease health care costs by reducing "over treatment" of patients. Additionally, biomarkers could prevent drug toxicity in susceptible patient populations. The perceived savings in drug development and the reduction of late-stage therapeutic failures of current pharmaceuticals are important drivers to identify and validate cancer biomarkers.

Desirable as effective cancer biomarkers may be, it is clear that the present capacity to discover candidate biomarkers exceeds by far the capacity to validate and effectively deploy these tests [5,6,7]. Barriers to development of cancer biomarkers include biologic factors such as heterogeneity of cancers and patient populations [8,9], variable presence of exogenous substances that affect biomarker presence and concentration, clinical pathologic factors that limit the precision of classifying the cancer type, grade, and stage, imprecise relationships between analytical detection and biologic significance, as well as the natural conservatism of health services, which place greater cost benefit demands on innovation than on existing technologies. For molecular signature biomarkers, analytical and bioinformatics technologies are current limitations that require the establishment of large biobanks containing patient data and specimens, as well as the development of clinical consortia capable of large-scale clinical trials.

A biomarker can be defined as a phenotypic parameter that can be objectively measured and evaluated as an indicator of normal or pathologic biological processes, or as an indicator of pharmacologic response to therapy [10,11,12,13]. Broadly considered, biomarker classification can include clinical symptoms, signs of disease, physiologic parameters, laboratory tests for histologic, biochemical, immunologic or molecular (genetic and genomic) markers and imaging [14]. More specifically related to molecular signatures, biomarkers can be classified as a molecule or a set of molecules that can be identified and quantitated *in vitro* or *in vivo* or accessed and displayed in an image (histologic or radiologic) with quantifiable characteristics specific for disease assessment [15,16,17]. Currently, there is an active search for molecules or sets of molecules specific for disease assessment, which can be imaged [18] to achieve organ, tissue or cellular localization. For histologic studies, this extends identification of cancer field components beyond morphology to the demonstration of molecular characteristics in specific cells within spatial tissue domains. For *in vivo* studies, this combines imaging and laboratory medicine to provide non-invasive biomarker assessment, which can be repeated in the patient to observe changes over time.

While there are many ways to categorize biomarkers, biomarkers can be classified as either prognostic or predictive [10,12,13,19,20]. Prognostic (natural history) biomarkers measure aspects of disease status, which can be used to measure burden of disease (genetic predisposition and environmental susceptibility), clarify diagnosis, assess stage, prognosis or outcome, and monitor natural history or therapy [21]. In theory, prognostic biomarkers are generated by comparison of patient data associated with a natural history of disease with data from patients given standard treatment. In practice, prognostic biomarkers are evaluated in comparison to our accumulated prognostic knowledge of specific cancers as characterized by histologic type, histologic grade, macroscopic size, clinical stage, and conventional treatment. For screening and early detection, the natural history of populations without cancer is compared to accumulated clinical knowledge of patients with familial or acquired predisposition to cancer. For early detection, the comparison is to knowledge that includes clinical pathological assessment of early neoplasia and its assessment by cytologic and histologic techniques. Predictive (drug activity) biomarkers are used to describe drug activity, such as proof of concept, dosage, optimal drug combinations, drug response and retardation of disease, progression in the presence of drug, as well as drug safety [12,13,16]. Predictive biomarkers separate populations that are candidates for treatment from those that are not, based on clinical outcome knowledge of previous clinical study populations exposed to both the cancer and the therapy. As the markers guide serious therapeutic choices, , the validation and qualification processes for predictive biomarkers are necessarily much more rigorous than for prognostic biomarkers.

Analytical molecular signatures require consistent preservation of the analytes within the samples collected and maintenance of these conditions throughout the analytical processes. Image molecular signatures require assessment from a consistent histologic or radiologic image plane. Both approaches require careful attention to the bioinformatics methodology used to discriminate signal from noise and validated methodology to associate the biomarker with the specific cancer feature. The properties of an ideal molecular signature cancer biomarker are listed in table 25-1.

Like other tests, biomarkers should have high sensitivity and high specificity. To be deployed widely, the biomarker must be cost effective and to be useful, tests must be repeatable over time. This implies that procedures should be minimally or non-invasive to the patient.

Cancer biomarkers can be generated by several analytical strategies including genomics, transcriptomics, proteomics and metabolomics [13]. Candidate biomarkers may be used individually, multiplexed or as groups to generate a signature, which indicates the state of a specific disease feature [16,22].

Table 25.1. Requirements for Molecular Signatures as Useful Cancer Biomarkers

General Properties	Analytical Requirements	Image Requirements
High sensitivity	Well preserved in samples	Precise imaging criteria
High specificity	Easily extracted, detected, analyzed	Easily detectable and quantifiable
Cost effective	Easily reproducible	Easily reproducible
Repeatable over time	√	√
Minimal patient invasion	√	√

In developing cancer biomarkers, it is relevant to ask why the search should be concentrated on "molecular" markers, and what are the advantages of "molecular signatures"? "Molecular" markers in the narrowest sense include heritable genetic mutations or polymorphisms that are associated with specific cancers, as well as genomic alterations that are restricted in specific clonal subsets of cancer cells. Indicators of the genomic change may be detected directly from extraction analysis of DNA or RNA or, alternatively from histologic assessment by *in situ* hybridization using fluorescence or colorimetric techniques. By extension, the molecular abnormality may be seen by detection of the abnormal gene product as RNA (transcriptomics), as protein (proteomics) or lipid (lipidomics) [23], or by dysfunction of the gene product in metabolic pathways (metabolomics). As cancer is characterized by progressive genomic changes, with or without an underlying genetic abnormality, it is reasonable to seek out biomarkers of the earliest genomic changes as key characteristics of cancer predisposition or preclinical detection.

However, once cancers are established, the key cell characteristics that determine cell replication rate, propensity to invasion, capacity to metastasize, as well as secondary reactions such as tumor-associated inflammation are determined by the added complexity associated with epigenetic changes, such as gene methylation [24] or histone modification [25,26,27,28], which regulate gene expression, as well as by posttranslational protein modifications, which alter protein activity [29](table 25-2). This complexity presents considerable challenge to the detection of specific biomarkers.

Gene methylation occurs preferentially in gene promoter regions in short genomic sequences termed CpG islands. As an example of particular interest, gene hypermethylation has the effect of downregulating or "silencing " tumor suppressing oncogenes [24]. Clinically, hypermethylation of PITX2 gene in a 4-member panel has been shown to increase the risk of breast cancer recurrence [30]. Hypermethylation of selected genes and downregulation in mRNA expression are being used to characterize biologic aggressiveness of urothelial carcinomas [31].

Molecular signature biomarkers of gene methylation have promise because methylation is confined to defined DNA regions; methylation of some genes is specific to genes associated with cancers in specific tissues, and gene methylation is associated with genes that predispose to neoplasia. Further, hypermethylated genes can be detected in blood [24]. Most proteins on the cell surface are glycosylated as are most circulating proteins[29]. Accordingly in established cancers, assessment of phenotypic biomarkers that reflect cell surface properties may be as effective as genotypic markers for prognostic assessment.

There are both biologic and empirical reasons to consider molecular signatures preferentially as cancer biomarkers. Biologically, cancer is a complex disease in which progressive genomic-based cellular derangements are aligned to the biologic aggressiveness and cancer stage. Therefore, the biologic activity of the cancer may be more easily inferred by assessment of a genomic marker signature than by a single or few salient markers. As well, bioinformatics operation on the molecular signature may yield additional information about the dynamic equilibrium of the signaling pathways that may prove clinically useful. Recently, Taylor [32], using public domain molecular signature data of breast cancers, demonstrated that the prognostic value of the markers could be increased if the association/disassociation of the markers as coherent networks was measured. Greater dissociation implied greater discoherence of metabolic networks indicating incremental biologic aggressiveness and worse prognosis. Empirically, molecular data sets incorporating large numbers of genes have been analyzed through the association of specific cancer features with molecular signatures composed of hundreds or even thousands of genes [33]. In some cases, these signatures have been deployed as clinical tests of prognosis while the underlying biologic mechanisms still remain to be discovered.

Table 25.2. Epigenetic and Post-translational Molecular modifications in cancer development

Modification	Compound	Example
1. Epigenetic Modification		
Methylation	DNA	5' regulatory region of glutathione-S-transferase in prostate adenocarcinoma
Methylation	Histone Proteins	Histone 3 lysine 4 Methyl transferase in leukemia
Acetylation	Histone Proteins	Histone acetylase CBP mutation in leukemia
2. Posttranslational Modification		
Glycosylation	Proteins	GP73 in hepatocellular carcinoma
Phosphorylation	Proteins	Tyrosine kinase substrates in breast cancer

Evaluation, validation and qualification are terms used commonly and interchangeably in the biomarker literature. Evaluation is a general term to describe assessment of methodologic processes throughout biomarker discovery development and implementation. Recently, the term "biomarker validation" has been reserved for evaluation of technical methods, especially analytical methods, whereas "biomarker qualification" is used as the term to evaluate clinical utility. Both biomarker validation and qualification processes are determined with reference to "fit-for-purpose" criteria [12,13,15,16,17,34,35,36].

Biomarker validation and qualification studies use many of the same analytical methods as biomarker discovery, but each type of study is distinguished by purpose-specific methodologic issues.

Discovery studies are exploratory and hypothesis-driven. These studies are carried out to identify genetic classifiers associated with specific disease properties. Validation studies are performed to confirm association of the biomarker with its purpose and to assess analytical reliability and reproducibility.

Qualification studies are performed to demonstrate the clinical utility of developed classifiers. These studies require patient cohorts, which are coherent for disease type, extent, and therapy [17].

Once biomarkers are qualified, reduction to practice requires a further process, biomarker standardization. Biomarker standardization implies that CLIA approved and laboratory developed tests from different laboratories would provide results of quantitatively comparable sensitivity and specificity.

25.2. Molecular Signature Biomarkers: Discovery

In general, cancer biomarkers are discovered by comparing samples from two different populations, one healthier or with benign disease and the second with the type of cancer of interest. To discover a candidate, biomarker, molecules are separated, identified, quantified and the marker defined by its unique expression pattern associated with the disease. There are two basic approaches to biomarker discovery. In the biologic approach, biomarker candidates based on their known association with cancer phenotype, such as structural features or metabolic pathways are assessed in comparison with cancer specific features or a group of related features. In the empirical approach, high throughput analytical methods for detection of genes, proteins, metabolites or their components, are applied using samples derived from patients with a reference specific cancer phenotype (cancer type, grade, stage, features). In both approaches, molecular signatures composed of multiple components are utilized.

After analysis, bioinformatics association amongst the biomarker components and between the components and the cancer's specific phenotype are determined. The molecular signature is further refined to determine the smallest signature with the highest association with the cancer feature. Both methods are predicated on the cancer's specific feature and the cancer population being sufficiently coherent biologically, a substantial challenge as the specified conditions under study (age, gender, cancer type, grade, stage, previous therapy, etc.) are increased.

The techniques for cancer biomarker discovery are continuing to evolve rapidly with genomic, proteomic and other methods trending towards higher throughput, greater detection sensitivity with more complex bioinformatics embedded in the bioanalytical processes [29,37]. Only a small fraction of proposed cancer biomarkers are based on molecular signatures [38,39,40,41]. Genetic and genomic biomarkers can be discovered through analysis of DNA or RNA molecular profiling, as well as the emerging technology of genome wide association studies (GWAS) [42].

Molecular profiling utilizes the global expression patterns of genes and collections of genes that are associated with specific cancer features or pathways [43,44,45,46]. Quantitative molecular expression profiling can be assessed by qPCR techniques. Again, fundamental analytical issues include knowledge of sample source, quality of DNA/RNA extraction and reproducibility of qPCR or other means of expression detection. One major methodologic issue is the 80% discordance rate between mRNA expression and protein abundance [47].

Recently, strategies have been deployed to extend the use of molecular signatures as predictive biomarkers to determine therapy for molecular breast cancer types [37]. In this work sensitivity profiles were generated for Luminal B and Basal subtypes of breast cancer for the drugs Cytoxan, Adriamycin, Taxol, Doctaxel, 5-FU, Topotecan and Etoposide. However, these profiles were found to be heterogeneous. Drug sensitivity was also linked to signal pathway activation i.e. Her1, SRC or RAS within these subtypes. Many subtypes (with the exception of Luminal A) are characterized by the activation of multiple pathways adding to the complexity of the analysis. This illustrates the difficulty of defining a molecular signature biomarker set, where multiple cancer subtypes, multiple pathway markers and multiple therapeutic options are involved.

For genomic studies blood samples can be used, but for genomic biomarkers tumor cells are usually obtained by either cytologic or biopsy methods. The detection of RNA transcripts can reflect differential expression of genes at time of sampling and, therefore, can be a better indication of biomarker activity in disease than DNA. Further, through RNA splicing, linked polymorphisms may be detected, increasing the potential number of candidate biomarkers. These methods require RNA preservation initially and through the extraction and analysis phases. Methods that can extract and detect RNA transcripts within the same process are on the near horizon and have promise to increase the sensitivity of RNA-based biomarkers [48]. Gene microarrays, commonly used in the genomics approach are often validated by reverse transcription PCR [49]. Chromosomal alterations can be detected with comparative genomic hybridization arrays. Subsequently, immunoassays are used to assess protein biomarkers and the multiplexing of these assays can increase throughput but are limited by the loss of sensitivity and the need to standardize assay conditions [16].

In the assessment of proteomic markers, challenges arise due to the complexity of the proteome in biologic samples. For example, the presence of highly abundant proteins can mask the presence of other less abundant proteins. Further, the incomplete understanding of molecular pathways of development and disease can make difficult the interpretation of protein fragments detected.

Protein biomarkers are discovered using technology such as gel electrophoresis, various forms of mass spectrometry and tissue arrays. Two-dimensional differential gel electrophoresis has been commonly used for discovery of protein biomarkers. Proteins are separated first by isoelectric focusing followed in the second dimension by separation by molecular weight. Gels are then stained, the spots excised and identified by mass spectrometry. Adaption of this technique includes the use of fluorophore labeling which allows normalization to a common internal reference [50]. However, this technique is not sensitive to proteins with extreme isoelectric points, proteins with large molecular weights, poor solubility or low copy numbers. Mass spectrometry has become a method of choice in the discovery of novel proteins, as it does not require antibodies for identification [29,51,52,53]. Preanalytical methods such as matrix-associated laser absorption and ionization (MALDI) have been used to preferentially concentrate proteins with particular physical characteristics prior to mass spectrometry, thereby increasing sensitivity [54]. Mass spectrometry can also be applied to histologic sections using laser microdissection [43,55]. In this technique, samples are taken from defined locations across patient sections and mass spectrometry is then performed on the samples removed. The data can then generate two-dimensional maps, which can be compared to maps from histologic tissue samples. These techniques have produced consistent protein signatures, but definitive identification of proteins requires further protein digestion and further analysis by advanced techniques, such as quadrapole mass spectrometry (MMS) and multiple reaction monitoring (MRM)[52]. Electron transfer dissociation mass spectroscopy is a novel technique, which is particularly useful in the study of proteins which are post-translationally modified either by glycosylation or phosphorylation [50]. The combination of liquid chromatography and mass spectrometry used in metabolomics for biomarker discovery is currently limited by the lack of metabolite databases and low throughput. Recently, combining transcriptive and proteomic approaches to cancer biomarker discovery are providing new insights into protein and protein network biomarkers [56]. As expected, DNA/RNA studies are best for discovering gene biomarkers involved in genes regulating protein expression and signal transduction processes, whereas protein methods are most useful for biomarkers relating to enzymes, transport proteins, cell mobility components and structural molecules. Selecting the optimal molecular signature in the biomarker discovery process is a very considerable bioinformatics challenge even assuming the analytes are extracted and detected completely and accurately. Four principal bioinformatics processes towards developing the molecular signature for candidate biomarkers have been discussed extensively by Simon [17]. These processes are:

1. Feature selection: detection of differentially expressed genes. In this assessment, distinction should be made between class comparison analyses where the objective is to identify differently expressed genes and class prediction analyses where the objective is to understand biologic mechanisms involving specific genes, particularly mechanisms, which may govern response to particular therapies. Major questions related to molecular signatures include: How many components are optimal? How many genes are sufficient? How many gene classes should be assessed? If too few compounds or too few gene classes are assessed, key associations amongst components that may determine biomarker utility might be missed. If too many components are placed in the algorithm, noise from components that contribute in only a small way to discrimination of the cancer feature can disrupt the integrity of the biomarker "signal". As well, analytical expense limits the practicality of very large signature sets. For optimal strategy in most studies, 10-100 components are thought to be optimal [57]. Accordingly, the trend is to find signatures with as few components as possible, typically on the order of five to 20 components.
2. Selection of the prediction model. This is the algorithm used to predict association of the biomarker with the disease feature.
3. Fitting the prediction model to the training data. This supposes an accurate model and an adequate training set in quality and patient numbers.
4. Estimating prediction error: This component predicts the margin of error of the biomarker and the cancer feature association in future use with independent data sets. This involves sample size planning and, to some extent, requires prior assessment of prediction error in existing data sets. For validation, the development of appropriate algorithms is a science itself and is dependent on the association that is being predicted, the number and types of features to be discriminated, and the practical strategy used to analyze large data sets [33,58].

The key bioinformatics methodologic issues revolve around the capacity to replicate the association findings with subsequent data on the same feature, and the detection of various classes of genes by a common standard so that different and independent data sets can be assessed in similar ways.

25.3. Molecular Signature Biomarkers: Validation

Candidate biomarkers for common cancers are numerous. Ultimately, the relatively few biomarkers that will prove useful clinically will have their association with a specific cancer feature or a well-validated therapy.

Biomarker validation is particularly challenging for molecular signatures or other pattern-based analysis, as large numbers of variables are assessed for small numbers of outcomes. Under these conditions, the possibility of "overfitting", finding a discriminatory pattern by chance, must be overcome [15]. This can be addressed by study design to account for bias, by deployment of sufficiently large data sets, and by comparison of the biomarker cancer feature association with independent data sets for reproducibility.

Within this overall framework, biomarker validation has two components: analytical validation and biologic validation.

1. *Analytic Validation:* The assay must measure the molecules of interest, reproducibly. Analytical validation includes chemistry, tissue microarrays, and bioinformatics. Assay parameters such as accuracy, precision, and range must be well defined. Validation of molecular and molecular signature biomarkers is similar to validation of other chemical biomarkers. The specific analytical issues have been described in detail [6,7,16,59]. A critical issue is the exclusion of signature components related to the presence of inflammation or coagulation or other acute phase reactants to injury [60].

Special challenges for analytical validation of molecular markers relate to DNA/RNA preservation and extraction, detection, and quantitation of multiple markers in same specimen, and the multiple steps required for pre-analytical and analytical methods as well as post-analytical statistical assessment.

Tissue microarray, the technique whereby candidate biomarkers (single or multiple) can be applied to a slide containing hundreds of different tissue samples is an important biomarker validation technology [61,62,63,64,65]. While originally applied using antibodies to protein biomarkers, with hybridization techniques, tissue microarrays can detect and localize gene probes on RNA transcripts within tumor cells. Combined studies to co-localize genomic and protein probes are feasible if fluorescent markers are used. The availability on the same slide of a tumor sample from multiple patients substantially reduces errors related to sequential staining, as well as reducing analysis costs [66].

Validation challenges for imaged molecular biomarkers within cancer cells include adequate localization of biomarkers, preservation of the association between the reporter label and the molecular biomarkers as well as the exclusion of markers associated with active inflammatory cells or tissue repair. For in vivo biomarker imaging, comparison of images over time can be challenging as tissues can be distorted by the effects of disease progression.

Validation methods assess the assay in terms of its reproducibility and accuracy and examine the optimal conditions to generate high performance[16]. Further, analytical validation requires compilation and sharing of data between laboratories, as well as a defined process for assay assessment. Statistical validation requires both internal and external validation [36]. Typically, with internal validation, the study set is split into two groups, a subset to generate the model and a subset to test the prediction of the model. External validation is more rigorous as it applies the model to an independent new data set.

2. *Biologic Validation:* Preferably, biomarkers should be firmly linked to a biological mechanism. This is desirable because association of a biomarker and a clinical feature does not necessarily represent causation. Association without causation is

likely to be coincidental and not likely to withstand validation scrutiny for large data sets [15,17].

A powerful approach to biology validation is the bioinformatics comparison of different molecular signatures from different studies to determine commonality and difference in identifying molecular pathways, and the connections amongst the signature components for each pathway [67,68,69]. The definitive test for biologic validation of biomarker is that a known compound, which blocks or enhances the biologic mechanism affects both the cancer biology and the presence and concentration of the biomarker.

25.4. Molecular Signature Biomarkers: Qualification

Biomarker qualification links the biomarker to both the biologic process and the clinical endpoints [70]. Biomarker qualification is a term reserved for clinical validation and involves the determination of biomarker clinical utility in disease assessment or therapy prediction.

For biomarker qualification, it is necessary to collect clinical data under Good Clinical Practice (GCP) guidelines and to perform the laboratory assays under GLP guidelines. These guidelines assure provenance of each step, as well as independent verification of each process step. Clinical validation requires appropriate clinical trials designed to optimize the amount of information gained. Targeted (or enriched) clinical trials select patients who are pre-screened in the presence or absence of specific marker. The data studied is used to determine the benefit of a treatment in a selected group of patients. In unselected clinical trials, all patients of a disease type or stage are eligible for study. This type of trial requires larger numbers of patients but may yield additional information about the effect of specific treatment [71]. Biomarker qualification involves extensive fit-for-purpose assessment. This is especially true for predictive biomarkers for drug efficacy and drug safety. Selected molecular signature cancer biomarkers, which are qualified and are used to assess therapy, are presented in table 25-3.

Table 25.3. Qualified "Molecular Signature" Predictive Biomarkers (examples)

Disease	Molecular Signature Biomarker	Drug
Breast cancer	HER2	Trastuzumab
Breast cancer	Cytochrome P450 variants	Tamoxifen
Gastrointestinal stromal tumour (GIST)	cKit mutations (exon 9 or 11)	Imatinib
Colorectal cancer	K-ras mutations	EGFR inhibitors (panitumumab, cetuximab)
Non small cell lung cancer	EGFR mutations	Gefinib
Chronic myelogenous leukemia	Ph chromosome	Imatinib

Her2 amplification selects patients for Trastuzumab breast cancer therapy [72,73]. Cytochrome P450 variants affect Tamoxifen exposure and toxicity in breast cancer [74]. c-KIT mutations within exon 11 or exon 9 predict sensitivity to imatinib [75,76,77]. K-RAS mutations confer resistance to EGFR inhibitors panitumumab and cetuximab in colorectal cancer [78,79,80]. Epidermal growth factor receptor (EGFR) mutations increase response to Gefitinib in non-small cell lung cancer [81] and in colorectal cancer, a polymorphism in EGFR results in increased progression-free survival in patients treated with Cetuximab [82].

Even with qualified predictive biomarkers, response to therapy can be complex. For example, Philadelphia chromosome positive patients with chronic myelogenous leukemia respond to Imatinib, but responses are better in those patients that do not have clonal evolution characterized by additional cytogenetic variants [83,84,85]. Similarly in acute lymphoblastic leukemia, patients in the otherwise unfavorable Philadelphia chromosome/BCR-ABL positive subgroup respond to Imatinib when added to other combination therapy [86].

In rare diseases, the small patient populations, the complexity of the molecular signatures, the multiple therapeutic options are factors, which challenge the capacity to demonstrate clinical utility of biomarkers.

Molecular signature prognostic biomarkers are exemplified by introduction of Mammaprint© [87,88] and Oncotype Dx© [89] for breast cancer assessment. Despite relatively high uptake by affected patients, direct evidence for clinical utility remains to be determined [90]. There is optimism that more refined assessment of the data can lead to better predictive value and hence more useful clinical application [32,33,65].

For each biomarker, the time course from discovery to validation, and from validation to qualification has been long. Further qualification of diagnostic methods is often required even after biomarkers have been incorporated into practice. As an example, there remains a critical need for HER2 testing to more accurately predict trastuzumab responders and non-responders. Perhaps the prototype of molecular markers, it is only recently that a molecular signature consisting of HER2 and the reference chromosome marker CEP17 has been deployed [91].

As well, HER2 amplification occurs by two biologic mechanisms, observed with FISH as clustered or non-clustered signals [92,93]. Whether there is a significant difference in clinical response between these two amplification mechanisms, remains to the established. Similarly, the clinical significance of HER2 genomic heterogeneity in tumor tissue domains remains to be assessed [94].

An even more compelling case can be made for molecular signature biomarkers in Tamoxifen therapy. The efficacy of Tamoxifen is reduced in 10% of the population with the cytochrome P450 variant CYP2D6 [74]. With CYP2D6 mutations, patients cannot metabolize Tamoxifen to the active agent Endoxifen.

While Tamoxifen therapy is common, cytochrome P450 molecular signature profiles for Tamoxifen metabolism are rarely tested, perhaps, because it is only recently that such testing is feasible on a routine basis [95,96,97]. Tamoxifen resistance extends beyond CYP2D6 variants to involve Tamoxifen interactions with estrogen receptor types and the coactivation or corepression of estrogen receptor [98]. Molecular signature biomarkers have been developed to address this problem [99,100].

25.5. Molecular Signature Biomarkers: Standardization

Once biomarkers have been accepted into clinical use, it is common that competitive tests emerge, which aspire to be more sensitive or specific. Comparison amongst biomarkers are subject to specific guideline criteria formulated by local, national and international specialty groups [101].

Molecular signature biomarkers pose a specific standardization challenge. For example, even if the signatures are analyzed in the same way, the bioinformatics algorithms employed by different laboratories are likely to be proprietary so that inter-laboratory comparisons cannot be performed easily. Accordingly, the Federal Drug Administration, USA (FDA) developed a guideline for *in vitro* diagnostic multivariate assays (IVDMIA) tests that combine values of multiple analytical variables into a complex computation to yield a single result [102].

Table 25.4. College of American Pathologists Laboratory-Developed Test Oversight Model

Classification	Determining Factors	Oversight	Examples
Low Risk	The test result is often used in conjunction with other findings to establish diagnosis. No claim that test result indicates prognosis or direction of therapy. The test presents low risk to patients.	The laboratory internally performs and reviews validation prior to offering for clinical testing. The accreditor during the normally scheduled inspections will verify that the laboratory performed appropriate validation studies.	Cytokeratin Fragile X
Moderate Risk	The test result is often used for predicting disease progression or identifying whether a patient is eligible for a specific therapy. The laboratory may make claims about clinical accuracy or clinical utility. The test has higher risk to patients.	The laboratory must submit validation studies to the accreditor for an external review prior to offering the test clinically.	KRAS HER2
High Risk	The test result predicts risk, progression, patient eligibility for a specific therapy, AND; The test uses proprietary algorithms or computations such that the test result cannot be tied to the methods used; or inter-laboratory comparisons cannot be performed. The test poses potentially significant risk to patients.	The laboratory must submit a high-risk test to FDA for review prior to offering the test clinically.	Oncotype Dx®

In vitro diagnostic multivariate assays tests would be considered as either Class II (510K) or Class III devices, depending on the clinical consequences from test interpretation and level of control to assure safety and effectiveness. In 2009, the College of American Pathologists (CAP) issued recommendations on laboratory developed tests (LDT)[103]. These are tests used for patient care that are neither FDA cleared nor FDA approved. Because of the evolving regulatory climate, it is likely that molecular signature biomarkers will be developed as LDT for the foreseeable future. The CAP has recommended that LDT oversight be stratified according to clinical level of risk to the patient.

The highest level of risk is assigned to predictive IVD's or LDT's that utilize proprietary algorithms or computation such that the test result cannot be directly compared to the analytical methods used (table 25-4). The current regulatory trend in 2010 is to link the diagnostic marker to the therapeutic risk, implying that markers that definitively guide chemotherapy would be considered as Class III devices.

Conclusion

Molecular signature biomarker development involves extensive processes of translational research and reduction to practice. The introduction of *K-RAS* mutation testing as a predictive marker for epidermal growth factor receptor (EGFR) inhibition therapy in metastatic colorectal cancer is particularly illustrative of these issues [104]. In the 1980's, *RAS* oncogene mutations associated with promoting tumor growth were detected in several human tumor types [105]. A variety of *K-RAS* mutations associated with colorectal carcinoma were subsequently identified but specific clinical application of this knowledge was elusive [106].

In 2006, during clinical trials of the EGFR inhibitor, cetuximab, it was discovered that the approximately 35% of patients who had a molecular signature set of seven particular *K-RAS* mutations were resistant to therapy [80,107]. Subsequently, this was shown to be true also for patients receiving panitumumab, another EGFR inhibitor in the same class [78,79].

Clinical uptake of *K-RAS* mutation testing was extremely rapid, in part because the drug toxicity and the high drug expense could be avoided in 35% of the patient population and, in part, because the selected 65% of the patient population with wild-type *K-RAS*, showed much better response to therapy. This led to considerable discussion amongst regulators as different methods (sequencing, qPCR kit) and different tests involving more mutations could be used to assess therapy.

In an effort towards standardizing the diagnostics, the American Society of Clinical Oncology issued a provisional opinion on testing for *K-RAS* mutations [108]. *K-RAS* mutation testing is an example of a fully qualified biomarker, yet the need for a further step, standardization, remains.

The objectives and key methodologic issues for discovery and development of molecular signature biomarkers are summarized in table 25-5. It is clear that as molecular signature biomarkers progress towards clinical standard of care, progressively extensive and costly analytical and bioinformatics barriers appear. Strategies to reduce these barriers include development of more robust multivariate analytical techniques, as well as more transparent and simpler bioinformatics algorithms.

Most of all, strategies to reduce the variables such as number of probes/signature and a more precise definition of biomarker utility will accelerate the application of molecular signatures into clinical practice.

Table 25.5. Molecular Signature Biomarkers: Discovery and Development Processes

Process	Objective	Key Methodologic Issues
Discovery	Association of biomarker with cancer feature Association with candidate biologic mechanisms	Precision of cancer feature definition Reproducible analytic techniques Availability of candidate biologic mechanisms
Validation	Demonstration of association with independent data set Demonstration of biologic mechanism	Availability of comparable independent data sets Analysis and bioinformatic assessment under Good Laboratory Practice conditions
Qualification	Demonstration of clinical utility in cancer predisposition, screening, diagnostics or therapeutics	Comparable clinical data sets Objective assessment of biomarker utility compared to utility of other biomarkers or standard of care previous to biomarker
Standardization	Demonstration that each method for assessment of particular biomarker is comparable in sensitivity, specificity, to originally qualified biomarker Demonstration of safety and efficacy of biomarker in clinical practice	Availability of biomarker for routine clinical use (ease of use, cost) Quantitative comparison of test methods for the biomarker with similar biomarkers for sensitivity, specificity, cost/benefit

References

[1] Dakubo GD, Jakupciak JP, Birch-Machin MA, Parr RL (2007) Clinical implications and utility of field cancerization. *Cancer Cell Int.* 7: 2.

[2] Nelson HD, Huffman LH, Fu R, Harris EL (2005) Genetic risk assessment and BRCA mutation testing for breast and ovarian cancer susceptibility: systematic evidence review for the U.S. Preventive Services Task Force. *Ann. Intern. Med.* 143: 362-379.

[3] Venkitaraman AR (2009) Linking the cellular functions of BRCA genes to cancer pathogenesis and treatment. *Annu. Rev. Pathol.* 4: 461-487.

[4] Lynch HT, Lynch JF, Attard TA (2009) Diagnosis and management of hereditary colorectal cancer syndromes: Lynch syndrome as a model. *CMAJ* 181: 273-280.

[5] Pritzker KPH (2002) Cancer biomarkers: easier said than done. *Clin. Chem.* 48: 1147-1150.

[6] Pritzker KPH, Azad A (2004) Genomic biomarkers for cancer assessment: implementation challenges for laboratory practice. *Clin. Biochem.* 37: 642-646.

[7] Pritzker KPH, Azad A (2005) Bringing biomarkers to clinical practice. *Clinical Lab. International* 25: 24.

[8] Chigira M, Shinozaki T, Shimizu T, Noda K (1990) No correlation between tumor markers and prognosis under polygenic control systems. *MedHypotheses* 32: 245-247.

[9] Rubin H (1990) The significance of biological heterogeneity. *Cancer Metastasis Rev.* 9: 1-20.

[10] Biomarkers Definitions Working Group B (2001) Biomarkers and surrogate endpoints: preferred definitions and conceptual framework. *Clin. Pharmacol. Ther.* 69: 89-95.

[11] Negm RS, Verma M, Srivastava S (2002) The promise of biomarkers in cancer screening and detection. *Trends Mol. Med.* 8: 288-293.

[12] Wagner JA, Williams SA, Webster CJ (2007) Biomarkers and surrogate end points for fit-for-purpose development and regulatory evaluation of new drugs. *Clin. Pharmacol. Ther.* 81: 104-107.

[13] Niedbala RS, Mauck C, Harrison P, Doncel GF (2009) Biomarker discovery: validation and decision-making in product development. *Sex Transm. Dis.* 36: S76-80.

[14] Schulte PA (1989) A conceptual framework for the validation and use of biologic markers. *Environ. Res.* 48: 129-144.

[15] Ransohoff DF (2004) Rules of evidence for cancer molecular-marker discovery and validation. *Nat. Rev. Cancer* 4: 309-314.

[16] Chau CH, Rixe O, McLeod H, Figg WD (2008) Validation of analytic methods for biomarkers used in drug development. *Clin. Cancer Res.* 14: 5967-5976.

[17] Simon R (2008) Development and Validation of Biomarker Classifiers for Treatment Selection. *J. Stat. Plan Inference* 138: 308-320.

[18] Parker A, McCaffery I, Patterson S (2009) Examining molecular biology in humans. *Biotechniques* 46: 358-360.

[19] Mildvan D, Landay A, De GV, Machado SG, Kagan J (1997) An approach to the validation of markers for use in AIDS clinical trials. *ClinInfectDis.* 24: 764-774.

[20] Bauer DC, Hunter DJ, Abramson SB, Attur M, Corr M, et al. (2006) Classification of osteoarthritis biomarkers: a proposed approach. *Osteoarthritis Cartilage* 14: 723-727.

[21] Duffy MJ (2007) Role of tumor markers in patients with solid cancers: A critical review. *Eur. J. Intern. Med.* 18: 175-184.

[22] Shinozaki T, Chigira M, Kato K (1992) Multivariate analysis of serum tumor markers for diagnosis of skeletal metastases. *Cancer* 69: 108-112.

[23] Fernandis AZ, Wenk MR (2009) Lipid-based biomarkers for cancer. *J. Chromatogr. B. Analyt. Technol. Biomed. Life Sci.*.

[24] Duffy MJ, Napieralski R, Martens JW, Span PN, Spyratos F, et al. (2009) Methylated genes as new cancer biomarkers. *Eur. J. Cancer* 45: 335-346.

[25] Gelato KA, Fischle W (2008) Role of histone modifications in defining chromatin structure and function. *Biol. Chem.* 389: 353-363.

[26] Armstrong SA, Golub TR, Korsmeyer SJ (2003) MLL-rearranged leukemias: insights from gene expression profiling. *Semin. Hematol.* 40: 268-273.

[27] Mistry AR, Pedersen EW, Solomon E, Grimwade D (2003) The molecular pathogenesis of acute promyelocytic leukaemia: implications for the clinical management of the disease. *Blood Rev.* 17: 71-97.

[28] Lehrmann H, Pritchard LL, Harel-Bellan A (2002) Histone acetyltransferases and deacetylases in the control of cell proliferation and differentiation. *Adv. Cancer Res.* 86: 41-65.

[29] Schiess R, Wollscheid B, Aebersold R (2009) Targeted proteomic strategy for clinical biomarker discovery. *Mol. Oncol.* 3: 33-44.

[30] Hartmann O, Spyratos F, Harbeck N, Dietrich D, Fassbender A, et al. (2009) DNA methylation markers predict outcome in node-positive, estrogen receptor-positive breast cancer with adjuvant anthracycline-based chemotherapy. *Clin. Cancer Res.* 15: 315-323.

[31] van der Kwast TH, Bapat B (2009) Predicting favourable prognosis of urothelial carcinoma: gene expression and genome profiling. *Curr. Opin. Urol.* 19: 516-521.

[32] Taylor IW, Linding R, Warde-Farley D, Liu Y, Pesquita C, et al. (2009) Dynamic modularity in protein interaction networks predicts breast cancer outcome. *Nat. Biotechnol.* 27: 199-204.

[33] Sun Y, Goodison S (2009) Optimizing molecular signatures for predicting prostate cancer recurrence. *Prostate* 69: 1119-1127.

[34] Lee JW, Devanarayan V, Barrett YC, Weiner R, Allinson J, et al. (2006) Fit-for-purpose method development and validation for successful biomarker measurement. *Pharm. Res.* 23: 312-328.

[35] De Gruttola VG, Clax P, DeMets DL, Downing GJ, Ellenberg SS, et al. (2001) Considerations in the evaluation of surrogate endpoints in clinical trials. summary of a National Institutes of Health workshop. *Control ClinTrials* 22: 485-502.

[36] Taylor JM, Ankerst DP, Andridge RR (2008) Validation of biomarker-based risk prediction models. *Clin. Cancer Res.* 14: 5977-5983.

[37] Bild AH, Parker JS, Gustafson AM, Acharya CR, Hoadley KA, et al. (2009) An integration of complementary strategies for gene-expression analysis to reveal novel therapeutic opportunities for breast cancer. *Breast Cancer Res* 11: R55.

[38] Gupta AK, Brenner DE, Turgeon DK (2008) Early detection of colon cancer: new tests on the horizon. *Mol. Diagn. Ther.* 12: 77-85.

[39] Pavlou M, Diamandis EP (2009) The search for new prostate cancer biomarkers continues. *Clin. Chem.* 55: 1277-1279.

[40] Makarov DV, Loeb S, Getzenberg RH, Partin AW (2008) Biomarkers for Prostate Cancer. *Annu. Rev. Med.*

[41] Sotiriou C, Pusztai L (2009) Gene-expression signatures in breast cancer. *N. Engl. J. Med.* 360: 790-800.

[42] Easton DF, Eeles RA (2008) Genome-wide association studies in cancer. *Hum. Mol. Genet.* 17: R109-115.

[43] Best CJ, Gillespie JW, Englert CR, Swalwell JI, Pfeifer J, et al. (2000) New approaches to molecular profiling of tissue samples. *AnalCell Pathol.* 20: 1-6.

[44] Rai AJ, Kamath RM, Gerald W, Fleisher M (2009) Analytical validation of the GeXP analyzer and design of a workflow for cancer-biomarker discovery using multiplexed gene-expression profiling. *Anal. Bioanal. Chem.* 393: 1505-1511.

[45] Saleh EM, El-Awady RA, Abdel Alim MA, Abdel Wahab AH (2009) Altered Expression of Proliferation-Inducing and Proliferation-Inhibiting Genes Might Contribute to Acquired Doxorubicin Resistance in Breast Cancer Cells. *Cell Biochem.* Biophys.

[46] Emmert-Buck MR, Strausberg RL, Krizman DB, Bonaldo MF, Bonner RF, et al. (2000) Molecular profiling of clinical tissue specimens: feasibility and applications. *Am. J. Pathol.* 156: 1109-1115.

[47] Tian Q, Stepaniants SB, Mao M, Weng L, Feetham MC, et al. (2004) Integrated genomic and proteomic analyses of gene expression in Mammalian cells. *Mol. Cell Proteomics* 3: 960-969.

[48] Rautio JJ, Kataja K, Satokari R, Penttila M, Soderlund H, et al. (2006) Rapid and multiplexed transcript analysis of microbial cultures using capillary electophoresis-detectable oligonucleotide probe pools. *J. Microbiol. Methods* 65: 404-416.

[49] Estilo CL, P Oc, Talbot S, Socci ND, Carlson DL, et al. (2009) Oral tongue cancer gene expression profiling: Identification of novel potential prognosticators by oligonucleotide microarray analysis. *BMC Cancer* 9: 11.

[50] Wong SC, Chan CM, Ma BB, Lam MY, Choi GC, et al. (2009) Advanced proteomic technologies for cancer biomarker discovery. *Expert Rev. Proteomics* 6: 123-134.

[51] Hood BL, Stewart NA, Conrads TP (2009) Development of high-throughput mass spectrometry-based approaches for cancer biomarker discovery and implementation. *Clin. Lab. Med.* 29: 115-138.

[52] McIntosh M, Fitzgibbon M (2009) Biomarker validation by targeted mass spectrometry. *Nat. Biotechnol.* 27: 622-623.

[53] Simpson KL, Whetton AD, Dive C (2009) Quantitative mass spectrometry-based techniques for clinical use: biomarker identification and quantification. *J. Chromatogr. B. Analyt. Technol. Biomed. Life Sci.* 877: 1240-1249.

[54] Li G, Zhang W, Zeng H, Chen L, Wang W, et al. (2009) An integrative multi-platform analysis for discovering biomarkers of osteosarcoma. *BMC Cancer* 9: 150.

[55] Cadron I, Van Gorp T, Amant F, Vergote I, Moerman P, et al. (2009) The use of laser microdissection and SELDI-TOF MS in ovarian cancer tissue to identify protein profiles. *Anticancer Res.* 29: 1039-1045.

[56] Seliger B, Dressler SP, Wang E, Kellner R, Recktenwald CV, et al. (2009) Combined analysis of transcriptome and proteome data as a tool for the identification of candidate biomarkers in renal cell carcinoma. *Proteomics* 9: 1567-1581.

[57] Dudoit S, Fridlyand J (2003) Classification in microarray experiments. In: Speed T, editor. Statistical Analysis of Gene Expression Microarray Data. New York: Chapman and Hall, CRC Press. pp. 93-158.

[58] Sun Y, Urquidi V, Goodison S (2009) Derivation of molecular signatures for breast cancer recurrence prediction using a two-way validation approach. *Breast Cancer Res.* Treat.

[59] Veltri RW, Miller MC, An G (2001) Standardization, analytical validation, and quality control of intermediate endpoint biomarkers. *Urology* 57: 164-170.

[60] Nosov V, Su F, Amneus M, Birrer M, Robins T, et al. (2009) Validation of serum biomarkers for detection of early-stage ovarian cancer. *Am. J. Obstet. Gynecol.* 200: 639 e631-635.

[61] Hoos A, Urist MJ, Stojadinovic A, Mastorides S, Dudas ME, et al. (2001) Validation of tissue microarrays for immunohistochemical profiling of cancer specimens using the example of human fibroblastic tumors. *Am. J. Pathol.* 158: 1245-1251.

[62] Hewitt SM (2009) Tissue microarrays as a tool in the discovery and validation of tumor markers. *Methods Mol. Biol.* 520: 151-161.

[63] Camp RL, Neumeister V, Rimm DL (2008) A decade of tissue microarrays: progress in the discovery and validation of cancer biomarkers. *J. Clin. Oncol.* 26: 5630-5637.
[64] van der Vegt B, de Bock GH, Hollema H, Wesseling J (2009) Microarray methods to identify factors determining breast cancer progression: potentials, limitations, and challenges. *Crit. Rev. Oncol. Hematol.* 70: 1-11.
[65] Lexe G, Monaco J, Doyle S, Basavanhally A, Reddy A, et al. (2009) Towards improved cancer diagnosis and prognosis using analysis of gene expression data and computer aided imaging. *Exp. Biol. Med.* (Maywood) 234: 860-879.
[66] Fons G, van der Velden J, Burger M, ten Kate F (2009) Validation of tissue microarray technology in vulvar cancer. *Int. J. Gynecol. Pathol.* 28: 76-82.
[67] Lucas JE, Carvalho CM, Chen JL, Chi JT, West M (2009) Cross-study projections of genomic biomarkers: an evaluation in cancer genomics. *PLoS One* 4: e4523.
[68] Reyal F, van Vliet MH, Armstrong NJ, Horlings HM, de Visser KE, et al. (2008) A comprehensive analysis of prognostic signatures reveals the high predictive capacity of the proliferation, immune response and RNA splicing modules in breast cancer. *Breast Cancer Res.* 10: R93.
[69] Sole X, Bonifaci N, Lopez-Bigas N, Berenguer A, Hernandez P, et al. (2009) Biological convergence of cancer signatures. *PLoS One* 4: e4544.
[70] Wagner JA (2002) Overview of biomarkers and surrogate endpoints in drug development. *Dis. Markers* 18: 41-46.
[71] Mandrekar SJ, Sargent DJ (2009) Clinical trial designs for predictive biomarker validation: one size does not fit all. *J. Biopharm. Stat.* 19: 530-542.
[72] Slamon DJ, Leyland-Jones B, Shak S, Fuchs H, Paton V, et al. (2001) Use of chemotherapy plus a monoclonal antibody against HER2 for metastatic breast cancer that overexpresses HER2. *N. Engl. J. Med.* 344: 783-792.
[73] Vogel CL, Cobleigh MA, Tripathy D, Gutheil JC, Harris LN, et al. (2002) Efficacy and safety of trastuzumab as a single agent in first-line treatment of HER2-overexpressing metastatic breast cancer. *J. Clin. Oncol.* 20: 719-726.
[74] Wu X, Hawse JR, Subramaniam M, Goetz MP, Ingle JN, et al. (2009) The tamoxifen metabolite, endoxifen, is a potent antiestrogen that targets estrogen receptor alpha for degradation in breast cancer cells. *Cancer Res.* 69: 1722-1727.
[75] Hornick JL, Fletcher CD (2007) The role of KIT in the management of patients with gastrointestinal stromal tumors. *Hum. Pathol.* 38: 679-687.
[76] Cassier PA, Dufresne A, Arifi S, El Sayadi H, Labidi I, et al. (2008) Imatinib mesilate for the treatment of gastrointestinal stromal tumour. *Expert Opin. Pharmacother* 9: 1211-1222.
[77] Lasota J, Miettinen M (2008) Clinical significance of oncogenic KIT and PDGFRA mutations in gastrointestinal stromal tumours. *Histopathology* 53: 245-266.
[78] Mack GS (2009) FDA holds court on post hoc data linking KRAS status to drug response. *Nat. Biotechnol.* 27: 110-112.
[79] Sheridan C (2008) EGFR inhibitors embrace KRAS. *Nat. Biotechnol.* 26: 839-840.
[80] Lievre A, Bachet JB, Boige V, Cayre A, Le Corre D, et al. (2008) KRAS mutations as an independent prognostic factor in patients with advanced colorectal cancer treated with cetuximab. *J. Clin. Oncol.* 26: 374-379.

[81] Sequist LV, Martins RG, Spigel D, Grunberg SM, Spira A, et al. (2008) First-line gefitinib in patients with advanced non-small-cell lung cancer harboring somatic EGFR mutations. *J. Clin. Oncol.* 26: 2442-2449.

[82] Goncalves A, Esteyries S, Taylor-Smedra B, Lagarde A, Ayadi M, et al. (2008) A polymorphism of EGFR extracellular domain is associated with progression free-survival in metastatic colorectal cancer patients receiving cetuximab-based treatment. *BMC Cancer* 8: 169.

[83] Druker BJ (2003) Imatinib alone and in combination for chronic myeloid leukemia. *Semin. Hematol.* 40: 50-58.

[84] Deininger MW (2003) Cytogenetic studies in patients on imatinib. *Semin. Hematol.* 40: 50-55.

[85] Jabbour E, Cortes J, O'Brien S, Giles F, Kantarjian H (2007) New targeted therapies for chronic myelogenous leukemia: opportunities to overcome imatinib resistance. *Semin. Hematol.* 44: S25-31.

[86] Gokbuget N, Hoelzer D (2009) Treatment of adult acute lymphoblastic leukemia. *Semin. Hematol.* 46: 64-75.

[87] Buyse M, Loi S, van't Veer L, Viale G, Delorenzi M, et al. (2006) Validation and clinical utility of a 70-gene prognostic signature for women with node-negative breast cancer. *J. Natl. Cancer Inst.* 98: 1183-1192.

[88] Brauch H, Murdter TE, Eichelbaum M, Schwab M (2009) Pharmacogenomics of tamoxifen therapy. *Clin. Chem.* 55: 1770-1782.

[89] Paik S, Tang G, Shak S, Kim C, Baker J, et al. (2006) Gene expression and benefit of chemotherapy in women with node-negative, estrogen receptor-positive breast cancer. *J. Clin. Oncol.* 24: 3726-3734.

[90] EGAPP (2009) Recommendations from the EGAPP Working Group: can tumor gene expression profiling improve outcomes in patients with breast cancer? *Genet. Med.* 11: 66-73.

[91] Bartlett JM, Campbell FM, Mallon EA (2008) Determination of HER2 amplification by in situ hybridization: when should chromosome 17 also be determined? *Am. J. Clin. Pathol.* 130: 920-926.

[92] Chibon F, de Mascarel I, Sierankowski G, Brouste V, Bonnefoi H, et al. (2009) Prediction of HER2 gene status in Her2 2+ invasive breast cancer: a study of 108 cases comparing ASCO/CAP and FDA recommendations. *Mod. Pathol.* 22: 403-409.

[93] Rogers M, Dore JH, Grunkin M, Pritzker KPH. Advancing breast cancer HER2 FISH quality by image analysis (abstract) 2009 December 9-13, 2009; San Antonio, Texas, USA.

[94] Vance GH, Barry TS, Bloom KJ, Fitzgibbons PL, Hicks DG, et al. (2009) Genetic heterogeneity in HER2 testing in breast cancer: panel summary and guidelines. *Arch. Pathol. Lab. Med.* 133: 611-612.

[95] Goetz MP, Knox SK, Suman VJ, Rae JM, Safgren SL, et al. (2007) The impact of cytochrome P450 2D6 metabolism in women receiving adjuvant tamoxifen. *Breast Cancer Res Treat* 101: 113-121.

[96] Jin Y, Desta Z, Stearns V, Ward B, Ho H, et al. (2005) CYP2D6 genotype, antidepressant use, and tamoxifen metabolism during adjuvant breast cancer treatment. *J. Natl. Cancer Inst.* 97: 30-39.

[97] Punglia RS, Burstein HJ, Winer EP, Weeks JC (2008) Pharmacogenomic variation of CYP2D6 and the choice of optimal adjuvant endocrine therapy for postmenopausal breast cancer: a modeling analysis. *J. Natl. Cancer Inst.* 100: 642-648.

[98] Girault I, Bieche I, Lidereau R (2006) Role of estrogen receptor alpha transcriptional coregulators in tamoxifen resistance in breast cancer. *Maturitas* 54: 342-351.

[99] Jansen MP, Foekens JA, van Staveren IL, Dirkzwager-Kiel MM, Ritstier K, et al. (2005) Molecular classification of tamoxifen-resistant breast carcinomas by gene expression profiling. *J. Clin. Oncol.* 23: 732-740.

[100] Meijer D, Jansen MP, Look MP, Ruigrok-Ritstier K, van Staveren IL, et al. (2009) TSC22D1 and PSAP predict clinical outcome of tamoxifen treatment in patients with recurrent breast cancer. *Breast Cancer Res. Treat.* 113: 253-260.

[101] Sturgeon CM (2001) Tumor markers in the laboratory: closing the guideline-practice gap. *Clin. Biochem.* 34: 353-359.

[102] FDA (2007) Draft guidance for industry, clinical laboratories, and FDA staff: in vitro diagnostic multivariate index assays. In: Administration FD, editor: FDA.

[103] CAP (2009) Laboratory-developed test oversight model.

[104] Monzon FA, Ogino S, Hammond ME, Halling KC, Bloom KJ, et al. (2009) The role of KRAS mutation testing in the management of patients with metastatic colorectal cancer. *Arch. Pathol. Lab. Med.* 133: 1600-1606.

[105] Bos JL (1989) ras oncogenes in human cancer: a review. *Cancer Res.* 49: 4682-4689.

[106] Ko JM, Cheung MH, Wong CM, Lau KW, Tang CM, et al. (1998) Ki-ras codon 12 point mutational activation in Hong Kong colorectal carcinoma patients. *Cancer Lett.* 134: 169-176.

[107] Lievre A, Bachet JB, Le Corre D, Boige V, Landi B, et al. (2006) KRAS mutation status is predictive of response to cetuximab therapy in colorectal cancer. *Cancer Res.* 66: 3992-3995.

[108] Allegra CJ, Jessup JM, Somerfield MR, Hamilton SR, Hammond EH, et al. (2009) American Society of Clinical Oncology provisional clinical opinion: testing for KRAS gene mutations in patients with metastatic colorectal carcinoma to predict response to anti-epidermal growth factor receptor monoclonal antibody therapy. *J. Clin. Oncol.* 27: 2091-2096.

In: Field Cancerization: Basic Science and Clinical Applications ISBN 978-1-61761-006-6
Editor: Gabriel D. Dakubo

Chapter 26

Chemoprevention Targeting Epigenetic Changes in Cancer

Fiona S. Poke and Adele F. Holloway

Abstract

The contribution of epigenetic changes to cancer development and progression is now well recognized. A myriad of altered epigenetic states have been found between normal and cancer cells, contributing to the aberrant gene expression patterns associated with cancer. The enzymes involved in catalyzing these epigenetic modifications have become prime targets for therapeutic intervention. The discovery of a range of natural and chemically synthesized inhibitors of these enzymes has shown enormous promise in restoring altered gene expression patterns by re-establishing the correct epigenetic information. In this chapter we describe epigenetic information and how it can be linked to cancer, the enzymes responsible for the coordination of the epigenetic state found within a cell, and the range of inhibitors that have been developed to target these enzymes as well as their use in cancer treatment.

26.1. Introduction

Epigenetic information encompasses all the physical and chemical modifications to chromatin, but excludes changes to the DNA sequence itself. Epigenetic information can be generated in two ways: through the methylation of cytosine residues in the DNA sequence; or through a range of chemical modifications or physical remodeling of the histone proteins which package DNA into chromatin. This information can be somatically, and in some cases meiotically, inherited. The contribution of genetic changes to cancer development and progression has long been recognized, and now the involvement of epigenetic changes is becoming increasingly apparent. Epigenetic modifications can influence gene expression in normal cells, and changes to the epigenetic information can lead to the aberrant gene expression patterns seen in cancer cells. Epigenetic modifications can generally be reversed and therefore offer a potential therapeutic target for the treatment and prevention of cancer. Considerable effort is therefore being given to the development of therapies targeting the epigenetic changes that are associated with cancer.

26.2. Epigenetic Modifications

Within the nucleus, DNA is packaged into a nucleoprotein complex called chromatin. Approximately 147 base pairs of DNA is wrapped around an octamer of four histone proteins, H2A, H2B, H3 and H4, to form a nucleosome, the fundamental unit of chromatin [1]. This linear array of nucleosomes is compacted further to form chromosomes. Chromatin is composed of highly compacted regions called heterochromatin that generally contains silenced genes, and more loosely compacted regions called euchromatin, which contains the more actively transcribed genes. These states are highly dynamic within a cell and are capable of changing rapidly, and therefore contribute to the regulation of gene expression in response to cellular signals. Changes to chromatin are facilitated by protein complexes, which modify the core histone proteins or physically remodel nucleosomes. DNA can also be methylated which can alter the chromatin environment so as to allow transcription factor binding and gene transcription to occur.

26.2.1. DNA Methylation

The methylation of DNA involves the covalent addition of a methyl group to a cytosine residue that is positioned 5' to a guanine residue (CpG) by a family of enzymes called DNA methyltransferases. The 5' regions of genes are associated with a high density of CpGs, called CpG islands, and these are for the most part unmethylated [2]. There is a strong link between the methylation of CpG islands in promoters and gene silencing. The methylation of DNA can lead to the direct blocking of transcription factor binding or can act as a binding site for methyl-CpG binding proteins which are associated with repressive chromatin complexes [2]. There is growing evidence to suggest that there is a connection or cross talk between DNA methylation and histone modifications in regulating gene expression [reviewed in 3].

26.2.2. Histone Modifications

Eight different histone modifications have been described that primarily occur at residues in the N-terminal of histone tails. These modifications include acetylation, methylation, phosphorylation, ubiquitination, sumoylation, ADP ribosylation, deimination and proline isomerisation [4]. While the majority of these modifications are poorly understood, it is known that they affect chromatin structure and function. The best-studied histone modifications are the acetylation of lysine residues and the methylation of lysines and arginines.

Histones can be acetylated on lysine residues only. Histone acetylation is generally correlated with a transcriptionally permissive chromatin environment. Acetylation of lysine neutralizes the positive charge of the highly basic histone tails, changing the interaction between histones and the negatively charged DNA [5]. This directly affects chromatin packaging and increases accessibility to transcription factor binding sites, so that a transcriptionally competent conformation is created.

Histone methylation correlates with different functional states depending on the residue methylated and the number of times it is modified. Both lysine and arginine residues can be methylated with up to three methyl groups potentially being added to lysine and one or two groups to arginines. Histone methylation does not affect the charge of the histone tails but alters basicity, hydrophobicity and the affinity for anionic molecules such as DNA as well as proteins such as transcription factors. A myriad of histone methylation marks have been associated with gene activation including tri-methylation of lysine 4 (H3K4me3) and mono-methylation of lysine 9 (H3K9me1) and 27 (H3K27me1) on histone H3. However, conversion of the H3K9me1 and H3K27me1 marks to di- and tri-methylation (H3K9me2/3 and H3K27me2/3) is associated with gene repression.

Many of the modified histone residues act as anchor sites for proteins and protein complexes, which are able to modify chromatin structure and function. This allows the formation of certain chromatin conformations as well as the propagation of this state to neighboring regions. The concept of histone modifications influencing DNA functioning in this way has been termed the 'histone code' [4]. The proteins that bind to modified histone residues include a host of chromatin remodeling complexes, which are large multi-subunit complexes containing up to 12 proteins [reviewed in 6]. The best described of these are the SWI/SNF and NURD complexes. These complexes have either a bromodomain or a chromodomain, which allows them to bind to acetylated histones or methylated histones, respectively. These complexes also have a central ATPase component, which utilize the energy of ATP hydrolysis to physically remove or slide the histones from DNA, increasing DNA accessibility to regulatory proteins and/or transcription factors, and thereby influencing gene activity.

Epigenetic modifications appear to act in concert to facilitate a particular outcome. For example, silenced genes in heterochromatin are generally characterized by DNA hypermethylation, histone hypoacetylation and H3K9 trimethylation. These modifications have also been found to be associated with gene silencing in euchromatin.

26.3. Epigenetic Changes Associated with Cancer

Many studies have demonstrated an association between epigenetic changes and cancer [reviewed in 7,8]. Differences in the epigenetic information, including histone marks and DNA methylation patterns, have been observed between normal and cancer cells. Changes in DNA methylation patterns have been observed in virtually all cancers studied. In many cases the epigenetic changes in cancer cells result in the activation of oncogenes and the aberrant silencing of genes such as tumor suppressor genes, anti-apoptotic genes and genes functioning as part of the DNA repair machinery. In colorectal cancer for example, H3K9 methylation, H3K9 deacetylation and DNA hypermethylation correlate with the silencing of tumor suppressor genes [9,10]. However, DNA hypomethylation has also been linked to cancer by generating genomic instability [11]. These changes in cancer cells are often strongly correlated with a change in expression of the enzymes that generate the epigenetic modifications. For example HDAC expression is upregulated in many cancer types [reviewed in 12]. The contribution of epigenetic changes to cancer development and progression, and the potential for reversing them makes them a prime target for therapeutic intervention.

26.4. Epigenetic Targets for Therapy

Given that epigenetic modifications are reversible, the enzymes that catalyse these modifications are targets for therapeutic intervention. Recent studies have shown that epigenetic alterations are likely promoted through an association between the enzymes that generate the epigenetic modifications and oncogenic proteins [reviewed in 13]. For example, gene silencing in Acute Promyelocytic Leukemia has been attributed to the leukemia-promoting PML-RAR fusion protein recruiting DNA methyltransferases, histone methyltransfereases (SUV39H1), HDAC3 and methyl CpG binding protein MBD1 to target promoters, leading to hypermethylation, an increase in the repressive H3K9me3 mark and reduced histone acetylation [14,15,16]. The best-studied epigenetic modifications are DNA methylation, and histone acetylation and methylation, and therefore the enzymes, which catalyze these processes, are well studied.

26.4.1. DNA Methylation

DNA methylation transpires in two different ways during development. First is de novo methylation that occurs during embryogenesis and cell differentiation, and this is where methylation patterns become rearranged. Second is the maintenance of these methylation patterns in adult cells, particularly across cell division. Different DNA methyltransferases (DNMTs) carry out the DNA methylation involved in these processes. DNA methyltransferases are a family of enzymes that work by transferring a methyl group from a donor molecule such as S-adenosylmethionine (SAM) to position 5 of the pyrimidine ring of a cytosine. In humans, DNMTs 1 and 2 are responsible for DNA methylation maintenance and 3a and 3b for de novo DNA methylation, although functional redundancy has been demonstrated [2].

26.4.2. Histone Acetylation

The acetylation of lysine residues in histones is the best studied of the histone modifications and concordantly so are the enzymes, which catalyse the addition or removal of acetyl groups. Histone acetyltransferases (HATs) are responsible for the transfer of acetyl groups from acetyl coenzyme A to lysine residues, while removal is facilitated by histone deacetylases (HDACs). The acetylation status of genes and therefore their expression is determined by the competing action of these enzymes [17]. Many HATs have been described, and many previously described transcriptional coactivators have now been shown to possess HAT activity [18]. Many of these are highly specific in the genes they target and the lysine residues they modify. The role of HATs in cancer is complicated as they have been demonstrated to be tumor suppressors and activators depending on the type of tumor and stage of growth [reviewed in 19].

At least 18 HDACs have been described in humans. Histone deacetylases can be divided into four classes: class I which are primarily nuclear and relatively ubiquitous; class II which shuttle between the nucleus and cytoplasm and are cell type specific; class III which are evolutionary distinct and are NAD-dependent; and class IV which contains a novel protein HDAC11 that is structurally related to class I and II HDACs [reviewed in 12]. Class I and II HDACs are similar in that they contain a conserved core deacetylase domain of around 400 amino acids, are zinc dependent and have considerable functional redundancy. Histone deacetylases also have restricted substrate specificity similar to HATs. The association of these enzymes with the abnormal acetylation and gene expression profiles seen in cancer is now well recognized [20,21]. Class I and II HDACs have been shown to be associated with oncogenic proteins in leukaemia, contributing to aberrant gene expression [22,23]. The best-studied human class III HDACs is the sirtuin family (Sirt1 and Sirt2). These enzymes have a highly conserved approximately 275 amino acid catalytic domain and use NAD hydrolysis to deacetylate lysine residues. Altered expression profiles of the sirtuins have been found associated with cancer [24]. For example, Sirt1 is overexpressed in prostate cancer cells compared to normal cells, and in prostate cancer tissues compared to adjacent normal tissue [25,26]. These enzymes are prime targets for therapeutic intervention in cancer.

26.4.3. Histone Methylation

More than 29 histone-methylating enzymes have been described in humans [27]. These can be divided into three general classes: SET domain lysine methyltransferases; non-SET domain lysine methyltransferases; and arginine methyltransferases. These enzymes all transfer methyl groups from SAM to the lysine or arginine residue, but do so in a highly specific manner, with each generally only modifying one particular residue. For example, SMYD3 has been shown to have specific H3 lysine 4 methyltransferase activity [28]. Many of the known histone methyltransferases are shown to have altered expression profiles in cancer [recently reviewed in 27]. SMYD3 for example is overexpressed in colorectal and hepatocellular carcinomas as well as breast cancer cells, and its knockdown has been found to inhibit cancer cell growth [28,29,30]. Overexpression of another histone methyltransferase, EZH2, has been found associated with breast cancer, prostate cancer, multiple myeloma and lymphoma [31,32].

While lysine methylation was initially thought to be a stable modification, several histone lysine demethylases have also been identified [reviewed in 33]. There are two main types: the amino oxidase lysine demethylase 1 (LSD1) and the Jumonji domain proteins. Lysine demethylase 1 can demethylate both active and repressive mono- and di-methylation marks, as well as non-histone proteins. The Jumonji proteins additionally target tri-methylated marks but different members of this protein family show specificity in the residue as well as the methylation state that they target [33]. Histone lysine demethylases appear to be part of large complexes and are likely to cooperate with other histone modifiers to regulate gene activity.

Although less is known about the enzymes involved in regulating histone methylation, they have been implicated in cancer and have good potential as targets for cancer treatment.

26.5. Therapeutic Agents for Chemoprevention

Over recent years, considerable advancement has been made in the identification and development of inhibitors that are primarily directed against the enzymes involved in DNA methylation (DNMTs), histone deacetylation (HDACs) and histone methylation (histone methyltransferases) (figure 26-1). These modifications are the best targets for therapeutic intervention in cancer as they are relatively well characterized, as are the enzymes that catalyze them. Epigenetic modifications both vary and overlap between different cells and cell types, and are also highly dynamic in response to changing cellular signals, therefore tailoring treatment specifically to cancer cells alone will be difficult to achieve. In addition, toxicity of some of these compounds will be a concern. However, many inhibitors have surpassed laboratory testing and are now in the advanced stages of clinical trials offering promising results for cancer treatment [recently reviewed in 19,34,35,36]. Research into this type of treatment for cancer has primarily concentrated on haemotological malignancies such as leukemia, however the focus on solid tumors is increasing.

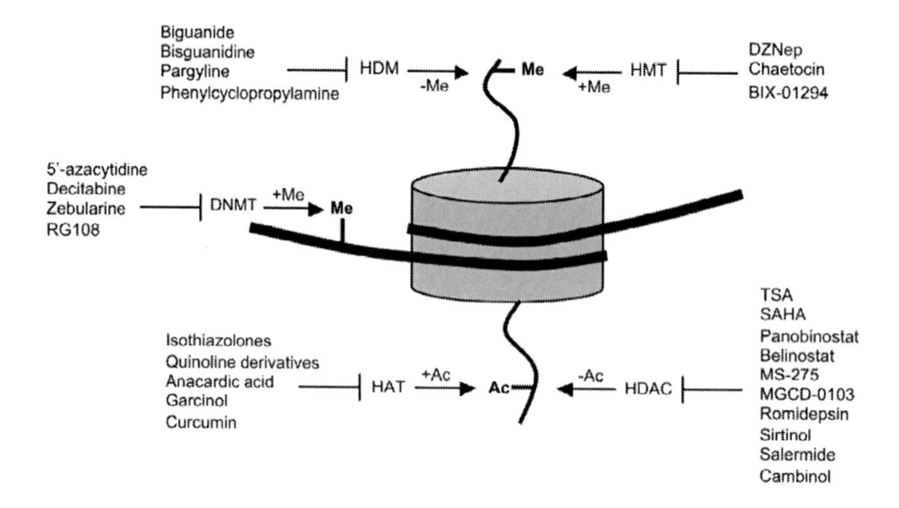

Figure 26.1. Inhibitors targeting epigenetic changes in cancer. Me = methyl group, Ac = acetyl group, DNMT = DNA methyltransferase, HAT = histone acetyltransferase, HDAC = histone deacetylase; HMT = histone methyltransferase, HDM = histone demethylase.

26.5.1. DNA Methyltransferase Inhibitors

The majority of DNMT inhibitors are nucleoside analogues. The best known of these is 5'-azacytidine. It is a ribose nucleoside that is converted within the cell to deoxynucleoside triphosphate, which can be incorporated into the DNA sequence during replication in place of cytosine. Similar to cytosine, it can be methylated by DNMTs, however, its modified pyrimidine ring prevents the methyl group from being transferred and the DNMT becomes covalently bound to the DNA [37,38]. Consequently the pool of DNMTs is reduced within the cell and DNA becomes progressively demethylated, as newly synthesized DNA cannot be methylated. While this mode of inhibition is particularly effective, the covalent trapping of DNMTs is toxic to the cell. RNA viability is also compromised as 5'-azacytidine can be incorporated into RNA. However, the effectiveness of this compound in reducing DNA methylation and reactivating silenced genes in cancer cells has been demonstrated, and in 2004 5'-azacytidine was approved by the US Food and Drug Administration (FDA) for the treatment of myelodysplastic syndrome and acute myeloid leukemia. 5'-azacytidine is also in the advanced stage of clinical trials for the treatment of other cancers, however success against solid tumors has been limited [34].

Many derivatives of 5'-azacytidine have been explored as alternatives to overcome the issues of instability and toxicity. One of these compounds, the deoxyribose analogue 5'-aza-2'-deoxycytidine (decitabine) is far less toxic and more specific than 5'-azacytidine because it is not incorporated into RNA. Decitabine has also been approved by the USFDA for use in the treatment of myelodysplastic syndrome and acute myeloid leukemia. More stable and less toxic cytidine analogs such as 5,6-dihydro-5-azacytidine, 5-fluoro-2'-deoxycytidine and zebularine (1-beta-D-ribofluranosyl-2(1H)-pyrimidinone) are currently in phase I and II studies. However, all these cytidine analogues reduce DNA methylation through incorporation into the DNA and formation of a covalent complex with DNMTs, thereby depleting DNMT levels. Therefore the toxicity associated with DNMTs permanently binding DNA is still a concern.

While 5'-azacytidine and its analogues are effective inhibitors of DNMTs, non-nucleoside inhibitors have been developed to address toxicity concerns associated with their use. These inhibitors bind and block the DNMT catalytic site and are not incorporated into DNA. Compound databases can be screened for suitable inhibitors using computer-generated models of the DNMT catalytic site. This method has identified a number of potential inhibitors including RG108, which binds the catalytic site in competition with cytosine [39]. These compounds are indene-base heterocycles linked by a three-carbon bond. *In vitro* assays with RG108 have found that it does indeed result in demethylation of DNA and in reactivation of tumor suppressor genes [40,41]. Toxicity of these compounds also appears to be lower than their nucleoside counterparts in human cells, offering a useful mode of inhibiting DNA methylation in cancer cells. RG108 is hydrophobic and therefore the development of more soluble derivatives will enhance its value as a cancer treatment.

26.5.2. Histone Acetyltransferase Inhibitors

Inhibitors of HATs have either been synthetically designed for this purpose or are natural products, which have been identified to have inhibitory properties. The synthetic inhibitors such as Lys-CoA and H3-CoA-20 are generally based on bisubstrate analogues and have been shown to have selective inhibition. However, their lack of cell permeability and instability renders them unsuitable for cancer therapy and they are therefore most useful for *in vitro* assays [42]. A few small molecules including isothiazolones and quinoline derivatives have been found to have HAT inhibitory roles and show antiproliferative properties against colon and ovarian tumour cell lines and leukemia cells [43,44]. Three natural inhibitors with *in vitro* and *in vivo* HAT inhibitory activity and increased cell permeability have been identified: anacardic acid from cashew nut shells [45]; garcinol, a polyisoprenylated benzophenone derivative isolated from *Garcinia indica* fruit that was shown to induce apoptosis in HeLa cells [46]; and curcumin a component of turmeric which was found to block hyperacetylation in prostate cancer cells and peripheral blood lymphocytes [47,48]. Curcumin is the most promising of these inhibitors and has been shown to have anti-tumour activities [49]. The discovery of HAT inhibitors is still in its infancy however several of the above compounds show promise for use in cancer treatment.

26.5.3. Histone Deacetylase Inhibitors

Histone deacetylase inhibitors inhibitors are by far the most well studied inhibitors for use in cancer treatment [reviewed in 50]. A large number of HDAC inhibitors have now been discovered mostly directed at the class I and II HDACs. These inhibitors are a range of natural and chemically synthesized compounds that act via the highly conserved HDAC catalytic domain and therefore target both class I and II HDACs but not class III. The class I and II HDAC inhibitors are generally of five types: small-molecule hydroxamates; short-chain fatty acids; cyclic peptides; electrophilic ketones; and benzamides, although there are a few other hybrid and miscellaneous molecules. Compounds representing all of these classes have been shown to inhibit HDAC activity, with several in the advanced stages of clinical trials for the treatment of cancer.

The hydroxamate class of inhibitors generally involves a hydroxamic acid moiety linked to a bulky hydrophobic cap. These inhibitors, while potent, have reversible effects. The first and best described of these inhibitors are trichostatin A (TSA) and suberoylanilide hydroxamic acid (SAHA). Although TSA has a wide range of anticancer effects, it has not been used in clinical trials due to its side effects. SAHA was approved in 2006 by the USFDA for the treatment of cutaneous T-cell lymphoma and is in advanced stage clinical trials for the treatment of other cancers. Crystallographic studies of the inhibitors bound to the HDAC have helped elucidate their mode of action, which appears to work via the inhibitor blocking the catalytic pocket of the HDAC [51,52,53]. The potency of the inhibitor is determined by how well it fits into the catalytic pocket, with TSA proving to be a much stronger inhibitor than SAHA due to its "tight" fit. While the bottom of the catalytic pocket is well conserved among class I and II HDACs, other parts are more variable and therefore there is potential to design inhibitors against these regions to obtain greater specificity for targeting particular HDACs. It is likely that the other classes of inhibitors work in a similar way, increasing the scope for designing inhibitors with more specific effects. Two other hydroxamate type inhibitors, panobinostat (LBH-589) and belinostat (PXD-101), are in phase I-III clinical trials. Panobinostat is being trialled for the treatment of chronic myeloid leukemia, refractory cutaneous T-cell lymphoma, and multiple myeloma, and belinostat for hematological malignancies as well as several types of solid tumors [54,55,56,57].

Two benzamide derivatives have shown promising results in cancer treatment. These compounds have a 2'-aminoanilide moiety, which likely chelates zinc or contacts key amino acids within the active site of the HDAC. MS-275 was found to induce apoptosis of acute myeloid leukemia cells, B-chronic lymphocytic leukemia cells, Jurkat lymphoblastic T cells and prostate cancer cells [58,59,60]. MGCD-0103 is in phase II clinical trials for the treatment of hematological malignancies and phase I/II for the treatment of solid tumors [61].

Romidepsin (FK-228, depsipeptide) is a cyclic peptide that inhibits class I and II HDACs [62]. It is converted to its active form within the cell whereby its mode of inhibition is through the sulfhydryl group interacting with the zinc in the catalytic pocket of the HDAC. Romidepsin induces cell cycle arrest and apoptosis in a range of human cancer cells and is being clinically trialed for the treatment of chronic myeloid leukemia, acute myeloid leukemia and cutaneous T-cell lymphoma [63,64,65]. Depsipeptide has been shown to reactivate many silenced genes in lung, colon and pancreatic cancer cells through demethylation of the promoters, with diminished recruitment of DNMT1 and decreased expression of histone methyltransferases G9A and SUV39H1, reducing H3K9 di- and tri-methylation around promoters [66]. These findings suggest that HDAC inhibitors may have a range of effects within the cell, including indirectly influencing methylation states.

The short chain fatty acid inhibitors are generally not very potent in their HDAC inhibition and require high concentrations for inhibition, and as such they are less useful for clinical purposes. Butyrate and valproic acid are the best-known inhibitors in this group and can inhibit cancer cell growth and induce apoptosis *in vitro* and *in vivo*.

Inhibitors of class III HDACs are becoming increasingly well studied with several molecules showing potential for use in cancer therapy. Several small molecules have been identified which do not interfere with NAD hydrolysis and so are more likely to be specific towards class III HDACs and not affect other NAD dependent enzymes. Several compounds are being investigated including sirtinol, salermide, splitomicin, cambinol and dihydrocoumarin. Sirtinol has been shown to inhibit class III HDACs (Sirt1) but not class I, and induce senescence in human breast and lung cancer cell lines [67]. In addition it has been found to inhibit the growth and viability of prostate cancer cells, while having no apparent effect on normal prostate cells [25]. Salermide appears to inhibit Sirt1 but not Sirt2 leading to tumor-specific death in a wide range of human cancer cell lines [68]. The ability of salermide to cause apoptosis in cancer cells was attributed to its ability to reactivate proapoptotic genes that were epigenetically repressed exclusively in cancer cells by Sirt1 [68]. Cambinol is an inhibitor of Sirt1 and 2 and has been shown to induce apoptosis in Burkitt lymphoma cells through acetylation of BCL-6 and p53 [69]. Sirtuin inhibitors have demonstrated great potential for use in cancer treatment.

Specificity is a primary concern with the use of HDAC inhibitors as therapeutic agents in the treatment of cancer. It was initially thought that these inhibitors would have extensive effects on gene expression, however, studies have shown that these effects are relatively specific with only a proportion of genes having altered expression in the presence of the inhibitor [70,71,72,73]. These studies also revealed that different HDAC inhibitors influence gene expression in different ways, most likely by inhibiting different HDACs. This raises the need for more knowledge on the roles of the different HDACs so that inhibitors can be tailored to achieve specific changes in gene expression.

26.5.4. Histone Methyltransferase Inhibitors

In comparison to the other enzymes responsible for epigenetic modifications within the cell, inhibitors of histone methyltransferases are poorly studied [recently reviewed in 27]. Some of the compounds that have been found to inhibit histone methyltransferases are SAM analogues including methylthio-adenosine, S-adenosyl-homocysteine (SAH) and the bacterial isolate sinefungin, and therefore they also inhibit other SAM-dependent enzymes including DNMTs. This lack of specificity is undesirable when identifying enzymes suitable for cancer treatment and therefore more specific inhibitors of histone methyltransferases have been explored.

Several histone lysine methyltransferase inhibitors have been identified that show promise as cancer drugs. The S-adenosyl-homocysteine hydrolase inhibitor, 3-deazaneplanocin A (DZNep) has been shown to inhibit H3K27 methylation (but not H3K9 methylation) leading to gene reactivation without affecting DNMT levels [74]. 3-deazaneplanocin A induced the apoptotic death of a range of cancer cells including breast, colorectal, prostate and hepatoma, with no obvious death in normal cells [74]. Chaetocin is a fungal mycotoxin that effectively inhibits SUV39H1 proteins and weakly inhibits other K9 histone methyltransferases such as G9a [75]. Chaetocin has exhibited anticancer properties against multiple myeloma [76], however cell toxicity is a concern. Its mode of action is as a competitive inhibitor of SAM, preventing H3K9 methylation but not the methylation of other lysine residues *in vivo*. This suggests the SAM-binding site is not conserved among SET domain histone methyltransferases and that specific inhibitors directed towards certain histone methyltransferases could be achieved. Supporting this, another study screened 125,000 compounds for potential histone methyltransferase inhibitors, and of the seven found, BIX-01294 did not compete with SAM and selectively inhibited G9a histone methyltransferase, while SUV39H1 or the arginine methylase PRMT1 were unaffected [77]. This inhibition resulted in the impairment of H3K9me2 generation while not affecting H3K9me3 or H3K9me1 states or methylation at other lysine positions *in vitro*.

The development of inhibitors of arginine methyltransferases is in its infancy. Arginine methyltransferases appear to have quite high specificity in the residues they methylate suggesting that specific inhibition could be achieved. A range of inhibitors such as AMIs (a group of compounds named simply as arginine methyltransferase inhibitors) [78], stilbamidine, allantodapsone and RM65 [79,80] are in the early stages of investigation and some are being used as models to scan for other inhibitory molecules. There is good potential for designing specific inhibitors against certain histone methyltransferases which could be used for more tailored treatment of cancer.

26.5.5. Histone Demethylase Inhibitors

While knowledge on lysine demethylases remains limited, research into their inhibition is very much in the early stages. To date only a handful of inhibitors of lysine-specific demethylase 1 (LSD1) have been described. Two drugs, pargyline and phenylcyclopropylamine have been shown to inhibit LSD1, although not specifically [81,82,83]. Two polyamine analogues, biguanide and bisguanidine, were found to be potent inhibitors of LSD1 in colon cancer cells, which resulted in the re-expression of many genes which were aberrantly silenced, through an increase in H3K4me2 [84]. Histone demethylases are therefore likely to be suitable targets for inhibition leading to the reversal of aberrant gene expression associated with cancer, and as knowledge of these enzymes increases, so will the discovery of further inhibitors.

26.5.6. Combined Therapy for Cancer Treatment

A drawback of using the inhibitors discussed above in cancer treatment is the potential for the epigenetic modifications to revert after the inhibitor has been removed. There is some evidence to suggest that a combination of inhibitors or their use in conjunction with conventional drugs is likely to be more effective by targeting cancer cells at several levels. The combination of DNMT and HDAC inhibitors has been clinically trialed in myelodysplastic syndrome and acute myeloid leukemia with promising results [85]. Histone deacetylase inhibitors have been shown to be highly effective in cancer treatment when used in conjunction with other drugs. For example, HDAC inhibitors used in combination with a tyrosine kinase inhibitor have been found to induce apoptosis in non-small cell lung cancer, ovarian cancer and leukemia cells [86]. Similar positive effects have been observed when using inhibitors alongside chemotherapeutic drugs. For example, decitabine has been shown to enhance the susceptibility of bladder carcinoma cells to cisplatin [87].

Conclusion

The development of a range of inhibitors targeting the epigenetic changes associated with cancer development and progression has shown considerable promise in cancer treatment strategies over recent years. Many of these inhibitors are in the advanced stages of clinical trials or have already been approved by the USFDA for use in cancer treatment. These have been shown to be effective alone or in combination with other similar inhibitors that target epigenetic modifications, as well as standard cancer treatments such as chemotherapy. As additional knowledge is obtained on the aberrant epigenetic profiles associated with cancer and the enzymes responsible for this, there will be great potential for identifying further useful inhibitors as well as tailoring drugs to target certain epigenetic changes. While this field is in its infancy it is showing considerable promise as a mode of treatment for cancer.

References

[1] Kornberg RD, Lorch YL (1999) Twenty-five years of the nucleosome, fundamental particle of the eukaryote chromosome. *Cell* 98: 285-294.

[2] Bird A (2002) DNA methylation patterns and epigenetic memory. *Genes and Development* 16: 6-21.

[3] Vaissiere T, Sawan C, Herceg Z (2008) Epigenetic interplay between histone modifications and DNA methylation in gene silencing. *Mutation Research-Reviews in Mutation Research* 659: 40-48.

[4] Kouzarides T (2007) Chromatin modifications and their function. *Cell* 128: 693-705.

[5] Brower-Toland B, Wacker DA, Fulbright RM, Lis JT, Kraus WL, et al. (2005) Specific contributions of histone tails and their acetylation to the mechanical stability of nucleosomes. *Journal of Molecular Biology* 346: 135-146.

[6] Vignali M, Hassan AH, Neely KE, Workman JL (2000) ATP-dependent chromatin-remodeling complexes. *Molecular and Cellular Biology* 20: 1899-1910.

[7] Esteller M (2008) Molecular origins of cancer: Epigenetics in cancer. New England *Journal of Medicine* 358: 1148-1159.
[8] Jones PA, Baylin SB (2007) The epigenomics of cancer. *Cell* 128: 683-692.
[9] Kondo Y, Shen LL, Issa JPJ (2003) Critical role of histone methylation in tumor suppressor gene silencing in colorectal cancer. *Molecular and Cellular Biology* 23: 206-215.
[10] Frigola J, Song J, Stirzaker C, Hinshelwood RA, Peinado MA, et al. (2006) Epigenetic remodeling in colorectal cancer results in coordinate gene suppression across an entire chromosome band. *Nature Genetics* 38: 540-549.
[11] Ehrlich M (2006) Cancer-linked DNA hypomethylation and its relationship to hypermethylation. DNA Methylation: Development, Genetic Disease and Cancer. Berlin: Springer-Verlag Berlin. pp. 251-274.
[12] Witt O, Deubzer HE, Milde T, Oehme I (2009) HDAC family: What are the cancer relevant targets? *Cancer Letters* 277: 8-21.
[13] Di Croce L (2005) Chromatin modifying activity of leukaemia associated fusion proteins. *Human Molecular Genetics* 14: R77-R84.
[14] Di Croce L, Raker VA, Corsaro M, Fazi F, Fanelli M, et al. (2002) Methyltransferase recruitment and DNA hypermethylation of target promoters by an oncogenic transcription factor. *Science* 295: 1079-1082.
[15] Villa R, Morey L, Raker VA, Buschbeck M, Gutierrez A, et al. (2006) The methyl-CpG binding protein MBD1 is required for PML-RAR alpha function. *Proceedings of the National Academy of Sciences of the United States of America* 103: 1400-1405.
[16] Carbone R, Botrugno OA, Ronzoni S, Insinga A, Di Croce L, et al. (2006) Recruitment of the histone methyltransferase SUV39H1 and its role in the oncogenic properties of the leukemia-associated PML-retinoic acid receptor fusion protein. *Molecular and Cellular Biology* 26: 1288-1296.
[17] Kuo MH, Allis CD (1998) Roles of histone acetyltransferases and deacetylases in gene regulation. *Bioessays* 20: 615-626.
[18] Grant PA, Berger SL (1999) Histone acetyltransferase complexes. *Seminars in Cell and Developmental Biology* 10: 169-177.
[19] Zheng YG, Wu J, Chen ZY, Goodman M (2008) Chemical regulation of epigenetic modifications: Opportunities for new cancer therapy. *Medicinal Research Reviews* 28: 645-687.
[20] Kim DH, Kim M, Kwon HJ (2003) Histone deacetylase in carcinogenesis and its inhibitors as anti-cancer agents. *Journal of Biochemistry and Molecular Biology* 36: 110-119.
[21] Marks PA, Jiang XJ (2005) Histone deacetylase inhibitors in programmed cell death and cancer therapy. *Cell Cycle* 4: 549-551.
[22] Lin RJ, Nagy L, Inoue S, Shao WL, Miller WH, et al. (1998) Role of the histone deacetylase complex in acute promyelocytic leukaemia. *Nature* 391: 811-814.
[23] Follows GA, Tagoh H, Lefevre P, Hodge D, Morgan GJ, et al. (2003) Epigenetic consequences of AML1-ETO action at the human c-FMS locus. *Embo Journal* 22: 2798-2809.
[24] Zhou W, Feng X, Li H, Wang L, Zhu B, et al. (2009) Inactivation of LARS2, located at the commonly deleted region 3p21.3, by both epigenetic and genetic mechanisms in nasopharyngeal carcinoma. *Acta Biochim Biophys Sin* (Shanghai) 41: 54-62.

[25] Jung-Hynes B, Nihal M, Zhong W, Ahmad N (2009) Role of sirtuin histone deacetylase SIRT1 in prostate cancer: A target for prostate cancer management via its inhibition? *The Journal of Biological Chemistry* 284: 3823-3832.

[26] Kojima K, Ohhashi R, Fujita Y, Hamada N, Akao Y, et al. (2008) A role for SIRT1 in cell growth and chemoresistance in prostate cancer PC3 and DU145 cells. *Biochemical and Biophysical Research Communications* 373: 423-428.

[27] Spannhoff A, Sippl W, Jung M (2009) Cancer treatment of the future: Inhibitors of histone methyltransferases. *International Journal of Biochemistry and Cell Biology* 41: 4-11.

[28] Hamamoto R, Furukawa Y, Morita M, Iimura Y, Silva FP, et al. (2004) SMYD3 encodes a histone methyltransferase involved in the proliferation of cancer cells. *Nature Cell Biology* 6: 731-740.

[29] Wang SZ, Luo XG, Shen J, Zou JN, Lu YH, et al. (2008) Knockdown of SMYD3 by RNA interference inhibits cervical carcinoma cell growth and invasion in vitro. *Bmb Reports* 41: 294-299.

[30] Hamamoto R, Silva FP, Tsuge M, Nishidate T, Katagiri T, et al. (2006) Enhanced SMYD3 expression is essential for the growth of breast cancer cells. *Cancer Science* 97: 113-118.

[31] Kleer CG, Cao Q, Varambally S, Shen RL, Ota L, et al. (2003) EZH2 is a marker of aggressive breast cancer and promotes neoplastic transformation of breast epithelial cells. *Proceedings of the National Academy of Sciences of the United States of America* 100: 11606-11611.

[32] Varambally S, Dhanasekaran SM, Zhou M, Barrette TR, Kumar-Sinha C, et al. (2002) The polycomb group protein EZH2 is involved in progression of prostate cancer. *Nature* 419: 624-629.

[33] Cloos PAC, Christensen J, Agger K, Helin K (2008) Erasing the methyl mark: histone demethylases at the center of cellular differentiation and disease. *Genes and Development* 22: 1115-1140.

[34] Dario LS, Rosa MA, Mariela E, Roberto G, Caterina C (2008) Chromatin remodeling agents for cancer therapy. *Reviews on Recent Clinical Trials* 3: 192-203.

[35] Mai A, Altucci L (2009) Epi-drugs to fight cancer: From chemistry to cancer treatment, the road ahead. *International Journal of Biochemistry and Cell Biology* 41: 199-213.

[36] Gronbaek K, Treppendahl M, Asmar F, Guldberg P (2008) Epigenetic changes in cancer as potential targets for prophylaxis and maintenance therapy. *Basic and Clinical Pharmacology and Toxicology* 103: 389-396.

[37] Michalowsky LA, Jones PA (1987) Differential nuclear-protein binding to 5-azacytosine-containing DNA as a potential mechanism for 5-aza-2'-deoxycytidine resistance. *Molecular and Cellular Biology* 7: 3076-3083.

[38] Santi DV, Norment A, Garrett CE (1984) Covalent bond formation between a DNA-cytosine methyltransferase and DNA containing 5-azacytosine. *Proceedings of the National Academy of Sciences of the United States of America* 81: 6993-6997.

[39] Siedlecki P, Boy RG, Musch T, Brueckner B, Suhai S, et al. (2006) Discovery of two novel, small-molecule inhibitors of DNA methylation. *Journal of Medicinal Chemistry* 49: 678-683.

[40] Brueckner B, Boy RG, Siedlecki P, Musch T, Kliem HC, et al. (2005) Epigenetic reactivation of tumor suppressor genes by a novel small-molecule inhibitor of human DNA methyltransferases. *Cancer Research* 65: 6305-6311.

[41] Schirrmacher E, Beck C, Brueckner B, Schmitges F, Siedlicki P, et al. (2006) Synthesis and in vitro evaluation of biotinylated RG108: A high affinity compound for studying binding interactions with human DNA methyltransferases. *Bioconjugate Chemistry* 17: 261-266.

[42] Lau OD, Kundu TK, Soccio RE, Ait-Si-Ali S, Khalil EM, et al. (2000) HATs off: Selective synthetic inhibitors of the histone acetyltransferases p300 and PCAF. *Molecular Cell* 5: 589-595.

[43] Mai A, Rotili D, Tarantino D, Ornaghi P, Tosi F, et al. (2006) Small-molecule inhibitors of histone acetyltransferase activity: Identification and biological properties. *Journal of Medicinal Chemistry* 49: 6897-6907.

[44] Stimson L, Rowlands MG, Newbatt YM, Smith NF, Raynaud FI, et al. (2005) Isothiazolones as inhibitors of PCAF and p300 histone acetyltransferase activity. *Molecular Cancer Therapeutics* 4: 1521-1532.

[45] Balasubramanyam K, Swaminathan V, Ranganathan A, Kundu TK (2003) Small molecule modulators of histone acetyltransferase p300. *Journal of Biological Chemistry* 278: 19134-19140.

[46] Balasubramanyam K, Altaf M, Varier RA, Swaminathan V, Ravindran A, et al. (2004) Polyisoprenylated benzophenone, garcinol, a natural histone acetyltransferase inhibitor, represses chromatin transcription and alters global gene expression. *Journal of Biological Chemistry* 279: 33716-33726.

[47] Balasubramanyam K, Varier RA, Altaf M, Swaminathan V, Siddappa NB, et al. (2004) Curcumin, a novel p300/CREB-binding protein-specific inhibitor of acetyltransferase, represses the acetylation of histone/nonhistone proteins and histone acetyltransferase-dependent chromatin transcription. *Journal of Biological Chemistry* 279: 51163-51171.

[48] Marcu M, YJ J, S L, Chung E, MJ L, et al. (2006) Curcumin is an inhibitor of p300 histone acetyltransferase. *Medicinal Chemistry* 2: 169-174.

[49] Shishodia S, Chaturvedi MM, Aggarwal BB (2007) Role of curcumin in cancer therapy. *Current Problems in Cancer* 31: 243-305.

[50] Emanuele S, Lauricella M, Tesoriere G (2008) Histone deacetylase inhibitors: Apoptotic effects and clinical implications. *International Journal of Oncology* 33: 637-646.

[51] Finnin MS, Donigian JR, Cohen A, Richon VM, Rifkind RA, et al. (1999) Structures of a histone deacetylase homologue bound to the TSA and SAHA inhibitors. *Nature* 401: 188-193.

[52] Somoza JR, Skene RJ, Katz BA, Mol C, Ho JD, et al. (2004) Structural snapshots of human HDAC8 provide insights into the class I histone deacetylases. *Structure* 12: 1325-1334.

[53] Vannini A, Volpari C, Filocamo G, Casavola EC, Brunetti M, et al. (2004) Crystal structure of a eukaryotic zinc-dependent histone deacetylase, human HDAC8, complexed with a hydroxamic acid inhibitor. *Proceedings of the National Academy of Sciences of the United States of America* 101: 15064-15069.

[54] Khan N, Jeffers M, Kumar S, Hackett C, Boldog F, et al. (2008) Determination of the class and isoform selectivity of small-molecule histone deacetylase inhibitors. *Biochemical Journal* 409: 581-589.

[55] Qian XZ, Ara G, Mills E, LaRochelle WJ, Lichenstein HS, et al. (2008) Activity of the histone deacetylase inhibitor belinostat (PXD101) in preclinical models of prostate cancer. *International Journal of Cancer* 122: 1400-1410.

[56] Steele NL, Plumb JA, Vidal L, Tjornelund J, Knoblauch P, et al. (2008) A phase 1 pharmacokinetic and pharmacodynamic study of the histone deacetylase inhibitor belinostat in patients with advanced solid tumors. *Clinical Cancer Research* 14: 804-810.

[57] Buckley MT, Yoon J, Yee H, Chiriboga L, Liebes L, et al. (2007) The histone deacetylase inhibitor belinostat (PXD101) suppresses bladder cancer cell growth in vitro and in vivo. *Journal of Translational Medicine* 5: 12.

[58] Lucas DM, Davis ME, Parthun MR, Mone AP, Kitada S, et al. (2004) The histone deacetylase inhibitor MS-275 induces caspase-dependent apoptosis in B-cell chronic lymphocytic leukemia cells. *Leukemia* 18: 1207-1214.

[59] Nebbioso A, Clarke N, Voltz E, Germain E, Ambrosino C, et al. (2005) Tumor-selective action of HDAC inhibitors involves TRAIL induction in acute myeloid leukemia cells. *Nature Medicine* 11: 77-84.

[60] Qian DZ, Wei YF, Wang XF, Kato Y, Cheng LZ, et al. (2007) Antitumor activity of the histone deacetylase inhibitor MS-275 in prostate cancer models. *Prostate* 67: 1182-1193.

[61] Fournel M, Bonfils C, Hou Y, Yan PT, Trachy-Bourget MC, et al. (2008) MGCD0103, a novel isotype-selective histone deacetylase inhibitor, has broad spectrum antitumor activity in vitro and in vivo. *Molecular Cancer Therapeutics* 7: 759-768.

[62] Itoh Y, Suzuki T, Miyata N (2008) Isoform-selective histone deacetylase inhibitors. *Current Pharmaceutical Design* 14: 529-544.

[63] Byrd JC, Marcucci G, Parthun MR, Xiao JJ, Klisovic RB, et al. (2005) A phase 1 and pharmacodynamic study of depsipeptide (FK228) in chronic lymphocytic leukemia and acute myeloid leukemia. *Blood* 105: 959-967.

[64] Piekarz RL, Frye AR, Wright JJ, Steinberg SM, Liewehr DJ, et al. (2006) Cardiac studies in patients treated with depsipeptide, FK228, in a phase II trial for T-cell lymphoma. *Clinical Cancer Research* 12: 3762-3773.

[65] Piekarz RL, Robey R, Sandor V, Bakke S, Wilson WH, et al. (2001) Inhibitor of histone deacetylation, depsipeptide (FR901228), in the treatment of peripheral and cutaneous T-cell lymphoma: a case report. *Blood* 98: 2865-2868.

[66] Wu LP, Wang X, Li L, Zhao Y, Lu SL, et al. (2008) Histone deacetylase inhibitor depsipeptide activates silenced genes through decreasing both CpG and H3K9 methylation on the promoter. *Molecular and Cellular Biology* 28: 3219-3235.

[67] Ota H, Tokunaga E, Chang K, Hikasa M, Iijima K, et al. (2005) Sirt1 inhibitor, Sirtinol, induces senescence-like growth arrest with attenuated Ras-MAPK signaling in human cancer cells. *Oncogene* 25: 176-185.

[68] Lara E, Mai A, Calvanese V, Altucci L, Lopez-Nieva P, et al. (2009) Salermide, a Sirtuin inhibitor with a strong cancer-specific proapoptotic effect. *Oncogene* 28: 781-791.

[69] Heltweg B, Gatbonton T, Schuler AD, Posakony J, Li HZ, et al. (2006) Antitumor activity of a small-molecule inhibitor of human silent information regulator 2 enzymes. *Cancer Research* 66: 4368-4377.

[70] Glaser KB, Staver MJ, Waring JF, Stender J, Ulrich RG, et al. (2003) Gene expression profiling of multiple histone deacetylase (HDAC) inhibitors: Defining a common gene set produced by HDAC inhibition in T24 and MDA carcinoma cell lines. *Molecular Cancer Therapeutics* 2: 151-163.

[71] Mitsiades CS, Mitsiades NS, McMullan CJ, Poulaki V, Shringarpure R, et al. (2004) Transcriptional signature of histone deacetylase inhibition in multiple myeloma: Biological and clinical implications. *Proceedings of the National Academy of Sciences of the United States of America* 101: 540-545.

[72] Peart MJ, Smyth GK, van Laar RK, Bowtell DD, Richon VM, et al. (2005) Identification and functional significance of genes regulated by structurally different histone deacetylase inhibitors. *Proceedings of the National Academy of Sciences of the United States of America* 102: 3697-3702.

[73] Van Lint C, Emiliani S, Verdin E (1996) The expression of a small fraction of cellular genes is changed in response to histone hyperacetylation. *Gene Expression* 5: 245-253.

[74] Tan J, Yang XJ, Zhuang L, Jiang X, Chen W, et al. (2007) Pharmacologic disruption of polycomb-repressive complex 2-mediated gene repression selectively induces apoptosis in cancer cells. *Genes and Development* 21: 1050-1063.

[75] Greiner D, Bonaldi T, Eskeland R, Roemer E, Imhof A (2005) Identification of a specific inhibitor of the histone methyltransferase SU(VAR)3-9. *Nature Chemical* Biology 1: 143-145.

[76] Isham CR, Tibodeau JD, Jin W, Xu RF, Timm MM, et al. (2007) Chaetocin: a promising new antimyeloma agent with in vitro and in vivo activity mediated via imposition of oxidative stress. *Blood* 109: 2579-2588.

[77] Kubicek S, O'Sullivan RJ, August EM, Hickey ER, Zhang Q, et al. (2007) Reversal of H3K9me2 by a small-molecule inhibitor for the G9a histone methyltransferase. *Molecular Cell* 25: 473-481.

[78] Cheng DH, Yadav N, King RW, Swanson MS, Weinstein EJ, et al. (2004) Small molecule regulators of protein arginine methyltransferases. *Journal of Biological Chemistry* 279: 23892-23899.

[79] Spannhoff A, Heinke R, Bauer I, Trojer P, Metzger E, et al. (2007) Target-based approach to inhibitors of histone arginine methyltransferases. *Journal of Medicinal Chemistry* 50: 2319-2325.

[80] Spannhoff A, Machmur R, Heinke R, Trojer P, Bauer I, et al. (2007) A novel arginine methyltransferase inhibitor with cellular activity. *Bioorganic and Medicinal Chemistry Letters* 17: 4150-4153.

[81] Metzger E, Wissmann M, Yin N, Muller JM, Schneider R, et al. (2005) LSD1 demethylates repressive histone marks to promote androgen-receptor-dependent transcription. *Nature* 437: 436-439.

[82] Schmidt DMZ, McCafferty DG (2007) trans-2-phenylcyclopropylamine is a mechanism-based inactivator of the histone demethylase LSD1. *Biochemistry* 46: 4408-4416.

[83] Yang MJ, Culhane JC, Szewczuk LM, Jalili P, Ball HL, et al. (2007) Structural basis for the inhibition of the LSD1 histone demethylase by the antidepressant trans-2-phenylcyclopropylamine. *Biochemistry* 46: 8058-8065.

[84] Huang Y, Greene E, Stewart TM, Goodwin AC, Baylin SB, et al. (2007) Inhibition of lysine-specific demethylase 1 by polyamine analogues results in reexpression of aberrantly silenced genes. *Proceedings of the National Academy of Sciences of the United States of America* 104: 8023-8028.

[85] Gore SD, Baylin S, Sugar E, Carraway H, Miller CB, et al. (2006) Combined DNA methyltransferase and histone deacetylase inhibition in the treatment of myeloid neoplasms. *Cancer Research* 66: 6361-6369.

[86] Yu CR, Friday BB, Lai JP, McCollum A, Atadja P, et al. (2007) Abrogation of MAPK and Akt signaling by AEE788 synergistically potentiates histone deacetylase inhibitor-induced apoptosis through reactive oxygen species generation. *Clinical Cancer Research* 13: 1140-1148.

[87] Shang DH, Liu YT, Matsui Y, Ito N, Nishiyama H, et al. (2008) Demethylating agent 5-aza-2 '-deoxycytidine enhances susceptibility of bladder transitional cell carcinoma to cisplatin. *Urology* 71: 1220-1225.

Contributors

Jorge Albores-Saavedra, MD
Instituto Nacional de Ciencias Medicas y Nutricion, Salvador Zubiran, Mexico City

Beste M. Atasoy, MD, MSc
Marmara Universitesi Hastanesi, Radyasyon Onkolojisi AD, Tophanelioglu cad., No:13/15 Altunizade – Uskudar, 34660, Istanbul, Turkey,

Kristen Batich, BA
The George Washington University Cancer Institute, Office of Cancer Prevention and Control, Washington, DC

Marco Bisoffi, PhD
University of New Mexico School of Medicine, Albuquerque, NM, USA

Russell Broaddus, MD
Department of Pathology, University of Texas M.D. Anderson Cancer Center, Houston, Texas

Miguel H. Bronchud, MA (camb), BMBCh (Oxon), MRCP (UK), DM (Oxon), PhD,
Hospital General of Granollers, Granollers, Barcelona, Spain
E-mail: mhbronchud@telefonica.net

Maximilian Burger, MD, FEBU
Oberarzt, Klinik für Urologie, Universität Regensburg, Landshuterstr. 65, 93053, Regensburg,
E-mail: maximilian.burger@klinik.uni-regensburg.de

J. Andrew Carlson, MD, FRCPC
Divisions of Dermatopathology and Dermatology, Department of Pathology, Albany Medical College, Albany, NY, USA
E-mail: CarlsoA@mail.amc.edu

Jonathan Castillo
Science Faculty. Biochemistry Institute. Biochemistry and Tumoral Pharmacology Laboratory. Universidad Austral de Chile.

Gabriel D. Dakubo, BSc(Hons), MBChB
Mito-Onc Consultancy, 1016 Brannan Lane, Thunder Bay, Ontario, Canada, P7J 1H7
E-mail: gabrieldakubo@gmail.com

Rostam D. Farhadieh, BSc(Med)Hons, MBBS, MD
St Vincent's Hospital, Melbourne, Australia; Prince of Wales Hospital, University of New South Wales, Sydney, Australia.
E-mail: rostam74@yahoo.com.au

Liviu Feller, DMD, MDENT
Department of Periodontology and Oral Medicine, School of Dentistry, Faculty of Health Sciences, University of Limpopo, Medunsa Campus, Medunsa Republic of South Africa
E-mail: Lfeller@ul.ac.za

Michael C. Frühwald, MD, PhD
Chefarzt I. Klinik für Kinder und Jugendliche, Klinikum Augsburg, Stenglinstr. 2 86156 Augsburg
Email: michael.fruehwald@klinikum-augsburg.de

Donald Gallup, MD
Department of Obstetrics and Gynecology, Mercer University School of Medicine, Savannah, Georgia 31403-3089

Jian-Xin Gao, MD, PhD
Department of Pathology and Comprehensive Cancer Center, Medical Center, Ohio State University, Columbus, OH, 43210 USA
E-mail: gao.49@osu.edu

Jeffrey K. Griffith, PhD
University of New Mexico School of Medicine, Albuquerque, NM, USA
E-mail: JKGriffith@salud.unm.edu

Girish Gupta, MB ChB, FRCP
Department of Dermatology, Lanarkshire Acute Hospitals NHS Trust, Lanarkshire, Scotland
E-mail: girish.gupta@lanarkshire.scot.nhs.uk

Tomonori Habuchi, MD
Department of Urology Akita University Graduate School of Medicine 1-1-1 Hondo, Akita 010-8543, Japan
E-mail: thabuchi@doc.med.akita-u.ac.jp

Arndt Hartmann, MD
Department of Pathology, University of Erlangen, Krankenhausstr. 12, 91054, Erlangen, Germany

Christopher M. Heaphy, PhD
The Johns Hopkins Medical Institutions, Baltimore, MD, USA

Donald E. Henson, MD
Department of Pathology and the Office of Cancer Prevention and Control, The George Washington University Cancer Institute, Washington, DC, USA
E-mail: patdeh@gwumc.edu

Adele Holloway, PhD
Menzies Research Institute. School of Medicine University of Tasmania Private Bag 58 Hobart, Tasmania 7001 Australia
E-mail: A.F.Holloway@utas.edu.au

Yi Lisa Hwa
Department of Internal Medicine, Mayo Clinic, Rochester, MN 55905, USA,

Anuja Jhingran, MD
Department of Radiation Oncology, Division of Radiation Oncology, The University of Texas M. D. Anderson Cancer Center, Houston, Texas

Shi-Wen Jiang, MD, MSc
Department of Biomedical Science, Curtis and Elizabeth Anderson Cancer Institute, Mercer, University School of Medicine at Savannah4700, Waters Avenue, Savannah, Georgia 31404, USA
E-mail: jiang_s@mercer.edu

Tadao Kakizoe, MD
National Cancer Center, 5-1-1 Tsukiji, Chuo-Ku, Tokyo, Japan

Makoto Kammori, MD
Tokyo Women's Medical University Institute of Endocrine Center, Department of Endocrine Surgery, Medical University, Tokyo, Japan
E-mail: mkammori@endos.twmu.ac.jp

Devendar Katkoori, MD
Department of Urology, Miller School of Medicine, University of Miami, Miami, FL, USA

Jun Kato, MD
Second Department of Internal Medicine, Wakayama Medical University, 811-1, Kimiidera, Wakayama-City, Wakayama, 641-0012, Japan
E-mail: katojun@wakayama-med.ac.jp

Kornelius Kerl, MD
University Children´s Hospital Muenster, Department of Pediatric Hematology and Oncology, Muenster, Germany

Sevil Kılçıksız, MD
Gaziantep Universitesi Tip Fakultesi Radyasyon Onkolojisi AD, 27310, Gaziantep, Turkey
E-mail: sevilkilciksiz@gmail.com

Ann Klopp, MD, PhD
Department of Radiation Oncology, Division of Radiation Oncology, The University of Texas M. D. Anderson Cancer Center, Houston, Texas
E-mail: AKlopp@mdanderson.org

Yutaka Kondo, MD, PhD
Division of Molecular Oncology, Aichi Cancer Center Research Institute, 1-1 Kanokoden, Chikusa-ku, Nagoya 464-8681, Japan
E-mail: ykondo@aichi-cc.jp

Ulrich Lehmann, PhD
Dipl.-Biochem. Institute of Pathology, Medizinische Hochschule Hannover, Carl-Neuberg-Str. 1, D-30625 Hannover, Germany
E-mail: Lehmann.Ulrich@MH-Hannover.de

Johan Lemmer, BDS, HDipDent, FCD(SA)OMP, FCMSAae, HonFCMSA
Deparmtent of Periodontology and Oral Medicine, School of Dentistry, Faculty of Health Sciences, University of Limpopo, Medunsa Campus. Emeritus Professor of Oral Medicine and Periodontology University of Witwatersrand, Johannesburg, Republic of South Africa.

Jinping Li, MD
Department of Biomedical Science, Mercer University School of Medicine at Savannah, 4700, Waters Avenue, Savannah, Georgia 31404, USA

Murugesan Manoharan, MD, FRCS, FRACS
Department of Urology, University of Miami Miller School of Medicine, P.O. Box 016960, (M814), Miami, Fl 33101
E-mail: mmanoharan@med.miami.edu

Eduardo Moreno, PhD
Department of Molecular Oncology, Spanish National Cancer Research Centre (CNIO), Melchor Fernández Almagro, 3, E-28029 Madrid, Spain
E-mail: emoreno@cnio.es

Michael Murphy, MD
Department of Dermatology, MC-6230, University of Connecticut Medical Center, Framington, CT 06030

Takeshi Obara, MD
Gastroenterology and Hematology/Oncology, Asahikawa Medical College, 2-1-1-1 East Midorigaoka, Asahikawa, Hokkaido, Japan 078-8510,

Fiona S. Poke, PhD
Menzies Research Institute, University of Tasmania, Hobart, Tasmania 7001, Australia

Laura B. Pritzker, PhD
YorkMedTech Partners Inc., 565 Bay Street, Suite 1204, Toronto, Ontario, Canada M5G 2C2

Kenneth P H Pritzker, MD, FRCPC
Laboratory Medicine and, Pathobiology; Surgery University of Toronto, Pathology and Laboratory Medicine, Mount Sinai Hospital 600 University Avenue Toronto, Canada, M5G 1X5
E-mail: kpritzker@mtsinai.on.ca

Juan Ren, MD
Cancer center, First Affiliated Hospital of Xi'an Jiao Tong University, 76 Yan Ta, West Road, Xi'an, Shaan' Xi Province, P. R. China, 710061

Christa Rhiner, PhD
Department of Molecular Oncology, Spanish National Cancer Research Centre (CNIO), Melchor Fernández Almagro, 3, E-28029 Madrid, Spain.

Juan C. Roa, MD
Department of Pathology. Molecular Pathology Laboratory. Universidad de la Frontera, Temuco. Chile. Scientific and Technological Bioresource Nucleus (BIOREN)
E-mail: jcroa@ufro.cl

Arnold M. Schwartz, MD, PhD
Department of Pathology, The George Washington University Medical Center, Washington, DC

Kave Shams, MBChB, MRCP
Department of Dermatology NHS Lanarkshire, Scotland

Rakesh Singal, MD
Department of Medicine, Miller School of Medicine, University of Miami, Miami, FL, USA

Andrzej Slominski, MD, PhD
Department of Pathology and Laboratory Medicine, University of Tennessee Health Science Center, 930 Madison Ave, Memphis, TN 38163

Davide Soldini, MD
Department of Pathology, University Hospital Zurich, Schmelzbergstrasse 12
8091 Zürich, Switzerland.

Sabrina L. Spencer, BS, BA, MS, PhD
Department of Systems Biology, Harvard Medical School, Boston, MA

Satoshi Tanno, MD, PhD
Gastroenterology and Hematology/Oncology, Asahikawa Medical College, 2-1-1-1 East Midorigaoka, Asahikawa, Hokkaido, Japan 078-8510,
E-mail: tanno1se@asahikawa-med.ac.jp

Tracy Tipton, BS
Department of Biomedical Science, Mercer University School of Medicine at Savannah, 4700, Waters Avenue, Savannah, Georgia 31404, USA,

Celestine S Tung, MD, MPH
Department of Gynecologic Oncology, MD Anderson Cancer Center, 1155 Herman Pressler, Unit 1362, Houston, TX 77030
E-mail: ctung@mdanderson.org

Toshikazu Ushijima, MD, PhD
Carcinogenesis Division, National Cancer Center Research Institute, 5-1-1 Tsukiji, Chuo-ku, Tokyo, Japan 104-0045
E-mail: tushijim@ncc.go.jp

Vincent L. Wilson, PhD
Department of Environmental Sciences, Louisiana State University and Veterinary Medical School, Baton Rouge, LA 70803

Kwong-Kwok Wong, PhD
Department of Gynecologic Oncology, Division of Surgery, The University of Texas M. D. Anderson Cancer Center, Houston, Texas

Takeichi Yoshida
Carcinogenesis Division, National Cancer Center Research Institute
5-1-1 Tsukiji, Chuo-ku, 104-0045, Tokyo, Japan

Index

B

C

D

E

F

G

H

I

J

K

L

M

N

Q

R

S

T

U